Occupational Therapies without Borders

Cover photograph by Ricard Parra and used with many thanks.

Commissioning Editor: Rita Demetriou-Swanwick
Development Editor: Catherine Jackson
Project Manager: Nancy Arnott
Designer: Stewart Larking
Illustration Manager: Merlyn Harvey

Occupational Therapies Without Borders: Volume 2

Towards an Ecology of Occupation-Based Practices

Frank Kronenberg BSc(OT) BA(Ed)

International Guest Lecturer in Occupational Therapy, Formal affiliations with Zuyd University, the Netherlands; University of the Western Cape, South Africa; Universidad Andres Bello, Chile; University of Salford, UK.

Director, Shades of Black Works, Cape Town, South Africa

Nick Pollard BA DipCOT MA MSc(OT) PGCE

Senior Lecturer, Sheffield Hallam University, Sheffield, UK

Dikaios Sakellariou MSc BSc(OT)

Lecturer, Cardiff University, Cardiff, UK

Forewords by

Desmond Tutu

Marilyn Pattison

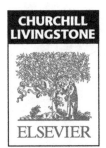

CHURCHILL LIVINGSTONE

ELSEVIER

Edinburgh London New York Oxford Philadelphia St Louis Sydney Toronto 2011

CHURCHILL
LIVINGSTONE
ELSEVIER

© 2011 Elsevier Ltd. All rights reserved.

First edition 2011

ISBN 978 0 7020 3103 8

British Library Cataloguing in Publication Data
A catalogue record for this book is available from the British Library

Library of Congress Cataloging in Publication Data
A catalog record for this book is available from the Library of Congress

ELSEVIER your source for books,
journals and multimedia
in the health sciences

www.elsevierhealth.com

Working together to grow
libraries in developing countries

www.elsevier.com | www.bookaid.org | www.sabre.org

 ELSEVIER BOOK AID International Sabre Foundation

The
Publisher's
policy is to use
**paper manufactured
from sustainable forests**

Printed in China

Contents

Contents

Contents

Having been privileged with opportunities to learn how to be of service to people in need, occupational therapists are committed to making themselves available as a relevant resource in the societies where they find themselves. The contributions to this book bear evidence that occupational therapists see a need to extend their involvement beyond their traditional clientele and employment settings. They seem to know that the promotion of all people's health and wellbeing goes hand in hand with struggles for social justice.

Your particular approach to advancing our wellbeing and health strikes me as both unique and easily taken for granted. While you value and work with medical understandings, your main aim seems to go beyond these. You seem to enable people to appreciate more consciously how what we do to and with ourselves and others on a daily basis impacts our individual and collective wellbeing.

If this is indeed your vision, then it connects with a particular human characteristic that we call *ubuntu* in Africa. It is akin, for example, to the Hindu notion of *dharma* and the Islamic concept *ummah* and it is also relevant to advancing the Western idea of *human rights*. Too often do we think of ourselves as just individuals, separated from one another, whereas we are connected and what we do affects the whole world. When we do well together, it spreads out; it is for the whole of humanity.

However, the Universal Declaration of Human Rights does not work like a magic wand in bringing about social justice and peace, and neither do *ubuntu* and its global local counterparts. These merely offer pointers to how human beings can do well together. Acting accordingly requires a renewal of hearts and minds that are rooted in a firm belief in and understanding of the common good, followed by a mobilization of hands-on involvements. As occupational therapists you have a significant contribution to make ... be inspired by Vivienne Budaza's explanation of occupational justice as *'doing well together'* (See Chapters 1 and 21), allowing people from all walks of life to contribute meaningfully to the wellbeing of others.

God bless you.

Desmond Tutu
Archbishop Emeritus of Cape Town
March 2010

Social injustice is killing people on a grand scale. Achieving health equity within a generation is achievable, it is the right thing to do, and now is the right time to do it (WHO 2008) and occupational therapists are the right people to be involved.

It gives me great pleasure to introduce this landmark book containing contributions from occupational therapists and colleagues from around the globe. It captures the essence of entrepreneurship which is 'a vision of empowerment for occupational therapists' (Pattison 2006). Occupational therapists need to move beyond traditional boundaries and be leaders of progress. The authors in this exciting publication demonstrate the many active roles that occupational therapists can play. The World Federation of Occupational Therapists (WFOT) is the key international representative of occupational therapists and occupational therapy and it links 66 countries (WFOT website n.d.) worldwide. The federation believes that occupational therapy has a valuable contribution to make to occupational performance as it affects the health and wellbeing of people. The federation maintains that it can positively influence health, welfare, education, and vocation at an international level, combined with the development of excellence within the profession.

As occupational therapists we need to develop the capacity and power to construct our own destiny. For some, reading this book might not be a comfortable journey. How can we effectively work with others if we have undercapitalized our own potential? We spend our careers enabling and assisting people to meet their maximum potential and the first section of the book – Discourses without borders – challenges occupational therapists to be the very best that we can be. It demands that we challenge our thinking, our constructs, and our sphere of influence. Being included in the society in which one lives is vital to the material, psychosocial, and political aspects of empowerment that underpin social wellbeing and equitable health (WHO 2008).

Entrepreneurship involves innovation. An entrepreneur searches for change, responds to it and exploits it as an opportunity (Drucker 1985). An entrepreneurial approach to practice is about thinking outside of the square, and finding increasingly innovative ways to deliver services and make a difference to people's lives, health, and wellbeing.

Occupational therapists' increasing involvement in community-based rehabilitation, disaster preparedness and response, among other emerging areas of practice, is based on the concept of social entrepreneurship. Working directly with communities on projects that are meaningful to each community, having influence on local and higher health and policy makers, and working with nongovernmental organizations (NGOs) position occupational therapists as having a unique contribution to the goals of a civil society. Occupational therapists need to understand the vital role they play in what makes populations healthy, and the second section of the book – Practices without borders – urges us to move beyond our traditional boundaries. What business entrepreneurs are to the economy, social entrepreneurs are to social change. They are the driven, creative individuals who question the status quo, exploit new opportunities, and refuse to give up – and remake the world for the better (Bornstein 2004). WFOT through its position papers and publications – on human rights, community-based rehabilitation, and cultural diversity, and the WFOT Minimum Standards for the Education of Occupational Therapists (2000) – supports this social contract.

The third section of the book – Education and research without borders – highlights the changing focus in education and research and mirrors the philosophical basis of the WFOT Minimum Standards for the Education of Occupational Therapists (2002). These standards have been written 'to encompass educational programmes that address occupation's potential to build healthy communities, as well as the potential to enhance wellness by helping people to develop personal skills in choosing and performing occupations in ways that will support well-being' (WFOT 2002).

The World Health Organization (WHO) endorses the situating of occupational therapy education in the context of understanding the social determinants of health as it supports the WHO's goals in monitoring, researching, and training in the social determinants of health.

I absolutely commend this book and my colleagues who have been involved in its development. It supports us as we strive to take our rightful place as agents of social change and equity.

The future is not someplace we are going, but one we are creating. The paths are not to be found, but made, and the activity of making them changes both the maker and the destination

Marilyn Pattison
Executive Director, World Federation of
Occupational Therapists
March 2010

References

Bornstein D: Quoted in: Drayton W, Brown C, Hillhouse K 2006 Integrating social entrepreneurs into the 'health for all' formula, *Bull World Health Organ* 84:591, 2004.

Drucker PF: *Innovation and Entrepreneur: Practice and Principles*, New York, 1985, Harper & Row.

Pattison M: OT – Outstanding talent: An entrepreneurial approach to practice. *Australian Occupational Therapy Journal* 53:166–172, 2006.

Schaar J: Futurist, n.d, 2010: Online. Available at: http://thinkexist.com Accessed February 20, 2010.

World Federation of Occupational Therapists: *Minimum Standards for Education of Occupational Therapists*, Forrestfield, Australia, 2002, World Federation of Occupational Therapists.

WFOT website: n.d., Online. Available at: http://www.wfot.org. Accessed July 5, 2010.

World Health Organization: *Commission on the Social Determinants of Health*, Final Report: Executive Summary. Geneva, 2008, World Health Organization. Online. Available at: http://www.who.int/social_determinants/thecommission/finalreport/en/. Accessed February 20, 2010.

What if?

We allowed ourselves to be inspired by the scenarios of ...

Jean Giono (2005), who through his story of a fictional person Elzéard Bouffie – *The Man Who Planted Trees* – succeeded in realizing his goal and most cherished idea 'to make planting trees likeable' (1957) ...

Peter Senge (Senge et al 2005, p. 2) who posed: 'It's common to say that trees come from seeds. But how could a tiny seed create a huge tree? Seeds do not contain the resources needed to grow a tree. These must come from the medium or environment within which the tree grows. But the seed does provide something that is crucial: a place where the whole of the tree starts to form. As resources such as water and nutrients are drawn in, the seed organizes the process that generates growth. In a sense, the seed is the gateway through which the future possibility of the tree emerges.' ...

... then we might appreciate this book to present a 'collection of seeds', ideas about alternative futures of occupational therapy, to take root and spread across our globe, hopefully 'helping to overcome inertia and denial that can so easily make the future a dangerous place' (Scearce & Fulton 2004, p. 2). Not all of them will attract or speak to all readers' interests, predispositions, and needs. It is therefore up to them, following Elzéard Bouffie's example, to find, identify, select, and plant those that seem most relevant to and viable in their daily life contexts. This may then also contribute to the cultivation of new generations of 'seeds'. The goal we share with our readers and colleagues might be to plant seeds that will flourish into a consciousness of how our daily occupations can influence our individual and collective wellbeing and that of our environments. This essentially calls for engagements in the service of a purpose that is larger than the advancement of our profession's interests. Chambers' (2009, p. 375) reflections on anthropology may offer some appropriate pointers in this regard, which resonate with the spirit of this book:

Anthropology is a choice. It is an invention. Like virtually any other discipline, we are burdened by our profession, which always seems to be cautioning us against getting overly inventive. After all, we need some enduring foci to define us, to prescribe our core values, to distinguish us from others. So we do our changing (just as we do our professing) at the margins ... Even so, the changes can be profound, although they might go largely unrecognized. I might be deluding myself here, but the only thing about us that really seems to endure is a position we take in the world. It is where we locate ourselves and just as often it is where we are put. It is on the margins, some distance from home, where we are at our best when we just listen and witness and practice our invisibility.

Background to this new volume

Surpassing both the publisher's and the authors' own expectations, the first volume of *Occupational Therapy Without Borders: Learning from the Spirit of Survivors* (Kronenberg et al 2005), which this text complements, had a worldwide impact and reached both traditional and nontraditional occupational therapy readers.

This book was also translated in Spanish *Terapia Ocupacional sin Fronteras: Aprendiendo del Espiritu de Supervivientes* (Kronenberg et al 2007) and it inspired the publication of *A Political Practice of Occupational Therapy* (Pollard et al 2008) and *Disaster and Development: An Occupational Perspective* (Thomas & Rushford, in press). The international informal network of proactive occupational therapists who contributed to and/or worked with the book also influenced and informed the landmark World Federation of Occupational Therapists (WFOT) position statements on community-based rehabilitation' (2004), human rights (2006), and cultural diversity (2010).

Frank & Zemke (2008, p. 112) identified 'occupational therapists without borders' (OTwB) to be part of what constitutes a 'movement', because its ideas and activities have arisen independently and

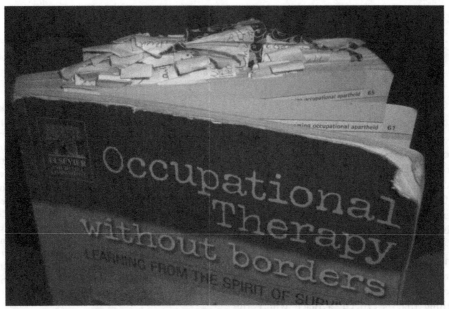

May the second volume prove to be as valuable resource as the original book.

heterogeneously, operating through social networks, rather than from any single, centralized source (Diani & McAdam 2003, McAdam et al 1996). Therefore, it seems both appropriate and useful to situate the movement OTwB in relation to Santos' depiction of the World Social Forum (WSF) as a 'new social and political phenomenon' (Santos 2003). He described the WSF as a 'set of initiatives – of transnational exchange among social movements, NGOs and their practices and knowledge of local, national or global social struggles against the forms of exclusion and inclusion, discrimination and equality, universalism and particularism, cultural imposition and relativism, that have been brought about or made possible by the current phase of capitalism known as neoliberal globalization' (Santos 2003, p. 236, see Chapter 1). As Frank & Zemke pointed out, OTwB also is not structured according to any of the models of modern political organization, be they democratic centralism, representative, and/ or participatory democracy. It came about in response to a need among some occupational therapists within the international community to establish a forum that allows and encourages constructive critique of professional practice. Besides raising theoretical, analytical, and epistemological questions, OTwB poses a political issue, which is perhaps best captured by the utopian motto 'Other

Occupational Therapies are Possible!'. This book therefore seems aligned with the WSF as critical utopia, advancing an epistemology of the South, and emergent politics (see Chapter 1).

Although greatly encouraged by the knowledge of a guaranteed and seemingly growing audience and platform for critically constructive discourses and practices, when Elsevier invited us to work on a second volume of the book, the decision to take this on did not come about easily. Apart from the fact that such a project is hugely time and energy consuming, our personal and professional life stories had undergone some significant changes. Hence, this book could not just be about revising and updating its original chapters. It would have to somehow reflect the evolving narrative of OTwB. A key point of contention was the appropriateness of the central focus on 'occupational therapy'. Acknowledging that the book's main audience consists of occupational therapy students and educators, we questioned to what extent our own local practices (as editors) could still be called 'occupational therapy', regardless of the intention to broaden its traditional scope by adding the qualification 'without borders'. We agreed that 'occupations as vehicles for bringing about meaningful and sustainable change' were still at the heart of our alternative vision and ideas of practice, but that the timing may not (yet) be right for a more radical shift in focus, e.g., 'Occupations without Borders', also inviting contributions by groups other than occupational therapists.

What can also be regarded as evidence of the impact of the original book was the coming out of 'new' colleagues worldwide who indicated their strong identification with the OTwB vision and who wished to share their 'without borders' perspectives and experiences in the new book. Their volume of interests to contribute rapidly outgrew the availability of chapter spaces. Although this volume offers an additional nine chapters, unfortunately not all proposals could be accommodated.

During a conversation about 'without borders' interpretations of our 'professional identity' and situated contexts, our Chilean colleague Alejandro Guajardo pointed out that it seems to make more sense to speak of 'occupational therapies' than its conventional singular form 'occupational therapy'.

This realization resonated well with our assertion that what 'occupational therapy' is to be about resists being universally predefined or 'bordered'. Instead its contributions ought to be largely informed and guided by unique possibilities in the local contexts in which practitioners engage with people and what matters most to them. Indeed, this is where the full meaning and purpose of the notion 'without borders' come in to play, providing the basis for constructing a plurality (or ecology) of occupation-based practices. These then are inclusive of but not limited to traditionally conceived (occupational) therapy (see Chapter 1).

Although the intention of the original book was to interpret the notion 'without borders' beyond geopolitical perspectives, readers' feedback often indicated that OTwB was understood as an nongovernmental organization that takes occupational therapists from so called privileged societies on 'rescue' or 'development' missions to 'developing countries' in the southern hemisphere. This impression was strengthened by the tendency of our practice chapters to represent Western professionals' perceptions of engagement in

community-based rehabilitation. Some of our colleagues have legitimately criticized this. Their point was that Westerners can count on a listening and supportive audience for work they did in challenging contexts in the South, whereas the work done by occupational therapists from the South is rarely presented as having the same weight. A 'without borders' practice as we see it, is about reciprocation, negotiation, and mutuality in the sharing of occupation-based and needs-oriented collaborations, rather than a one-way street for Western expertise. In an attempt to rectify this, this volume includes mostly 'without borders' chapters that share perspectives and experiences from the authors' own 'backyards'. This also makes good sense given the fact that our rapidly changing world is characterized by the massive uprooting and relocation of populations and resources.

The second editor of the original book Salvador Simó Algado decided to withdraw from the editorial team in order to focus his vision and energies on building the innovative 'without borders' practice-education-research project 'Jardin Miquel Martí i Pol' at the University of Vic in Cataluña, Spain (see cover page and Chapter 38) and the project Human, Social and Ecological Sustainability, related to occupational justice and ecology. Based on his invaluable editorial contributions to *A Political Practice of Occupational Therapy* (Pollard et al 2008), Dikaios Sakellariou was welcomed to complete the editorial OTwB team of 'three muskOTeers'.

We can only wish that this publication triggers a similarly generous wave of free and critically constructive engagements with occupation-based discourses and practices of change as its predecessor did.

Frank Kronenberg
Nick Pollard
Dikaios Sakellariou
2010

References

Chambers E: In both our possibilities: anthropology on the margins, *Hum Organ* 68:374–379, 2009.

Diani M, McAdam D: *Social Movements and Networks: Relational Approaches to Collective Action*, Oxford, 2003, Oxford University Press.

Frank G, Zemke R: Occupational therapy foundations for political engagement and social transformation. In Pollard N, Sakellariou D, Kronenberg F, editors: *Political Practice of Occupational Therapy*, Edinburgh, 2008, Elsevier Science, pp 111–136.

Giono J: *Letter to the Waters & Forests Manager of Digne, Mr. Valdeyron*, 1957. Online. Available at: http://www.pinetum.org/GionoUK.htm Accessed January 5, 2010.

Giono J: *The Man Who Planted Trees*, White River Junction, 2005, Chelsea Green Publishing.

Kronenberg F, Algado SS, Pollard N, editors: *Occupational Therapy Without Borders: Learning from the Spirit of Survivors*, Edinburgh, 2005, Elsevier/Churchill Livingstone.

Kronenberg F, Algado SS, Pollard N, editors: *Terapia Ocupacional sin Fronteras: Aprendiendo del Espiritu de Supervivientes*, Madrid, 2007, Panamericana.

McAdam D, McCarthy JD, Zald MN: *Comparative Perspectives on Social Movements: A Political Opportunities, Mobilizing Structures, and Cultural Framings*, Cambridge, 1996, Cambridge University Press.

Pollard N, Sakellariou D, Kronenberg F, editors: *A Political Practice of Occupational Therapy*, Edinburgh, 2008, Elsevier Science.

Santos BdS: *Challenging Empires. The World Social Forum: Toward A Counter-Hegemonic Globalization. Part I –Toward a Counter Hegemonic Globalization*, 2003. Online. Available at:http://www.choike.org/documentos/wsf_s318_sousa.pdf Accessed January 7, 2010.

Scearce D, Fulton K: *What If? The Art of Scenario-Thinking for Non-Profits*, 2004, Global Business Network Community Online. Available at:http://www.musicandmedia.org/standard/pdf/what_if_1.pdf Accessed January 5, 2010.

Senge P, Scharmer CO, Jaworski J, Flowers BS: *Presence: Exploring Profound Change in People, Organizations, and Society*, London, 2005, Nicholas Brealey.

Thomas K, Rushford N: *Disaster and Development: An Occupational Perspective*, Sydney, in press. Elsevier Churchill Livingstone.

World Federation of Occupational Therapists: *Position Paper on Community-Based Rehabilitation*, Forrestfield, Australia, 2004, World Federation of Occupational Therapists Online. Available at: https://www.wfot.org/office_files/CBRposition%20Final%20CM2004%282%29.pdf Accessed January 7, 2010.

World Federation of Occupational Therapists: *Position Statement on Human Rights*, Forrestfield, Australia, 2006, World Federation of Occupational Therapists Online. Available at: https://www.wfot.org/office_files/Human%20Rights%20Position%20Statement%20Final%20NLH%281%29.pdf Accessed January 7, 2010.

World Federation of Occupational Therapists: *Position Statement on Cultural Diversity*, Forrestfield, Australia, 2010, WFOT. World Federation of Occupational Therapists.

Dedication

To Elelwani, Masana Nelly and Isha Tshiala – for providing me with a deep sense of belonging, and to South Africa – for becoming home, where what must be done by all who live here matters … way beyond its national borders.

Frank

To my wife Linda especially for her tolerance, and to Sally, Molly, Joshua and Daisy for holding the fort while I bashed the computer.

Nick

To my family.

Dikaios

Acknowledgments

A sincere expression of gratitude is extended to the worldwide community of readers and users of the original book. Your very positive responses have been and continue to be a great source of encouragement and inspiration. Your spirit allowed numerous meaningful engagements to come about, making the unfolding journey of 'occupational therapists without borders' a true example of collective story-making.

We wish to express a special word of thanks to the international contributors who committed themselves to generously share their views and experiences in the chapters of this book. It has once again been a privilege to walk and learn with you as colleagues and editors.

We thank our editorial team at Elsevier/Oxford, Rita Demetriou-Swanwick, Catherine Jackson, Nancy Arnott, and Lotika Singha for their valuable support.

Dikaios also wishes to acknowledge the supportive environment of the Department of Occupational Therapy, Cardiff University, which enabled his participation in this and numerous other projects.

Nick would like to thank his colleagues in the Occupational Therapy Team at Sheffield Hallam University for their support, and also his students for their interest, enthusiasm, and willingness to discuss ideas.

Frank first acknowledges the space, patience, and support that his wife and daughters afforded him. It literally meant that at times, family matters were put on hold to allow book project issues to be attended to. *Ndi a livhuwa, bedankt*, thank you Elelwani, Masana, and Isha. Second, high fives to all global and local colleagues (to be) who enthusiastically participated in 'without borders' guest lectures, workshops, courses, and those who engaged through emails and Facebook. Your sharing of what you were 'occupassional' about often times kept me going. In this regard I wish to express a special word of gratitude to students and colleagues at Zuyd University, Heerlen, the Netherlands – the regular program and the German Bachelorstudiengang; University of the Western Cape in Cape Town/South Africa; Universidad Andres Bello, Santiago de Chile/Chile; and University of Salford in the Greater Manchester area in the United Kingdom.

Daniela Alburquerque MS OT
Occupational Therapist, Director of Rehabilitation
Movement Disorder Center (CETRAM), Medicine Science
Faculty, University of Santiago
Santiago, Chile

Mami Aoyama PhD OTR (Japan)
Professor and Head, Department of Occupational Therapy
Nishikyushu University (University of West Kyushu)
Kanzaki, Japan and Coordinator Human Activity and
Sustainability Group

Karen Barney PhD MS BS OTR/L FAOTA
Associate Professor and Chairperson
Department of Occupational Science and
Occupational Therapy
Doisy College of Health Sciences, Saint Louis University
St Louis, MO, USA

Denise Dias Barros PhD (Sociology) Master (Social Sciences-
Anthropology) OT
Professor of Occupational Therapy
Universidade de São Paulo: Member of the Metuia Project:
Member of Casa das Africas Project
Brazil

Althea Barry BSc (OT)
Programme Developer
Grandmothers Against Poverty and AIDS (GAPA)
Cape Town, South Africa

Peter Beresford BA (Hons) PhD AcSS FRSA
Professor of Social Policy and Director of the
Centre for Citizen Participation
Brunel University
Middlesex, UK

Mary Black MS OTR/L
Occupational Therapist
Heartland Alliance Marjorie Kovler Center
Chicago, IL, USA

Pamela Block PhD
Clinical Associate Professor, Occupational Therapy
Program
Stony Brook University
New York, NY, USA

Wendy Bryant PhD MScOT BSc (Hons) Dip COT FHEA
Lecturer, Occupational Therapy
Brunel University
West London, UK

Imelda Burgman PhD MA (MotLearn) PGDipSc (AnatSc)
BAppSC (OT) OTR AccOT
Lecturer, School of Health Sciences
University of Newcastle
New South Wales, Australia

Grace Patricia Mary Cairns BSc (OT)
Occupational Therapist
Rehabilitation Department (Vocational Rehabilitation)
West Vaal Hospital, Anglo Gold Ashanti Health Ltd
North West, South Africa

Pedro Chana MD
Director and Associate Professor Neurologist
Movement Disorder Center (CETRAM)
Medicine Science Faculty
University of Santiago
Santiago, Chile

Melina T Czymoniewicz-Klippel MHSt BOcc Thy(Hons)
Doctoral Candidate, Social Science and Health
Research Unit
School of Psychology and Psychiatry
Monash University, Melbourne, Victoria, Australia
and
Lecturer and Global Health Minor coordinator,
Department of Biobehavioral Health,
Pennsylvania State University
Pennsylvania, USA

Teresa Cassani Danner MS OTR/L
Occupational Therapist
Baylor Our Children's House in Grapevine
Fort Worth, TX, USA

Jo-Celéne De Jongh PhD MPhil B (OT)
Senior Lecturer, Department of Occupational Therapy
University of the Western Cape
Cape Town, South Africa

R Lyle Duque MSc (OT) OTRP FOTAP
Editor, *Philippine Journal of Occupational Therapy*
and
Program Director, Life Skills Therapy Center
Philippines

Hanif Farhan BOT (Hons)
Occupational Therapist, Faculty of Allied Health Sciences,
Universiti Kebangsaan
Kuala Lumpur, Malaysia

Louise Farnworth BAppSc (OT) GradDipCrim MA PhD
Associate Professor and Head of Department of
Occupational Therapy
Monash University
Victoria, Australia

Farhana Firfirey BSc (OT)
Lecturer, Department of Occupational Therapy
University of the Western Cape
Cape Town, South Africa

Gillian Frost
Member of Voluntary Development Team, Director
Founder Member and Ex Joint Coordinator
Pecket Learning Community
West Yorkshire, UK

Sandra Maria Galheigo PhD M Ed OT
Assistant Professor, Faculty of Medicine
University of São Paulo
São Paulo, Brazil

Roshan Galvaan PhD MSc BSc (OT)
Senior Lecturer, Division of Occupational Therapy
Faculty of Health Sciences
University of Cape Town, South Africa

Débora Galvani MSc PhD Student
Occupational Therapist, Department of Physical Therapy
Speech Therapy and Occupational Therapy
University of São Paulo, Brazil

Rosie Garland MA BA (Hons) PGCE
Writer, Performer
Manchester, UK

Maria Isabel Garcez Ghirardi OT PhD
Lecturer in Undergraduate Studies, Occupational
Therapy Department
University of São Paulo
São Paulo, Brazil

Toby Ballou Hamilton MPH PhD OTR/L
Assistant Professor, University of Oklahoma
Health Sciences Center
Oklahoma City, OK, USA

Erin C Hanrahan Med BSc MOTR/L
Occupational Therapist
Greater Minneapolis — St Paul Area
Minnesota, USA

Joan Healey MA BA (Hons) PGCE DipCOT
Senior Lecturer in Occupational Therapy, Faculty of
Health and Wellbeing
Sheffield Hallam University
Sheffield, UK

Carmen Gloria de las Heras MS OTR
Professor of Undergraduate and Postgraduate Programs,
School of Occupational Therapy
University Andrés Bello
Santiago, Chile

Lucia Hess-April PGD (Disability Studies) MPH BSc (OT)
PhD Student and Lecturer
Department of Occupational Therapy
University of the Western Cape
Cape Town, South Africa

Mark J Hudson PhD
Professor of Anthropology
Department of Occupational Therapy
Nishikyushu University (University of West Kyushu)
Kanzaki, Japan and Coordinator,
Human Activity and Sustainability Group

Moses N Ikiugu PhD MA BA (Magna Cum Laude) DipOT
DipCounselling Psychology OTR/L
Associate Professor and Director of Research,
Occupational Therapy
University of South Dakota
Vermillion, SD, USA

Michael K Iwama PhD MSc BSc (Human Performance), BSc OT,
OT(C), OT Reg (Ont)
Associate Professor, Graduate Department of
Rehabilitation Sciences and Department of Occupational
Science and Occupational Therapy
Faculty of Medicine, University of Toronto
Ontario, Canada

Avital Kaufman MS BSOT
Occupational Therapist Head
Department of Occupational Therapy
Hogar de Ancianos Villa Israel
Santiago, Chile

Gary Kielhofner DrPH OTR FAOTA
Professor and Wade-Meyer Chair
Department of Occupational Therapy, College of
Applied Health Sciences
University of Illinois at Chicago
Chicago, IL, USA

Debbie Kramer-Roy PhD MA (Education and International Development), BSc (OT)
Advanced Paediatric Occupational Therapist
Ealing Services for Children with Additional Needs
Ealing, UK

Frank Kronenberg BSc(OT) BA(Ed)
International Guest Lecturer
Formal affiliations with Zuyd University, the Netherlands
University of Salford, UK
Universidad Andres Bello, Chile
University of the Western Cape, South Africa
and
Director, Shades of Black Works
Cape Town, South Africa

Barbara Lavin MOT NZROT
Occupational Therapist, Older Person's
Mental Health Team
Hutt Hospital
Hutt Valley, New Zealand

Kee Hean Lim MSc DipOT PG Cert in Learning and Teaching in Higher Education
Lecturer and Researcher in Occupational Therapy
Brunel University, School of Health Sciences and Social Care, Middlesex, UK

Roseli Esquerdo Lopes PhD (Education) Med OT
Professor, Department of Occupational Therapy
Universidade Federal de São Carlos
Member of the Metuia Project
Brazil

Alexander Lopez JD OT/L
Clinical Assistant Professor
Executive Director PAR FORE
Stony Brook University
New York, NY, USA

Rona M Macdonald PhD Candidate MSc (OT)
BHSc OT Reg (Ont)
Graduate Department of Rehabilitation Science
University of Toronto
Toronto, Ontario, Canada

Hazel Mackey PhD MA DipCOT PGCE
Localities Manager
Stoke on Trent Primary Care Trust, UK

Anne MacRae PhD OTR/L BCMH FAOTA
Professor, Department of Occupational Therapy
San Jose State University
San Jose, CA, USA

Amy Marshall MS OTR/L
Assistant Professor, Department of Occupational Therapy
Eastern Kentucky University
Richmond, KY, USA

Elizabeth McKay PhD MSc OT BSc (Hons) DipCOT FHEA
Reader/Director of Occupational Therapy
Brunel University
West London, UK

Elisabeth Gómez Mengelberg
Occupational Therapist, Head of Occupational Therapy,
Psychiatric Hospital Dr José T. Borda
Buenos Aires, Argentina

Candice Joy Mes BSc (OT)
Occupational Therapist
Pro-Practicum School for Vocational Training
Johannesburg, South Africa

Jaime Philip Muñoz PhD OTR/L FAOTA
Associate Professor, Department of Occupational Therapy
Duquesne University
Pittsburgh, PA, USA

Alison Nelson PhD MOccThy (research) BOccThy
Associate Lecturer
Department of Occupational Therapy
University of Queensland
Brisbane, Australia

Pauline Nugent
Member, Pecket Learning Community
West Yorkshire, UK

Shirley Peganoff O'Brien PhD OTR/L FAOTA
Professor, Department of Occupational Therapy
Eastern Kentucky University
Richmond, KY, USA

Liliana Paganizzi BSc (OT) MSc (Public Health)
Lecturer, Clinical Supervisor, Universidad Nacional
de San Martin
San Martín, Provincia de Buenos Aires, Argentina

Stephen Parks PhD
Associate Professor of Writing and Rhetoric
Syracuse University
Philadelphia, PA, USA

Neha Patel MSc (OT)
Occupational Therapist
Willesden Health & Care
Harrow, UK

Suzanne M Peloquin PhD OTR FAOTA
Professor, Department of Occupational Therapy
School of Health Professions
The University of Texas Medical Branch at Galveston
Galveston, TX, USA

Mershen Pillay DEd MSpPath BSp & HearTher
Audiologist and Speech-Language Pathologist
University of Cape Town, South Africa
and Mafraq Hospital
Abu Dhabi, United Arab Emirates

Nick Pollard BA DipCOT MA MSc (OT) PGCE
Senior Lecturer in Occupational Therapy
Sheffield Hallam University
Sheffield, UK

Gina Marie Prioletti MS OTR/L
Staff Therapist
Canonsburg General Hospital
Pittsburgh, PA, USA

Elelwani Ramugondo PhD (OT)
Head of Division
Occupational Therapy School of Health & Rehabilitation
University of Cape Town
Cape Town, South Africa

Pamela K Richardson PhD OTR/L FAOTA
Professor and Post-Professional Program Co-ordinator
Department of Occupational Therapy
San Jose State University
San Jose, CA, USA

Sandra Rogers PhD OTR/L
Associate Professor, Pacific University of Oregon,
College of Health Professions
School of Occupational Therapy
Hillsboro, Oregon, USA

Charlotte Royeen PhD OTR/L FAOTA
Dean, Edward and Margaret Doisy College
of Health Sciences
Professor of Occupational Science and
Occupational Therapy
Saint Louis University
Saint Louis, MO, USA

Matin Royeen PhD (OT)
Senior Civilian Advisor to the US Military,
Kabul, Afghanistan

Nancy A Rushford MSc (OT) MA (Counselling Psychology)
Doctoral Student and Postgraduate Fellow, Faculty of
Health Sciences
University of Sydney
Sydney, New South Wales, Australia

Dikaios Sakellariou MSc BSc (OT)
Lecturer, Cardiff University
Cardiff, UK

Anne Shordike PhD OTR/L
Professor, Department of Occupational Therapy
Eastern Kentucky University
Richmond, KY, USA

Salvador Simó
PhD candidate, Master in Inclusive Education, Master in
Translation and Interpretation Studies, BOT
and
Lecturer, Universitat de Vic
Department of Human Development and
Community Action
Co-ordinator of the Research Group
Occupational Science and the project Sustainability
human, ecological and social (SHES)

Pat Smart
Member, Pecket Learning Community
West Yorkshire, UK

Neeltjé Smit BOccTher MBA BOccTherHons
Doctoral Candidate in Social Sciences
Senior Lecturer, Occupational Therapy
Stellenbosch University
Tygerberg, South Africa

Yolanda Suarez-Balcazar PhD
Head and Professor, Department of Occupational Therapy
University of Illinois, Chicago
and
Associate Director, Center for Capacity Building for
Minorities with Disabilities Research, Chicago, IL, USA

Rachel Thibeault PhD MSc BSc(OT)
Full Professor, Occupational Therapy Programme
School of Rehabilitation Sciences,
Faculty of Health Sciences
University of Ottawa
Ottawa, Canada

Kerry A Thomas BSc (OT) GradDip (Health Science)
Director, *inter*part and Associates (International Partners in
Action, Research and Training)
and
Adviser with the WFOT Disaster Preparedness
and Response Project
Australia

Nicole A Thomson PhD Candidate MSc (OT) BHSc OT Reg
(ONT)
Graduate Department of Rehabilitation Science
Faculty of Medicine, University of Toronto
Toronto, Ontario, Canada

Elizabeth Townsend PhD OT(C) RegNS FCAOT
Professor Emerita
School of Occupational Therapy,
Dalhousie University
Nova Scotia, Canada

Geraldine Vacher
Borough Lead OT
Hillingdon Hospital
Hillingdon
London, UK

Hanneke van Bruggen BSc HonDscie FWFOT
Executive Director of ENOTHE (European Network of
Occupational Therapy in Higher Education),
Hogeschool van Amsterdam,
Netherlands

Lana van Niekerk PhD M(Arb) b(Arb)
Division Occupational Therapy
School of Health and Rehabilitation Sciences
Cape town, South Africa

Jesse Vogel OT
Occupational Therapist
Coney Island Hospital
Brooklyn
New York, USA

Sarah R Walsh MOT OTR/L
Adjunct Instructor, Saint Louis University
Department of Occupational Science
and Occupational Therapy,
Saint Louis, MO
and
Occupational Therapist
Peter and Paul Community Services
Saint Louis, MO, USA

John A White PhD OTR/L
Director and Professor, Pacific University School of
Occupational Therapy
Hillsboro, Oregon, USA

Gail Whiteford PhD MHSc BAppSc
Professor and Pro Vice Chancellor (Social Inclusion)
Macquarie University
Sydney, New South Wales, Australia

Introduction: courage to dance politics

Frank Kronenberg   Nick Pollard   Elelwani Ramugondo

OVERVIEW

Of the multiple challenges that face occupational therapists, the biggest one may be collectively living up to *our* full potential. This is particularly significant because at the *heart* of our profession's value proposition to society, potential is critical. In response to this challenge, we must be tuned into our own music – the art of being ourselves and doing what we are really called to do. A raised occupational consciousness may help cultivate a critical understanding of the influences of internalized hegemony on our everyday practice, and how this impacts on our ability to advance individual and collective wellbeing.

In this chapter, Santos' 'epistemological operations of the South' – sociologies of absences and emergences, are used as lenses through which to critically explore and juxtapose monocultural expressions of occupational therapy against an ecology of occupation-based practices, suggesting that these are at play on a continuum of hegemonic and alternative or counter-hegemonic practices.

Clues of emergent alternative occupational therapies are identified and described: to encourage and remind people and society to understand, build and maintain working relationships through collective occupations (purpose); people's ability to positively influence their wellbeing, humanity's and the planet's through doing well with others and the environment (premise); a political possibilities-based practice with people from all walks of life in real-life contexts (occupation-based approaches); using eclectic modes of productivity (sustainAbilities).

The chapter does not intend to be directive or prescriptive regarding what occupational therapy is (to be) about, but instead freely shares ideas to inspire and to invite dialogue and debate.

Tuning into the music of occupational therapy

In the 1980 documentary film *From Mao to Mozart* the late violinist Isaac Stern said of music: 'The instrument is not that important, it is only a means to an end, in other words, you don't use music to play the violin you use the violin to play music.' As he played he added 'dancing', with his violin, body, and soul all acting as one (Stern 1979). If occupational therapy is an instrument, occupation may be the music. Occupation becomes powerful when there is coherence between what people collectively wish to do and who people are, and hope to become. This is as relevant for occupational therapists as it is for everyone else. The practice of occupational therapy is not separate from all other occupations occupational therapists engage in. As occupational therapists aspiring to realize our full potential, we might ask ourselves to what extent are we in tune with the music or the art of occupational therapy? This question of value has been a critical theme in the profession's reflections on itself. Occasionally these reflections have had a tinge of anxiety (Wilcock 2002). The anxiety becomes significant as our profession's contributions towards global healthcare are currently being challenged by factors such as competition for limited resources, other professions widening their practice, and pressure for generic rather than specialist workers (Wilding 2010). A further challenge is the emerging political awareness among occupational therapists reflecting on and questioning traditional modes of practice – including education and research – in terms of its accessibility to the

DOI: 10.1016/B978-0-7020-3103-8.00010-9

majority of the world's populations and relevance to their local contexts (Kronenberg et al 2005, Pollard et al 2008b, Thibeault 2006, World Federation of Occupational Therapists (WFOT 2004, 2006, 2010, Whiteford 2007).

Suppose that we were to assess our personal and professional status of wellbeing (Doble & Santha 2008) from an occupational perspective. We could ask whether we are 'living life to its fullest' (American Occupational Therapy Association (AOTA) 2008). As occupational therapists or occupational scientists we could ask: to what extent are we doing justice to what matters most to us, personally and professionally through our daily practices? A further question is: to what extent are we conscious or sensitive to the impact of our actions on the planet and its ecological systems (Ikiugu 2008, Morin 1999, Thibeault 2002)? Honoring one of our profession's core principles that 'every human being is unique' implies that we acknowledge that a diversity of people represents diversity in values (Wilcock 2002). These values feed both conflict and cooperation, which the Dutch political scientist Van der Eijk identified as 'the motor of all political engagement' (Kronenberg & Pollard 2006, p. 69). They also suggest a deep responsibility at the *heart* of occupational therapy, which entails the practice of respect for people's differences (see Chapter 7). This practice is based on the premise that people's experiences of health and wellbeing are influenced by opportunities, as well as their own abilities to be true to themselves, in order to be in tune with the music of their lives. Occupational therapists are, however, often challenged either to effectively operationalize these responsibilities, or to critique the frequently ethnocentric premises they are founded on (Hammell 2009a,b).

Occupational consciousness

It can be difficult for professional workers to find an objective position that is not tangled up in the ideology and the interests of the dominant order which frame their actions. Even activities that appear to be counter to the prevailing system may be tolerated in order to vent dissident expression in a way that does not present a serious challenge. By their nature professionals and the professional bodies to which they belong adhere to the principles and structure of the dominant social order to build and preserve their power; change can represent a threat to the operational privileges that have been carefully negotiated over

> # Box 1.1
>
> ## Occupational consciousness – working definition
>
> An ongoing awareness of the dynamics of hegemony, an appreciation of the role of personal and collective occupations of daily life in perpetuating hegemonic practices, and an appraisal of resultant consequences for individual and collective wellbeing.

time. However, representing the interests of a profession entails conflict as well as cooperation, and it is inevitable that in this process occupational therapists have to develop strategic and tactical reflections (Pollard et al 2008a, see Chapters 8 and 14). In her doctoral thesis, Ramugondo (2009) introduced the notion *occupational consciousness* (Box 1.1) which is rooted in the notions of political consciousness advanced by Fanon (1963) and Biko (1987).

What value can our discourses and practices of change and the process of raising occupational consciousness bring to the struggles of people with experiences of disability, poverty, and social exclusion, and whose social position is often limited by the hegemonic exercise of power? Occupational consciousness and 3P Archaeology (3PA) (Kronenberg et al 2005, 2010, Pollard et al 2006, Pollard & Kronenberg 2008, see Chapter 33) may serve to illustrate how our values as well as individual and collective everyday doing are critically intertwined with hegemony. 3PA is a tool that allows individuals and collectives to engage in critical in-depth introspection, deconstruction, and reaffirmation of their enacted values. Its key questions offer lenses to focus and reflect on our *personal* and *professional* values – what we stand for, 'our talk', and in terms of exercising our *politics*; to what extent are we putting these values into practice – what we stand for, 'our walk'? Everyday occupational therapy practice presents opportunities where the 3Ps of 3PA are expressed. The extent to which occupational therapists are conscious of how their everyday actions perpetuate hegemonies (occupational consciousness) that may negatively impact the lives of the people we aim to serve is critical (Morin 1999, see Chapters 6, 8, 13–15, 17, and 27). It appears therefore that there is a conceptual and practical goodness of fit between raising occupational consciousness and engaging with the 3PA as part of reflecting on how we are doing in living up to our potential (also see 'critical occupational therapy' in Chapter 8).

Towards an ecology of occupation-based practices

Occupational therapy education describes a process of being socialized voluntarily into the privileged realm (social status, influence, compensation) of professions (Box 1.2), a process which may actually serve to exclude students from a working-class background through simply failing to acknowledge either their occupational experiences (Beagan 2007) or that of the communities around them (see Chapter 42). The acknowledgment that professions are essentially instruments of hegemony (Box 1.2) has been little discussed within the profession, though some of the central planks of its holistic and client-centered ethos are coming under scrutiny (Hammell 2007, 2009a,b, Pollard et al 2005, 2008b, Pollard & Sakellariou 2009, see Chapters 14 and 15). Understanding what this is about may at least partly explain some of our struggles to articulate and enact the holistic ethos we claim, through strategies and tactics that may be perceived as counter-hegemonic (Box 1.2).

As explained with more detail in the Preface of this book, 'occupational therapy without borders' (the movement) came about in response to a need among some occupational therapists within the international community to establish a forum that allows

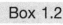

Box 1.2

Definitions: profession, hegemony, counter-hegemony

Profession: 'A vocation founded upon specialized educational training, the purpose of which is to supply disinterested counsel and service to others, for a direct and definite compensation, wholly apart from expectation of other business gain' (Rugland 1993:224).

Hegemony: The political, economic, ideological, or cultural power exerted by a dominant group over other groups, regardless of the explicit consent of the latter (Gramsci 1978).

Counter-hegemony: Counter-hegemony implies alternatives to existing configurations of power (Abbot & Worth 2002, Cox 1981, 1983). 'Counter-hegemonic processes are typically based on three complementary features: challenging the hegemonic status quo; contesting hegemonic legitimacy, and; the creation of alternatives. A counter-hegemonic strategy is usually twofold: resistance to hegemonic pressures (reactive) and the building-up of a counter-hegemonic alternative strategy (active)' (Cascao 2008:17).

and encourages critique of professional practice, acknowledges and confronts 'negativity', and engages with that to which they aspire, or 'positivity'. The book's title, *Occupational Therapies without Borders: Towards an Ecology of Occupation-based Practices*, suggests that occupational therapy does not and cannot constitute a monocultural practice – defined by a rather narrow, imposed, and exclusive set of rational criteria that are mainly rooted in Western modernity. Instead it argues for a plurality of interpretations (Morin 1999), including those that serve hegemonic interests. Continuing with the metaphor of music and borrowing from Senge et al (2005), the authors consider that most of what we (collectively) have written in the past, at best, may have described the words but left the music of 'occupation' largely in the background. We may have been too preoccupied with what we do and how we do it, instead of connecting with who we are and the inner place or source from which we operate both individually and collectively, trusting that here we may encounter values that unite us in our diversity. The 'without borders' discourses, practices, education, and research chapters illustrate this diverse stance. Next we will explore in more detail some of the tendencies that characterize hegemonic and possibly alternative or even counter-hegemonic practices that influence definitions and manifestations of occupational therapy. The contributions to this book may have been 'pushed' by the limitations posed by the former and 'pulled' by the possibilities that are offered by the latter.

Occupational therapists mostly operate in and serve a minority within the global population, in countries that are able to afford complex health and social care services. Even within some of those wealthy countries occupational therapy services are not available to all who might have need of them (Hammell 2009a,b, Kronenberg et al 2005, Kronenberg & Pollard 2006, Pollard et al 2008b, Thibeault 2006, Watson & Swartz 2004). Through the pursuit of trade, countries such as Britain, United States, Australia, Canada, and a number of European states became economically and politically powerful. As a consequence of their waxing and waning dominance through history they have disseminated knowledge, science, technology, and culture to the rest of the world. A characteristic of that dominance has been the privilege given to market forces in determining international relationships; in many cultures, and not only Western ones, trade, profit, and greed have been a key principle behind the pursuit of political dominance and empire building (Ferguson 2004,

Hobsbawm 1987, 1994). These issues are also evident in newer economic relationships: the importance of oil in the Middle East in financing unsustainable developments and governmental elites; the importance of gas in central European politics among former Soviet bloc countries; China's developing interest in bargaining for African raw materials to supply its industrial demands. Because market-based globalization has been the pattern of historical development over hundreds of years, it has been assumed that it is the only way to organize international relationships. It is also an assumption that maintenance of a global market is the right way to assure political stability, as was proven by the consequences of the 1930s slump (Hobsbawm 1994). In the current international financial crisis economic interventions have been aimed at maintaining the market. This serves a hegemonic position that maintains its credibility by threatening catastrophe if it is threatened. Any rival knowledge can be discounted because the consequences would be inefficiency and incoherency, destabilizing hegemonic assumptions of the natural equilibrium of world trade and the scientifically proven law of the market (Santos 2003).

This position, almost ingrained in the popular consciousness to the point of being common-sensical, is challenged by the World Social Forum (WSF, see Preface). The WSF proposes an alternative 'epistemology of the South' (Santos 2003, p. 236) that there is no global social justice without global cognitive justice, a principle based in human conscience. There are two main ideas behind this. The first is that even if science is 'objective', it is not neutral. Scientific research is mostly funded on the basis that the outcomes will be profitable or will enhance military power. These objectives support the global hegemony, but do not serve the majority of people. If science was to be truly neutral, it might as well develop research into outcomes that do not serve the hegemony. The second is that although science serves the hegemony, there is little to suggest that the hegemony itself is supported by scientific knowledge, since its practices are based on tacit, often unscientific, undertakings. Most of what we actually do in our lives is based on tacit, vernacular forms of knowledge, despite our technical and scientific understanding and the use of tools and economic or ergonomic systems, and materials that are derived from these (Gramsci 1971, Morin 1999, see Chapter 15). Tacit and unscientific practices have to be made credible in order to give hegemonic power a valid basis in knowledge. This would also give credibility to

counter-hegemonic practices (Santos 2003, Soares & de Lima 2007), except that hegemonies have the means to determine what can be perceived as valid or invalid knowledge. Human occupation is characterized by its complexity, which makes it difficult to encapsulate in the tick-boxes and categorizations (Harries 2007) afforded by hegemonic and technico-scientific forms of knowledge (Santos 2003). These are often unable to take account of other forms of knowledge. Occupational therapists' concern with client-centeredness is often about addressing personal, individual, and community needs, recognizing these as important to the way people live their lives (Creek 2007, Pollard et al 2008a). These organic, tacit elements of doing, being, becoming, and belonging are the underpinning components of culture, economics, science, and politics, enhancing their richness and diversity (Pollard et al 2008b, Santos 2003). Concepts such as rationality and efficiency serve to contain counter-hegemonic practices or to deny them any purchase in the overriding logic of hegemonic goals (Santos 2003).

Hegemonic practices, sociology of absences and monocultural occupational therapy

Santos (2003) uses the terms *sociology of absences* and *sociology of emergences* (Box 1.3) to identify the epistemological processes, or 'five logics or modes of production of non-existence' (p. 238) by which nonhegemonic and potentially counter-hegemonic

Box 1.3

Epistemological operations of the South (from Santos 2003)

Sociology of absences: an inquiry that aims to explain that what 'does not exist' is, in fact, actively produced as nonexistent, or described as a noncredible alternative to what exists. Its goal is to identify and valorize those social experiences in the world that are declared nonexistent by hegemonic rationality.

Sociology of emergences: an inquiry into the alternatives that are contained in the horizon of concrete possibilities. Its goal is to identify and enlarge the signs of possible future experiences, under the guise of tendencies and latencies that are actively ignored by hegemonic rationality and knowledge.

Table 1.1 Logics or modes of production of nonexistence

Hegemonic monocultures	Produce social forms of nonexistence	Replace by ecologies
Knowledge and rigor of knowledge	Scientific versus the ignorant	Knowledges
Linear time	Advanced versus the residual	Temporalities
Classification and naturalization of difference	Superior versus the inferior	Recognition
The universal and the global	Global versus the local	Trans-scale
Criteria of capitalist productivity and efficiency	Productive versus the nonproductive	Productivity

Adapted from Robertson (2006).

social experiences (or individual, personal, or community needs) are invalidated. Through their concern with human occupation at both a clinical and institutional level and an individual and community level occupational therapies have a place on the continuum of hegemonic and counter-hegemonic practices. However, these 'five logics or modes of production of non-existence' are expressed by hegemonic monocultures, for example the monoglossias that pose limits to occupational therapy's claim to holism (Pollard & Sakellariou 2008), which can be replaced by counter-hegemonic 'ecologies' (Santos 2003, p. 239, see Table 1.1). These will be briefly explained and juxtaposed with examples on how they may play out in the daily practices of occupational therapists.

Knowledge versus knowledges

Where modern science – *empiricism!* – is privileged as a monoculture it becomes the sole criteria of truth, and where high culture privileges itself as a monoculture it becomes the only arbiter of esthetic quality. This process establishes a canon that is then used to determine values of, for example, truth, ignorance, or esthetic worth (Santos 2003, Soares & de Lima 2007), despite the reality that science progresses and cultures develop, so these values are not necessarily static. One example can be found in the AOTA Centennial Vision: 'We envision that occupational therapy is a powerful, widely recognized, science-driven, and evidence-based profession with a globally connected and diverse workforce meeting society's occupational needs' (AOTA 2007, p. 613, Schwartz 2009). The qualifiers 'powerful', 'science-driven', 'evidence-based', seem to indicate monocultural criteria of what constitutes knowledge, although such a

statement may also indicate strategic values. Failing to echo the priorities of the hegemonies that control the healthcare market might damage occupational therapists' professional interests and practices. However, Whiteford (2007) identified the discourse that surrounds evidence-based practice (EBP) agenda as 'an institutional threat to the development of diversity in occupational therapy', suggesting that 'the way in which EBP [evidence-based practice] is currently framed most certainly privileges particular knowledge paradigms and particular types of research – reifying quantitative (randomized controlled trials) and rejecting qualitative approaches, which would put us at risk of delimiting our ability to develop our knowledge base' (p. 23). Iwama (2005) alerts us that if we start accepting constructions such as hierarchies of evidence, we are immediately in conflict with our beliefs about people and the most appropriate means through which we understand the diversity of occupation (also see 'critical occupational therapy' in Chapter 8).

Santos' (2003) ecology of knowledges offers a way of negotiating such experiences through the exposition of credible tacit bases for critical knowledge and understanding. The identification of these can be used to counter monocultural logic, for example in the way that the experience of disability can sometimes be used to challenge medical or clinical judgments (see Chapter 4), in the way that organic and tacit experiences of learning can be used to confront hegemonic educational practice (see Chapter 2), or that cultural and other occupations can be organized around local needs (Pollard et al 2008b, see Chapters 15, 18 and 19). In practice occupational therapists are open to and value the lived experiences (see Chapters 2–5 and 19) of the people they work with. Occupational therapists may consider their

5

profession's strong narrative component of discourses of practice and reflection (Whiteford 2007) as a key source of knowledge and experiential expertise that informs their practice and decision making. However, for occupational therapy to present itself as both an art and a science (Clark & Lawlor 2008, Peloquin 2005), an openness to and appreciation of other sources of knowledge than science have to be robust. As Greenhalgh (2009) points out, the story contributed by the expert patient can be significant but is only one aspect of a complex array of social, political, and geographic factors that influence the environment and context inhabited by both the patient and the healthcare professional.

Here it is appropriate and useful for occupational therapists to tap into and contribute to the emerging field of transdisciplinary knowledge construction. It is based on the premise that argues that 'knowledge guided by reason, linear logic and science, is only one way or avenue for solving global problems' ... 'the other is the way of understanding; the way of intuition, imagination, spirituality, and discovering shared truth' (Alsop et al 2006, p. 266, Max-Neef 2004, McGregor 2005, Nicolescu 2006, see discussion on social responsiveness, p. 12).

Linear time versus temporalities

Santos' second logic is the 'monoculture of linear time' (2003, p. 238). This assumes a staged timetable of development, represented for example by such rites of passage as an industrial revolution through which core countries of the 'developed world' are in 'advance' of the rest. Through the assumption of this linear progress other countries can be classed as 'backward', premodern, underdeveloped, etc. They are presented as nonexistent because the monoculture of linear time supposes that development relates to economic productivity. Occupational therapy is at risk of perpetuating a monocultural perspective too, although this has been challenged by our previous books (Kronenberg et al 2005, Pollard et al 2008b) and others (Ikiugu 2008, Iwama 2006) as well as other calls for diversity (e.g. Hammell 2009a,b, Whiteford 2007, WFOT 2004, 2006, 2009, 2010). There might be a similar concern with regard to the narrow base of occupational science, which perhaps could be harnessed to *doing something*, knowledge transfer, and knowledge exchange as part of the process of investigating the science of doing (see Chapter 8, Pollard et al 2010).

Santos' (2003, p. 239) 'ecology of temporalities' recognizes the diversity in conceptions of time. Linear time (perhaps represented by the simple figure of an arrow) arose in the West in the past 200–300 years with industrial development, but the duration of time, or pace, varies considerably between different Western cultures (Poole 2000, Roeckelein 2000). Other, earlier conceptions of time, such as circular time or cyclical time, oriented to seasons, coexist in the same cultures, whereas other cultures have very different concepts in which the past, present, and future may be indistinguishable (Poole 2000). Cultural conventions, such as modern films or novels, do not always present time in a linear way, but use flashbacks or even flashes forward to unfold a narrative. Thus the past or the future may be a component of the present and our understanding of it in the narrative testimony we share with others; this individual, experiential oriented understanding of our personal lives contributes to a polyphony – a multitude of voices through which occupation-based actions are negotiated (Pollard & Sakellariou 2008). The consequences of these perspectives disrupt the hegemonic perspective of sociology, the monocultural view of development that presents African or Asian peasants as 'backward' and the activities of Western farmers with modern agricultural machinery and scientific farming methods as 'advanced'. Rather, Santos' (2003) sociology of absences considers all social practices as forms of autonomous development that reflect local needs and cultural priorities, which are in turn influenced by the surroundings. From this perspective, irrespective of where they occur, all human activities are contemporaneous.

Western occupational therapists may struggle to reconcile their concept of linear time with local understandings of time when they find themselves in contexts that might be externally labeled or even branded 'underdeveloped'. In many cultures time is not as important as relationships, and therefore it is not possible to waste time, and a drive to do things by the clock so dominant in Western outcome-oriented culture may impede opportunities for slower paced learning, thinking, and reflecting that might lead to improvements in efficiency in the longer term, because outcomes have been negotiated in terms of local needs (Poole 2000). The WFOT minimum standards (2002) acknowledge that occupational therapy must be closely informed by the needs and particularities of people in their local context. However, curriculums may still have a way to go to reflect these standards since the majority of texts available to occupational therapy students and their educators are produced in the West (Hammell 2009a,b).

Classification and naturalization of difference versus recognition

Although science has often been a criterion for notions of truth or even the truth of uncertainty (Fernandez-Armesto 1997), Santos' third logic, the 'monoculture of classification and naturalization of difference' (Robertson 2006, p. 8), concerns a popular concern of science in the establishment of hierarchical differences by ranking and classifying them (see Chapters 10, 14, 19, and 40). Occupational therapists engage in this process by responding to categories such as psychiatric diagnoses, or through their own processes of assessment. The 'monoculture of classification' consists of distributing populations according to categories, for example in the way that science has historically been used to underpin unscientific sexist, racist, or eugenic ideas (Hobsbawm 1987, Ferguson 2004). These categories then emerge as fixed, 'natural' hierarchies. Fanon (1963) attacked the way in which racist approaches to the medical treatment of Algerian patients were based on a Western science of eugenic principles that suggested the Algerian patients were inferior beings to their French counterparts. For much of its history, Western capitalism has harnessed scientific explanations to the racist ideologies that supported its lucrative business of slavery (Balibar & Wallerstein 1991, Boulle 1988, Quijano 2000) and the continued exploitation of migrant and colonial labor (Ferguson 2004, Ramdin 1987).

The combined monocultural logic of the hegemonic perspective is potentially funneled through the narrow socioeconomic class, gender, and geocultural base of the occupational therapy profession (Frank & Zemke 2008, Pollard & Sakellariou 2009, Sakellariou & Pollard 2008). For example, its narrow conceptualization of occupation (see Chapter 7) and the limited scope for intervention afforded by the profession's dependency on medicine's scientific reductionism (Frank & Zemke 2008) may restrict the capacity and power of therapists to construct or negotiate practices in terms of the needs of the people they are working with, a concern of many of the contributors to this book. Equipping occupational therapy's ability to resource people around the globe requires the building of a workforce that represents the world's diversity (Hammell 2009a,b, Whiteford 2007, WFOT 2009, 2010).

The 'ecology of recognition' (Santos 2003, p. 240) is a means of opposing the colonial mentality of race and unequal sexuality implicit in the 'monoculture of classification'. An ecology of differences can develop through mutual recognition on a principle of equality. Once difference is understood to be equal there can be no ethical basis for differences in power and material differences become a problem (Santos 2003). This is recognized through a core value of occupational therapy, that all people have the potential to contribute to the advancement of the health and wellbeing of others and themselves, and is implicit in the WFOT position papers on community-based rehabilitation (2004), human rights (2006) and the guiding principles on diversity and culture (2010). It is also an implication of a move towards creating a broader political awareness of the significance of access to the means of meaningful doing through concepts such as occupational justice, occupational deprivation, and occupational apartheid (Kronenberg et al 2005, WFOT 2004, see Chapters 8 and 40).

The universal and global versus trans-scale

The 'monoculture of the universal and the global' is Santos' (2003, p. 239, Robertson 2006) fourth logic of the production of nonexistence. It operates through historical power asymmetries that have often led to the privileging of 'global and universal' epistemologies and ways of knowing at the expense of existing 'particular and local' knowledges. So violent have these impositions been that some scholars refer to the process as one of 'epistemicide' (Coleman & Johnson 2008, p. 1). If the global and the universal are always understood to be more significant, then the particular and local can never be presented as credible interests. For occupational therapy the unwitting assumption of this monoculture can result in the failure to provide services which meet local needs, and is reinforced again by the narrow bases of the profession as we have just discussed, particularly the way the dominance of English as the *lingua franca* tends to prioritize evidence and theory in English over other sources, rendering the profession monoglossic because it cannot access other evidence (Pollard & Sakellariou 2008, see Chapter 6).

Santos' 'ecology of trans-scale' (2003, p. 240) emphasizes the particular and the local, identifying them as representing values that have not been ordered by hegemonic globalization. In many examples in this book local cultures and local social practices are encouraged as examples of diversity and alternatives to global culture (Kronenberg et al 2005, Pollard et al 2008a,b, see Chapters 2, 11, 15, 18, 19, 27, and 41). For example, globalization encourages local franchises of international businesses, serving a global community of shareholders and investors concerned principally with their own profits and economic returns. An ecology of trans-scale is concerned with the development of local businesses or cooperatives. These both serve local needs and retain the economic benefits in the immediate community.

Much of the content of this book and its predecessors, combined with the rising debate about occupation and rights, may serve as an example of an attempt to connect with and honor what matters most to people where they live, and develop practices that remind people of who they are and what works for them. Allowing for polyphony (Pollard & Sakellariou 2008), developing critical perspectives such as occupational literacy (Pollard 2008) and occupational consciousness (Ramugondo 2009), are some possible strategies that may facilitate the operationalization of Santos' ecology of trans-scale, and caution in adopting values that are often aggressively introduced by globalization. The African ethic of *ubuntu* (see the Foreword by Tutu and Chapter 21) is another example of recuperating a local 'logic' that is not the result of hegemonic globalization. South African occupational therapists consider that this value ought to inform and guide the further development or transformation of their services (Lorenzo et al 2006, Ramugondo 2009, Watson & Swartz 2004). Van Binsbergen (2002, p. 6) summarizes Ramose's (1999) argument on globalization and *ubuntu* as follows:

> The globalization process in which the modern world is increasingly drawn, amounts to the ascendance of a market-oriented economic logic of maximalization, in which the value, dignity, personal safety, even survival of the human person no longer constitute central concerns. This process is reinforced by the North Atlantic region's drive for political and cultural hegemony. African societies have suffered greatly in the process, but their lasting value-orientation in terms of ubuntu holds up an alternative in the sense that it advocates for a renewed concern for the human person.

Ubuntu is already applied in the peripheral contexts of villages and kin groups in southern Africa today, but it is also capable of inspiring the wider world, where it may give a new and profound meaning to the global

debate on the Western concept of human rights (Ramose 1999), along with other cultural perspectives, for example the Hindu notion of *dharma* and the Islamic concept of *umma* (Coleman & Johnson 2008). To prevent us from falling into the trap of polarizing different cultural perspectives, the authors agree with Van Binsbergen (2002) and Santos (2007), who advocate for intercultural dialogue that is based on acknowledgment of the reciprocal incompletenesses and weaknesses of cultures. This is not the place to address these cultural concepts in depth and critically, but the authors want to caution against applications that may either over-romanticize or that aim to commodify (in a Marxist sense, Blunden 2010) these sociocultural philosophies.

Criteria of capitalist productivity and efficiency versus alternative productivities

Finally, Santos' fifth logic concerns the 'monoculture of the criteria of capitalist productivity and efficiency' (2003, p. 239). This is a strong underpinning logic for the profession, with its philosophical origins in Christian socialism and the mental hygiene movement (Frank & Zemke 2008), the need for a critical perspective on the purposes of vocational rehabilitation (Holmes 2007), and pressure to deliver services to budget. Santos' 'monoculture of the criteria of capitalist productivity and efficiency' applies as much to nature, where sterility is a negative quality, as it does to market forces, where it is understood that people who cannot work are described as lazy or lacking skills, and products that do not yield profit are dumped.

Although occupational therapists make a claim to 'client-centered practice' on the grounds that it suggests informed choice (Hammel et al 2007), this is often in a way that fails to address a critique to the capitalist orthodoxy this term implies. Clients, or even *consumers*, as they are identified in many occupational therapy documents, are people who have the means to buy access to services, and this logic derives from working in environments where people can and do choose the clinical services they buy (Kronenberg & Pollard 2006, Kronenberg et al 2005). Our professional codes of ethics, which state that we do not withhold treatment to anyone on discriminatory grounds, can only be upheld if this principle is extended to those who cannot pay. Much of the time access to an occupational therapist is determined through referral from other clinicians, but many health professionals work under conditions that are determined by an ethic of care framed within an ethic of profit. Of course, there are limits to the extent that healthcare can be afforded, and it makes little sense to offer interventions that are disproportionate in terms of cost and outcome. However, the balance of priorities between people who can argue effectively for expensive forms of treatment and many people unable to argue for occupation-based engagements from which they might benefit should be critically considered (see Chapter 16).

The 'ecology of productivity' (Santos 2003, p. 240) counters the monoculture of the criteria of capitalist productivity and efficiency through its emphasis on alternative systems of production, popular economic organizations, workers' cooperatives, self-managed enterprises, solidarity economy, useful unemployment (Illich 1980) etc., all which have been hidden or discredited by the capitalist orthodoxy of productivity. One of the central ideas or myths behind global capitalism is that development and economic growth are infinite. This has already been shaken by economic events in the past century and has for some time been understood to be unsustainable in an aging global population (Hobsbawm 1994). The other is that accumulation is better than distribution, a short-term logic that has also taken little account of historical events such as the collapse of empires (Ferguson 2004).

For occupational therapists the implications of an ecology of productivity are that they might – as is already evident through emerging role opportunities and authors contributing to this book such as Alburquerque et al, Barros et al, Lopez and Block, Paganizzi and Mengelberg – become more active in developing other avenues of making their services relevant and available. This could mean working through nongovernmental organizations (see Chapters 16, 17, 19, and 20), governments (Garcia 2003, 2005), or social entrepreneurship (see Chapter 21).

Sociology of emergences and alternative or counter-hegemonic occupational therapies

Santos (2003) says that existence can be considered in three modal terms of reality, necessity, and possibility. While the first two are the focus of hegemonic forms of rationality and knowledge, there is

something of a hegemonic aversion to possibility because it involves risk to the status quo. Consequently Santos' sociology of emergences focuses on possibility. 'Possibility is the world's engine'... which has three strokes, turning through the moments of ... 'want (the manifestation of something lacking), tendency (process and meaning), and latency (what goes ahead in the process). Want is the realm of the Not, tendency the realm of the Not Yet, and latency the realm of the Nothing and the All, for latency can end up either in frustration or hope' (Santos 2003, p. 241).

The future represents latent possibilities for 'concrete social experiences' (Santos 2003, p. 242) which give 'clues' to new practices. Although the chapters in this book represent perspectives of occupational therapy without borders, all of them are situated along a spectrum of more or less hegemonic or counter-hegemonic views and practices of occupational therapy in which clues for innovation can be made out (Table 1.2). These chapters offer clues to the possibilities for practices and the future forms the profession may develop, they express the latency of occupational therapy (Santos 2003) which may be expressed in the ideal of occupational justice.

Table 1.2 Clues of emerging pathways for alternative futures of occupational therapy

Purpose – what we want to do?	Encourage and remind people and society to understand, build and maintain working relationships through collective occupations
Premise – why we do what we do?	People can positively influence their wellbeing, and that of humanity's and the planet's, through doing well with others and the environment
Occupation-based approaches – how and where do we translate our intent into real action?	A political possibilities-based practice with people from all walks of life in real-life contexts
SustainAbilities – how can we sustain what we do?	Eclectic modes of productivity: from paid work to involvements that are not monetarily compensated, social entrepreneurship, and social responsiveness

Purpose – what we want to do?

The purpose of alternative occupational therapy is to encourage and remind people and society to understand, build, and maintain working relationships through collective occupations (see Chapters 2–4, 16–22, 24, 26, 29, 30–33, 35, 38, 39, and 42). We acknowledge that none of the clues offered here are sure recipes for bringing about sustainable social and/or environmental changes. These approaches or strategies are only as good as the intentions, the capacities, and the power of the people who choose to work with them.

Although the assertion 'human beings are social animals' may be widely recognized, it points to a human quality that is often taken for granted. It is also generally acknowledged that success in any sphere of life often hinges on relationships that work. Yet, it seems there is no single profession that specifically focuses on how to build and maintain working relationships. This may partly be because the modern world, including the occupational therapy profession, appears to have largely bought into, entrenched, and promoted individualism. This worldview stresses that the interests of an individual should take precedence without regard to how this may impact on the social health of the collective. Collective goals seem to have been mostly ignored or seen to be in competition with the advancement of the individual (Ramugondo & Kronenberg 2010). In his introductory address at an occupational science symposium in Cork, MacLachlan (2005) pointed out that occupational therapists could help society to create new ways of promoting social cohesion, identify common values, and to work toward common goals. Wilcock (1998) acknowledged 'the critical moral importance of occupation in human life' and argued that 'occupational therapy is a neglected source of community re-humanization' which 'can be more effectively utilized if it is not limited to being a service solely for sick people' (p. 222). In Africa, it is the ethic of *ubuntu* focusing on people's allegiances and relations with each other which holds potential for informing culturally appropriate practices in order to meet collective local needs (see the Foreword by Tutu and Chapter 21).

Premise – why we do what we do?

The premise on which alternative occupational therapy is based is that people from all walks of life can positively influence their wellbeing, and that of humanity's and the planet's, through doing well with others and the environment (see all chapters, particularly Chapters 16, 23, 26, and 38). It is informed by sociocultural practices that value 'reciprocal obligations and harmonious relationships' (Hammell 2009a, p. 10) and social relationships, interdependence, reciprocity, mutual obligation, and belonging (Iwama 2006, Lim 2004, see Chapters 9 and 11). This vision also connects with what Bunting (2004, p. 322) contended that 'we are all interdependent, and it is in that web of dependence that we find our deepest contentment'. Hammell (2009a) pointed out that contrary to Western egocentric ideology, research demonstrates that interdependence is 'an indispensable feature of the human condition' (Reindal 1999, p. 354), and that the ability to contribute to others is associated with lower levels of depression, higher self-esteem, and fewer health problems (e.g., Anson et al 1993, Schwartz & Sendor 1999, Stewart & Bhagwanjee 1999), suggesting that occupations that promote interdependence contribute positively to wellbeing. Gladwell's (2008) opening story, 'The Roseto Mystery' in *Outliers – the story of success* also affirms the proposed vision, when he concludes that to fully understand health and wellbeing requires 'looking beyond the individual's personal choices or actions in isolation' (p. 10).

Questions that are critical in advancing the proposed vision are for example: Within any collective occupations, are everybody's interests considered and respected? How are relationships built and maintained? How do these relationships advance the collective good? The phrase 'doing well with others' was coined by Vivienne Budaza, and represents her interpretation of occupational justice (see Chapter 21). Lang-Etienne's core questions are also relevant and useful: 'What do you need to do in order to remain centered and compassionate? What are the social consequences of your professional decisions? And what are their environmental consequences?' (Thibeault 2002, p. 200).

Occupation-based approaches – how and where do we translate our intent into real action?

Alternative occupational therapy constitutes a *political possibilities-based practice* that engages with what matters most to people from all walks of life (including but not limited to those living with an illness or disability) in their *real-life contexts*. The latter refers to the actual places and spaces where people live, work, love, play, and so on, and this includes cyber space.

Occupation-based approaches explicitly acknowledge that human beings are political animals and interact as such (Kronenberg & Pollard 2006, Kronenberg et al 2005, Kronenberg 2009, Pollard et al 2008, see Chapter 33). A *political possibilities-based practice* is driven by the art in the 'art and science of occupational therapy' (Clark & Lawlor 2008, Peloquin 2005, see Chapter 7). This is not the place to delve into the question, What is politics? However it might be helpful to clarify our view with a phrase by the nineteenth-century German statesman Otto von Bismarck, who said: 'Politics is not a science, it is an art. Politics is the art of the possible' (Thaysen 2007, p. 2–3). A political possibilities-based practice of occupational therapy is to enable practitioners to 'make things work' when they perceive themselves to be in conflict with the hegemony. It is about exercising what Joseph Nye coined as 'soft power' – *getting others to want what you want*, vis-à-vis 'hard (command) power' – *getting others to do what you want*, which can rest on inducements (carrots) or threats (sticks), i.e., military power and economic power. 'Soft power' co-opts whereas 'hard power' coerces (Joseph 2002). Nye (2002, 2003, p. 552) said:

> Soft power rests on the ability to set the political agenda in a way that shapes the preferences of others. It is one source of influence, and more than persuasion or the ability to move people by argument, it rests on the ability to entice and attract, which often leads to acquiescence or imitation.

Soft power arises in large part from our values (occupational consciousness and 3PA), which are the motor of a political possibilities-based practice of occupational therapy.

Additionally with regards to a possibilities-based practice, 'at any given moment there is a limited horizon of possibilities, and so it is important not to waste the unique opportunity of a specific change offered by the present' (Santos 2003, p. 241). In order to bring about any sort of transformation you need to start working with current realities, before you can pursue what you might wish for – in the world, in others, in yourself. A possibilities-*based* practice is what generates practice-*based* evidence, to complement evidence-*based* practice.

Occupation-based approaches acknowledge that effective communication and negotiation across diversity in languages, culture, and media require mutual open curiosity and shared reflection. This can happen simultaneously in the communication process, but requires all participants to assume that their understanding may be found to be tenuous, rather than firm. The process is not one which is directed, but reconciled. For instance, it appears to make good sense for practitioners to use their local language to name occupational therapy and its core construct 'occupation' if this allows for more effective negotiations of values. Perhaps it could be considered to acknowledge English to be the 'mother tongue' of our profession, and allow its 'offspring' to exist by different names. Occupation-based approaches can also make more and better use of mobile communication technologies accessible in the local context to maximize these as a resource.

SustainAbilities – how can we sustain what we do?

Alternative occupational therapies can be sustained by eclectic or heterogeneous modes of productivity, from paid work – increasingly within civic and non-governmental organizations (see Chapters 16, 17, 19, 20, 22, and 24) to other involvements that are not monetarily compensated. Many of the people involved are motivated directly by their personal experiences of adversity, and their capacity for leadership derives from a personal experience of survival (see Chapters 2, 5, 17–19, 21, 29, and 38). On this continuum lie various other modes such as social entrepreneurship (see Chapters 17 and 21) and social responsiveness initiatives (see Chapters 30, 34, 38, and 39).

Going beyond monocultural interpretations of 'productivity', here we embrace an ecology of productivities, to discover 'doings that work'. The play on the word 'sustainAbilities' is meant to emphasize that in order to advance the purpose of the original term (sustainabilities), those who acknowledge its value must put it into practice. Apart from a deep curiosity into who human beings are and what matters most to them, this requires an openness and drive to acquire the necessary set of abilities (e.g., creative networking, putting business plans together, cultivating personal leadership, political lobbying, debating, media training, etc.). Occupational therapy education primarily prepares students for the job market, for example in the United Kingdom the number of places at universities are determined by agreements with regional health authorities. The filling of anticipated vacancies does not allow for sustaining what occupational therapists may be inspired to do, guided by the principles of the profession if they decide to work in areas outside statutory health and social care. Following are some pointers to possible pathways towards sustainAbilities.

We can start by reviewing our *everyday occupational engagements*. The full potential of occupational therapy at times appears to be realized in these spheres of life vis-à-vis our professional settings. The restrictions of the workplace, for example, generic demands, the need to meet workplace targets for numbers of client contacts, and budgetary limitations at times inhibit the realization of occupational therapy's full potential. Occupational therapists have often not been in a position to exercise the power to determine ways of engaging with people that are better suited to professional aims rather than those of the employing institution (Pollard et al 2010). Therapists who review their own lives may realize how through their everyday engagements they may be advancing professional values unique to occupational therapy in their immediate communities or the larger society. As individuals many of us are involved in such activities that lie beyond the confines of our job. It is through this kind of personal reflection that opportunities through which alternative practices can be negotiated may emerge.

Social entrepreneurship, which is by its nature essentially bound by the social mission and theory of change (Sinha 2009a), allows for a multitude of ways to sustain alternative practices of occupational therapy (Pattison 2010, see the Foreword by Pattison, and Chapters 17 and 21). Rather than leaving societal needs to the government or business sectors, social entrepreneurs act as change-agents for society. They find what is not working, seize opportunities others miss, improve systems, invent new approaches, create and spread solutions, and even persuading entire societies to take new leaps (Ashoka 2010). A social entrepreneur uses *earned income* strategies to pursue a social mission, creating and *sustaining* not just private but social value. The factor 'earned income' distinguishes social entrepreneurship from nonprofits, which are often primarily reliant on philanthropy, grants, and voluntarism (Sinha 2009b). Furthermore, rather than wealth generation (compare business entrepreneurs), mission-related impact is the criterion for measuring one's value creation. Wealth is only a means to an end for social entrepreneurs (Dees 1998, Martin & Osberg 2007). Bornstein (2007)

identified the following characteristics in excellent social entrepreneurs – they demonstrated a willingness to:

- self-correct – 'this inclination stems from the attachment to a goal rather than to a particular approach or plan' (p. 234)
- share credit – 'there is no limit to what you can achieve if you don't care who gets the credit' (p. 235)
- break free of established structures – the word 'entrepreneur' comes from French, originally meaning 'to take into one's own hands'
- cross disciplinary boundaries – 'one of the primary functions of the social entrepreneur is to serve as a kind of social alchemist: to create new social compounds; to gather people's ideas, experiences, skills, and resources in configurations that society is not naturally aligned to produce' (p. 236)
- work quietly – working for years on their ideas in relative obscurity before they become recognized
- express a strong ethical impetus – their motivation came down to a clear sense of what is right and what is wrong, which apparently was not only evident in their work, but also in how they lived their lives.

These qualities in themselves suggest that social entrepreneurship is not an easy road to take, and derives from necessity, difficulty, and vision. Our experience can be that difficulties continue to arise through the negotiation of projects, and the strong ethical impetus and other skills that Bornstein identifies are important in maintaining the gains made.

Another way to help sustain alternative occupational therapies is through involvement in universities' *social responsiveness* initiatives (see Chapters 25, 26, 29, 30, 32, 34–36, 38, and 42). In our ever more engaged world, increasingly, higher education institutions are intentionally connecting academic work to the public good through socially responsive academic engagement with a range of external constituencies (excluding academic constituencies) as a core element of their role in society (University of Cape Town 2008a). Hall (2009a) in this regard, speaks of 'community engagement as a key public good in what is increasingly being understood as the "third sector" (e.g. from formal NGOs [nongovernmental organizations] through special interest groups and networks to informal organizations and alliances), filling the space between the private sector, on the one hand, and the role of the state in providing infrastructure and social transfers, on the other' (Hall 2009a, p. 26), and he foresees that 'In the future, it is probable that such networks of engagement will come to define Higher Education' (Hall 2009b, p. 5). Although there are a multitude of definitions of social responsiveness, one definition espouses it as 'the production and dissemination of knowledge for public benefit, demonstrating engagement with external constituencies and showing evidence of externally applied scholarly activities' (University of Cape Town 2008a, p. 15). Forms of social responsiveness can be: socially engaged service and learning (link with the formal curriculum, e.g., community-based education); socially engaged research (e.g., knowledge dissemination, collaborative research involving active participation of external constituencies, the research project should not only lead to advances in knowledge, but also have an intentional public purpose); socially engaged research and teaching (transformation of curriculum based on knowledge generated through social engagement, development of new forms of pedagogy and the generation of new knowledge predicated on social engagement); and civic engagement with no link to the formal curriculum e.g., student voluntary or compulsory community service (University of Cape Town 2008a, b).

Courage to dance politics

The following anecdote may serve to remind occupational therapists that our art – values, music – may be best expressed through a particular action, accepting that it may provoke certain anxieties, but trusting that we can overcome them:

> At an international conference on religion in Japan, an American delegate, a social philosopher from New York, said to a Shinto priest, 'We've been now to a good many ceremonies and have seen quite a few of your shrines. But I don't get your ideology. I don't get your

theology.' The Japanese paused as though in deep thought and then slowly shook his head. 'I think we don't have ideology,' he said, 'We don't have theology. We dance.'

Campbell & Moyers (1988, p. XIX)

For occupational therapists to live up to *their full potential* – which may require that we go beyond monocultural expressions of occupational therapy, towards an ecology of occupation-based practices – we must have the courage to *dance politics*. Remember Von Bismarck's phrase 'politics is the art of the possible', which connects with the art of occupational therapy, and is essentially constituting a possibilities-based practice. To *dance politics* (see Chapters 16–19, 21–24, 29–33, 38, and 39) then refers to learning the art of exercising *soft power* through *attraction*, which refers to the ability to get others to want the same things that we want. What do we want to do? We want to promote individuals' and collective wellbeing by exposing people and society to the music of their human potential. Enough said, let's dance ...

Acknowledgments

We wish to thank Elizabeth Townsend, Mershen Pillay, and Sandra Galheigo for reading and offering valuable comments on the final draft. And *dankie* to Madeleine Duncan for having acted as a 'sparring partner' during the writing process of this chapter. A special word of gratitude goes to the participants in 'political reasoning and a political practice of occupational therapy' courses at Zuyd University, Netherlands (2007), University of the Western Cape (2006), Cape Town, South Africa, Universidad Andres Bello, Santiago de Chile, Chile, Touro College, New York, United States (2008–2010), particularly for their constructive feedback on engaging with 3P Archaeology.

References

Abbot JP, Worth O: *Critical Perspectives on International Political Economy*, Basingstoke, 2002, Palgrave.

Alsop A, Duncan M, Lorenzo T, et al: Looking ahead: future directions in practice education and research. In Lorenzo T, Duncan M, Buchanan H, et al: editors: *Practice and Service Learning in Occupational Therapy*, Chichester, 2006, Wiley, pp 263–274.

American Occupational Therapy Association: AOTA's centennial vision and executive summary, *Am J Occup Ther* 61:613–614, 2007.

American Occupational Therapy Association: OT brand: 'living life to its fullest', 2008: Online Available at: http://www.aota.org/brand.aspx. Accessed January 7, 2010.

Anson CA, Stanwyck DJ, Krause JS: Social support and health status in spinal cord injury, *Paraplegia* 31:632–638, 1993.

Ashoka: *What is a social entrepreneur?* 2010, Online. Available at: http://www.ashoka.org/social_entrepreneur. Accessed January 8, 2010.

Balibar E, Wallerstein IM: *Race, Nation, Class: Ambiguous Identities*, New York, 1991, Verso Books.

Beagan BL: Experiences of social class: learning from occupational therapy students, *Can J Occup Ther* 74:125–133, 2007.

Biko S: *I Write What I Like. Volume 217 of African Writers Series*, Heinemann, London, 1987, Aelred Stubbs.

Binsbergen van W: *Ubuntu and the globalisation of Southern African thought and society*, 2002, Online. Available at: http://www.shikanda. net/general/ubuntu.htm. Accessed July 5, 2010.

Blunden A, editor: *Commodification. Encyclopedia of Marxism*, Online. Available at: http://www.marxists. org/glossary/terms/c/o.htm. Accessed February 2, 2010.

Bornstein D: *How to Change the World: Social Entrepreneurs and the Power of New Ideas*, Updated edition. USA, 2007, Oxford University Press.

Boulle PH: In defense of slavery: eighteenth century opposition to abolition and the origins of a racist ideology in France. In Krantz F, editor: *History From Below*, Oxford, 1988, Blackwell, pp. 219–246.

Bunting M: *Willing Slaves. How the Overwork Culture is Ruling Our Lives*, London, 2004, Harper-Collins, p 322.

Campbell J, Moyers B: *The Power of Myth*, New York, 1988, Doubleday, p XIX.

Cascao AE: Ethiopia – challenges to Egyptian hegemony in the Nile basin, *Water Policy* 10(Suppl 2):17, 2008.

Clark F, Lawlor M: The making and mattering of occupational science. In Crepeau EB, Cohn ES, Boyt Schell BA, editors: *Willard and Spackman's Occupational Therapy*, ed 11, USA, 2008, Lippincott Williams & Wilkins, pp 2–14.

Coleman WD, Johnson NA: *Building dialogue on globalization research: what are the obstacles and how might these be addressed?* Paper prepared for presentation to the workshop on Building South-North Dialogue on Globalization Research: Phase II. Waterloo, Ontario, Canada, 2008, Centre for International Governance Innovation, Online Available at: http://www.globalautonomy.ca/global1/servlet/Dialogue2pdf?fn=SN08_ColemanJohnson. Accessed February 2, 2010.

Cox R: Social forces, states and world orders. Article republished. In Cox R,

Sinclair T, editors: *Approaches to World Order*, 1996, Cambridge, 1981, Cambridge University Press, pp 85–123.

Cox R: Gramsci, hegemony and international relations. In Cox R, Sinclair T, editors: *Approaches to World Order*, Cambridge, 1983, Cambridge University Press, pp 124–143.

Creek J: The thinking therapist. In Creek J, Lawson-Porter A, editors: *Contemporary Issues in Occupational Therapy*, Chichester, 2007, Wiley, pp 1–21.

Dees JG: *The meaning of 'social entrepreneurship'*, 1998, Kauffman Center for Entrepreneurial Leadership. Online. Available at: http://www.fntc.info/files/documents/The%20meaning%20of%20Social%20Entreneurship.pdf. Accessed January 8, 2010.

Doble SE, Santha JC: Occupational well-being: Rethinking occupational therapy outcomes, *Can J Occup Ther* 75:184–190, 2008.

Fanon F: *The Wretched of the Earth*, New York, 1963, Grove.

Ferguson N: *Empire, How Britain Made the Modern World*, London, 2004, Penguin.

Fernandez-Armesto F: *Truth, a History and a Guide for the Perplexed*, New York, 1997, Thomas Dunne.

Frank G, Zemke R: Occupational therapy foundations for political engagement and social transformation. In Pollard N, Sakellariou D, Kronenberg F, editors: *A Political Practice of Occupational Therapy*, Edinburgh, 2008, Elsevier, pp 111–136.

Garcia Ruiz AS: *Rehabilitacion cumunitaria Bogota – Colombia*, Bogotá, 2003, Secretaria Distrital de Salud Direccion de Salud Publica Julio de, 2003.

Garcia Ruiz AS: Community based rehabilitation, strategy of human rights and quality of life for the people with disabilities, *World Federation of Occupational Therapists Bulletin* 51:16–22, 2005.

Gladwell M: *Outliers: the Story of Success*, London, 2008, Penguin.

Gramsci A: *Selections from the Prison Notebooks* (Hoare Q, Nowell-Smith G, editor and translator), London, 1971, Lawrence and Wishart.

Gramsci A: *Selections from Political Writings, 1921–26* (Hoare Q, translator and editor), London, 1978, Lawrence and Wishart.

Greenhalgh T: Patient and public involvement in chronic illness: beyond the expert patient, *Br Med J* 17:338, 2009.

Hall M: *Universities do serve communities*, South Africa, 2009a, Mail & Guardian, p 26.

Hall M: *Installation address Martin Hall, Vice-Chancellor*, 2009b, University of Salford. Online. Available at: http://www.corporate.salford.ac.uk/leadership-management/martin-hall/wp-content/uploads/whiteness.pdf. Accessed January 15, 2010.

Hammel J, Magasi S, Heinemann A, et al: What does participation mean? An insider perspective from people with disabilities, *Disabil Rehabil* 30:1445–1460, 2007. Online. Available at:http://dx.doi.org/10.1080/09638280701625534. Accessed December 17, 2009.

Hammell KW: Client-centred practice: ethical obligation or professional obfuscation? *British Journal of Occupational Therapy* 70:264–266, 2007.

Hammell KW: Sacred texts: A sceptical exploration of the assumptions underpinning theories of occupation, *Can J Occup Ther* 76:6–13, 2009a.

Hammell KW: Contesting assumptions in occupational therapy. In Curtin M, Molineux M, Supyk-Mellson J, editors: *Occupational Therapy and Physical Dysfunction: Enabling Occupation*, Edinburgh, 2009b, Churchill Livingstone/Elsevier, pp 39–54.

Harries P: Knowing more than we can say. In Creek J, Lawson-Porter A, editors: *Contemporary Issues in Occupational Therapy*, Chichester, 2007, Wiley, pp 161–188.

Hobsbawm EH: *The Age of Empire, 1875–1914*, London, 1987, Weidenfeld and Nicholson.

Hobsbawm EH: *Age of Extremes, the Short Twentieth Century*, London, 1994, Michael Joseph.

Holmes J: *Vocational Rehabilitation*, Oxford, 2007, Blackwell.

Ikiugu M: *Occupational Science in the Service of Gaia. An essay describing a possible contribution of occupational scientists to the solution of prevailing global problems*, Baltimore, 2008, Publish America.

Illich I: *The Right to Useful Unemployment*, London, 1980, Marion Boyars.

Iwama M: Occupation as a cross cultural construct. In Whiteford G, Clair Wright-St. V, editors: *Occupation and Practice in Context*, Sydney, 2005, Churchill Livingstone.

Iwama M: *The Kawa Model: Culturally Relevant Occupational Therapy*, Edinburgh, 2006, Churchill Livingstone Elsevier.

Joseph JA: Public values in a divided world: a mandate for higher education, *Liberal Education* 88:6–15, 2002.

Kronenberg F: From an apolitical practice to a political practice of occupational therapy, *Ergoscience* 4:22–23, 2009.

Kronenberg F, Pollard N: Political dimensions of occupation and the roles of occupational therapy. Plenary address at the 2006 AOTA conference in Charlotte/NC, *Am J Occup Ther* 60:617–625, 2006.

Kronenberg F, Algado SS, Pollard N: *Occupational Therapy Without Borders. Learning from the Spirit of Survivors*, Edinburgh, 2005, Elsevier/ Churchill Livingstone.

Kronenberg F, Wouda P, Harren M, et al: *Self-empowerment of OT students through political reasoning at Zuyd University in the Netherlands*. Paper presented at the 15th Congress of the World Federation of Occupational Therapists, Santiago, Chile, 2010.

Lim KH: Occupational therapy in multicultural contexts. Letter to the editor, *British Journal of Occupational Therapy* 67:49–50, 2004.

Lorenzo T, Duncan M, Buchanan H, et al: *Practice and Service Learning in Occupational Therapy: Enhancing Potential in Context*, Chichester, 2006, John Wiley & Sons.

McGregor SLT: Transdisciplinarity and a culture of peace, *Culture of Peace Online Journal* 1:1–12, 2005. Online. Available at:http://www. consultmcgregor.com/documents/ research/ transdisciplinarity_and_culture_of_ peace.pdf. Accessed January 16, 2010.

MacLachlan M: *The cultural dynamics of health. Introductory address at 4th Occupation UK and Ireland Occupational Science Symposium.*

Culture and Health – an occupational perspective, 8–9 September, Cork, Ireland, 2005.

Martin RL, Osberg S: *Social entrepreneurship: the case for definition. Stanford social innovation review*, 2007. Online Available at: http://www.skollfoundation.org/ media/skoll_docs/2007SP_feature_ martinosberg.pdf. Accessed January 8, 2010.

Max-Neef M: Foundations of transdisciplinarity, *Journal of Ecological Economics* 53:1–145, 2004. Online. Available at: http://www. max-neef.cl/download/Max_Neef_ Foundations_of_transdisciplinarity. pdf. Accessed January 16 2010.

Morin E: *Seven complex lessons in education for the future*, Paris, 1999, UNESCO. Online. Available at: http://unesdoc.unesco.org/images/ 0011/001177/117740eo.pdf. Accessed January 16, 2010.

Nicolescu B: *Transdisciplinarity—past, present and future. Moving worldviews—Reshaping sciences, policies and practices for endogenous sustainable development*, Holland, 2006, COMPAS Editions. Online. Available at: http://www.compasnet. org/afbeeldingen/Books/Moving% 20worldviews/Nicolescu.pdf Accessed January 16, 2010.

Nye JS: Limits of American power, *Political Science Quarterly* 117:552, 2002–2003.

Pattison M: Entrepreneurial opportunities in the global community. In Curtin M, Molineux M, Supyk-mellson J, editors: *Occupational Therapy and Physical Dysfunction: Enabling Occupation*, ed 6, Oxford, 2010, Churchill Livingstone, Elsevier, pp 329–338.

Peloquin SM: The art of occupational therapy: engaging hearts in practice. In Kronenberg F, Simo Algado S, Pollard N, editors: *Occupational Therapy Without Borders. Learning from the Spirit of Survivors*, Edinburgh, 2005, Elsevier/Churchill Livingstone, pp 99–109.

Pollard N: When Adam dalf and Eve span: occupational literacy and democracy. In Pollard N, Sakellariou D, Kronenberg F, editors: *A Political Practice of Occupational Therapy* Edinburgh, 2008, Elsevier Science, pp 39–51.

Pollard N, Sakellariou D: Facing the challenge: a compass for navigating the heteroglossic context. In Pollard N, Sakellariou D, Kronenberg F, editors: *A Political Practice of Occupational Therapy*, Edinburgh, 2008, Elsevier Science, pp 237–244.

Pollard N, Sakellariou D: Is doing 'good' good? *Asian-Pacific Disability and Rehabilitation Journal* 20:53–65, 2009.

Pollard N, Alsop A, Kronenberg F: Re-conceptualizing occupational therapy, *British Journal of Occupational Therapy* 68:524–526, 2005.

Pollard N, Sakellariou D, Kronenberg F: Political competence in occupational therapy. In Pollard N, Sakellariou D, Kronenberg F, editors: *A Political Practice of Occupational Therapy*, Edinburgh, 2008a, Elsevier Science, pp 21–38.

Pollard N, Kronenberg F, Sakellariou D: A political practice of occupational therapy. In Pollard N, Sakellariou D, Kronenberg F, editors: *A Political Practice of Occupational Therapy*, Edinburgh, 2008b, Elsevier Science, pp 3–20.

Pollard N, Sakellariou D, Lawson-Porter A: Will occupational science facilitate or divide the practice of occupational therapy? *International Journal of Therapy and Rehabilitation* 17:648–654, 2010.

Poole BS: On time: contributions from the social sciences, *Financial Services Review* 9:375–387, 2000.

Quijano A: Colonialidad del poder y classificacion social, *Journal of World Systems Research* 6:342–386, 2000.

Ramdin R: *The Making of the Black Working Class in Britain*, Aldershot, 1987, Wildwood House.

Ramose MB: *African philosophy through ubuntu*, Harare, 1999, Mond Books.

Ramugondo EL: *Intergenerational shifts and continuities in children's play within a rural Venda family (early 20th to early 21st century)*, Doctoral dissertation, Cape Town, South Africa, 2009, University of Cape Town.

Ramugondo EL, Kronenberg F: *Collective occupations: a vehicle for building & maintaining working relationships*. Paper presented at the 15th Congress of the World Federation of Occupational Therapists, Santiago de Chile, 2010.

Reindal SM: Independence, dependence, interdependence: Some reflections on the subject and personal autonomy, *Disability and Society* 14:354, 1999.

Robertson SL: Absences and imaginings: the production of knowledge on globalisation and education, *Globalisation, Societies and Education* 4:303–318, 2006.

Roeckelein JE: *The concept of time in psychology: a resource book and annotated bibliography*, Westport CT, 2000, Greenwood.

Rugland W: *Assuming the mantle of professionalism. Valuation Actuary Symposium Proceedings. Luncheon address*, 1993, Online. Available at: http://www.soa.org/library/proceedings/valuation-actuary-symposium-proceedings/1985-99/1993/january/vasp935.pdf. Accessed.

Sakellariou D, Pollard N: Three sites of conflict and cooperation: class, gender and sexuality. In Pollard N, Sakellariou D, Kronenberg F, editors: *A Political Practice of Occupational Therapy*, Edinburgh, 2008, Elsevier Science, pp 69–90.

Santos BdS: *Challenging empires. The world social forum: toward a counter-hegemonic globalization (Part I—toward a counter hegemonic globalization)*. Edited version of a two-part paper presented at the XXIV International Congress of the Latin American Studies Association, March 27–29, 2003 Dallas, USA, 2003. Online Available at: http://www.choike.org/documentos/wsf_s318_sousa.pdf. Accessed January 7, 2010.

Santos BdS: Human rights as an emancipator script? Cultural and political conditions. In Santos BdS, editor: *Another Knowledge is Possible: Beyond Northern Epistemologies*, London, 2007, Verso.

Schwartz CE, Sendor M: Helping others help oneself: Response shift effects in peer support, *Soc Sci Med* 48:1563–1575, 1999.

Schwartz KB: Reclaiming our heritage: connecting the founding vision to the centennial vision (Eleanor Clarke Slagle lecture), *Am J Occup Ther* 63:681–690, 2009.

Senge P, Scharmer CO, Jaworsky J, et al: *Presence: exploring Profound Change in People, Organizations and Society*, London, 2005, Nicholas Brealey.

Sinha S: *Social entrepreneurship: definition and example*, 2009a. Online. Available at: http://www.pluggd.in/social-entrepreneurship-definition-and-examples-297. Accessed January 8, 2010.

Sinha S: *Understanding social entrepreneurship and traits of a social entrepreneur*, 2009b. Online. Available at: http://www.pluggd.in/social-entrepreneurship-definition-297. Accessed January 8, 2010.

Soares R, de Lima: Absences and emergences: production of knowledge and social transformation, *Matrizes* 1:231–235, 2007. Online Available at: http://www.usp.br/matrizes/img/01/Resenha3Rosana_en.pdf. Accessed January 15, 2010.

Stern I: *Mao to Mozart: Isaac Stern in China. Documentary film by Murray Lerner*, 1979. Online. Available at: http://www.youtube.com/watch?v=moJbjMoD26k&feature=related. Accessed January 5, 2010.

Stewart R, Bhagwanjee A: Promoting group empowerment and self-reliance through participatory research: A case study of people with physical disability, *Disabil Rehabil* 21:338, 1999.

Thaysen U: *Politik als Kunst: Bewaehrung in der eheren Dichotomien der Politik*, 2007, Online. Available at: http://www.swp-berlin.org/en/common/get_document.php?asset_id=4122. Accessed January 8, 2010.

Thibeault R: In praise of dissidence: Anne Lang-Etienne (1932–1991). Muriel Driver Memorial, *Can J Occup Ther* 69:197–204, 2002.

Thibeault R: Globalization, universities and the future of occupational therapy: Dispatches for the majority world. WFOT 2006 Congress: keynote speech, *Australian Occupational Therapy Journal* 53:151–172, 2006.

University of Cape Town: *Social responsiveness policy framework*, 2008a, Online. Available at: http://www.socialresponsiveness.uct.ac.za/about/policy_framework/. Accessed January 15, 2010.

University of Cape Town: *Social responsiveness report: portraits of practice*, 2008b, Online. Available at: http://www.socialresponsiveness.uct.ac.za/usr/social_resp/reports/SR_report_2008.pdf. Accessed January 15, 2010.

Watson R, Swartz L: *Transformation Through Occupation*, London, 2004, Whurr.

Whiteford G: The Korn unfurls: The emergence of diversity in occupational therapy thought and action, *New Zealand Journal of Occupational Therapy* 54:21–25, 2007.

Wilcock AA: *An occupational perspective of health*, 1998, Slack, Thorofare, p. 222.

Wilcock AA: *Occupation for Health, volume 2. A Journey from Prescription to Self Health*, London, 2002, College of Occupational Therapists.

Wilding C: Defining occupational therapy. In Curtin M, Molineux M, Supyk-Mellson J, editors: *Occupational Therapy and Physical Dysfunction: Enabling Occupation*, Edinburgh, 2010, Churchill Livinstone/Elsevier, pp 3–15.

World Federation of Occupational Therapists: *Revised minimum standards for the education of occupational therapists*, Australia, 2002, WFOT, Forrestfield.

World Federation of Occupational Therapists: *Position paper on community-based rehabilitation*, 2004, Online. Available at: https://www.wfot.org/office_files/CBRposition%20Final%20CM2004%282%29.pdf. Accessed January 7, 2010.

World Federation of Occupational Therapists: *Position statement on human rights*, 2006. Online. Available at: https://www.wfot.org/office_files/Human%20Rights%20Position%20Statement%20Final%20NLH%281%29.pdf. Accessed January 7, 2010.

World Federation of Occupational Therapists: *Guiding principles on diversity and culture*, Forrestfield, Australia, 2009, WFOT.

World Federation of Occupational Therapists: *Position statement on cultural diversity*, Forrestfield, Australia, 2010, WFOT.

Section 1

Discourses without borders

Pecket Learning Community

2

Pat Smart   Gillian Frost   Pauline Nugent   Nick Pollard

OVERVIEW

In Pecket Well College, no one is written off ... we encourage people to be proud of themselves. We are adults with a voice and a will to be heard.

Joe, a founder member

Like a Jack-in-the-box, we're not put in a box. We spring from courses to voluntary work for the college, to management, to running workshops, to paid work! From coming in the front door as strangers, we become the host and hostess. It's like a bouncing ball – our strengths and confidence then encourage others, and so it goes on.

Peter, a founder member

Living with reading, writing, and maths difficulties

Pecket Well College (now Pecket Learning Community), West Yorkshire, United Kingdom, has been running free community-based day courses and residential weekends since 1985 for people tackling reading, writing, and communication problems. Some of the people involved have participated in the evolving history of residentials and other special events and activities in adult basic education since the late 1970s. The story of Pecket as an adult learning community that is run by its own learners, many of whom have disabilities, is one of struggle as well as success and inspiration. People come to Pecket Learning Community to pass on their skills to others, but often pick up many more skills and go away feeling better about themselves. Not only that, they pass on the 'Pecket way' to others they go on to work with.

Reading, writing, and maths are increasingly essential skills for everyday life. So much occupational choice depends on access to the written word. For people with low levels of these skills employment opportunities have vastly diminished; modern banking systems and cash retrieval systems have become impossible to use for those with severe difficulties with reading; communication technologies have replaced face-to-face contact and assume high levels of numeracy and literacy. While for some the new technologies make life easier, many are more occupationally disadvantaged than ever. Low levels of basic skills are also associated with a range of other difficulties in life that contribute to social and occupational deprivation – poverty, unemployment, poor housing, poor health, living in communities deprived of resources, likelihood of periods in prison, and disaffected youth (Whiteford 2000).

In the United Kingdom, 26 million people have inadequate levels of basic literacy and numeracy skills (Department for Education and Skills (DfES) 2001). Seven million people have severe difficulties with reading, writing and numeracy (Moser 1999). At the age of 30, people with poor numeracy were over twice as likely to be unemployed than those with competent numeracy (Carpentiari 2007). An estimated 136 000 people aged 16–60 in West Yorkshire have either lower or very low literacy skills and 182 000 have lower or very low numeracy skills, while 63 wards out of 126 in West Yorkshire rank in the poorest 25% nationally for educational deprivation (West Yorkshire Economic Partnership 2005).

Those with the lowest skills and greatest barriers need outreach and creative/flexible provision, which the voluntary sector is well placed to deliver. Pecket Learning Community aims to promote greater equality of opportunity and social inclusion for people in these most disadvantaged groups. People need support to deal with day-to-day concerns such as money management, benefits, housing, health, and other welfare issues. Their difficulties are compounded by the stigma associated with having problems with the written word and numeracy. The stress involved in the constant vigilance and effort necessary to hide and find ways round these difficulties is enormous. The fear of exposure is ever present, some even hiding their difficulties from their own families.

For nearly a quarter century, Pecket Learning Community has used creative activity as an effective method in building people's confidence to tackle these problems. People have the opportunity both to write and to see their words in print (through life stories, poetry, ideas, research), magazine and book production being at the heart of our activities, along with the creative expression of individuals and groups, in song writing, and often in the wall hangings and art work which adorn the college walls. Drama is also a popular and powerful medium at Pecket in which individuals and groups work out problematic issues and transform shame into pride, secrets into assertive advocacy.

People often find that their lives have changed as a result of these courses and they become involved themselves as volunteers, not only in their own education but in their own communities. This improves their opportunities in gaining work. Volunteering is essential to the college, and an essential part of the learning process. Pecket Learning Community has maintained its resilience through this wealth of voluntary workers who kept the college going through the normal funding crises of the voluntary sector. Participants have amassed valuable experience in outreach work to encourage others like themselves into education, in planning, running courses, doing publicity and running the college. They can become directors, and/or attend meetings, make decisions, decide on policy, and help with administration and outreach work. One of the potential parallels with occupational therapy is the similarity between this approach and that of the settlement movement led by the Barnetts at what became Toynbee House in London, and was the predecessor of the Hull House movement in Chicago. Wilcock (2006) describes how the settlement movement offered new migrants to the United States a program of voluntary and cooperative approaches to what is now recognized as community development including adult education.

Pecket Learning Community also encourages participants to contribute to building up the capacity and sustainability of their own local community environment through training, developing skills, work experience, and progression routes. Partnership projects have been set up to target specific groups and areas. Pecket Learning Community promotes wider access for all, especially those groups less likely to take up formal, traditional educational routes and those lacking in basic skills. Teaching materials are developed jointly so that they are flexible and responsive to people's needs and the issues relevant to them. Difficulties faced in everyday life are tackled in our provision in reading, writing, maths, and information and computer technology, along with a staggering range of interests to pursue once asked, given encouragement and the opportunity to develop them.

A residential weekend on healthy eating included workshops on likes and dislikes, writing about foods, quizzes, practical cooking sessions (all meals scratch cooked by a rota of participants working with a tutor in the kitchen) with foods that many participants had not tried before, social events, and a workshop from a dietician. Each person began the weekend identifying their 'toffee twin' – taking a diabetes-friendly sweet from a basket and opening it to find a random number assigned to them and another participant. Toffee twins agree to look out for each others' needs during the whole weekend.

Who are we? Where did we spring from?

Pecket members don't fit in one box nor do our difficulties with reading and writing. Some of us were not taught to read and write for cultural reasons; some of us have specific or other learning difficulties. Some have dyslexia, didn't have much schooling, or had disrupted childhoods. Some have other disabilities and because of these, we were not expected to learn or do things for ourselves. Some were made to feel stupid at school or were put down by our parents who did not understand our difficulties so needed to rebuild our confidence. Some used to be able to read and write but have lost the ability for a variety of reasons –

often linked to trauma. We made a choice not to use the names 'tutor' or 'student' among ourselves because those labels made us feel like kids, instead we generally refer to ourselves as 'members' or 'Pecketwellians'. This helps those who experienced trauma at school to move forward. A few of us have worked as tutors in adult basic education or community education or community arts but wanted to work side by side with those who have experience of tackling difficulties with the written word.

For many of us, the starting point is fear, shame and a disabling sense of failure. Having been labeled stupid, lazy or disruptive throughout our schooling, and having to deal with commonly held prejudices about our difficulties on a daily basis, making a start to tackle our difficulties needed all our courage. Participants have said: 'I have tried other classes but never got on like I do at Pecket', 'I am ashamed and don't let on I can't read and write', 'I am just thick', 'When I go to other classes I am the one who never gets anywhere' (Pecket Well College 2006). But coming to Pecket, or being involved in the group who set it up, has enabled us to see ourselves differently. We see dyslexia and other difficulties with the written word as a difference associated with strengths as well as weaknesses, an ability as well as a disability.

Pecket Learning Community is a service user-led organization that came together in 1984, from a group of adults from Calderdale who attended a week's residential course organized by the 'Write First Time Collective', which also produced a national adult basic education students paper. The course, a writing week held at Nottingham University, was for people like ourselves from all over the country. During the course, one of the founder members wrote a poem, 'The progression of learning', which includes the lines 'I found a way/ Of wearing the flag of illiteracy/ With pride' (Goode 1989). We all had different backgrounds and life experiences but many things bonded us.

1. We all had difficulties with reading, writing and/ or numbers, had bad experiences of schooling and had faced our fear of education by joining the local adult education centre.
2. We had joined in with national and regional events and groups working on student and community writing and publishing (see Chapters 15 and 18) and other ways of students finding their voice and making themselves heard, encouraged, and supported by our tutor.
3. We had found a place within education that excited us and we wanted more but we had to stick together and fight to try to keep and protect this special thing we had found. We wanted to build on it, but it wasn't possible to develop what we wanted within the adult education centre we all went to.
4. We knew things could be better if we had more say in our learning and we were prepared to work hard to make this happen.
5. We had all worked closely with our tutor on a variety of projects to do with student writing and publishing. We knew we could work together side by side.

Our 'tutor' and some of the other 'tutors' we had met along the way were positive, encouraging and supportive but we were all trapped in the same system that set too many limits on what progress we could make together.

That shared experience in Nottingham gave us a dream and the courage and determination to stick together and to work alongside 'tutors' who wanted to work with us in equal partnership. The idea of Pecket was born on the train journey home! We were clear and determined from day 1 that we, as learners, must be involved in everything and at every stage. Along with our 'tutor' and another 'tutor' from the adult education centre who had experience of setting up cooperatives, we formed a group to set up a residential centre. None of us had ever started a 'group' or 'organization' before but we had all been involved in various community groups and writing groups and we knew that together we could do it. We always found the people with the other skills needed who were willing to help us.

One of the 'tutors' offered us free use of the dining room in her home as an office base, and of an unoccupied old co-op shop and warehouse which was also part of the same lovely old building. It was above a famous beauty spot in the heart of the Pennines, in Pecket Well, near Hebden Bridge in West Yorkshire. We also worked out in the community wherever we could find a free space. We met in each other's homes, community rooms, rooms in pubs, the Irish Club, and labor club rooms – whatever was offered to us for free. We traveled all over the country and in this and other ways we got immense encouragement and support from people and groups we met and wrote to, and from funders too.

Pat Smart (long-term friend of Pecket, volunteer and ex-outreach worker, member of voluntary development team)

With help and fundraising Pecket converted the building into a welcoming and accessible residential centre. Development work, outreach, residential, and other courses continued. In 1985 Pecket became a registered charity, and in 1988 a company limited by guarantee. Its management committee of between seven and 25 elected trustees has a majority membership (over 51%) of people with experience of basic skills difficulties, recruited from participants and volunteers along with supporters with different expertise as advisers and/or directors. In 1992 Pecket opened a residential centre for adult basic and community education. Finally in 1999, a lottery grant enabled the purchase of the whole building. Pecket now owned the first residential centre for adult basic and community education in the United Kingdom, set up and run by 'service users' or 'beneficiaries'.

Pecket participants have included groups of East European asylum seekers, an Asian women's mental health group, community groups, and statutory organizations such as the West Yorkshire Fire and Rescue

Service. Recent computer courses have targeted the older person in the community, generating demands for further courses to be run. The transformational possibilities of the residential experience were demonstrated dramatically with the drug users' project. From a group of 12, two came off drugs, realized their personal ambitions, and became involved as volunteers for Pecket.

In the late 1990s 'Pecketwellians' played both host and tutor to Egyptian adult basic education providers and their tutors for residential courses and workshops on working with, and especially including, adult learners. The 'Pecket approach' has influenced other adult education projects in Spain, Denmark, Sweden, Germany, and Greece as well as the United States and Canada. Like many other community-based organizations, recent national changes in funding trends and education policy have had a huge impact on Pecket Learning Community. The word 'college' has become misleading and limited. Pecket has relaunched itself. As a user-led holistic adult educational project Pecket Learning Community now covers many areas including basic education, residential education, arts, disability, self-advocacy and empowerment, health, and volunteering. It targets people from communities experiencing disadvantages in many areas, while being open to all adults, from whatever background, with difficulties with the written word, numeracy, language, and communication as well as community education groups. In occupational terms, Pecket Learning Community is enacting 'doing, being, becoming and belonging' (Wilcock 1998) through user-led education.

'We are adults with a voice and a will to be heard'

Pecket Learning Community has had to develop a flexible approach that takes account of changing conditions, while remaining true to its roots. Courses and education materials are adapted so that they are appropriate to the needs of individual participants or groups. Many workshop leaders have taught in mainstream colleges, adult and community education but come prepared to take risks and work in different ways; listening and learning to share power is often the opposite of how they have been prepared to 'teach'. We have all learnt from Pecket 'a long hard

lesson/ to learn something/ as simple/ as/ our humanity/ bursting out/ from behind/ the cardboard/ cut-outs of/ 'tutor'/ 'student' (Frost 1994, p 8). 'Learners' are usually expected to respond to 'tutors' questions (rather than think and question); at Pecket Learning Community they are supported and encouraged to find their own voice and questions, and to let go of frustrations, fear, embarrassment, and sometimes anger – all of which can bring power too. They have to take some responsibility and be prepared to try different ways of learning before discovering how to become participants in their own education.

For many, it is the first time in their lives that they are asked what they want.

> When you can't read or write, other people have a 'power' or 'authority' over us that they are often unaware of. Their skills give others access to information that we do not have. We have to give up our privacy and ask others to read intimate and personal papers – as well as constant junk mail. Everybody benefits: Pecket Well College asked for my help (with computers) so I became a volunteer ...
> I had no formal qualifications yet found myself passing on what I knew to others, to people who had ... no voice in the community
>
> Pat Smart

Pecket encourages skills-sharing so that participants can become workshop leaders, whether working alongside a 'tutor' or in their own right. Workshop leaders and those working in education outside of Pecket Learning Community can become participants in members' training workshops.

John Glynn was possibly the first adult basic education student employed on an adult basic education project. He was one of the founder workers of the Gatehouse Project, which encouraged student writing, and published books by adult basic education students. John's strengths with art and layout were invaluable, and because of the cooperative structure of Gatehouse, he had experience of all aspects of the work of the project. He took part in a writing development pack project (Frost et al n.d.) in which, through writing, he came to understand the process by which he had been failed by the education system (see his telling indictment of the education system in 'School a Wasted Childhood') (Glynn n.d., p. 1–12). In this way, his confidence and skills grew, and eventually he became a worker for Pecket, as a workshop leader of the magazine group and as a finance worker. The 'student' became 'the tutor'.

Arguing for basic education needs

Directors are aware of the real risk that Pecket could become 'funding led' – bowing to pressures to slot into existing patterns of education provision, but the users have a strong voice. Pecket has in the past maintained a high local profile aimed at encouraging active involvement in adult learning or community activities through its learners participating in contacts with local radio, national and local press, national and regional TV, published material, tapes, CDs, video, and the internet. Pecket Learning Community believes in volunteering at all levels of organization as an essential part of the learning and of the personal development processes, and a peer approach as the most effective way of reaching people. People listen to others like themselves and can be inspired by their confidence and enthusiasm, as well as identifying with their vulnerability. They are relieved to know there are others with the same difficulties and that awareness is the beginning of the process of change. All Pecket's policies and practices are informed by the experience of the users as a strategy of addressing barriers to access (Flanagan 1997, Woodin 2007) and consequently hit many of our own targets – and those of funders. Pecket Learning Community estimates that up to 1000 people will take part in community and other courses/training provisions over the next five years. Learners can obtain free courses, free transport, assistance to cover childcare and dependant care costs, necessary support workers, and adaptations to meet the needs of people with disabilities.

Pecket Learning Community must be one of the very few organizations to have resisted the move to accreditation. Fear is the greatest barrier for people working on reading, writing, and maths. Pecket's non-accredited courses aim to make learning as stress-free as possible. In other areas such as volunteering or directors' training, Pecket has no objection to accreditation as long as it is what the participants want.

Changes in both national funding trends and adult education policy in the United Kingdom have made commitment to nonaccredited learning extremely challenging. Provision has moved from small adult education centers to large colleges of further education, where most students are young people. Many older adults feel out of place or are intimidated by these large institutions, which can feel impersonal.

Colleges are under pressure from current funding arrangements to show results fast and cannot afford to work with the people who need the most help. Other provision is in Learndirect centers (http://www.learndirect.co.uk) which offer independent advice for basic education, but where generally people need to have some level of independence in working on computers. Small-scale innovatory projects in the voluntary sector among community groups and in prisons may indicate a suitable direction for the development of provision for people not catered for elsewhere (North Liverpool Citizens Advice Bureau n.d.).

It is sometimes difficult to imagine where the provision of 'basic' might actually start. Most of our learners feel that the education system let them down once before to the extent that they are terrified of learning. Having left school and lived their lives labeled as 'thick' they are reluctant to come back to education as an adult for more imposition of the same inflexible outcomes which do not meet their needs. Pecket has refused funding which makes these kinds of demands. Access to a college which 'is not like a school or other colleges, it is more like a big family', has to work on other criteria.

Many times someone has had to decline the chance of coming on a course because they had no dependant care. Even our offer to pay it for them was no use to them as they didn't have the carers to do it. As Pecket has fully disabled access we were able to tell one lady to bring her very aged mum along. She did, and her mum enjoyed it so much she came on a course herself. This left more time for the daughter to pursue looking for a job, while her mum eventually moved on to a further education class nearer home. Participants often bring along other people they know with similar needs as themselves, and this increases the need for more Pecket courses.

Pat Smart

There are still millions of people held back by problems with the written word/ communication/ number. Pecket specializes in ways of working that reach 'the hard to reach'. Sandra Breeze (2008) writes: 'we like to give all our participants free drinks and biscuits ... A lot of our participants are very nervous at first, so having a cuppa plays a very important part, helps them to settle down and feel at home.' This is why the college tea urn is always on, and situated in a welcoming room on your left as you come into the building. It's a space where you can, if you need to, just hang around and get the feel of the place. Some people will need to sit there for a day or so before venturing into one of the learning rooms, and may take a while before they build up sufficient confidence to take part in a course. People come to Pecket Learning Community to realize it's not their fault they can't read, and soon begin work on their reading, writing and or maths without pressure and at their own pace. It's all right to feel you have had enough and want to have a cup of tea or go for a walk – and you won't be thrown off the course for going to have one in the middle of a session.

> We have to communicate to funders that mastering the skills of reading, writing and numeracy is a long process for those with the greatest difficulties, but well worth 'the investment' in terms of the improvements in employment opportunities, health, crime prevention, and many related areas of social problems. And we have to develop the center as a residential resource for groups within adult basic and continuing education, and community groups, in line with the original conception in establishing the center.
>
> Pat Smart

Unhappily, the culture of funding at present means that the spirit of cooperation that informed practice in the 1970s and 1980s started to change in the 1990s. Providers often see each other as competition, rather than as potential partners and fear 'poaching' of their students. Tutors have more and more pressure to show results through the accredited courses that are now the norm, and have little time to engage or support their students in engaging in other provision and activities. One of our biggest challenges is to try to overcome this sense of threat and work out ways in which providers can work together to offer progression routes to their participants. Pecket Learning Community's role is to start people off on their educational journey, helping to build their confidence and skills to access mainstream provision.

The beginning of the process

There remains very little provision for adults who have difficulties with the written word or numeracy. Pecket Learning Community is helping to raise public awareness of the issues and overcome the stigma which fundamentally affects their quality of life. Readers of this chapter will recognize these concerns as occupational as well as educational priorities. Our members are proud to be a public voice on this issue. The work they have done and continue to do for Pecket Learning Community ensures their confidence and pride, and makes them excellent ambassadors. In all this talk of disadvantage, deprivation and poverty, we never lose sight of the rich life experience of our participants, their talents and vast potential.

Sowing the seeds

Sow the seeds of words in fertile minds,
scatter them on the wind far and wide.
Words are life,
never fear of giving them to others.
Once the seeds are sown,
Feed often with encouragement.
Watch as the seedlings unfold
and the words are caressed by eager ears.
What a wonderful feeling when you see
the stem of knowledge blossom.
Spring, Summer, Autumn or Winter,
Whatever the season, sow those seeds.

Pat Smart

References

Breeze S: *Tea letter*, Pecket Well, 2008, Pecket Well College.

Carpentiari J, editor: *Five years on. Research, development and changing practice*, NRDC 2006–2007, London, 2007, National Research and Development Centre. For Adult Literacy and Numeracy. Online. Available at: http://www.nrdc.org.uk/download.asp?f=3913&e=pdf. Accessed November 11, 2008.

Department for Education and Skills: *Skills for life: Improving adult literacy and numeracy*, London, 2001, Department for Education and Skills. Online. Available at: http://www.dcsf.gov.uk/readwriteplus/bank/ACF35CE.pdf. Accessed November 11, 2008.

Flanagan J: *Looking back*, Halifax, 1997, Pecket Well College.

Frost G: Strange child. In Pecket Well College, editor: *Pecket Well College Opening Day Book*, Pecket Well, 1994, p 8.

Frost G, Hoy C, Glynn J, editors: *Opening time. A writing resource pack written by students in Basic Education*, Manchester, (n.d.), Gatehouse.

Glynn J: School a wasted childhood. In Frost G, Hoy C, Glynn J, editors: *Opening time. A writing resource pack written by students in Basic Education*, Manchester, (n.d.), Gatehouse, pp 1–12.

Goode P: *The Moon on the Window – The Book of Gobbledegook*, Open Township, 1989, Hebden Bridge.

Moser C: *Improving literacy and numeracy: a fresh start*, Sudbury, 1999, Department for Education and Employment.

North Liverpool Citizens Advice Bureau: *Financial literacy in prison*, (n.d.), Online. Available at: http://www.archive.basic-skills.co.uk/content/documents/?FileID=1311572160. Accessed November 11, 2008.

Pecket Well College: *Pecket survey 2006*, 2006.

West Yorkshire Economic Partnership: *West Yorkshire investment plan strategic economic assessment*, 2005, Online. Available at: http://www.fit4funding.org.uk/assets/uploads/files/sea%2020051.pdf. Accessed November 11, 2008.

Whiteford G: Occupational deprivation, global challenge in the new millennium, *British Journal of Occupational Therapy* 63:200–204, 2000.

Wilcock AA: Doing, being, becoming, *Can J Occup Ther* 65:248–257, 1998.

Wilcock AA: *An occupational perspective of health*, Thorofare, NJ, 2006, Slack.

Woodin T: 'Chuck out the teacher': radical pedagogy in the community, *International Journal of Lifelong Education* 26:89–104, 2007.

Meeting the needs for occupational therapy in Gaza

3

Barbara Lavin

Dear students

First of all let me offer you my sincere congratulations on your graduation! The obstacles to reaching this day have been many, more than we could possibly have anticipated when we very happily accepted you all to the program. When I reflect on the last two years particularly, I wonder how it was possible to proceed under such difficult and unpredictable circumstances and I must admit that there were times when it was not easy to find a way forward to avoid the latest obstacle. But as an occupational therapist I have been regularly amazed and delighted at the resilience of the human spirit, and the capacity to endure difficulties in order to reach a valued goal. And it seems that this resilience and perseverance has been very much in evidence in your journey of the last four years towards the completion of the program and this day. I suspect that more resilience and perseverance will be required as you develop your professional careers as occupational therapists in Gaza – but by now you have had lots of practice!

I am sorry that things didn't work out as planned. I am also sorry not to be able to share this day with you. That is quite a major disappointment for me. But I send you my greetings and best wishes not only for this graduation day but for your future. I hope to hear good things about your work with the people of Gaza who are very much in need of the services you can offer. I hope that you will continue to develop yourselves personally and professionally, to reflect on what you do and to support each other even if you are working in very different fields. Perhaps most of all I hope that you have the opportunity to do these things in an atmosphere of peace and stability.

Warm greetings and best wishes from Barbara

This letter was written from Wellington, New Zealand in March 2008 to be read at the graduation of 10 occupational therapy students living in Gaza. The students graduated on 27 March, 2008, more than five years from the time the initial idea to recruit students from Gaza to study occupational therapy at Bethlehem University was developed.

Introduction

Occupational therapists are very familiar with the power of the environment to shape, curtail, and enhance occupational performance. This is the story of how an environment, in all its dimensions but particularly an institutional environment, influenced the education of a group of occupational therapy students and the teachers responsible for the education. It is a story of obstacles overcome only to be replaced by obstacles of even greater magnitude. But it is also the story of how adversity develops strength and creativity, and less than ideal conditions optimize motivation and determination to succeed. Ultimately it is the story of a group of people who refused to give up and go away and eventually were able to realize their ambitions. The main people in the story are students and teachers in the occupational therapy program at Bethlehem University. All of us were changed by the experiences as the story unfolded. It required skills and strengths we didn't know we had and exposed weaknesses we would have preferred to keep hidden. The story also involved and affected parents, administrators, funders, and all others involved in the delivery of the program, other universities, lawyers, journalists, and the students' peers. In the course of this experience the occupation – that of student and that of teacher – also had to change. Traditional ways of teaching by face-to-face lectures and skill demonstrations could not be done and new ways were required. We learned to do new things when the old ways didn't work, we learned to make priorities when the time was restricted, and we learned to make compromises when what was needed could not be found.

© 2011, Elsevier Ltd.
DOI: 10.1016/B978-0-7020-3103-8.00012-2

The background to the story

Two places are crucial to this story: the Gaza Strip and Bethlehem in the West Bank. Physically, Gaza is separated from the West Bank by approximately 50 km, less than one hour's drive, although the journey from Bethlehem to Gaza can take two hours, 12 hours or might not be achieved at all. Not for nothing is Gaza often referred to (by those who live there and those who try to get in or out) as a prison. Access in and out of Gaza is restricted to two crossing points, Erez, the entry point into Israel, and Rafah, the entry point into Egypt. A 'safe passage' that would allow Palestinians to travel between Gaza and the West Bank without threatening Israel's security opened in 1999. By the time our project started it had long been closed and in spite of being frequently on the agenda for discussion has never reopened.

The Gaza Strip is one of the most densely populated areas in the world, 3881.6 persons per square kilometer in an area of 365 km (Palestinian Central Bureau of Statistics 2005), a total population of over 1.4 million. More than 41% of the population is aged under the age of 15. A report by the Palestinian Civil Society Consultancy Meeting in April 2006 (Palestinian Medical Relief Society (PMRS)) on social determinants of health provides a comprehensive summary of the social conditions affecting health in Palestine. These include, but are not limited to, the occupation and resultant oppression and conflict and restrictions on movement, poverty, social customs such as consanguineous marriage, and unemployment. Health is further influenced by factors such as lack of coordination between healthcare providers and the lack of implementation of laws such as the Disability Law 1999. Children, women, people with disabilities, and people with mental health problems were identified as being particularly disadvantaged in the current circumstances.

The Palestinian Central Bureau of Statistics (1997) has published statistics on the incidence of disability in the West Bank and Gaza as part of the population census. Using the North Gaza Governorate as an example, in a total population of 179 690, 2932 people are reported as having disabilities. The largest groups are mobility, mental, and visual disabilities. Of those of school age, less than 50% are attending school, and of those of working age less than 20% are employed. Given the current economic circumstances in Gaza since the start of the *intifada*, it is likely that even fewer people with disabilities are employed. These statistics give no indication of the extent to which people could be more independent if they had access to occupational therapy, however, they do indicate the extent of the need for services that address independence and participation in the community.

In 2003, access to occupational therapy services in Gaza was limited, there being only two foreign-trained (Greece and Jordan) Palestinian therapists. Other rehabilitation services such as physiotherapy were more readily available, and a rehabilitation hospital, Al Wafa, was well established in Gaza City.

The story begins

It seemed like such a good idea. A throwaway remark during a visit to Al Wafa led to the development of a plan to bring a group of students from Gaza to Bethlehem University to study occupational therapy. Since 1996 Bethlehem University has had a degree program in occupational therapy. As part of the university's mission statement is to address the needs of the disadvantaged members of the community, the need for occupational therapy services in Gaza fitted well.

Although 2003 had not so far been a good year with violence perpetrated by both sides in the form of suicide bombings and consequent retaliation by the Israeli Defense Forces (IDF) it didn't seem unrealistic to persevere with developing the scheme to bring the students to Bethlehem. Things moved quickly. Bethlehem University acknowledged that there was certainly a need and supported the process of recruitment. Organizations in Gaza indicated that they would be willing to employ graduates. A UK-based organization, Action Around Bethlehem Children with Disabilities (ABCD), and a Swedish organization, the Swedish Organization for Individual Relief (SOIR), offered scholarships. The applicants were informed that it was likely that they would have to spend the entire four years in Bethlehem as it was considered a risk for the students to return to Gaza for vacations given the frequency and unpredictability of the closures that would effectively trap them in Gaza. In June of 2003, a group of 40 applicants sat the university entrance exam at Al Wafa Hospital and were interviewed. At the end of the day 10 prospective students had been selected, seven men and three women, all Muslim.

As one of the students, Riham Al Muza'nin put it:

> I felt excited to be accepted on the program and waited for the moment when I would move to my university to start my academic life, join my colleagues in the regular classes and meet my new teachers who would provide me with the practical and theoretical skills to be an efficient therapist to help people with disabilities in Gaza become more independent. Unfortunately, this was only a dream that accompanied me through the four years and it didn't come true.

The first year – 2003/04

The first weeks of the academic year of 2003/04 came and went but there was no sign of the students. All had been refused the permits from the Israeli authorities necessary to leave Gaza and travel to Bethlehem. It seemed impossible to imagine that a group of students who were going to study a much-needed health profession would be refused the required permits, but in the words of Mohammad Al Rozzi, one of the students:

> The first challenge was the travel ban by the Israeli authorities on travel to Bethlehem University in the West Bank. The justification of the Israeli Army was very strange – 'potential terrorists'. It is not good for anybody to be labeled as a terrorist for trying to reach a university.

The first decisions needed to be taken. To proceed or to jettison the whole plan? We kept hoping and encouraged the students to try all the means at their disposal, including any influence they had with any authorities. I was reluctant to jettison the plan for a number of reasons. Many people had worked hard to get this far, organizations had made commitments and as we had made a commitment to the students we needed to follow through on that. The reality of the situation in Gaza remained: only two therapists and many needs. Any means of improving access to occupational therapy services was worth pursuing. The interim solution to the current problem was to identify the courses that could be provided by another institution and get the students enrolled. The Palestine College of Nursing in Khan Younis agreed to help and the students began studying anatomy, human growth and development, and healthcare. As the semester progressed and the students remained in Gaza the next problem was how to teach introductory occupational therapy courses. In the absence of organized occupational therapy services there were few role models and we believed that it was crucial to establish a sense of identity early on.

The Norwegian Occupational Therapy Association (NETF) came to the rescue and a Norwegian occupational therapist arrived in Gaza to teach the students for blocks of time from two to six weeks. We are grateful for the work done by Margrete Hoen who visited many times over the next year and took the students through the introductory courses, adult rehabilitation courses, and the first clinical fieldwork. The situation remained unpredictable and unstable. But the first steps had been taken. Of course, we all remained optimistic that this was only an interim arrangement until the students could come to Bethlehem.

The second year – 2004/05

I reorganized my workload and traveled twice a week to Gaza to teach courses in mental health. A hospital conference room was not the ideal place in which to lecture and to conduct practical skills training in group work but somehow we managed and Al Wafa Hospital tolerated the mess and disruption. The situation remained unstable and quite frequently classes were held while the sounds of shelling were heard alarmingly close. Mostly, somewhat surprisingly, I made it in and out of Gaza. Sometimes it took a long time. Nowhere is the power of authority more palpable than when trying to move from one place to another, be it Bethlehem to Gaza, Gaza to Egypt, or Bethlehem to Jordan. I had become accustomed to long delays getting in and out of Gaza, mostly getting out. Generally the delays left me sitting for hours at either the Palestinian side or the Israeli side, the latter being preferred because it had air conditioning. I learned early on to arm myself with occupations, a book, some marking, a Sudoku, although often there was a sense of camaraderie and the time was passed with chatting to others, foreigners and Palestinians, in the same situation.

Several times my waiting time was spent in the tunnel.

Let me describe the tunnel:
It is dusty, dirty, smells of sweat and urine, and is deserted at some times and unbearably crowded at others. After walking around 200 m you reach an electronic gate in front of which you must wait until the gate swings open. In my experience this could take from five minutes to nearly three hours but many others reported much longer waits. My privileged position as a foreigner probably expedited my progress through the gate. Sometimes, to my humiliation, I was allowed through but the Palestinians who had been

waiting much longer were not. After the gate was a turnstile, similar to those found in cattle and sheep yards and the feeling of squeezing through with a laptop, briefcase, and bag of books gave me a sense of kinship with animals being herded. Then comes an electronic check – this is all in the absence of humans, voices only, frequently misinterpreted as the sound was poor – and various requests to remove, lift, or otherwise manipulate parts of clothing. If I felt uncomfortable removing a shirt to reveal a skimpy camisole while a group of workers watched, it was much more humiliating for a woman to remove a head covering as was frequently requested for no apparent reason other than perhaps humiliation.

At this time we started experimenting with the use of videoconferencing for teaching some courses. The facilities at Bethlehem University were not operational but we were well-supported by the British Council, which allowed the use of their facilities in Ramallah and in Gaza City. Financially we were able to cope with the extra expenses through the generosity of the NETF. For a while the videoconferences went smoothly. Mostly the connection worked and the facilities at the British Council were adequate for our needs and the technical support was excellent. Then, a few days of rage and violence changed all that. The Council's facilities in Gaza were all but destroyed and other solutions had to be found. When Bethlehem University developed its own facilities for the first time the two groups of students who should have been one group were meeting face-to-face in the classroom. This was a challenge for the teachers and also for the students.

> I found it really difficult to attend lectures by videoconference. I hated this technology and my class participation decreased in these classes, even though I knew it was the only solution.
>
> Riham

The third year – 2005/06

In the Fall semester of 2005 we were joined by Lisa Henley, a Swedish occupational therapist. The plan for the Spring semester of 2006 was for Lisa to travel to Gaza twice a week to teach a theory and skills course. The situation was unstable once again and the occasional kidnapping of foreigners had made people wary of entering Gaza. We did as I had done before – made decisions on a day-to-day basis. A crash course in the use of a distance-learning program, e-class, meant that the theory course got off the ground with little delay. The students didn't like the medium much but it was a viable alternative to face-to-face teaching in the circumstances. The skills course posed another

problem altogether. We kept hoping that the situation would improve but of course it didn't. In the end we – Lisa, the students, and I – went to Cairo, to a small hotel in Zamalek which advertised having a conference room and assured us it had adequate teaching facilities. The conference room was small and strangely shaped, the teaching facilities were a whiteboard but the staff rallied around and were quite nonplussed with our requests – a bed in the conference room, certainly, use of a staff car to practice transfers, no problem. Looking back that first trip was idyllic in the number of things that went right. We didn't imagine that there would be two more trips, each progressively more difficult.

The fourth year – 2006/07

Nelly Husari from Ramallah and a graduate of the Jordan College of Occupational Therapy took the bulk of the responsibility for the occupational therapy courses in the final year. Videoconferencing with Gaza and Bethlehem students together continued, as did the use of the e-class and a new development, Ergonet. Some courses with practical components were a challenge for teacher and students. Kalman (2007) describes the somewhat surreal situation of Nelly in an empty lecture hall, directing her words to a screen and assessing a young girl in a wheelchair who is nervous because of the strange surroundings. For the students, still grappling with the shift from the habits of rote learning and memorization that they had developed since childhood and never really abandoned, the new styles of teaching and learning were a major challenge. An additional complication at this time was the electricity supply in Gaza, which was frequently restricted to a few hours a day and often didn't work at all.

In spite of the use of all available technology, some final face-to-face teaching of skills was required and so another trip to Cairo was planned. This trip, in the summer of 2007, was a nightmare from start to finish and for the students it didn't end when the classes were over and we had returned to Bethlehem. We agonized over this decision to go, weighing the pros and cons as well as we could in the circumstances and knowing that any changes in the situation were likely to be for the worse rather than the better. In the end that was the tipping point. If the situation got worse then who knew when we would be able to meet up with the students. We were so close to concluding the program that we couldn't contemplate a further, indefinite delay. So Nelly and I went, both traveling via Jordan as she was prohibited from using the airport. A few warning bells were ringing the day we left. Some of the students had been returned from the border already but as this had happened before we figured that if they tried again then it would work.

We arrived at the school on the first scheduled day of teaching to find four students, the girls and one boy. Another would arrive two days later after which we gave up hope of the others making it. The teaching went reasonably well. The nights were spent wrestling with the problem of the other students in Gaza who were all wishing they were with us. They didn't know it then but two weeks later they would be feeling very glad that they had remained in Gaza. The border was closed shortly after the fifth student arrived in Cairo. The situation in Gaza was chaotic with escalating fighting between the rival political factions, Hamas and Fatah. The students in Cairo were tormented by what was happening there and how it was impacting their families and friends. A constant topic of conversation was the border crossing – when would it reopen. The news was not encouraging but then, we also were accustomed to the situation on the ground changing very rapidly. Nelly and I said farewell to the students and returned to Bethlehem. It was the last time we would see them face to face. We tried not to think of the consequences of Rafah remaining closed. But it did, and for more than two months the students were unable to return to their homes and families. Surviving this period of 'enforced exile' was of course their major concern. Ours was what to do next as the circumstances in Gaza became more and more difficult and we waited for the group in Cairo to return home. From now until the students finally completed the program at the end of 2007, Nelly, from September the program coordinator as I had returned to New Zealand, would have to use all the ingenuity she possessed to deliver the remaining material to the students who were living in a highly unstable situation politically, economically, and in terms of availability of resources such as electricity.

People react differently to adverse conditions. In our case it seems that it brought out some creative solutions that went beyond the problem they were designed for. For example, the necessity of finding alternative methods to teach skills led us to the use of video for self and peer assessment. This circumvented the problem of lack of face-to-face teaching but also exposed the students to a higher level of critical self-reflection than they may otherwise have experienced. It also highlighted the difficulty of peer criticism and giving and receiving honest feedback. For us, as educators the constant need to find a new way to deliver material without compromising the standards of the program led to developments that will continue to enhance the program at Bethlehem University. The most important of these was the development of Ergonet, an online program using videos of clinical situations to enhance reflection, critical thinking, and problem solving, areas that were real challenges for the students. Modeled on a program originally designed to teach art history and then adapted for teaching physiotherapy in the north of Norway, Ergonet was the brainchild of Rita Jentoft, the coordinator of the Bethlehem project for NETF, specifically as a response to the problems with the Gaza students.

Throughout the project the students were not just passive participants in a process that was out of their control. Early on they had taken the initiative to contact an Israeli organization which focused on freedom of movement for Palestinians, Gisha. This was a very smart move. Although the Israeli Supreme Court ultimately rejected the petition presented by Gisha on behalf of the students and refused permission for them to travel to Bethlehem, it resulted in a lot of publicity in newspapers, other publications, and on television. The solid support from Gisha, particularly from Sari Bashi, the Director, maintained and sustained the students' hopes and dreams over the years. Perhaps this time the court would find in their favor. It never happened but it is interesting to speculate on the role of hope in this process. We will never know to what extent this hope of success contributed to all of us continuing on with a project that often appeared doomed and not worth the effort required to persevere and solve yet another problem. Another lesson learned – hope is crucial even when the objective and intellectual assessment of the situation deems it hopeless.

> Always I had a daydream imagining life at the university. These thoughts and daydreams helped me a lot to forget our reality and the obstacles we faced. Many days passed when I was in a depressed mood since I was concentrating all my thoughts on the decision of the court (to allow us to travel to Bethlehem). But then I looked around me and found that my situation was not so bad because the university stood beside us and didn't give up. They suggested many solutions and alternatives and we coped and continued.
>
> Riham

And so we arrive at the end and my letter to the students on the occasion of their graduation, some nine months after their peers. A videoconference graduation, but nevertheless a joyful occasion for everyone concerned.

The final words belong to Mohammad:

I believe we were given an opportunity to discover ourselves. For me, I discovered many bright and beautiful sides in my character. Patience and determination to achieve goals were among things which I learned through the program.

Mohammad

References

Bethlehem University: Online. Available at: http://www.bethlehem.edu. Accessed April 3, 2008.

Gisha: Online. Available at: http://www.gisha.org/. Accessed April 27, 2008.

Kalman M: *For college students in Gaza, choices are few*, 2007, Chronicle of Higher Education, 4 May.

Palestinian Central Bureau of Statistics: *Disability statistics*, 1997. Online. Available at: http://www.pcbs.gov.ps/Portals/_pcbs/phc_97/phc_t10.aspx. Accessed April 9, 2008.

Palestinian Central Bureau of Statistics: *Population statistics*, 2005, Online. Available at: http://www.pcbs.gov.ps/Portals/_pcbs/populati/demd1.aspx. Accessed; Online. Available at: http://www.pcbs.gov.ps/DesktopDefault.aspx?tabID=3820&lang=en. Accessed April 9, 2008.

Palestinian Medical Relief Society: *Report of Palestinian Civil Society Consultancy Meeting*, 2006. Online. Available at: http://www.pmrs.ps/last/pdfs/palestian%20Social%20determinants%20of%20health%20report.pdf. Accessed April 9, 2008.

Palestinian National Authority: *Palestinian Disability Law*, 1999, Online. Available at: http://siteresources.worldbank.org/DISABILITY/Resources/Regions/MENA/PalestinianDisLaw.pdf. Accessed April 10, 2008.

Manchester Survivors Poetry and the performance persona Rosie Lugosi

4

Rosie Garland

OVERVIEW

This chapter provides an overview of Manchester Survivors Poetry, a UK-based user-led project focusing on self-advocacy through the occupation of creative writing. Reflecting on how the project provided a supporting role in the creation and development of the performance persona Rosie Lugosi the Vampire Queen: poet, cabaret performer, and parodist of popular song. The chapter then examines issues of performance as an integrative tool, finding (and using) a voice, the representation of women, queer performance, exploring personal darkness, defining and reclaiming space as an outsider artist, as well as challenging preconceptions of what survivors look like, act like, can achieve, and are capable of artistically.

Manchester Survivors Poetry

I begin with an introduction to Manchester Survivors Poetry, a group I have been involved with in various ways for 10 years: as a participant, a user, a volunteer fundraiser, a coordinator, and a workshop facilitator. Perhaps a good place to start is the group's Mission Statement (2004):

> Manchester Survivors Poetry provides weekly writing workshops by and for Survivors of mental distress, providing support, self-advocacy, creative development, emancipation, networking, learning opportunities and the breakdown of isolation.
>
> We also provide performance opportunities, the validation of Survivors' experiences, and aim to break down prejudice and stigma.

The important features of Manchester Survivors Poetry are that it is a grassroots, locally run and entirely user-led initiative offering therapeutic support to survivors of the mental health system. Manchester Survivors Poetry is community focused. It is proud of its cooperative links with Survivors UK and other regional survivors groups. Manchester Survivors Poetry attracts participants from across the Greater Manchester area. As it is the only group of its kind in the North West of England, Survivors are prepared to travel from all parts of Greater Manchester (and further afield) to attend meetings, readings, workshops, and social events.

Time to pause again, this time for a definition of survivor, taken from Survivors' UK, based in London:

> A survivor is a person with a current or past experience of psychiatric hospitals, recipients of ECT [electroconvulsive therapy], tranquillisers and other medication, users of counselling and therapy services, survivors of sexual abuse, child abuse, drug and alcohol addiction and other survivors who have empathy with our experience.

The support offered at Manchester Survivors Poetry focuses on self-advocacy through creative writing. This is the activity, or occupation, which the group experiences as therapeutic – the core construct and medium of support, nurturance, and change. The group holds free weekly workshops as well as organizing readings and social events in order to give survivors regular opportunities to process experiences, recover from trauma and gain confidence. The workshops focus on creative development, as well as providing learning and networking opportunities. A special feature of Manchester Survivors

Poetry is that it is noninstitutionalized. And, from experience, it helps to keep users of the group out of institutions.

The group's activities are governed by what the group wants. Group members choose the structure of weekly workshops, versus other formats such as drop-in or advice center. Neither the organization nor the activities are managed by professionals, whether occupational therapists, community psychiatric nurses or other outsiders. This is not in any way to trivialize or to deny the importance of such professionals – it is a recognition that there are different strata of support. The fact that this group is user-led is its strength. It is one of the keys to the group's staying power, despite drawbacks. Manchester Survivors Poetry is part of the picture of community support for marginalized people. It is 'a', not 'the', model. The point needs stressing: I am not asserting that 'user-led' is better. But group members have experienced professionals who struggle to deal with the concept that a user might not 'need' him or her, all or any or part of the time. In other words, users don't know what's best for them, and clever professionals do.

As survivors have lived through a wide range of trauma and abuse, including institutionalization, the process of recovery is lonely and difficult. Manchester Survivors Poetry raises self-esteem, creates camaraderie and a sense of community through group support. As a result of the group's activities, participants discover and experience validation of their stories, histories, and experiences. It is more than being given a voice. We take and assert our voices.

What Manchester Survivors Poetry aims to do is move survivors of mental distress from isolation, stigma and dependence into active community involvement, increased self-reliance and a sense of self-worth. Manchester Survivors Poetry is about hidden regeneration within a local community of interest. It takes individual survivors from 'invisible victim' to active participant. For example, service users are encouraged and supported to be a part of the life of the group, through activities such as facilitating workshops and reading at public events. These activities and the self-confidence they engender enable the survivors to operate more effectively within networks of families and local communities as partners and family members. Therefore, Manchester Survivors Poetry contributes to the process of bringing survivors from the stage of being nonparticipatory victims to becoming more active members of the community.

To sum up, Manchester Survivors Poetry helps to resolve issues of trauma and stress in a grassroots, noninstitutionalized way. This is done through the validation of life-stories, building self-esteem among some of the most vulnerable citizens and communities of Greater Manchester.

The creation of Rosie Lugosi, Lesbian Vampire Queen

(Fig. 4.1)

On a personal level, my involvement with Manchester Survivors Poetry has given meaning and focus to my creative expression. To say that creative writing is my 'occupation' does not do justice to its place in my life. I have 10 years of commitment to my writing, in all its guises. I am aware of its tasks and possibilities. My relationship with my writing is core to my identity; the lens through which I focus and filter my experience, giving meaning and color

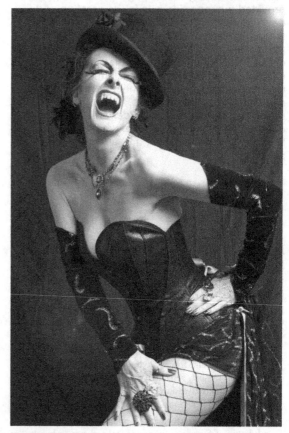

Figure 4.1 • Rosie Lugosi, Lesbian Vampire Queen. Photograph with permission of Holly Fairclough.

to the emotional landscape I inhabit. It provides me with passion, heartbreak, grief, and excitement, as well as quieter times when I just tread water – like any relationship. Therefore, it is of prime importance to me to look for effective ways to feed the motivation, courage, and sheer stubborn-mindedness that keeps me writing.

I use performance as an integrative tool, boosting self-esteem and finding my own voice. Manchester Survivors Poetry has provided support and validation to help develop the performance persona of Rosie Lugosi, Lesbian Vampire Queen, poet, cabaret performer, and parodist of popular song. I perform as a singer, performance poet, and Mistress of Ceremonies, and can be found in alternative arts venues, cabaret and burlesque shows, poetry slams, queer events, comedy festivals, TV and radio appearances, women's events, and literature festivals. I have a breadth of writing and performance experience, and have established a considerable national and international track record. This has taken me across Europe and the United States, and I have performed at events as diverse as the Cheltenham Festival of Literature, Europride, Femme 2008, BBC 3 Whine Gums, and the Great Labor Arts Exchange in Washington DC.

My writing includes short stories, nonfiction (e.g., Lugosi 1998), poetry (widely anthologized, as well as three solo collections) and songs. In addition, I have recently written a complete novel. I am also an experienced workshop facilitator, and have facilitated creative writing, poetry and performance workshops for organizations including Apples and Snakes, Survivors UK, Manchester Poetry Festival and the University of Philadelphia.

In this section I shall trace the sources and inspirations behind this alter-ego of Rosie Lugosi. She is 'The girl you never loved but always looked for'. In and through her I perform the monstrous-feminine.

Succubus

She breathes on you; swear you don't feel a thing
But the looking-glass is misting
Damp with her condensation.
She writes: *she 4 me, 4 eva, I love U, true*
These are the ghosts she promises you.
Vinegar dreams that make you stand up
And suck your fingers
Chew the salt that crusts beneath your nails.
She fills you with silk, sandpaper,

Bites that tattoo your back and legs
with crescents of scarlet stars.
And she sings:
Baby baby, daddy shall have a new master
Swinging your heart on the end of a ribbon. Sleepy yet?
Thumbs your eyelids till they
Sings in your ears until they
Pins your butterflies until they
Crouches on your ribs until they
Squeezes you until
Braids bits of seven-year-itch bitterness
Into the air that curls up from your tongue.
Writes: *she 4 me, 4 eva, I love U, true*
These are the ghosts she promised you.
She sings the blues
Purples you with a garden of rosy bruises
Small as her fists, wide as you can force it.
She is teeth and tongue and
Old enough to slip your window catches
The girl you never loved
But always looked for.
She never comes when you call. You cannot warm her.
She writes: *she 4 me, 4 eva, I love U, true*
These are the ghosts she promises you.
She sings black and blue murder
There's something she forgot to mention
If you could only speak her name
The one you keep forgetting.
She is no accident that just keeps happening.
She's the breath you gasp out,
She's your half-empty bed
The bottles rolling on the floor
Why you hate the weekends
Why it's just too hard to hold it all together
And why no other woman ever looks like her.
She 4 me, 4 eva, I love U, true
These are the ghosts she promised you.

Lugosi (2003)

Quintessential outsider

Rosie Lugosi is a Frankenstein creation, sewn together from worst nightmares and wildest dreams, and all the murky things we're not supposed to think about. She asks questions we are not supposed to ask. This section will be structured around the questions I get asked when I perform Rosie Lugosi and I'll start with the question I get asked most often: Why did you choose the image of the vampire to express yourself?

For a number of reasons. It's nothing to do with the wispy Anne Rice school of vampires, (Rice 1976) nor the passive Hammer Horrors (Sangster 1971) who got staked by Peter Cushing in the final reel (after everyone had got a good gawp at their cleavages). As a child I was afraid of the dark, and wanted something really effective to help me deal with it. Something that knew the geography of darkness and wasn't afraid. I wanted the most powerful invisible friends in the world, and I came up with vampires. They reveled in the dark. Vampires were the most powerful creatures in the world. Nothing scared them.

The vampire is the quintessential outsider: it exists outside society, challenging and outraging social mores. It 'does not respect borders, positions, rules and disturbs identity, system, order' (Kristeva 1982, p. 4). More than that, it disturbs and challenges those identity systems. It outrages social order. Yet 'normal' society is entranced, fascinated, obsessed. It wants not only to possess but also to destroy.

This abjectness, this lack of respect for rules and borders, has traditionally been viewed negatively. Female vampires in particular have been viewed as 'an expression of women's position as outsiders, women's social and cultural alienation' (Jackson 1981, p. 71).

But this misses an important point. I believe that the female vampire can be seen as an outsider through choice. She has not been thrown out of society: she defies it. She's a woman in rebellion against the family and expectations of sexual passivity, not merely ejected. Rosie Lugosi is not a leech on the patriarchal beast which is drawn to her yet tries to stake her. She gets her blood elsewhere. Therefore, she breaks the pattern of being hooked into patriarchy's push-me–pull-you relationship with powerful sexually active women.

Vampires are contradictory. They embody and make clear the breach between dualities (human and nonhuman, mad and sane, professional and nonprofessional . . .). They exist within the contradiction of needing to 'pass as human' so as to avoid getting staked every five minutes. They invite questions about what we accept unquestioningly.

Vampires don't fit. Neither did, nor do I. They don't have 'normal' families. They don't strive for the hetero-normative imperative of marriage plus children plus mortgage. They build alternative family groupings. They create new members of the group in a way that doesn't involve childbirth. They have families of choice, not families of origin. Oh, and they are sexy. I was attracted to their unconventional sexuality. As an isolated queer teenager it seemed radical to propose a form of sexual expression not focused entirely on male genitalia (it still does).

Therefore, the archetypal image of the vampire resonates with me in a powerful way. It links to my adolescent searching for a sense of self in a deeply conservative, rural home. Rosie Lugosi is 'not an icon but an inroad' (Young 1988) into self-awareness and what it means to be a performer who is queer and a survivor. I am looked at, still. But now I possess knowledge. I am able to look back.

Drag and dis-ease

The second question I get asked is 'Are you a man or a woman?'

The answer is that Rosie Lugosi is a female drag queen. In this I am unique. There are occasions when I am mistaken for a 'man' when I am dressed ('dragged up') as Rosie Lugosi. People, invariably women, have approached me and asked me to clarify my gender – even with a cleavage at eye level. Men seem to accept what is on show: hence mainstream jokes about men accepting the gender they 'see' in movies such as *Mrs Doubtfire* and *Tootsie*, to name but two.

I am confusing. I blur gender boundaries because, as they tell me, 'no real woman would ever act like you'. What they mean is that no 'real' woman would be so loud, sexually assertive, wear such exaggerated makeup, make such exaggerated gestures, be so confident, so fearless (and thereby so terrifying). Rosie Lugosi is so extreme a representation of the feminine that I just can't be a woman. I must be a man. It is drag.

Just as drag is about being an imposter, Rosie Lugosi appropriates drag, perverting notions of what makes a woman a real woman. When do her clothes become so extreme that she stops being female and becomes a drag queen, an imposter, a fake? Rosie Lugosi is a drag queen, therefore she is a fake woman. Or is she? Can we believe our eyes?

This false and deceptive dress is analogous to the nature of vampires – they pass as human, but they too are imposters. They are false humans. Of course, this links in to the very real stigma that survivors bear, that they too are not fully human. They are not fully accepted into human society. Like vampires, they too are marginal and therefore not to be trusted.

Body politic

I am not just a woman dressed as a woman. It goes further. Rosie Lugosi is not just about a soupçon of lipstick and a subtle dab of eyeliner. I am doing something far more disruptive. I am performing the 'feminine' and performing it all wrong. Rosie Lugosi is a perverse deployment of femininity. A caricature. Just as Rosie Lugosi parodies songs, she parodies femininity. I play with it, and have fun.

I play with the theme of forbidden female fruit. I dress the part and portray Rosie Lugosi as the *Radical Lesbian Separatist Dominatrix Bitch Goddess Top Femme Vampire Queen*.

It's a fine line. Try to name voluptuous, overtly sexual comediennes and you run out of steam pretty quickly. Mae West is one of the few examples that springs to mind. This reflects women's deeply troubled relationships with their bodies. Female comics struggle with making their bodies sexual, in case it distracts (it will), or they are dismissed as eye-candy (they are).

Rosie Lugosi is very much more in control of her tits. I make my body part of the act. It is an extreme body, and both personifies and encapsulates the whole ambivalence still felt about sexually active and confident women. Rosie Lugosi embodies the defiant and transgressive power of unconventional female sexuality – the predatory vampiric villainess who never gets staked. Six feet tall in six-inch stilettos, clad in a PVC catsuit, towering wig, fangs and hoisted cleavage, she transforms previous notions of what constitutes both gothic and queer performance. She is a spectacle, but not a passive spectacle to be consumed.

Through Rosie Lugosi I am performing the tensions that women feel about how 'real' women are represented in society and the media. Women are still under pressure to conform to a narrow range of acceptable presentations of woman. The 'acceptables' women are offered are about invisibility. Sensible shoes, beige, fleece, eyes down, humble. And that's only in white Western culture. We are told this will make us safe. However, my experience of living through the Yorkshire Ripper experience taught me early on that is not true. The lie that only whores in

short skirts are attacked persists. It's the same kind of lie as 'stranger danger' for kids. Anyone who has lived with domestic violence will tell you that no clothing or behavior can make you 'safe'.

So why bother? If neither clothing nor behavior can make us safe, why waste creative energy trying? Rosie Lugosi is my response to that question. In short, Rosie Lugosi performs the 'bad girl', reclaiming and redefining the notion of 'slut'.

How queer is queer? Lesbians shouldn't dress like that . . .

This links with the next question: 'But you don't look like a real lesbian', the title of one of my pieces.

Realesbian

But you don't *look* like a lesbian . . .
I am the double-take
The queerest of the queer
So secure in my sexuality
That tonight I'll wear a dress
Which hugs my waist and hips.
But you don't look like a *real* lesbian . . .
So you tell me what's real
While I shake out my hair
Kick off my heels
Peel off your shirt and tie
And push you into the pillows.
But you don't look like a *normal* lesbian . . .
You're damn right, I'm not normal
I'm a subverter of society
And all its expectations
So perverted, I love women
And that includes myself.

Lugosi (2000)

Rosie Lugosi transgresses notions and perceptions of how lesbians perform and present 'lesbianism' to straight and queer communities. There is still a tension, a hangover from 1980s feminism, that flamboyance is politically suspect. That 'dressing up' is letting the side down. I'm in agreement with Emma Goldman, who said 'If I can't dance, it's not my revolution'. (The history of this misquotation is to be found in Goldman (1934) and Shulman (1991).) And dressing up is subversive. It plays with notions of what we can be and what we are told we can't be. Clothing is an instrument of power, and I am appropriating it. Occupying it.

Through what Rosie Lugosi wears I am exploring clothing as an instrument of power. I am a direct descendant of the suffragettes who fought for the right to look and dress as they saw fit, some wearing red lipstick as an act of defiance. However, I'm not coming out with a trite 'this is a liberating choice to dress like Rosie Lugosi'. I wear no makeup when I'm not performing. That choice is just as challenging of how women should perform themselves as the makeup I wear as Rosie Lugosi.

Growing old disgracefully

This links with the next question I am asked: 'Should you be wearing that at your age?'

I've spotted that I am growing older, and I want to do it disgracefully. I have every intention of continuing to perform. I do not see performance as being limited to something that a woman does in her twenties, fresh from college. Why should we stop?

Rosie Lugosi throws out that challenge. She physically embodies the monstrous-feminine through the outward trappings of the dominatrix-vampire-crone. She transgresses age boundaries by challenging notions of how women are supposed to dress at a particular age. There is still a horror of older sexually active women. Of crones. Of witches. Rosie Lugosi is a radical response to that question. She will not start wearing beige. Part of my act is to say that 'I am 987, but don't look a day over 14th century'.

I do hope you are all sitting uncomfortably . . .

Finally, let us finish with sado-masochism and laughter. When I am performing, I use comedy to subvert notions of normative sexuality and gender-specific behaviors. To subvert notions of what constitutes appropriate female behavior. I know the power of humor over preaching (I am aware how this resonates with the activities of groups such as Payasos Sin Fronteras). I believe in the power of laughter to make people think.

Rosie Lugosi undermines the slander against feminists that they have no sense of humor, that politics are boring or unfashionable. Rosie Lugosi tells jokes, and is a joke personified. She embodies the 'howl of laughter that would ridicule and demolish any notion of the feminine that takes itself seriously' (Duggan & McHugh 2002). I'm proud to call myself a feminist – it would be nice if other feminists were as proud to hear me say it.

Conclusion

Performing Rosie Lugosi is about choice. Choosing to represent myself in this particular way. It is about finding a voice and using it, loudly. Through Rosie Lugosi I give expression to the unexpressed dark side of my self and my experiences. Naturally, Rosie Lugosi has similarities with myself, and draws upon aspects of my self (and that makes her lively). However, this is not necessarily in ways that the audience imagines.

The Rosie Lugosi material I write and perform is a mixture of humor and 'dark materials'. In Manchester Survivors Poetry we recognize that writing is a powerful tool and form of exploration of personal darkness. To quote one user of the group: 'without Survivors I wouldn't have written about my darkness. People want me to shut up about it.'

As Rosie Lugosi I am utilizing the image of predatory female and I am reclaiming it. Rosie Lugosi is not to do with looking or acting 'feminine' (the social construct of the disempowered and passive female). I'm reclaiming the power of being a show-off, that sign of ego and expression so much frowned upon in female children. Yes, I'm too big for my thigh-high PVC boots, and it's wonderful. By utilizing the classic image of the dominatrix as performance poet, I play with concepts of power: where and in whom it is situated, and how it is used by women.

Rosie Lugosi cannot be dismissed as a tart in high heels and a wig. She is a challenge. A challenge to what women are supposed to look like. To what women are and aren't allowed to do. To what women are and aren't allowed to say. How women are supposed to behave. And of course, what survivors are allowed to say. In addition I am breaking down stereotypes of what survivors look like, sound like, can be, and can achieve. What it means to be different and proud.

Rosie Lugosi embodies the power of a defiant and avenging angel. She says what she wants to say, wears what she wants to wear, and she does it for herself, not to please anyone. I examine what poetry is capable of; what it is and isn't supposed to do.

Traditionally, vampires are supposed to be the living dead. The paradox is that as a suppressed, passive, unintegrated, underconfident voiceless individual I was never nearer death. As Rosie Lugosi the Lesbian Vampire Queen, one that has survived stakes and stalkers, and anything else the world has thrown at me, I have never been more alive.

References

Duggan L, McHugh K: A Fem(me)nist Manifesto. In Rose CB, Camilleri A, editors: *Brazen Femme: Queering Femininity*, Vancouver, 2002, Arsenal Pulp Press, pp 165–170.

Goldman E: *Living My Life*, New York, 1934, Knopf.

Jackson R: *Fantasy, the Literature of Subversion*, London, 1981, Methuen.

Kristeva J: *Powers of Horror: an Essay on Abjection*, New York, 1982, Columbia University Press.

Lugosi R: Coming out at night. In *Acts of Passion*, New York, 1998, Haworth Press, pp 201–208.

Lugosi R: *Coming Out At Night*, Manchester, 2000, purpleprosepress.

Lugosi R: *Creatures of the Night*, Manchester, 2003, purpleprosepress.

Rice A: *Interview With The Vampire*, New York, 1976, Knopf.

Sangster J: *Lust For a Vampire*, UK, 1971, Hammer Films.

Shulman AK: Dances with feminists, *Women's Review of Books* 9:37, 1991.

Young S: Feminism and the politics of power. In Gamman L, Marshment M, editors: *The Female Gaze*, London, 1988, Women's Press, pp 173–188.

Further viewing

Websites

http://www.rosielugosi.com
http://www.myspace.com/rosielugosi
http://www.myspace.com/rosiegarland

Rosie Lugosi performance clips on YouTube:

http://www.youtube.com/watch?v=59RkU_btyz8
http://www.youtube.com/watch?v=gWBojBkzpdc

Payasos Sin Fronteras

http://www.clowns.org/

Further reading

Lugosi R: Tears for souvenirs. In *Queer Words*, Aberystwyth, 1997, Premiere Cymru, pp 85–96.

Lugosi R: *Hell and Eden*, 1997, Dagger Press, West Bromwich.

Lugosi R: The bones of Venice. In *In Blood We Trust*, London, 1999, Dark Angel Press, pp 66–73.

Lugosi R: You'll do. In *The Diva Book of Short Stories*, London, 2000, Diva Books, pp 173–186.

Lugosi R: Here be tygers. In *Cadenza*, Rugby, 2001, QWF Press, pp 9–13.

Lugosi R: The purple wallpaper. In *Groundswell*, London, 2002, Diva Books, pp 139–146.

Lugosi R: file>>corrupted. In *City Secrets*, Manchester, 2002, Crocus Press, pp 159–168.

Lugosi R: Terminus. In *Necrologue*, London, 2003, Diva Books, pp 181–190.

Lugosi R: A piece of her night. In *Va Va Voom*, London, 2004, Millivres Press, pp 209–215.

Lugosi R: My dear. In *Bitch Lit*, Manchester, 2006, Crocus Books.

Lugosi R: A trip to the zoo. In *Practice to Deceive*, Durham, 2007, Gemini Press, pp 7–10.

Lugosi R: Look both ways. In *The Art of Tying Knots*, Lancaster, 2007, Flax Books, pp 4–9.

Lugosi R: The vampire queen. In Volcano D, Dahl U, editors: *Femmes of Power*, London, 2008, Serpent's Tail, pp 124–127.

Lugosi R: Sadie Jones took me line dancing & heirloom quality. In *Discovering a Comet*, Abercynon, 2008, Leaf Books, pp 31–34.

Lugosi R: Room with a partial view. In *The Sandhopper Lover and other Stories*, Gwynedd, 2009, Cinnamon Press, pp 160–171.

Links

Europride, Manchester

http://www.manchesterpride.com

Femme 2008, Chicago

http://www.femmecollective.com

The great labor arts exchange, Washington DC

http://www.laborheritage.org/glaecco.htm

Whine gums, BBC3

http://www.babycow.co.uk/bc2003.swf

Treating adolescent substance abuse through a perspective of occupational cultivation

5

Jesse Vogel

OVERVIEW

Substance abusers, especially those who are within an orthodox Jewish community, often feel alienated, isolated, and looked down upon. Through my personal experiences, as well as my training as an occupational therapist, I have been able to successfully work with this population where others have struggled. The more traditional techniques of imposed abstinence as well as treatment in an artificial environment, such as a rehabilitation facility, are very often not effective with adolescents in the Jewish community. Rather, I find, joining individuals where they are and working together to develop their own strengths and skills can change the path that their lives are taking, for the better. Through the therapeutic use of myself, I am able to relate my life experiences to what they are going through and show that the potential exists for them to make something of themselves and become productive and valued members of society. I connect with the person, not the problem. It is through this borderless occupational therapy approach that this concept can be generalized on a global scale.

Introduction

I will explain why I chose to put a word as odd and seemingly out of place as 'cultivation' in the title with a parable that I have devised which explains my specific choice of words. There was once a very poor idealistic farm hand who had tremendous foresight who worked very hard to buy a piece of land. This particular plot of land hadn't borne fruit for some time and was considered to be both worthless and a waste of effort. The farm hand's reasoning for purchasing this piece of land was that with time, patience, and expert use of his unique skills that he had acquired through his own experiences, he would be able to work the land and cause it to not only bear fruit but to become an inspiration to its surroundings and hopefully inspire others to follow his lead and to make the world a more beautiful place, one plot of land at a time. I believe that this parable expresses the ideals of the borderless community. The ultimate satisfaction that a person who has had to struggle in his or her life to accomplish and achieve, is to inspire others who are either going through similar struggles to those that they had gone through or worse to be able to accomplish and thrive.

I recently took a course at Touro College of Health Sciences located in New York, United States, entitled Advanced Occupational Therapy Theory and Practice, by guest lecturer, Frank Kronenberg. The purpose of this course was to develop within the students a better grasp of contemporary occupational theories, as well as to improve their ability to put theory into practice in both traditional and up-and-coming areas of practice. In order to accomplish this goal, Kronenberg introduced the class to the theory of 3P archaeology, 'which describes an in-depth investigation of who we are at interrelated personal, professional, and political levels' (Kronenberg & Pollard 2006, p. 623).

Our final assignment was to open up our borderless eyes and to find an area that could be improved through thinking 'outside of the box'. The term 'borderless' in this context has a simple explanation. A typical occupational therapist treats specific diagnoses with somewhat predictable treatment modalities that vary based on their style and level of

DOI: 10.1016/B978-0-7020-3103-8.00014-6

experience. To me, borderless occupational therapy treats people whose disability doesn't fit into the medical model. Their problems stem from an unpredictable conglomerate of both internal and external situations, triggers, and influences. The treatment of these individuals doesn't come from a textbook, exercise regimen, or splinting protocol. Working with them has to transcend the 'borders' of the typical treatment regimen. Fortunately I have had many opportunities and experiences in my life to have something to write about. This chapter is a revised version of my final assignment.

I have chosen the topic of working with Jewish youth in religious communities who are considered to be youth at risk. I think that the whole idea of 'youth at risk' is a very comforting thought for people who like to dilute the truth in order to make it more palatable. People think that they will be working with children who are at risk before the risk takes over the children's lives. This is not the case. The youth who I have worked with have already been 'risked' before I came into the picture. Most of them are substance abusers who have juvenile records with correctional institutions. Because of my own life experiences, I am generally accepted and trusted by this population. I strongly believe that in this type of setting, with these types of issues, an occupational therapist is truly a 'jack of all trades' (Friedland 1998, p. 379).

I grew up in a typical middle-class neighborhood as a secular Jew who was both friends and accepted by pretty much everyone who lived in my neighborhood. My neighborhood had a dramatic shift in population that within two to three years became predominantly Muslim and Arabic. While this shift in population was occurring, I was becoming more in touch with my Jewish heritage and became orthodox. With this newly introduced cultural friction, I found myself being challenged for being a Jew almost on a daily basis as well as losing friends. I would be involved in multiple altercations per week and became quite good at it to the point that I have sent several people to the hospital. Around the same time, I was in an accident. I was rollerblading and went to cross the street without wearing a helmet or padding and was hit by a car. The aftermath of the accident was a fractured spine (L5–S1) and coccyx. I was given Vicodin (a combination of hydrocodone and acetaminophen) for the pain, which was quite intense. Unfortunately, back then, it was much easier to get prescription painkillers because of a lack of

oversight. One and a half years later, I was still on the Vicodin (addicted), but I was taking six 750 mg pills of Vicodin HP (high potency) three times per day. I noticed that when I would get into altercations I didn't feel any pain when I would get hit. I also noticed that I didn't care as much about the cultural clashes in my neighborhood that I was met with on a daily basis. Retrospectively, I think that the lack of social acceptance is what drove me to street drugs because I had built up such a tremendous tolerance to the Vicodin that I wanted something that would take me to the next level of high. I know that it sounds hypocritical to become more religious while at the same time being a chemical abuser, but I was young and in my head I was able to find a way to justify it. Although in my chemically induced years I did a lot of things that I am not proud of, in the end I was able to intellectualize my problems and end all of my drug use on my own, without the help of a drug rehabilitation program.

Due to my experiences with substance abuse and social rejection I have become a much stronger person and decided that I would use my experiences to try to help other people who were in the same situation as I was. I knew many people who were unable to pull themselves out of that situation and either ended up in jail or dead and I didn't want to let that happen to these kids. I felt and still feel like it is my duty as a survivor, who they will listen to because of what I have gone through, to help others who don't have the strength of character to fix their own lives. In occupational therapy, occupations 'include things people need to, want to, and are expected to do' (Frank & Zemke 2009, p. 111). There are a lot of expectations that are placed upon these kids from their friends, families, cultures, and by the world itself. Because I don't always deal with situations with the politically correct style (because it doesn't work), I am forced to deal with constant conflicts and count on cooperation to keep the process going.

Most people who are in the position to help these kids make an obvious and concrete distinction that they are different and in some way better than these kids, and that the kids needed to change who they are as people to come back to society to be able to thrive in the world. This concept is not only untrue but it also couldn't be more false and asinine. In every one of these kids is a person who is inherently good. Unfortunately they are misguided and made a right instead of a left at some moral juncture in their lives and haven't been able to backtrack. I want to be able to take their existing strengths, motivation (whether or not they have been used positively), and longing for social acceptance to allow them to make the decisions to improve their lives. We are all made up of the people who we have been. This is not a fancy way of talking about a person's collective conscious due to reincarnation. It means that every time we make a decision that alters our lives, we have become a different person. In other words we take aspects, concepts, and the things that we have learned through both positive and negative experiences that we have gone through in our past to mold who we are today. This notion is expressed in a lofty work called the Mishna, which is the oral expression and interpretation of the Torah (Old Testament). At the end of Makkos, one of the volumes of the Mishna, the text describes how a person should use potentially harmful aspects of their personality for good, even the negative character trait of blood lust by becoming a *shochait* (the person who slaughters the animals that are intended to be used for food) and by doing this, harness their character trait that could potentially be negative and harmful for a positive and constructive occupation.

Many of these kids are victims of occupational alienation. They are refused access to jobs, social recognition, and acceptance because of the activities that they participate in. This sounds a lot like 'The segregation of groups of people through the restriction of access to dignified and meaningful participation in occupations of daily life' (Kronenberg & Pollard 2005, p. 67) just because of the way they dress, talk, or use illegal drugs. Some of the problems that I have to contend with are lack of motivation to engage in positive occupations; identifying themselves as being alienated; poor internal self-esteem; past/present drug abuse; criminal history; involvement with gangs; impulsive behavior; and absence of interaction skills on an interpersonal level. I believe that between using my personal experiences and utilizing the borderless art/science of occupational therapy, my dynamic duo of skills is much more successful than someone who is utilizing either one or the other of these skills.

These youth feel alienated from the rest of their society. In the religious Jewish community, there is a strong core value of learning and fitting in. When a child has difficulties learning and or fitting into the 'mold', they often feel rejected, ashamed, and unable to 'experience satisfaction' (World Federation of Occupational Therapists (WFOT) 2004). In these children, either an occupational imbalance or deficit is often present. This can lead to rebellious behavior which unfortunately may lead them down the path of drugs and criminal behaviors. These children have the right to be different without being pitied.

When I am working with one of these children, I don't use the typical approaches because I feel that they usually are not effective. The typical approach is to make a clear and defined difference between the children and yourself. It is also to not allow any ingestion of alcohol, cigarettes, and drugs during the session. Our ethos tells us that a 'fresh perspective on current challenges is possible' (Peloquin 2005, p. 611) in order to be able to 'help meet the individual patient more on his own terms' (Peloquin 2005, p. 615) and who they need me to be to facilitate a more positive change in them. I have found that by making that distinction between them and you and by not allowing any of their bad habits to enter with them turns them off to anything you could say. The typical approach also has sessions in set environments that are controlled. I believe that if you can accomplish a goal in a controlled environment, it is a great thing. But it doesn't prepare them to transfer those accomplishments to the outside world where you cannot control the environment. I only meet with them in normal places such as a bus stop, a park, while shopping, at a fastfood restaurant, a bar, or any other place where they would usually hang out, as suggested by Hooper & Wood (2002) who state that you should take the treatment to the client. I also allow them to smoke or drink around me at first while we are building a relationship of trust, for two reasons: first, because to them there is no reason why they shouldn't, and, second, because it allows me to gain their trust and acceptance. We talk about everything and anything. It is important to have flexible boundaries with these kids because many times they will be testing your limits to see if you can be trusted and if you are truly who you present yourself to be.

Once I feel like I have gained their trust, I begin to plant seeds that will hopefully blossom in time. I start by making suggestions for places to meet in order to show them for example, that we can hang out the same way in Dunkin' Donuts as we did in the park or at a bowling alley instead of a bar where their friends hang out. If they are still either drinking or smoking in front of me, I begin to try to get them to do it less around me. For example, if they are smoking marijuana around me, then I blame myself and ask them to smoke less around me because when I smell it I want to have it again. This takes the blame off them, which throughout their lives is usually where the blame ends up and puts it solely on me and gives them the rare opportunity to help someone else. I have found that by removing the blame from them and accepting it on yourself, you are not only more accepted, but you are also more effective in positively affecting their life choices by enabling people-centered empowerment, as suggested by Kronenberg & Pollard (2005, p. 71). I have also noticed that understanding is both a means and an end. This technique is a 'means' in that spending social time together is an engagement tool. It is also an 'end' because the more they understand me, the more they understand that they can have a future if they turn their life around and choose to take the high road which still has traffic and potholes but the view is much more satisfying and fulfilling.

I find that many kids use drugs or drink because it allows them to transcend their problems and gain acceptance. I begin to show them how all it does is to not make them notice that they are spiraling out of control. I have lots of witty metaphors about flying a plane with a blindfold on or riding a bike with a blindfold on because there is always someone else who is better at doing something than you are so there is no reason why you should try (the full version would take up too much room) and just let yourself crash. Many of these kids are good with their hands as is commonly the case with habitual marijuana smokers. If that is the case I get some wood and some of my tools and we make something together using 'everyday occupation as a therapeutic entity' (Hasselkus 2006, p. 628) to give away to someone who needs it if possible. By showing them that they can do something when the chemicals are out of their system shows them that they can be restored to a productive life if they would be rehabilitated. It shows them that they can have a 'higher quality of life through preventing and overcoming obstacles' (American Occupational Therapy Association (AOTA) Centennial Vision 2009). One of the things that I hope to accomplish, as Hasselkus (2002) suggests, is to effectively change the features of everyday living that they build meaning from.

Eventually, when I start to see that my working with them is beginning to bear fruit, I start to incorporate 'occupational storytelling and occupational story making' (Clark 1993, p. 1074). We often do role playing to aid us with the storytelling and making. I have found that this is only truly effective if the client is chemical free and able to not only focus, but also to internalize the new information that they have learned in order to bring about change in their lives. I am using my personal experiences and empathy as well as showing them that they are not alone. Through probing and exploring their functional and dysfunctional areas of occupation, I formulate a plan of action which will hopefully be able to utilize their strengths and weaknesses to bring about a functional outcome. Through utilizing occupational perspective, we can treat the person as a whole. Utilizing the 3P approach (Kronenberg & Pollard 2005, 2006), I am able to give an explanation of who I am, where I come from, and what I stand up for on three interrelated levels. As a Person, I am able to offer my own experiences, which directly relate to their own and which will allow them to understand that they are not alone. It also shows them that if one person can overcome issues that are similar to theirs that hope still exists for them as well. On a Professional level, I am able to be more than just a mentor to them. I am able to assess the areas of occupation they are either void of or have an imbalance in and attempt to infuse their life with purposeful and meaningful occupations which will give them inherent self-driven motivation to gain new skills and to continue to grow. On a Political level, I will hopefully be able to, as we said in class, strategically engage in conflict and cooperation situations about people's capacities and power to construct and influence their destinies.

I am keen to see programs like this take off in every major city. I understand that there are mentor programs and other interventions of that nature, but they don't harness the limitless potential of occupational therapy without borders. I wish that more occupational therapists would feel more comfortable with and take advantage of the bold and exciting borderless world around us.

Acknowledgment

I would like to take the opportunity to thank the editors of this book for the opportunity to share my ideas with a greater audience, who will hopefully be able to utilize my thoughts to facilitate a positive change in the world, one troubled individual at a time.

References

American Occupational Therapy Association: *Centennial Vision*, 2009, Online Available at: http://www.aota.org. Accessed April 19, 2010.

Clark F: The 1993 Eleanor Clarke Slagle lecture – occupation embedded in a real life: Interweaving occupational science and occupational therapy, *Am J Occup Ther* 47:1067–1078, 1993.

Frank G, Zemke R: Occupational therapy foundations for political engagement and social transformation. In Pollard N, Sakellariou D, Kronenberg F, editors: *A Political Practice of Occupational Therapy*, Oxford, 2009, Churchill Livingstone-Elsevier, pp 111–136.

Friedland J: Occupational therapy and rehabilitation: An awkward alliance, *Am J Occup Ther* 52:373–379, 1998.

Hasselkus BR: *The meaning of everyday occupation*, Thorofare, NJ, 2002, Slack.

Hasselkus BR: The 2006 Eleanor Clarke Slagle lecture – the world of everyday occupation: Real people, real lives, *Am J Occup Ther* 60:627–640, 2006.

Hooper B, Wood W: Pragmatism and structuralism in occupational therapy: The long conversation, *Am J Occup Ther* 56:40–50, 2002.

Kronenberg F, Pollard N: Overcoming occupational apartheid, a preliminary exploration of the political nature of occupational therapy. In Kronenberg F, Simo Algado S, Pollard N, editors: *Occupational Therapy Without Borders. Learning from the Spirit of Survivors*,

Edinburgh, 2005, Elsevier/Churchill Livingstone, pp 58–86.

Kronenberg F, Pollard N: Plenary presentation, 2006: political dimensions of occupation and the roles of occupational therapy, *Am J Occup Ther* 60:617–625, 2006.

Peloquin SM: Embracing our ethos, reclaiming our heart, *Am J Occup Ther* 59:611–625, 2005.

World Federation of Occupational Therapists: *WFOT position paper on community based rehabilitation*, Forrestfield, Australia, 2004, World Federation of Occupational Therapists.

Occupational therapy in the social field: concepts and critical considerations

6

Sandra Maria Galheigo

To Heloisa Bevilacqua Penna Franca
dear mentor and friend
inspiration and wisdom,
a life lesson.

OVERVIEW

This chapter intends to initiate the reader to concepts and considerations for the constitution of a social field in occupational therapy from a critical standpoint. It starts by presenting the differences which have to be taken into account in the debate, from the occupational therapy's creation to the dynamics of the social field in countries central and peripheral to the world economic system. Next, the chapter introduces Squires's ideas of a social terrain and Bourdieu's concepts of *field* and *habitus*, which guide the argument throughout the text. Then, the chapter addresses how deprivation has been dealt with through the concepts of marginality, exclusion, apartheid, disaffiliation, and vulnerability, contextualizing them in historical and social terms. Finally, the chapter discusses the development of critical knowledge and practice in the social field. It points out the importance of developing an epistemic reflexivity by occupational therapists and occupational scientists working in the field, and it raises the possibility of combining hermeneutics and dialects in the development of research. In the conclusion, the chapter addresses the concept of occupation as human action and indicates the ideas of emancipation, empowerment, and the struggle for human rights as the ultimate contributions of the work in the social field.

Introduction

Occupational therapy originated during the early twentieth century and rapidly expanded from the United States to the United Kingdon, Sweden, Canada, Australia, New Zealand, South Africa, Israel, India, and Denmark. Since then occupational therapy has developed in various countries across the world. One of the first important expansions took place in the 1950s, when the United Nations encouraged the formation of social workers and rehabilitation professionals through the creation of schools in the poor countries which came to be crucial to the development of occupational therapy in Latin America (Hardiman & Midgley 1982, Soares 1991). This diffusion process was also stimulated by the International Rehabilitation Movement and the World Federation of Occupational Therapists.

In general, the countries initiating occupational therapy used reference material from the countries where the profession was well established. Nevertheless, this was not a taken-for-granted process. In a world polarized by the Cold War, the replication of Westernized policies and practices in the peripheral countries was controversial. Those who advocated diffusion, pointing out its benign influence, backed their views on modernization theory, which argued that developing countries should pass through the same stages of the advanced industrialized ones. Otherwise, those who viewed the idea of diffusionism as improper were backed by streams of thought, based on theories on imperialism or on dependency which pointed out that the issue was not a matter of economic growth, development, and modernization

DOI: 10.1016/B978-0-7020-3103-8.00015-8

of the less-developed countries. Instead, it was about understanding and fighting against their dependency on the world system (Midgley 1981, 1984).

Beyond the ideological factors, there were also criticisms concerning the indiscriminate incorporation of foreign knowledge and practices since it sometimes resulted in the use of concepts, practices, approaches, and methodologies that were not appropriate to that particular context (Midgley 1981, Soares 1991, Watson & Fourie 2004). Finally, the intensity of the assimilation of knowledge and practices also depended on other determining factors such as the nonexistence of significant language and culture barriers (English is the hegemonic language in occupational therapy publications), the access to journals and books (usually expensive to import and to translate, considered cost-ineffective by publishers), the possibility of regular contact with international groups and participation in world congresses and so forth.

The particular characteristics of occupational therapy expansion, briefly presented here, provided, on one side, a somewhat universal understanding of the profession but, on the other side, the existence of different constructions of knowledge and practices in occupational therapy worldwide. It would not be feasible to portray them all in this chapter. Nonetheless, it is reasonable to assume that nowadays occupational therapy largely depends on how new knowledge and practices are produced in order to attend local needs and policy-making demands. Also, on how they interact with historical, social and political contexts wherein they take place. On an international basis, communication and exchange of knowledge and practices have been deeply facilitated by the internet; international cooperation has been extremely improved, mainly in academic settings. Different areas of occupational therapy have benefited from this proximity, though the transference of concepts, frameworks, and methodologies is still problematic.

With regards to occupational science, a somewhat similar historical path applies. Originating in the United States in the late 1980s, occupational science has nowadays an International Society for Occupational Science (created in 1999) and associations in the Australia region, Canada, European Union (ECOTROS), Japan, United States, and United Kingdom and Ireland (ISOS 2009). Worldwide, many other people have expressed their self-professed interest in occupational science, most of them occupational therapists. The international occupational science dialogue may be facilitated because of its focus on the study of occupation and its application to health and community development, and because it does not involve the usage and transference of therapeutic methods from one place to another.

With reference to the practice of occupational therapy with people regarded as disadvantaged, excluded, marginalized, and so forth, the book *Occupational Therapy Without borders* (Kronenberg et al 2005) was an initiative that enabled the contact with many local experiences, which unveiled themselves to be, in some sense, globally connected. Like a kaleidoscope, the book displayed a portrait of different occupational therapy practices, their concepts, methods, and theoretical frameworks. At the same time, it offered a comprehensive picture of the contemporary scenario, which may be exchanged, combined, modified inasmuch as new syntheses are carried out.

Challenging the still present hegemonic medical model, the book makes it possible to gain insight into new concepts and ideas akin to sociological readings. The chapter 'Occupational therapy and the social field: clarifying concepts and ideas' (Galheigo 2005) sought to introduce the reader to the discussion of the role of occupational therapy in the social field from a critical standpoint, based on the author's academic and practical experiences in Brazil. In the process of rewriting the chapter for this edition, we realized that some changes needed to be made to enable a wider audience to connect with it. The processes related to social policy making, social organization and the struggle for human rights are socially, culturally, and politically embedded. As such, discussing their concepts, frameworks and methods is a difficult task due to the many possibilities of misinterpretation.

Taking the concept of citizenship, as an example, one may notice different and controversial usages across countries and, even, across political periods of a particular country. For example, during the 1980/1990s British Conservative Government era, the idea of 'active citizenship' implied the free acceptance of voluntary obligations to the community by its members. According to them, increasing young people's 'active citzenship' would contribute to their process of becoming adults (France 2007, Squires 1990). Some authors argue that a similar idea of citizenship was later used by the subsequent New Labour Government in the construction of youth policies for 'citizenship training' regarded as important due to youth apathy and social disengagement (France 2007, Lister et al 2005). In the same period in some Latin American countries, after decades of dictatorial regimes, the re-democratization process was under way. In Brazil, the 1980s was a period when major social movements arose, resulting in the 1988 Constitution, which granted new citizens' rights leading to the establishment of comprehensive social policies (Barros et al 2005, Paoli 1992). Thus, after the 1990s the concept of citizenship became largely apprehended by a large scope of social and political actors in Brazil (Assies et al 2002, Dagnino 1994). In South Africa, the 1980s was also a period of intense protesting against apartheid, which finally ended in 1990. Similar to the Brazilian Constitution, the 1996 South African Constitution 'encompass civil and political rights but also include the unique feature of rights of access (e.g. to water, food, health care, housing)' (Watson & Fourie 2004 p. 43). Consequently, the idea and usage of the concept of citizenship in Brazil and South Africa have a political and social relevance since they are identified as an encouraging result of the struggle of the civil society. Otherwise, the idea of the citizenship advocated by Thatcherism (France 2007, Squires 1990) and by the New Labour Government (France 2007, Lister et al 2005) concerning youth affairs may be identified as a disciplinary idea.

Political discourses are constructed by government, political parties, and social organizations, and they may be incorporated or discredited by people in general or by particular groups. Taking this in consideration, in this new edition, I seek to make use of concepts and ideas which may be shared in a transdisciplinary way by a larger audience, avoiding professional vocabulary and concepts that may carry strong local representations. The concept of 'social field' will be kept as central to the arguments in this chapter, being supported by Squires (1990) who makes use of:

> the adjective 'social' as a particular kind of constructed concept . . . having in mind 'the social' as an arena – society, or 'social' space, the 'social' terrain . . . a field of work or an area of activity . . . 'the social' is itself a field, a 'zone of intervention' or a 'political terrain'. It forms the battleside for a range of competing political programmes, it is the space for which they compete. And as victories are secured or defeats registered, or simply as the balance of power shifts in the conflicts running throughout 'the social', its meaning and significance is inflected in different directions. . . . So the social is constituted by power relations, formed by the ebb and flow of political forces. A second meaning involves understanding the 'social' not only as a terrain but also as a form of rationality, as a discourse or political language.
>
> Squires (1990, p. 7–9)

In order to reflect on the construction of knowledge and practices in occupational therapy from a critical standpoint, this chapter retakes some concepts presented previously and seeks to widen the ones in need of some revision. First, it intends to address the concept of field such as envisioned by Pierre Bourdieu to discuss what is at stake when the concept of field is brought on. Second, to display the life conditions and to identify the people regarded as excluded, the chapter will discuss concepts such as exclusion, marginalization, apartheid, disaffiliation, and vulnerability since they harbor implicit meanings which should be made clear. Finally, the chapter makes some propositions to consider occupational therapy's position in a 'social' field from a critical standpoint. It addresses the importance of those working in the field to develop epistemic reflexivity and it raises the possibility of combining hermeneutics and dialects in research development. Finally, the chapter addresses the concept of occupation as human action and indicates the ideas of emancipation, empowerment and the struggle for human rights as the ultimate contributions of working in the social field.

Considerations on Bourdieu's concepts of *field* and *habitus*: implications for the constitution of a social field

When occupational therapy addresses the life conditions of those with limited access to human rights, it enters another field of practice, different from healthcare and rehabilitation and closer to the welfare system. The latter may be considered a mix since it comprises the provisions of social benefits and services through administrative governmental institutions, market entrepreneurship, and agencies within civil society (in which funding and orientations come from very different economic, political, and ideologic agendas). Moreover, the welfare systems vary substantially from one country to another, and the theme is very contentious everywhere. Consequently, while a critical discussion of occupational therapy in the 'social' field may take into account some very different scenarios, it is possible to find a framework that may provide a broad support for analysis. Pierre Bourdieu's ideas may provide some useful theoretical contribution by conceptualizing the field we are addressing.

Bourdieu's work has provided interesting contributions to the understanding of many aspects of social life. In particular, the concepts of field and habitus have been the basis for studies in education, culture, politics, arts, and media among others (Bonnewitz 2003, Bourdieu 1993, 1996, Ortiz 2003, Peillon 1998). For Bourdieu, the social space is constituted by relatively autonomous social fields that organize and produce social life. The fields, in his view, are social microcosms with a specific logic, order, and needs. They do not have defined borders but articulate among themselves, guaranteeing the process of social differentiation in complex societies (Bonnewitz 2003, Ortiz 2003). Though his concept of social space breaks with the traditional hierarchical view based on a pyramidal idea of society, it is embedded in the notions of conflict and social stratification. Thus the characteristics, rules, and forms of a field vary in accordance to its practices, history, and the hegemonic and counter-hegemonic strategies used by its different members, namely institutions, professional corporations, internal groups, social agents, and so forth. The field for Bourdieu is dynamic, structured, and organized in networks. Its members may assume different roles, acting as producers, distributors, users/consumers, legitimizers, or regulators. From this position they produce and dispute capital and power. Bourdieu's social space is characterized by an unequal distribution of capitals, described as: economic capital (the aggregate of economic goods and production means; labor force); cultural capital (intellectual qualification produced by family and education; cultural goods); social capital (social mobilization of people, groups, and collectivities through various connections, such as social networks, membership); and symbolic capital (the aggregate of rituals related to honor, recognition of one's social value, legitimacy) (Bonnewitz 2003, Bourdieu 1993, 1996, Ortiz 2003, Peillon 1998).

Although the main focus in Bourdieu's studies was on education and culture, there have been some applications to other fields such as welfare studies. Peillon (1998), using Bourdieu's ideas, states that the first step is to understand the position of the welfare field in the social formation, since it involves the state, market mechanisms, and organizations of civil society. Consequently, people's access to resources varies greatly depending on the capability of accumulating and making use of one kind of capital. For instance, if groups or communities display important organization, accumulating significant social capital,

their position in terms of accessing benefits, rights and/or services is higher. Since their achievement is recognized as important and legitimate, there is a consequential increase in their symbolic capital. As such, the increase in capital accumulation implies a direct boost in power.

The access to the welfare system may take place in different forms which will affect the ways the agents and the recipients see themselves and relate one to the other. They may see a welfare benefit, social policy, service or program as a right any citizen deserves, something one may struggle for or something that only those legitimately entitled may receive. On the other side, the agents involved in delivering services may see their duties as a job, a political and social engagement or a personal mission. The representations that the users/consumers and agents have over their role and place in the welfare system and their hegemonic or counter-hegemonic actions are generated on the basis of their habitus.

A central concept in Bourdieu's theories, habitus is defined as a set of inculcated or incorporated dispositions, acquired through the process of socialization and through life experiences. This results in the embodied attitudes and tendencies of perceiving, thinking, feeling, and doing, which are seen as 'natural', working as if they are unconscious principles of action, perception, and reflection (Bonnewitz 2003, Peillon 1998). Consequently, the way agents and recipients will answer and act in a meaningful way to situations will depend on their habitus and, if I may say so, on the way they reflect about it.

The influence of the habitus explains the frequent occurrence of misrecognition, as for instance, when one describes his/her actions as care or empowerment when they are really operating as a means of social control. As a result, actions in the welfare field, as in any other field, occur amid conflict since the field is a site of struggle. Power and control may take different shapes; they may be implicit or ingrained in the form of micro-powers. They may be explicit in agendas of control and they may get replies in form of resistance, such as the call for action usually encompassed by social movements. They may appear as domination or be disguised by a patrimonial attitude. The field may intend to produce either mass loyalty/legitimacy to the status quo or to reduce social inequality and promote human rights. As it is, no action is taken for granted, it always implies political choices.

Thus, Bourdieu's ideas and Peillon's reflection on the welfare field may contribute to provide a critical frame of analysis for occupational therapy in the 'social' field. Working in this field is always a political endeavor. It entails a degree of reflexitivy, through a collective effort, to unveil socially conditioned configurations embedded in the production of knowledge and the development of practices in occupational therapy. For instance, some terms have been used, sometimes in an alternative way, to address people who have been excluded from access to human rights. The next section aims to make these terms clear.

Marginality, exclusion, apartheid, disaffiliation, and vulnerability: concepts of deprivation

Despite the common usage of some concepts related to the deprivation of life conditions or the lack of fulfillment of basic human needs, they are often used interchangeably as if their meanings were the same. This is the case of concepts such as marginality, inclusion/exclusion, apartheid, 'disaffiliation', and vulnerability. On the contrary, they have their meanings embedded in some major theoretical frameworks. Mixing them up may lead to inconsistencies in the comprehension of arguments and implementation of actions. Examining them may clarify the further analysis.

Marginality is a concept that has been used for a wide range of social conditions relating to urban poverty. Robert Park (1928) first used the concept of marginal man in the 1920s in his study of the behavior of migrant communities in Chicago. The marginal man, according to Park, was marked by instability since he lived in two different cultural realities and felt a stranger in both of them. However, whatever negative features one might see in this character, Park envisaged the marginal man as an opportunity to understand the processes of civilization and progress better. Consequently, at this point, the concept was associated with social change and nonconformity.

In Latin America, although marginality is commonly explained as a lack of integration, the two major streams of thought emerging from the 1970s differed on its causality (Quijano 1978). The structural-functionalist approach (associated with the theory of modernization) assumes that because society is a systemic organization and works on consensual

basis, marginality takes place when one of its members does not adapt to its rules. Marginality and the lack of integration here are reduced to the adaptation or not of someone to a given social structure (Quijano 1978). In contrast, according to the Marxist standpoint (associated with the theory of dependence), marginality is a result of the social relations of production, specific to the capitalist accumulation. Marginality is thus understood as a social conflict resulting from the marginal incorporation of the population in the labor market and is used to refer to dependent economies (i.e., typical of peripheral countries). This concept of marginality is still current nowadays. In Latin America, from the 1950s to the 1980s the notion of marginality came to be attributed to various circumstances related to urban poverty, poor living conditions in the slums, the lack of access to the benefits of the urban, industrialized society, and the unstable position of workers in the process of production (Escorel 1999). Also, it came to be seen as a way of transgressing the social order, which led to the stigmatization of the term in Brazil through the association of the term 'marginal' with 'troublemaker'.

Exclusion is a notion that started to be used, without particular emphasis, by Foucault (1978) to refer to the so-called Great Confinement. Then, those whose common feature was their incapacity for productive work, such as the insane, disabled, poor, and deviant, were confined in the Hôpital Général in Paris. Therefore, the term exclusion was primarily associated with the ideas of banishment, confinement and social control. Later, René Lenoir (1974), another French author, used the term to allude to the subjective dimension of being poor in the twentieth-century France, particularly in the 1970s and 1980s. Also, exclusion was used to refer to the instability of working relations and personal bonds in the contemporary world.

At the turn of the millennium, the process of exclusion may represent the collapse of ideas of inclusion and universality of human rights; a disintegration process by which an astonishing number of people come to be unquestionably accepted as disposable and become segregated either culturally, spatially, ethnically, or economically. The term exclusion thus expresses the disruption of social bonds, either material or symbolic. It may refer to different processes and groups, modes and causalities but it cannot be used to consign a specific event in a particular society. It goes beyond the condition of the unstable integration in the labor market and suggests a wide set of circumstances, which may affect identity, social cohesion and the sense of belonging (Escorel 1999).

Escorel, following Hannah Arendt's works, argues that social exclusion may reduce social groups to the condition of *animal laborans*, which means people whose main concern is exclusively the maintenance of their survival. These people are expropriated (excluded) from their condition of *homo faber* (which involves the human capacity of doing, creating and building the living world) and *bios politikos* (which involves the drive for interaction and participation in public life) (Escorel 1999).

The extensive and diffuse uses of the notion of exclusion have also given reason for criticism. First, if one takes diversity and plurality in contemporary societies as an example, one has to be careful not to mistake exclusion for difference, since not all difference leads to exclusion. Second, the concept of exclusion cannot be applied indiscriminately across all social systems, without considering each one's cultural attributes. Although one should think in global terms as far as universal human rights are concerned, one should take into account local realities, customs, beliefs and peculiarities in social stratification and social structure (see also Chapter 9).

Exclusion is also considered an inadequate notion to be applied for circumstances where, more than inequality or discrimination, there is a strict dividing line, restraining social mobility, religious, and ethnic relations and creating two disconnected worlds. In this case, the term apartheid or social apartheid is preferably used since it stresses difference and better defines a fragmented territory, a social fracture. The idea of social apartheid implies the existence of two separate and opposing worlds, each one with its internal solidarity principles and social dynamics (Buarque 1993, Escorel 1999).

Furthermore, Robert Castel (1999) points out that exclusion has become an all-encompassing term for all global miseries. He argues that the excluded is actually a *desaffilié*, whose path is made of series of disruptions in the balance of the previous living conditions. *Désaffiliation*, a French neologism freely translated here as *disaffiliation*, is a concept created by Robert Castel to approach, from another standpoint, the 'new social question', i.e., the result of the rise of unemployment and the growing vulnerability of working conditions in the 1990s in France. Castel (1991) chooses to approach it as an outcome of the intersection of two axes: the axis of integration/nonintegration in work and the axis of belonging/not belonging to a family sociability. The multiple combinations of these factors will define one's condition. This may deteriorate from integration, when there are satisfactory professional and family guarantees, to vulnerability, when there is some fragility both in work and family life, to disaffiliation, when a rupture occurs in both. By the end of the process of disaffiliation, a process of weakening and rupture of social bonds, economic loss becomes complete deprivation and disruption of affective ties becomes isolation (Castel 1995, Escorel 1999). This extreme condition is, for example, the one faced by homeless people, street children, and refugees around the world.

Vulnerability is actually a concept that has been used by disciplines such as sociology, economics, development studies, social policy, public health, nutrition, and environmental studies. In general terms, vulnerability is usually defined as a susceptibility to be hurt or harmed in some sense. Consequently, it has often been related to insecurity and risk, despite controversies. Economic studies usually view vulnerability as a household response to risk, given some underlying conditions. Although, considering the difficulties of measuring them in an aggregated form, they have settled to apply measures of vulnerability to each of the different outcomes (crime, poverty, and so on). Thus, this approach may be criticized by ruling out a comprehensive account of the complex concept of vulnerability and by supposing that all the vulnerability conditions may be measured in monetary or quantitative terms (Alwang et al 2001).

On the contrary, some sociological and development studies tend to support qualitative studies on vulnerability as an approach to the study of poverty since they argue that the latter may not be captured by quantitative measures. For them, one important aspect of vulnerability is that it addresses collective settings and contexts, displacing social issues from personal-centered approaches and enables them to explore through participatory research approaches, the coping strategies that people develop. Chambers argues that coping strategies vary greatly and those engaged in policy making and relief projects should take into account local people's views since there are no simple or universal solutions (Alwang et al 2001, Chambers 2006). In public health, vulnerability became a key concept when the Vancouver International Aids Conference in 1996 envisaged a new approach to the acquired immune deficiency syndrome (AIDS) epidemic, which replaced a perspective that stigmatized people by labeling them as members of risk groups with risky behaviors. This different approach led to the understanding that the chance of someone becoming sick is the outcome of individual, social, and contextual aspects, and resulted in a change of approach in policy making and intervention of the epidemic in some countries (Ayres et al 2003). The concept of vulnerability used in this social, contextualized, comprehensive perspective allows a more suitable approach to 'social questions' since it focuses on the need to recognize the influence of various contexts on the increase of susceptibilities to human suffering. Also, it provides knowledge about people's coping strategies, enabling them (and those involved in any kind of assistance or project) to create appropriate alternatives.

As shown above, marginality, exclusion, apartheid, disaffiliation, and vulnerability are concepts attached to particular theoretical frameworks and their origins are inscribed in specific social domains. Making them clear helps to reduce misrecognition and to promote a dialog among those acting in the social field, since such practices involve people from different professional and theoretical origins. It is important to stress that, although these concepts are useful as a point of departure, they still focus on negative features such as failure, the absence or the lack of something, or on deprivation. Other key concepts should be pursued to explore affirmative aspects and provide principles for action. Emancipation, self-determination, collective action, citizenship, human rights may be some of them. In the introduction, concepts, ideas and practices in the 'social' field were described as socially, historically and politically constructed. People in the field have to respond and engage in a reflective way that takes account of local contexts, as they are developed ahead.

Considerations for the development of critical knowledge and practice in the social field

The concepts presented earlier may provide some reference for those who work in the social field. This, like any field, has its own dynamics and organization, needs, and demands: theories, discourses, and controversies. Besides, matters should not be addressed on individual basis nor expected to be resolved in a straightforward way. Actions rarely have idealized outcomes, decision-making processes often involve controversies. Macro-politics has a constant impact on people's lives, on the policy-making process, and on the programs in progress, resulting in frequent setbacks. As a consequence, occupational therapists soon understand that their basic knowledge and practice in health and rehabilitation are not enough. New understandings and approaches are required. It becomes crucial for occupational therapists to decide which theories to make use of, how to implement their practices, produce knowledge, and establish a dialog with other contributors in the social field.

To answer these new challenges, it seems appropriate to answer the call of Kinsella & Whiteford (2008). When discussing theory and knowledge generation in occupational therapy based on the ideas of Bourdieu & Wacquant (1992), they argue 'for the need for occupational therapy to engage in epistemic reflexivity to make such processes [how epistemic communities choose theories and produce knowledge] more explicit, and to adopt a more critical stance in this regard' (Kinsella & Whiteford 2008, p. 7). Thus, occupational therapists, by becoming aware of their theoretical and epistemological choices, may make the production of knowledge and practices in occupational therapy gain in consistency and credibility in the social field.

One of the first questions to be addressed in this regard is: Why should knowledge and practice in the social field take a critical standpoint? The affirmative answer rests on the idea that occupational therapists should avoid developing knowledge and practices to maintain the social and political status quo. A critical perspective of the 'social question' understands social exclusion and its correlative, as elements of capitalism and, social conflict as a component of the dynamics of social relations. Although exclusion is more clearly seen in the peripheral countries, in contrast to the relatively stable conditions of those at the core of the economic system, the rise of neoliberalism, the decline of the systems of social welfare and the changes in contemporary labor relations have had an impact in living standards worldwide. These conditions should be understood on the basis of their global interconnection, although one must admit that the ordinary people of the peripheral countries have paid the major socioeconomic burden and they have vast social matters to take in hand.

Beyond this, other important questions concern the type of methodologies that should be used to tackle social matters. Important criticisms have already been made to the usage of patrimonialist, top-down approaches, where the 'agents' are considered instructed or enlightened and the 'receivers' are considered less bright and informed, in need of tutelage to deal with their own problems (Barros et al 2005). With regards to research, positivist methodologies have already been largely criticized for assuming a scientific 'neutrality' that is disconnected from social class, moral values, and the political positions of scientists. Because positivist research focuses on objectivity and precision, it is insufficient to deal with a variety of social matters that demand taking into account subjective aspects and the social actors' own views (Minayo 1999).

Critical understandings of social matters require combining a focus on the people as subjects of their own lives with the view that there is no personal, subjective understanding disconnected from history, culture, and the social macro-processes. Hence, some authors have argued for a methodology that combines hermeneutics and dialectics (Minayo 2002) or a critical hermeneutics (Kinsella 2006). The first states that hermeneutics, by an interpretive process, allows the apprehending of meaning in texts (in broad terms, including biographies, narratives) daily life events and historical facts. In this way, hermeneutics brings forward the Other and proposes intersubjectivity as the ground for scientific processes and human action (Minayo 2002). In a contrasting but complementary way, dialectics brings in dissent, change, and the influence of the macro-processes. Then, this allows difference, diversity, conflict, and the rupture of meaning to be critically emphasized and dealt with (Minayo 2002). Going further, Kinsella (2006), presenting critical hermeneutics and its contributions to qualitative research, argues that it may contribute to enable the creation of space for the oppressed and marginalized to articulate their histories and discourses, assisting them to become active interpreters.

Therefore, either in research or in the development of practices, it is essential to listen to people's stories and opinions, recognize their resilience and learn the strategies they develop to endure and survive life events, taking into account the historical, cultural, social, and political contexts where they are imbedded. For occupational therapists and scientists, it is crucial to study and better comprehend the dynamics of everyday life, inasmuch as it gives structure, form, and meaning to what people do, and to what people are (Berger & Luckmann 1991, Certeau 1994, Goffman 1969, Lefebvre 1971).

Occupation, activity, and praxis are some of terminologies used in occupation therapy and occupational science, and the existing controversies concerning professional terminology worldwide are acknowledged but will not be addressed here (Barros et al 2005, Nelson & Jonsson 1999, Lentin 2004a,b, Wilcock & Jakobsen 2001). However, it is worth mentioning Cutchin et al's statement (2008) that action is crucial for the understanding of occupation and their usage of Dewey's and Bourdieu's theories of human action. According to them, habitus, context, and creativity are crucial features of human action/occupation and not peripheral as they have been often considered. The processes of perceiving, thinking, feeling, and doing are as much personal as social, since they are the results of macro- and micro-processes that cannot be taken apart. In short, if working in the social field implies taking action in a transformative way, understanding occupation, activity or praxis as human action is crucial for the engagement of occupational therapy and occupational science in this field (see Chapter 34).

The final question refers to the ultimate goals of working in the social field from a critical standpoint. At first, it is important to recall that this sort of action supports non submission to oppressive acts, pledging for empowerment and social and political emancipation (Freire 1978, 1979a,b). Emancipation is mentioned here in terms of going beyond customs and conditions of hierarchical domination. It implies the struggle for the reduction of inequality, oppression and exploitation and aspires to the redistribution of power and resources. Thus it is a concept that follows the ethics of justice, equality, and participation. Empowerment is the process through which people experience opportunities to make decisions and contemplate new courses of action, and take notice of new demands as well as new life opportunities. Engaging in critical perspectives will require occupational therapy and occupational science to envision their actions as means of achieving these ultimate purposes.

References

Alwang J, Siegel P, Jorgensen S: *Vulnerability: a view from different disciplines*, Social Protection Discussion Paper Series No. 0115. Washington, DC, 2001, Social Protection Unit, Human Development Network, The World Bank. Online. Available at: http://www.wds.worldbank.org/external/default/main?pagePK = 64193027&piPK = 64187937&theSitePK = 523679&menuPK = 64187510&searchMenuPK = 64187283&theSitePK = 523679&entityID = 000094946_01120804004787&searchMenuPK = 64187283&theSitePK = 523679. Accessed January 5, 2009.

Assies W, Calderon MA, Salman T: Ciudadanía, Cultura Política y Reforma del Estado en América Latina, *America Latina Hoy* 32:55–90, 2002.

Ayres J, França I Jr, Calazans G, Saletti Filho H: O Conceito de vulnerabilidade e as práticas de saúde: novas perspectivas e desafios. In Czeresnia D, Freitas C, editors: *Promoção da Saúde*, Rio de Janeiro, 2003, Fiocruz, pp 117–139.

Barros D, Ghirardi MI, Lopes R: Social occupational therapy: a social-historic perspective. In Kronenberg F, Algado S, Pollard N, editors: *Occupational Therapy without Borders – Learning from the Spirit of Survivors*, London, 2005, Elsevier Churchill Livingstone, pp 140–151.

Berger P, Luckmann T: *The Social Construction of Reality: a Treatise in the Sociology of Knowledge*, London, 1991, Penguin.

Bonnewitz P: *Primeiras Lições Sobre a Sociologia de Pierre Bourdieu*, Rio de Janeiro, 2003, Vozes.

Bourdieu P: *Sociology in Question*, London, 1993, Sage.

Bourdieu P: *The Rules of Art. Genesis and Structure of the Literary Field*, Cambridge, 1996, Polity Press.

Bourdieu P, Wacquant L: *An Invitation to Reflexive Sociology*, Chicago, 1992, The University of Chicago Press.

Buarque C: O *Que é Apartação: o Apartheid Social no Brasil*, São Paulo, 1993, Brasiliense.

Castel R: De l'indingence à l'exclusion, la désaffiliation: précarieté du travail et vunerabilité relationelle. In Donzelot J, editor: *Face à l'exclusion – le modèle français*, 1991, Esprit, pp 137–168.

Castel R: *Les Métamorphoses de la Question Sociale: Une Chronique du Salariat*, Paris, 1995, Fayard.

Castel R: As armadilhas da exclusão. In Belfiore-Wanderley M, Bógus L, Yazbek MC, editors: *Desigualdade e a Questão Social*, São Paulo, 1999, EDUC, pp 15–48.

Certeau M: *A Invenção do Cotidiano: Artes de Fazer*, Petropolis, 1994, Vozes.

Chambers R: Editorial introduction: vulnerability, coping and policy, *IDS Bulletin* 37:33–40, 2006.

Cutchin M, Aldrich R, Bailliard A, Copolla S: Action theories for occupational science: the contributions of Dewey and Bourdieu, *Journal of Occupational Science* 15:157–165, 2008.

Dagnino E: Os movimentos sociais e a emergência de uma nova noção de cidadania. In Dagnino E, editor: *Os Anos 1990, Política e Sociedade no Brasil*, São Paulo, 1994, Brasiliense, pp 103–115.

Escorel S: *Vidas ao léu: Trajetórias de Exclusão Social*, Rio de Janeiro, 1999, Fiocruz.

Foucault M: *História da Loucura na Idade Clássica*, São Paulo, 1978, Perspectiva.

France A: *Understanding Youth in Late Modernity*, Maidenhead, 2007, Open University Press.

Freire P: *Ação Cultural Para a Liberdade e Outros Escritos*, Rio de Janeiro, 1978, Paz e Terra.

Freire P: *Pedagogia do Oprimido*, ed 7, Rio de Janeiro, 1979a, Paz e Terra.

Freire P: *Educação Como Prática da Liberdade*, ed 9, Rio de Janeiro, 1979b, Paz e Terra.

Galheigo SM: Occupational therapy and the social field: clarifying concepts and ideas. In Kronenberg F, Algado S, Pollard N, editors: *Occupational Therapy without Borders – Learning from the Spirit of Survivors*, London, 2005, Elsevier Churchill Livingstone, pp 87–98.

Goffman E: *The Presentation of Self in Everyday Life*, Harmondsworth, 1969, Penguin.

Hardiman M, Midgley J: *The Social Dimensions of Development: Social Policy and Planning in the Third World*, Chichester, 1982, John Wiley.

ISOS: *International Society for Occupational Science*, 2009. Online. Available at: http://isos.nfshost.com/links.html. Accessed January 5, 2009.

Kinsella E: *Hermeneutics and Critical Hermeneutics: exploring possibilities within the art of interpretation. Forum: Qualitative Social Research 7(3/19)*, 2006. Online. Available at: http://www.qualitative-research.net/index.php/fqs/issue/view/4. Accessed July 22, 2008.

Kinsella E, Whiteford G: Knowledge generation and utilisation in occupational therapy: towards epistemic reflexivity, *Australian Occupational Therapy Journal* 56:249–258, 2008.

Kronenberg F, Algado S, Pollard N, editors: *Occupational Therapy without Borders – Learning from the Spirit of Survivors*, London, 2005, Elsevier Churchill Livingstone.

Lefebvre H: *Everyday Life in the Modern World*, London, 1971, Allen Lane.

Lenoir R: *Les Exclus*, Paris, 1974, Seuil.

Lentin P: Occupational Terminology, *Journal of Occupational Science* 12:51–53, 2004a.

Lentin P: Occupational Terminology, *Journal of Occupational Science* 12:85–86, 2004b.

Lister R, Smith N, Middleton S, et al: Young people and citizenship. In Barry M, editor: *Youth Policy and Social Inclusion: Critical Debates with Young People*, London, 2005, Routledge, pp 33–50.

Midgley J: *Professional Imperialism: Social Work in the Third World*, London, 1981, Heinemann.

Midgley J: Diffusion and the development of social policy: evidence from the Third World, *J Soc Policy* 13:167–184, 1984.

Minayo MC: O *Desafio do Conhecimento: Pesquisa Qualitativa em Saúde*, Hucitec-ABRASCO, São Paulo, Rio de Janeiro, 1999.

Minayo MC: Hermenêutica-dialética como caminho do pensamento social. In Minayo MC, Deslandes S, editors: *Caminhos do Pensamento: Epistemologia e Método*, Rio de Janeiro, 2002, Fiocruz.

Nelson D, Jonsson H: Occupational terms across languages and countries, *Journal of Occupational Science* 6:42–47, 1999.

Ortiz R, editor: *A Sociologia de Pierre Bourdieu*, São Paulo, 2003, Olho d'água.

Paoli MC: Citizenship, inequalities, democracy and rights, *Social and Legal Studies* 1:143–159, 1992.

Park R: Human migration and the marginal man, *AJS* 33:881–893, 1928.

Peillon M: Bourdieu's field and the sociology of welfare, *J Soc Policy* 27:213–229, 1998.

Quijano A: Notas sobre o conceito de marginalidade social. In Pereira L, editor: *Populações 'Marginais'*, São Paulo, 1978, Duas Cidades, pp 11–71.

Squires P: *Anti-social Policy: Welfare, Ideology and the Disciplinary State*, London, 1990, Harvester Wheatsheaf.

Soares L: *Terapia Ocupacional: Lógica do Capital ou do Trabalho?*, São Paulo, 1991, Hucitec.

Watson R, Fourie M: International and African influences on occupational therapy. In Watson R, Swartz L, editors: *Transformation Through Occupation*, London, 2004, Whurr Publishers, pp 33–50.

Wilcock A, Jakobsen K: Occupational terminology, *Journal of Occupational Science* 8:25–31, 2001.

An ethos that transcends borders

7

Suzanne M. Peloquin

OVERVIEW

In discussing the power of occupation and a therapy built around it, founders and early supporters of occupation as therapy iterated central themes with visionary zeal. From their discussions, a professional ethos emerged: time, place, and circumstance open paths to occupation; occupation fosters dignity, competence, and health; occupational therapy is a personal engagement; caring and helping are vital to the work; and effective practice is artistry and science. Collectively, these beliefs capture that which many occupational therapists profess – declare and affirm – in the world. The occupational therapy ethos has shaped the character of the profession, established its reputation, and carried its spirit across changing times and myriad places.
Our ethos of origin restores our clearsightedness into what is essential about our character: we are pathfinders. We enable occupations that heal. We co-create daily lives. We reach for hearts as well as hands. We are artists and scientists at once. Rooted in a deep commitment to serve the underserved, the profession's ethos offers a perspective on personal empowerment that transcends societal borders and begs a more global practice.

Introduction

It is time to reclaim the occupational therapy profession's ethos of origin so as to liven and animate a more global practice (Peloquin 2005). The occupational therapy ethos is rooted in a deep commitment to serve the underserved and can thus shape a perspective on empowerment that transcends societal and

professional borders. In support of this assertion, I offer evidence of each ethologic belief as it emerged from early American history followed by an example of how the same belief is made manifest in more current and global occupational therapy practice.

As a first step in this excursion into the profession's ethos consider the meaning of the word. Definitions of the term *ethos* include these: a person's character or disposition; an individual's moral nature; the characteristic spirit or prevailing sentiment of a group; the genius – that extraordinary and distinctive capacity or aptitude – of a people or institution; the guiding beliefs, standards, or ideals that pervade and characterize a group; the spirit that motivates the ideas or practices of a community; the complex of fundamental values that permeate or actuate major patterns of thought and behavior (Simpson & Weiner 1989). A profession's ethos is thus an interlacing of sentiment, value, and thought that captures its character, conveys its genius, and manifests its spirit. An ethos carries beliefs so fundamental and sound that they endure, both supporting and transcending the particularities of diverse paradigms, protocols, and cultures.

The ethos of occupational therapy

The early decades of the twentieth century shaped the context from which a professional ethos for occupational therapy practice emerged in the United States. Early supporters of the use of occupation, the founders of the Society for the Promotion of Occupational Therapy (SPOT), and early occupational

© 2011, Elsevier Ltd.
DOI: 10.1016/B978-0-7020-3103-8.00016-X

workers drew from the context of the times and their experiences a common understanding: occupation could help. Needs that begged occupational interventions came from diverse realms. There were poor immigrants in city slums, soldiers with amputations and shell shock, hospitalized patients with disabling illnesses such as tuberculosis and stroke, men and children hurt by developing machinery, wealthy women with a sense of ennui, workers dulled and demoralized by factory routines, insane individuals whose days lacked a healthy rhythm. (Peloquin 2005).

In discussing the power of occupation and a therapy built around it, founders and early supporters of occupation as therapy iterated central themes with visionary zeal. From their discussions, five beliefs emerged with guiding potential, each a confluence of sentiment, value, and thought. Each had the capacity to shape character, establish reputation, and carry the profession's spirit across changing times and myriad places. Each survives to this day in spirited practice (Peloquin 2005). Because each ethologic belief captures a distinct and equally important dimension of occupation or occupational therapy, each relates to the others existentially rather than sequentially or hierarchically. The end result is this complex of guiding beliefs: time, place, and circumstance open paths to occupation; occupation fosters dignity, competence, and health; occupational therapy is a personal engagement; caring and helping are vital to the work; and effective practice is artistry and science. Taken together, these beliefs capture that which many occupational therapists profess – declare and affirm – in the world. Because these beliefs address the depth of human need, the profession's ethos transcends the boundaries of societal culture or professional models.

Time, place, and circumstance open paths to occupation

One guiding belief within our ethos is that time, place, and circumstance open paths to occupation, challenges notwithstanding. Situated in life circumstances of all kinds, persons *occupy* time and place (Reed & Sanderson 1999). Adolf Meyer (1922), a neuropathologist and early champion of the profession, saw time's path to occupation. Sharing his philosophy of occupational therapy as Professor of Psychiatry at Johns Hopkins University, he said: 'Man learns to organize time and he does it in terms

of *doing* things ... and one of the things he does we call work and occupation – we might call it the ingestion and proper use ... of time with its successions of opportunities' (p. 9–10).

Meyer (1922) cited philosopher Pierre Janet, noting that proper use of time is 'the realization of reality, bringing the very soul of man out of dreams of eternity to the full sense and appreciation of actuality'. If a person's use of time was a doing, it was also and more essentially a becoming, a realization of the soul (Peloquin 1990, 1997, Wilcock 1998). Honing in on a population of interest, he said that valuing time led to a 'conception of mental illness as *problems of living*' rather than as only problems with thinking, or diseases, or disorders of constitution (Meyer 1922, p. 4v).

Taking a complementary if more pragmatic view, Allan Cullimore (1921), Chief of Educational Service in Letterman Hospital in San Francisco, spoke of time's worth. He applauded occupational therapy's *real* work as therapeutic agent, cautioning against busy work. 'Occupational therapy planned to kill time', he said, 'stands in the same relation to the real occupational therapy as that of first aid to medical treatment based on examination and careful diagnosis' (p. 537). 'Occupations must lead somewhere', Cullimore said of the meaningfulness of occupation, 'and the patient must want to follow' (p. 538). Time and circumstance, we note, open paths to occupation. Place and circumstance do so as well.

Many places of the time called for occupations: hospitals for the insane; wards in general hospitals, from pediatric to psychopathic to orthopedic; hospital workshops; sanitaria for the treatment of tuberculosis; tents and army barracks, schools for defectives; institutions for the blind; convalescent homes; and private dwellings. Meyer's (1922) philosophy included an individual's harmonic engagement with place: 'Our conception of man is that of an organism that maintains and balances itself in the world of reality and actuality by being in active life and active use ... and acting its time in harmony with its own nature and the nature about it' (p. 5). He supported an 'orderly rhythm in the atmosphere' of hospitals, using among disturbed patients the habit training approach to life tasks – dressing, eating, working, playing – developed by Eleanor Clarke Slagle (Meyer 1922).

Thoughts about occupation's emergence as valuable from a convergence of time, place, and circumstance have endured. In Chapter 25, Munoz et al describe the manner in which therapists within four unique programs use occupation in correctional systems where offenders, said to be 'doing time', may perceive themselves as 'killing time'. Collectively, these community-university programs include occupation among incarcerated offenders who often experience occupational deprivation and imbalance that confound habits already proven to be maladaptive. Much like Slagle's early habit training, occupation in prisons can infuse meaningful rhythms into dispiriting atmospheres.

For offenders, awareness of the more balanced, productive, and harmonic time use that will be required in future places is a critical acquisition. Geena's situation is poignant: she is typical of imprisoned women who struggle to make a new life in the community, who strive to realize their dreams. If aspects of her occupational life fail, Geena may be homeless, jobless, and at risk for returning to violent relationships and drug use. Imprisonment time can become an opportunity for Geena to learn to manage problems of living.

Our ethos embraces a focus on occupation's capacity to lead somewhere, even in prisons, because of this longstanding belief: time, place, and circumstance open paths to occupation. Guided by an ethos that addresses problems of living, occupational therapy practitioners can be pathfinders among criminal offenders.

Occupation fosters dignity, competence, and health

Another guiding belief within our ethos is that occupation fosters dignity, competence, and health. Founder William Rush Dunton Jr (1919) conveyed his belief in the healing role of occupation in a creed that prefaced a book on wartime work, known as reconstruction therapy. He wrote:

> That occupation is as necessary to life as food and drink. That every human being should have both physical and mental occupation. That all should have occupations which they enjoy... That sick minds, sick bodies, sick souls, may be healed through occupation
>
> Dunton (p. 17)

Almost 10 years earlier, Robert Carroll, a physician in Asheville, North Carolina (1910), had noted the worth of occupation in terms of dignity and competence, confidently proposing a 'Law of Work' and asserting that 'work truly is life'. He said:

> The greatest influence, the true and lasting benefit in work as a therapeutic agent, rests in the moral uplift, the great mastering of self which comes when one is taught to work right, when one knows the joy and forgets the burden of doing, when self-mastery displaces indulgence, when doubt of one's strength is replaced by faith
>
> Carroll (1910, p. 2034)

Whether endorsed as moral creed or scientific law, the belief was this: occupation fosters dignity, competence, and health. Meta Anderson (1920) thus said that occupational therapy 'should inspire the feeling of pleasure and self-respect which comes from being useful, and the feeling of power which comes from progressive daily achievement' (p. 326). Most poignant is her story, told in the language of the day:

> An official was visiting the work of the feebleminded in a certain school. The teacher reported the good work done by the various schoolchildren. When she had finished, a low grade girl member of the class tugged at her sleeve and said, 'Tell him that I cleaned the garbage can.' She had cleaned the garbage can and had done it very well. She beamed over the praise given to her after she had called attention to her accomplishment. She had been useful and her joy was unbounded.
>
> Anderson (1920, p. 326)

One soldier gave this testimonial to occupation: 'I got a new vision of life ... [I] saw the dignity of labor made new and interesting, and even more powerful because of the handicap' (Cooper 1918, p. 24–25). Belief in the healing power of occupation – in its capacity to help individuals become hale and whole – has endured.

In Argentina today, belief in the healing power of occupation is enacted in ways described in Chapter 24. One intervention in particular, the Coming Back to School project reported by Elisabeth Gaziano, supported teens lacking education, an occupation considered primary in many cultures. If education can be seen as developing competence and healthy habits, it can also be seen as youthful work that fosters dignity. Some 58 teens participated in the year-long back-to-school project. They came from impoverished families whose parents received incomes from government programs, had only temporary work, or scavenged for food on rubbish piles. Several teens had had problems with the law, and some had not finished basic prerequisite studies.

The teens were included in regular planning and educational readiness meetings, enabling them to craft a new vision of their lives. Organizers of the program initially used an economic incentive of $50.

Teens earned the money only if involved in various educational activities. This effort resonates with Carroll's Law of Work (1910) that holds that individuals must learn how to work right. Some 86% of the teens finished school that year. Although the occupational therapist agrees that the money was the prime motivator at the start, by the program's end, engagement in education was the focus. A power came from progressive daily achievement.

Our ethos embraces a focus on improving the occupational lives of teens and their families because of this belief: occupation fosters dignity, competence, and health. Guided by an ethos that transcends societal and economic barriers threatening to exclude youth, occupational therapy practitioners enable impoverished youth to become hale and whole through education.

Occupational therapy is a personal engagement

A third guiding belief within our ethos holds that occupational therapy is a personal engagement. Engagement with others – the commitment to involve and occupy the self and be bound by mutual promise – was thought necessary for patient and therapist alike. George Barton (1920), an architect and founder informed by nursing courses and his own disability, clarified the aim of occupational work. Such engagement and co-creation were essentially and deeply personal:

> Not in the making of a product, but in the making of a MAN, of a man stronger physically, mentally, and spiritually than he was before, for just as his body can be strengthened by carefully graded exercise from week to week, as his mind can be strengthened and be improved in the same way, so also may his spirit be reborn in greater strength and purity by the effort for, and the realization of his triumph over disability and despair.
>
> Barton (p. 308)

Years earlier, Tracy (1913) had described the requisite engagement, noting of hospital work that occupational nurses 'are constantly being impressed with the fact that the technical and mechanical part of their work is but one aspect of their professional duty, that a broader conception must be attained – a sense of obligation to minister to the individual as well as to the disease' (p. 9) and to be 'thoughtful of the deeper needs of her patient' (p. 11). Therapeutic obligation included deep consideration.

Meyer (1922) spoke of the integrity implicit in such engagement: 'It takes rare gifts and talents and rare personalities to be real pathfinders in this work. There are no royal roads; it is all a problem of being true to one's nature and opportunities and of teaching others to do the same with themselves' (p. 7). Being true and real was important. Equally vital to the engagement were other ways of being endorsed by Kidner (1929) in an address to graduating students:

> May you realize in increasing measure the value of certain spiritual things which are the real making of life, but which we call by many common names. Kindness, humanity, decency, honor, and good faith – to give these up under any circumstances whatever, would be a loss greater than any defeat, or even death itself.
>
> Kidner (1929, p. 385)

Perceptions of occupational therapy as a personal engagement continue to empower therapists today. Within the Schizophrenia Campaign in Chile, occupational therapists were instrumental in facilitating three events, entitled 'Encounter with everybody', 'Art with everybody', and 'Sports with everybody', described in Chapter 28. Each event asked for personal engagement from stakeholders in the course of this illness. The astute use of the phrase *with everybody* helped assure inclusion of those living with the illness, their family members, community residents, healthcare workers, students and staff members at various facilities, government representatives, and members of the media. The occupational nature of events ranging from cultural displays to sports, reflected consideration of the deeper needs of this diverse group and invited participation and co-creation. Many joined in this promissory effort at improving the lives of those with mental illness, at triumphing over potential despair.

Our ethos embraces true and real alliances among those with schizophrenia because of this belief: occupational therapy is a personal engagement – a mutual commitment to involve and occupy the self and be bound by promise. Guided by an ethos of engagement, occupational therapy practitioners use kindness, humanity, and good faith to co-create life among those living with mental illness.

Caring and helping are vital to the work

A fourth guiding belief within our ethos is that caring and helping are vital to the work. Herbert Hall (Hall & Buck 1915), physician and early practitioner, spoke with deep feeling of any individual left idle or bereft. He said, 'Put yourself in that man's place – imagine the despair and the final degeneration that must sap at last all that is brave and good in life' (Hall & Buck 1915, p. viii).

Ora Ruggles (Carlova & Ruggles 1946), reconstruction aide during the First World War, enacted the empathy endorsed by Hall. She explained the caring effects of such empathy, 'I don't see what's missing. I see what's there. I see real manhood. I see great courage. I see tremendous strength. I see true spirit. That's what gives me courage, strength, and spirit. I gain as much or more as the men I try to help' (Carlova & Ruggles 1946, p. 76). She said that she had made a great discovery, simple, yet so effective: 'It is not enough to give a patient something to do with his hands', she said. 'You must reach for the heart as well as the hands. It's the heart that really does the healing' (Carlova & Ruggles 1946, p. 69). Early practitioners sought to develop traits that shaped such caring. Moodie (1919) valued, 'above all, infinite patience, the ability to teach and to criticize without causing offense or discouragement, the power of inspiring confidence in others, and last but not least an optimistic temperament and a sense of humor' (p. 314).

Hall (1922a) described the nature of our helping: 'Occupational therapy ... attempts to restore the general effectiveness of people who have become incapacitated through illness and who are not able to make satisfactory progress' (p. 163). Respect for personal dignity was central to such helping. Susan Wilson (1929), Chief Occupational Therapist at Brooklyn State Hospital, said that 'the patient's every moment is carefully supervised', but 'the treatment must not become too paternal, killing the patient's sense of responsibility for his own person' (p. 191). Similarly, Crane (1919) characterized our therapy as one which 'makes the patient a creator' (p. 64).

In Chapter 27, Iwama et al reveal their use of the Kawa (river) model with a variety of clients from five continents. In each instance of differing cultural context, the therapist explained in user-friendly language the metaphor of life as a river and asked clients to draw their life flow. They were invited to represent significant elements in that life flow as rocks, or walls, or driftwood. Supported by personal affirmations and optimistic expectations, clients drew their lives in significant ways, depicting both obstacles and smooth passages.

Clients then told stories of their rivers, empowered by caring therapists and freed by a model that transcends off putting values such as individualism, egocentricism, or able-ism. Each story elaborated a unique life, an elaboration that led each therapist to assess obstacles and discuss options for better flow. Our ethos enables the use of heartening strategies such as the Kawa model because of this belief: caring and helping are vital to our work. Guided by a caring ethos, occupational therapy practitioners press past cultural otherisms, through the Kawa model, to reach for hearts as well as hands (Peloquin 2002).

Effective practice is artistry and science

A fifth guiding belief within our ethos is that effective occupational therapy is at once artistry and science. As noted above, the interpersonal art is part of our ethos. A patient told Ruggles (Carlova & Ruggles 1946), 'You're an artist in the greatest medium of all. You're an artist in people' (p. 92). Supporting such artistry and vision, physician Addison Thayer (1908) of Portland Maine told a colleague using occupation, 'It is not so much the work as the way you inspire the person to take it up' (p. 1486).

Artistry of the apt intervention is also part of the ethos. As an example, an anonymous piece in *The Modern Hospital* in 1922 read, 'Every OT worker of experience has seen hard, rebellious men and women soften and become teachable under the influence of quiet work ... which may carry over into the machine life a new sense of humanity, a growing love of creative accomplishment' (Anonymous 1922, p. 374).

Science has been of equal value. Hall (1922b) called occupational therapy 'the science of prescribed work' (p. 245). Elizabeth Upham (1918), Director of the Art Department at Milwaukee Downer College, framed it more deeply as 'the science of healing by occupation' (p. 13). Calling for records and statistics in occupational therapy, Horatio Pollock (1929), Director of the Statistical Bureau of the New York Department of Mental Hygiene, regarded occupational therapy 'as a scientific effort for the restoration to health of the mentally and physically ill' (p. 416).

Barton's (1915) scientific hypotheses, thought extreme, included one that any medicine of the day listed in *materia medica* books had an occupational equivalent. If doctors prescribed benzol as a leukotoxin, he said, occupational therapists could engage the same patient in canning work so that benzine fumes could yield the same effect (Barton 1915). Signs of scientific pursuit were everywhere. Harry Mock (1919), a lieutenant-colonel, supported the Walter Reed way of noting motion gained. He included a photograph of a soldier flexing to view his measurements. The caption read, 'Visualizing results encourages the patient' (p. 13). The idea of an integrated practice based on art and science permeates cases published in our early years. The one included here is representative in that it reflects artful intervention combined with data gathering science:

> 'Private J. was studying law when he was drafted ... He was wounded by shrapnel in his left arm and a stiff, flexed elbow had resulted. Reading law books would hardly benefit his condition but J. was interested also in making mission furniture out of old boxes and lumber ... Using his left hand chiefly, he soon became adept at hammering, sawing, planing, and other movements which necessitated a certain amount of flexion and extension of the elbow joint. Every week the amount of motion in the joint was measured and a careful record made. When J. saw by actual measurement that his range of motion in this joint was increasing, he was indeed happy and redoubled his efforts. Practically full joint movement had been restored when he was finally discharged.'
> Mock (1919, p. 14)

Beliefs about practice as artistry *and* science have endured. In Chapter 42 Danner et al describe an educational strategy of city walking that helps students see cultural differences in a way that mitigates a negative bias. Educators launched a process of inviting students to walk unfamiliar streets, embedding that action within an institution-supported qualitative study. City walking implemented to foster cultural competence is an imaginative project. It also prompts the acquisition of knowledge through empirical observation and existential experience. The kinds of themes that emerged within focus groups revealed that students benefited from both the artistry and science inherent in the project. Students exposed to such an approach might be more aware of the superficiality of cultural borders.

Our ethos, grounded in a confluent ethos of art and science, invites educators to immerse learners in that confluence because of this belief: effective practice is artistry and science. Guided by an ethos within which cultural competence is seen as artistry *and* science, occupational therapy educators challenge artificial borders with approaches such as city walking.

Conclusion: the guiding power of our ethos

Consider the guiding potential of our ethos. Each belief is expressive, persuasive, and thoughtful. Each evokes the best of who we are; each plumbs the depth of what we do. Together they afford us this view: ours is an ethos of engagement – a commitment to involve and occupy ourselves and be bound by mutual promise. Were we to distill the complex of our guiding beliefs into one brief account, our ethos might be this: engagement for the sake of persons and their occupational natures. We engage so that others may also engage (Moyers 1999). This is our character; this is our genius; this is our spirit.

We can stand on the rock that is our ethos and from there proclaim a view that transcends artificial borders: time, place, and circumstance open paths to occupation. Occupation fosters dignity, competence, and health. Occupational therapy is a personal engagement. Caring and helping are vital to the work. Effective practice is artistry and science. Our profession takes this stand for the sake of persons and their occupational natures.

Mihaly Csikszentmihalyi (1993) a modern-day friend of occupational therapy, offered thoughts to guide a profession through this millennium. His thoughts reverberate with our ethos and with any effort designed to press our profession to realize itself more fully. 'You are a part of everything around you', he said. 'You shall not deny your uniqueness. You are responsible for your actions. You shall be more than what you are' (Csikszentmihalyi 1993, p. 289–290). This call to transcendent action is clear.

The ethos of occupational therapy restores our clearsightedness into what is essential about our character. We are pathfinders. We enable occupations that heal. We co-create daily lives. We reach for hearts as well as hands. We are artists and scientists at once. If we discern this in ourselves, if we act on this understanding every day, we will reclaim a magnificent heart and be more than what we are.

Acknowledgment

Permission to use segments from Peloquin SM 2005 Embracing our ethos, reclaiming our heart. American Journal of Occupational Therapy 59:611–625 was granted by the American Occupational Therapy Association.

References

Anderson ML: Mental reconstruction through occupational therapy, *Mod Hosp* 14:326–327, 1920.

Anonymous: What David Belasco said, *Mod Hosp* 18:373–374, 1922.

Barton GE: Occupational therapy, *Trained Nurse Hosp Rev* 54:138–140, 1915.

Barton GE: What occupational therapy may mean to nursing, *Trained Nurse Hosp Rev* 64:304–310, 1920.

Carlova J, Ruggles O: *The Healing Heart*, New York, 1946, Messner.

Carroll RS: The therapy of work, *Journal of the Medical Association* 54:2032–2035, 1910.

Cooper G: Re-weaving the web: A soldier tells what it means to begin all over again, *Carry On* 1:23–26, 1918.

Crane BT: Occupational therapy, *Boston Medical and Surgical Journal* 181:63–65, 1919.

Csikszentmihalyi M: *The evolving self: A psychology for the third millennium*, New York, 1993, Harper Collins.

Cullimore AR: Objectives and motivation in occupational therapy, *Mod Hosp* 17:537–538, 1921.

Dunton WR Jr: *Reconstruction therapy*, Philadelphia, 1919, Saunders.

Hall HJ: American Occupational Therapy Association, *Archives of Occupational Therapy* 1:163–165, 1922a.

Hall HJ: Science so-called, *Mod Hosp* 18:558–559, 1922b.

Hall HJ, Buck MM: *The Work of our Hands*, Yard, New York, 1915, Moffat.

Kidner TB: Address to graduates, *Occup Ther Rehabil* 8:379–385, 1929.

Meyer A: The philosophy of occupational therapy, *Archives of Occupational Therapy* 1:1–10, 1922.

Mock HE: Curative work, *Carry On* 1:12–17, 1919.

Moodie CS: The value of occupational therapy to the nursing profession, *Hospital Social Service Quarterly* 1:313–315, 1919.

Moyers P: The guide to occupational therapy practice, *Am J Occup Ther* 53:247–322, 1999.

Peloquin SM: Time as a commodity: Reflections and implications, *Am J Occup Ther* 45:147–154, 1990.

Peloquin SM: The spiritual depth of occupation: Making worlds and making lives, *Am J Occup Ther* 51:167–168, 1997.

Peloquin SM: Reclaiming the vision of reaching for heart as well as hands, *Am J Occup Ther* 56:517–526, 2002.

Peloquin SM: Embracing our ethos, reclaiming our heart, *Am J Occup Ther* 59:611–625, 2005.

Pollock HM: The need, value, and general principles of occupational therapy statistics, *Occup Ther Rehabil* 8:415–420, 1929.

Reed KL, Sanderson SN: *Concepts of occupational therapy*, Philadelphia, 1999, Lippincott Williams and Wilkins.

Simpson JA, Weiner ESC, editors: *The Oxford English Dictionary*, Oxford, 1989, Clarendon Press.

Thayer A: Work cure, *JAMA* 51:1485–1486, 1908.

Tracy SE: *Studies in invalid occupation*, Boston, 1913, Whitcomb and Barrows.

Upham E: *Rehabilitation of disabled soldiers and sailors – teacher training for occupational therapy. Training of teachers for occupational therapy for the rehabilitation of disabled soldiers and sailors*, 1918, Federal Board for Vocational Education: Washington Government Printing Office.

Wilcock AA: Reflections on doing, being, and becoming, *Can J Occup Ther* 65:248–256, 1998.

Wilson SC: Habit training for mental cases, *Occup Ther Rehabil* 8:189–197, 1929.

Participatory Occupational Justice Framework (POJF 2010): enabling occupational participation and inclusion

8

Gail Whiteford   Elizabeth Townsend

OVERVIEW

Our chapter on a participatory occupational justice framework (POJF) is designed to raise consciousness and critical, reflexive dialog among professionals who are engaged in *doing justice* in everyday life. To that end, we present POJF 2010 (updated from POJF in the first edition of this book) as *a conceptual tool for doing justice* – as opposed to only thinking about or feeling concerned about issues of equity and justice in everyday life. In guiding practice, the POJF 2010 also guides *knowledge translation* and *knowledge exchange* about occupation, enablement, and justice with professionals and the public. Evidence for the POJF 2010 is drawn from a critique of our own and others' real-life practice experiences, research findings, and philosophy.

We begin by highlighting the three main conceptual foundations of the POJF 2010: occupation, enabling, and justice. We then emphasize that use of the POJF 2010 requires: critical reflexivity; collaborative negotiation of power relations; a focus on context – notably the policy, funding, and legal contexts in which people live and participate; and, importantly, relentless optimism fueled by visions of possibility and hope for an occupationally just world.

The significance of this chapter is its emphasis on a justice of difference and social inclusion in everyday life occupations regardless of differences in ability, age, gender, or other characteristics – a justice for all to participate in those occupations that underpin economic, social, and cultural structures, and provide vehicles for the realization of individual and collective identity, potentiality, and transformative development. Naming occupational justice enriches our understanding of justice at the embodied level of real, everyday, lived experience.

While any professional may use the POJF 2010, we propose that occupational therapists who adopt the POJF 2010 are, because of its conceptual underpinnings and inherent processes, practicing *critical occupational therapy*. This term is congruent with critical education and critical or radical social work traditions, and applies particularly when practice is with disadvantaged or oppressed communities or populations and aims to advance their empowerment in processes of transformative change.

Introduction

To advance the development of occupational justice as a construct of real and pressing relevance for dialog (Townsend & Wilcock 2004, Wilcock & Townsend 2000), we highlight the three underlying concepts of occupation, enablement, and justice, and emphasize the necessity of critical reflexivity, and negotiated, collaborative power relations. Occupational justice is an evolving concept that describes a vision of society in which all populations have the opportunities, resources, privilege, and rights to participate to their potential in their desired occupations (Townsend & Wilcock 2004, Wilcock & Townsend 2000).

The cornerstone of the chapter is an updated Participatory Occupational Justice Framework (POJF 2010) to guide individualized and population-based practice. The POJF 2010 is a conceptual tool for professionals to use in *doing justice* in everyday life – a tool to guide practice processes and prompt *knowledge exchange* (sometimes called knowledge translation or transfer) about occupation,

© 2011, Elsevier Ltd.
DOI: 10.1016/B978-0-7020-3103-8.00017-1

enabling, and justice through active partnerships with professionals and the public in homes, schools, workplaces, and social and cultural institutions. This tool is congruent with the 1948 United Nations Universal Declaration on Human Rights and subsequent human rights positions taken by the United Nations and the World Health Organization (WHO); the 2006 position statement on human rights by the World Federation of Occupational Therapists (WFOT) which centralizes the pursuit of occupational justice as a primary vision for occupational therapy worldwide (WFOT 2006); and the International Classification of Functioning, Disability and Health (ICF) (WHO 2001) which is used in many fields to profile participation restrictions as injustice in everyday life.

The common elements of the POJF 2010 with other occupational therapy conceptual and process models and with some ecological–human interaction models in other fields are: a concern for equity of social participation in civic society as well as in personal and family life; a participatory process for social inclusion of individual, community or population voices in all planning, decision making, and evaluation; and, an explicit focus on the influences of environmental forces that produce injustice in everyday life.

We refer to the interdisciplinary research field of occupational science when discussing research on occupation, enabling, and justice; we locate practice implications for enabling occupational justice in the profession of occupational therapy. While the POJF 2010 may be used to guide any professional practice, we name occupational therapy practice with a participatory occupational justice lens as critical occupational therapy. As in critical education (Freire 1972) and critical or radical social work (Baily & Brake 1975), critical occupational therapy does not refer to practitioners criticizing others per se. Rather, a critical or radical practice in any profession focuses on changing the regulations, policies, laws, economic practices, media images, professional practices, and other forces that govern what people can do, want to do, and even imagine what is possible to do within the structural arrangements of society. Critical perspectives typically raise ethical, moral, civic, and philosophic questions about injustice and the tensions or gaps between ideals and the reality of communities or populations living everyday with inequitable disadvantages or oppression associated with age, ability, ethnicity, gender, race, sexual orientation, or socioeconomic status. In keeping with other critical professional practices, key features of critical occupational therapy would be:

- Article I. Occupational therapists engage in *critical reflexivity* to constantly challenge gaps between occupational therapy philosophy, ideas, theories, and the practical realities of everyday practice
- Article II. Occupational therapy practice is *collaborative and participatory* in all decision making processes from planning to evaluation and follow-up
- Article III. Occupational therapy goals and objectives are explicit on *enabling the social inclusion of disadvantaged or oppressed communities or populations*
- Article IV. Occupational therapy solutions and methods are through *engagement of people individually and collectively in necessary and desired occupations*
- Article V. Occupational therapy is known to emphasize social change as well as individual change in *transformation of the environment (context) to develop more equitable opportunities, resources, privilege, and enablement* for all to participate to their potential and to exert choice and control over what they do every day
- Article VI. Occupational therapists work in teams and partnerships with relentless optimism, visions of possibility, and hope for an occupationally just world.

Orienting language and ideas from Western occupational therapy epistemology

Recognizing that any profession may use the POJF 2010 and that the ideas, values, and beliefs may resonate in many professions, the POJF 2010 draws heavily on occupational therapy and occupational science epistemology: specifically the English language and Western ideas, values, and beliefs for three related concepts: occupation, enablement, and justice (Fig. 8.1). To profile WHAT concerns are addressed in using the POJF 2010, we identify occupational therapists' and occupational scientists' domain of concern for everyday life, described here as everyday occupations, and we name an occupational perspective as a lens for focusing on the positive or negative engagement in everyday occupations of individuals, families, groups, communities, organizations, and populations. To explain HOW any professionals using the POFJ 2010 may work

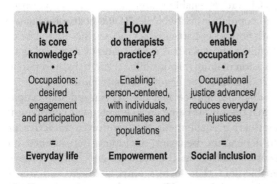

What	How	Why
is core knowledge?	**do therapists practice?**	**enable occupation?**
•	•	•
Occupations: desired engagement and participation	Enabling: person-centered, with individuals, communities and populations	Occupational justice advances/ reduces everyday injustices
=	=	=
Everyday life	**Empowerment**	**Social inclusion**

Fig. 8.1 • Three pillars of occupational therapy knowledge.

with communities, organizations, and populations, in particular and with individuals, families, and groups in some circumstances, we profile collaborative enabling approaches for enabling personal and social transformation through occupational engagement. In exploring WHY professionals might use the POJF 2010, we emphasize occupational therapists' implicit, historical social vision of everyday justice, a justice of difference and social inclusion. (Fig. 8.1).

With justice as a distinguishing feature, we emphasize that the POJF 2010 highlights the importance of engaging in critical reflexivity. Critical reflexivity is the habit of reflecting on the consistency between philosophy, knowledge, and action in practice (Aronson 1999, Bourdieu & Johnson 1998, Denton et al 2004, Sandywell 1996). We have named enabling approaches to raise consciousness to power relations, hierarchical versus collaborative decision making, and in justice from an occupational perspective (Townsend 2003a, Wilcock 2006). Our aim in presenting the POJF 2010 is to strengthen occupational therapists' and other professionals' abilities to consistently raise consciousness of, articulate, and defend, both philosophically and theoretically, a transformative vision of a more occupationally just world (Stadnyk et al 2010, Wilcock & Townsend 2009), and to engage in knowledge translation and knowledge exchange about occupation, enabling, and justice in everyday professional practice.

Occupation – what is the domain of concern and perspective?

Concerns about occupational injustice start with a focus on everyday life, described by occupational therapists and occupational scientists in English

using the broad concept and language of occupation. By adopting an occupational perspective, professionals would look particularly at what people do every day on their own and collectively; how people live to seek identity, satisfaction, and autonomy; how people organize their habits, routines, and choices to promote health; and how people collectively have organized systems such as education and health to support (or not) what all populations need and want to do in their occupations to live well and be healthy. An occupational perspective is the lens for engaging individuals, families, groups, communities, organizations, and populations in negotiated processes, actions, and critical reflection to facilitate contextually meaningful modes of occupational participation (Law et al 2002, Townsend & Polatajko 2007, Whiteford & Wright 2005, Yerxa et al 1990).

Occupational therapy and occupational science research is increasingly informing us that occupation is as necessary for human existence as air, food, and water, and that the power of occupational engagement can be used therapeutically to heal the body, form community connections, and organize what people do. In recognizing the centrality of occupation for humans, occupational therapists and occupational scientists have begun to advocate that societies define and protect occupational rights. Proposed rights include rights to meaningful occupational engagement, enrichment and growth through occupational engagement, choice, control, and autonomy around occupational engagement, and balanced occupational engagement with neither too much nor too little to do over a lifetime and in particular circumstances. An occupational perspective and occupational rights will, *and should*, look and be described in different languages and be experienced differently depending on the site, setting, and specific sociocultural and political milieus (Iwama 2003, 2005, Jarman 2010). Consistent with a stance of critical reflexivity on difference and inclusion, we emphasize here the complex and interconnected weave of structural factors in society that enable and preclude participation in occupations of meaning, necessity, and obligation.

Clearly, the POJF 2010 guides practice and knowledge exchange that extends beyond occupational therapy processes for enabling components of individual occupational performance, a professional focus we argue has hitherto delimited the social contribution of occupational therapy. Occupational therapy's historic roots in activism and social reform through occupational engagement are most visible on the margins since the profession aligned itself with medicine with its emphasis on the biomedical functions and structures of the body. Occupational therapists have complied with structures that have truncated our ability to work within a collectivist orientation to understanding and addressing the social and economic determinants of occupational participation by communities and populations (Wilding & Whiteford 2007a, Yerxa 1992).

Enabling and enablement: how professionals practice

In addition to the focus on occupation, everyday practice following the POJF 2010 is distinguished by culturally attuned, participatory, collaborative enabling approaches, sometimes described using the noun *enablement* (Polatajko 2001, Townsend & Landry 2004, Townsend et al 2007a). An enabling approach means that practitioners employ participatory, empowerment-oriented methods of working in partnership with people and organizations – what the occupational therapy profession has described for over 25 years as client-centered practice contrasted with profession-expert, prescriptive practice (Canadian Association of Occupational Therapists (CAOT) 1991, 1993, 1998/2002, Townsend & Polatajko 2007). There are many complex, problematic tensions in the governance and power relations of client-centered practice (Townsend et al 2003). As well, the linguistic standpoint is troublesome in that the term *client* is not universally applicable (especially cross-culturally) and it has a commercial orientation. Although client has been used in occupational therapy literature to emphasize a relationship based on collaboration, we refer hereafter in this chapter to person-centered practice with communities or populations, consistent with the philosophy underpinning critical occupational therapy.

Enabling may be oriented to change with individuals, or to social change with families, groups, communities, organizations, or populations (Townsend et al 2007b, c), although the POJF 2010 focuses most on practice with communities and populations. Enabling as an approach and core occupational therapy competency is complex because enabling approaches encompass an array of participatory practices that differ in different contexts. Importantly, enabling approaches favor partnership over autocratic, hierarchical relationships. Accordingly, a collaborative, enabling approach *with* communities and populations is ideologically and politically aligned with notions of participatory citizenship. Requisite to enabling approaches is a transparency and sharing of decision making responsibilities and risks, and public accountability for negotiated outcomes.

Enabling approaches are recognized in occupational therapy as being on an enablement continuum: ineffective enablement that reinforces addictive or co-dependent behavior, including dependence on professionals, is at the opposite end from effective enablement that fosters empowerment and transformative change (Townsend & Polatajko 2007, p. 83–171). With ineffective enablement, good intentions may go astray or actually do harm if well-meaning practitioners take over where collaborative planning, decision making, and evaluation should prevail. Ineffective enablement is displayed when practitioners assume to know best without consultation with those involved, or put policies, protocols, and other governance structures in place that prescribe standards without listening and learning what will work in a particular sociocultural context with a particular population. With effective enablement, individuals, communities or populations are full partners in enabling occupational justice.

Occupational justice – why occupational therapists enable occupation

The vision underpinning occupational therapists' concern for occupation and the use of enabling approaches appears to be an implicit or expressed commitment to everyday justice, specifically social inclusion in the occupations of a society. Concerns for occupational justice are likely implicit and unconsciously underpinning occupational therapy when the implied or stated goals and objectives are to increase their participation in everyday occupations (Townsend & Wilcock 2004). Explicit, immediate concerns may be to enable a person's desired body function and organizational skills to improve self-care, but the implicit purpose of occupational therapy should differ from physiotherapy or other body-function professions, and should enable persons to participate equitably in occupations as a valued member of society. Other immediate, explicit concerns may be to make local environmental changes, such as installing a ramp for wheelchair use or to negotiate with an employer to introduce routine 'time out' for stress management. The implicit purpose in both examples should differ from the carpenter's interest in building ramps and the psychological consultant's interest in stress management. The occupational therapists' purpose in both examples would be to enable environmental change, i.e., social change, to structure opportunities, resources and privileges that would enable socially excluded persons to participate more equitably in occupations as valued members of society.

Conversely, occupational justice is occupational therapy's implied social vision when the consequences of *not* providing occupational therapy are restricted participation and social exclusion, for instance, when people are unable to find employment while being dependent on others for self-care, wheelchair lifting, or stress management. Occupational therapists would implicitly recognize the values, beliefs and assumptions that occupation is necessary to human existence and it seems to be injustice to deny people the right to experience meaning, growth, choice, autonomy, and equitable privileges with others to participate in occupations.

Clearly, one of the most significant outcomes in working toward occupational justice would be the achievement of an occupationally just world – that is to say, greater equity worldwide for everyone to choose and participate to their potential in their desired occupations (Townsend & Wilcock 2004, Wilcock & Townsend 2000). Although occupational therapists are fairly new at using the language of justice or rights, we know that injustice exists in everyday life when participation is barred, confined, segregated, prohibited, undeveloped, disrupted, alienated, marginalized, exploited, or otherwise devalued for some more than others (Townsend 2003b). It follows that enabling occupational justice, as a matter of social inclusion, extends beyond enabling individual wellbeing to enabling more equitable opportunity, resources, privilege, and occupational rights.

Importantly, at the level of internationally accepted nomenclature, the framing or construction of the concept and practice of occupational injustice is congruent with positions on human and civil rights expressed for over 60 years by the United Nations and the WHO, including the WHO ICF (WHO 2001). Occupational therapists have expressed a profession-wide concern for justice by profiling the concept of participation restrictions in the 2006 statement on human rights by the WFOT.

Alignment of language, ideas, and philosophy: occupational justice and critical reflexivity

In framing occupation, enabling, and justice as pillars of occupational therapy knowledge, there are consequences for the profession; one of the most important is the requirement to interrogate the alignment between occupational therapy epistemological foundations, the stated philosophy, and the profession's enactment of these foundations in society. In other words, we need to critically consider whether what we think, say, and do is consistent with what we believe. This requires more than mere reflection; it requires critical reflexivity.

Reflexivity has been defined (Sandywell 1996) as the 'act of interrogating interpretive systems' (p. xiv). In reflexivity, things are understood as significations, that is, as the outcome of social and cultural constructions. In considering the need for critical reflexivity in occupational therapy and other fields, the work of Bourdieu (Bourdieu & Wacquant 1992) is particularly salient. His term *epistemic reflexivity* was developed in order to denote critical reflection on the social conditions under which disciplinary knowledge comes into being and gains credence. Enacting epistemic reflexivity within a discipline or profession, such as occupational therapy, means identifying and understanding how social traditions and prevailing discourses contribute to knowledge construction over time. The focus of epistemic reflexivity is to do the detective work within the discipline or profession, to consider the invisible assumptions underpinning everyday theorizing and practice, and from this location to interrogate what exists and what may be possible.

What might this critical, reflexive approach mean when considering occupational justice? Considering whether occupational justice is, in fact, fundamental as a guiding philosophy and knowledge foundation in everyday practice is an important starting point. Certainly the extent to which the occupational therapy knowledge base is informed by relevant research is important and in this respect we would argue that, while other sciences, including the biologic, managerial, social and psychological sciences, inform occupational therapy, occupational science is fundamental to the profession's knowledge and practice developments. Interestingly, a science of occupation is still not universally accepted as being the most important science underpinning occupational therapy practice of enabling occupation; this is perhaps reflective of the broader social reality in which basic sciences (and in the case of occupational therapy, biomedical sciences in particular) are reified or privileged in institutions and discourses (Whiteford & Wilcock 2001).

The problem associated with biomedical science being accorded greater status than occupational science and occupational therapy knowledge is that a disconnect occurs. One cannot simultaneously prioritize both biologic needs and occupational needs. Each will predicate actions that may be entirely incompatible. In health institutions, such as hospitals and clinics, it is most often the occupational needs that are neglected. This has been highlighted by Wilding in an action research study that considered how the everyday practices and language usage of a group of occupational therapists in a hospital served to reinforce the dominant biomedical paradigm rather than enable autonomous decision making about occupational issues (Kinsella & Whiteford 2009, Wilding & Whiteford 2007b). The neglect of occupation – occupational therapists' core domain of concern (WHAT we know) – is reflective of attendant power dynamics which shape HOW occupational therapists attempt to enable occupational participation, and WHY our vision of occupational justice has global implications. Not only is there neglect of occupational issues, occupational therapists may not explicitly profile our broad spectrum of enablement skills, and practitioners without an explicitly stated and documented occupational focus may be unaware of why this profession might be included in organizations and in interactions with other professions and the public. A lack of critical, reflexive engagement on behalf of the profession (as suggested previously), tends to reinforce and further entrench occupational therapists' long-standing, institutional dynamics as an 'allied health profession' dependent on medical sponsorship (Wilding & Whiteford 2007a).

As well as the politics of governance and power within institutions and between professional groups, there are also power relations and a politics of power in occupational therapy's relations with individuals, families, groups, communities, organizations or populations (Byrne 1999, Deegan 1997, Kronenberg et al 2005). When any professionals, including occupational therapists, structure programs and implement and evaluate them, careful attention is needed to the negotiation of power. We note that occupational therapists' and occupational scientists' conception of occupational justice as a concern for

social inclusion taking difference into account is necessarily aligned with postmodern interests in multiple perspectives, distributed and collaborative power, diversity, and critiques of universal theories (Habermas 1995, Kuhn 1989, Rolfe 2001).

A participatory occupational justice framework (POJF 2010)

Highlights of the POJF 2010

As Table 8.1 illustrates, occupational justice is contrasted yet aligned with social justice. Occupational justice is distinguished by a concern for inclusive, embodied participation in the real-life occupations that people decide are necessary or meaningful for them; and by the optimistic vision of possible societies in which all populations have *equitable opportunity*, *resources*, *privilege*, and *occupational rights* for meaningful, occupational engagement. These concerns differ from distributive justice concerns for equal access to and distribution of services, goods or equal pay for equal work, and restorative justice concerns for fair compensation for harm against persons or society and the rehabilitation of those identified as offenders.

To make occupational justice explicit in everyday, professional practice, we introduced the POJF in the first edition of this book and have updated the chapter to incorporate critical reflexivity and updated literature. The POJF 2010 (Fig. 8.2) makes occupational justice explicit in the occupational therapy tradition of ongoing naming and framing of practice processes (Polatajko 1992). This framework uses the language and ideology of collaborative, occupational enablement that is gaining international, occupational therapy and occupational science usage (CAOT 1998/2002, Kinsella & Whiteford 2009, Law et al 2002, Polatajko 1992, Townsend 2003b, Townsend & Landry 2004, Townsend & Polatajko 2007, Townsend & Wilcock 2004, Whiteford & Wilcock 2001, Whiteford & Wright 2005, Wilcock & Townsend 2000, Wilding & Whiteford 2007a, b). This POJF 2010 draws on the 2007 guidelines for *Enabling Occupation II: Advancing a Vision of Health, Well-being and Justice Through Occupation* (Townsend & Polatajko 2007), particularly the Canadian Practice Process Framework (CPPF) (p. 174–272), and the Canadian Model of Client-Centred Enablement (CMCE) (p. 88–171).

Table 8.1 Concepts of justice

| | Social justice | | | Occupational justice |
	Procedural	Distributive	Restorative	Participatory
Concerns	Processes of dispute resolution	Having or acquisition	Repair or renewal	Meaningful engagement in valued, chosen occupations
Contested Terrain	Equality of voice, unequal human and financial resources	Measurement and comparison of assets and deficiencies of social groups	Credibility of perpetrators and victims, measurement of damage and fair compensation of goods or rights	Occupational classification; social versus economic value of occupations, competing needs for opportunities and resources
Aims	Equal voice and procedural rights	Equal rights to and equal responsibility for goods, services, privileges	Restoration of perpetrators, restitution to victims	Enablement of different opportunities and resources, taking differences into account in social structures
Issues of power	Individual defendants and prosecutors to be heard without bias	All social groups to have equal advantages for participation in daily life	Individual defendants to be exonerated, individual or class victims to be compensated	Different opportunities and resources to enable full citizen participation by all individuals, families and social groups
Actions for justice	Equal procedural processes	Equal distribution or allocation	Confession of guilt, compensation to victims	Enablement of difference for social inclusion

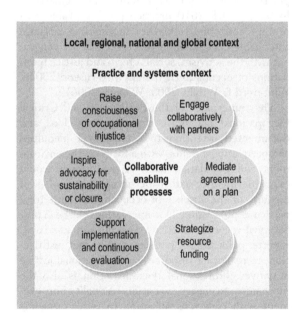

Fig. 8.2 • Participatory occupational justice framework (POJF 2010)

Although it was designed with occupational therapists in mind, the POJF 2010 may be used by any professional interested in practice with a commitment to advance occupational justice. Vertical shading with the left darker than the right in each process circle in Figure 8.2 implies a partnership: professionals will practice in a collaborative instead of a traditional, hierarchical professional relationship with persons who are members of communities or populations. The POJF 2010 names professional opportunities, responsibilities, and power relations in enabling occupational justice. Although there are mutual opportunities and responsibilities for all partners in collaborative practice, the occupational therapist has a professional, ethical, moral, civic, and financial responsibility – and opportunity – to enable individual and/or social change when funding is committed to include a professional, such as an occupational therapist.

In describing justice as a social vision of occupational therapy and of the POJF 2010, we emphasize community development and population approaches, occupational participation, and, inter alia, a constant vigilance to power and inequity in everyday life. Use of an occupational justice lens stretches professional practice beyond individualized, technical or instrumental goals (i.e., goals for improving individual body function, using technical supports). This means taking into account in setting goals the presence of power, social structures, and important differences between groups in a range of contexts, rather than attempting to set goals that standardize and universalize what everyone does in life or in a service context (Stadnyk et al 2010, Townsend 2003a, Townsend & Wilcock 2004, Wilcock 2006, Wilcock & Townsend 2000, 2009).

The POJF 2010 (see Figure 8.2) is portrayed as a circle of interconnected processes for enabling collaborative planning, evaluation, and decision making. The circle of collaborative enabling processes in Figure 8.2 is embedded and interconnected within a Practice and Systems Context that refers to such processes as staffing, professional frames of reference and scope of practice, professional regulation, interprofessional power relations, labor unions, ethics, workloads, budgets, protocols, policies, accountability, and liability. Processes identified with a practice and systems context are, in turn, embedded and interconnected within the local, regional, national and global context of economic policies, public and private control of education, health and social network supports, sociocultural beliefs, habits and routines, telecommunications and transportation, industry standards, primary resource policies, and more.

While the processes are nonlinear, the typical starting point for a professional is to become conscious and raise consciousness in others of occupational injustice. The typical closing process for professionals is to inspire advocacy for collaborative decision making about sustainability or closure of professional relationships or of programs and services. The other four processes are typical in program planning, implementation and evaluation, except for naming key enablement skills in collaborating, mediating, supporting, and inspiring advocacy. While resource finding is typically not distinguished as a process separate from planning, finding new or reorganized economic and human resources is an essential departure from occupational therapists' tendency of making do with very little within existing systems even when resources are available for other professions or projects. Processes may be repeated or adjusted as needed depending on where practice starts, partner readiness, resource conditions, and other factors. The essence of enabling occupational justice is enabling change in everyday occupations through engagement in everyday occupations for doing justice reflexively in local, global, and practice contexts.

POJF 2010 processes are named to profile six key enablement skills that are markers of collaborative partnerships informed by a vision of occupational justice (Table 8.2): raise consciousness, engage

Table 8.2 Enablement skills profiled in the participatory occupational justice framework

Six enablement skills profiled in the participatory occupational justice framework (POJF 2010)
Raise consciousness of occupational injustices
Engage collaboratively with partners
Mediate agreement on a plan
Strategize resource finding
Support implementation and continuous evaluation of the plan
Inspire advocacy for sustainability or closure

collaboratively, mediate, strategize, support, and inspire advocacy. The POJF 2010 is intended for use by professionals enabling occupation with individuals, families, groups, communities, organizational, or populations (Townsend & Polatajko 2007): the emphasis in this chapter and in enabling occupational justice is on working with communities and populations, recognizing that an occupational justice practice may begin with individuals. Questions for each POJF 2010 practice process (Table 8.3) prompt epistemic reflexivity in choosing language and enablement skills for processes that are congruent with the activism, social reform and justice foundations of occupational therapy (Townsend 2003b, Whiteford & Wright 2005, Wilcock 2006).

The centerpiece of the POJF 2010 and Critical Occupational Therapy is the overt, conscious, and documented attention to occupational inequities and occupational rights, with a focus on the environment and population data. A practitioner would explicitly identify and name occupational issues of inequity or the absence of occupational rights for a particular population. Documentation may be in professional records, practice protocols and standards, reports, publications, policies, and budget justifications to reallocate resources for occupational justice initiatives. Professional documentation is also the mechanism to engage in continuous quality improvement with conscious attention to reduce ongoing injustice: e.g., to document narrative and statistical data on injustice, to communicate with all partners in all processes, to chart the resources used or sought, and to visually profile responses to the plan and the evaluation of outcomes from multiple standpoints. One would also document occupational injustice in publicly accessible forms, using

Table 8.3 Critical occupational therapy practice processes, reflexivity and power relations in a participatory occupational justice framework (POJF 2010)

Practice Processes	Critical Reflexivity and Attention to Power Relations
Non-linear & interrelated processes between Start and Conclude	
Raise consciousness of occupational injustices	Become aware of occupational injustice as a concern for social inclusion in everyday life: Is a particular community or population inequitably excluded from participating in typical occupations? What forms of consciousness raising are culturally appropriate? What forms of early collaboration will include those with diverse perspectives in raising consciousness of occupational injustice? How is social exclusion experienced as an everyday, embodied injustice? Alienation, hopelessness, or meaningless? Being overoccupied with too much to do or underoccupied with too little to do? Prolonged occupational deprivation? Marginalization? Persistent and historical dependence in daily life occupations? Occupational segregation etc.? What documentation is being created to illustrate and make publicly explicit injustices in everyday occupations in a particular context for a particular population? What is the knowledge transfer or mutual knowledge exchange strategy? How will narratives and other data on injustice be accessible to others, e.g., website, brochures, reports?
Engage collaboratively with partners	Respond to a request, referral, contract offer, or other arrangement, or initiate a partnership: What population or community is of central concern, and what issues have sparked a link with occupational therapy? How ready are all partners to participate, and how resilient do they hope to be for the process? What conflicting and congruent beliefs, values, cultural, and power issues need attention? What education, mediation, or negotiations will actively show respect for the worth, dignity, and rights of all? How will the designated client and other partners participate, e.g., by verbal interaction, written documents, third party reports, nonverbal expression in photographs and other objects, talking circles, focus groups? What documentation is being created? How will the partnership and agreed justice frameworks be documented? What is the knowledge translation and knowledge exchange strategy? How will all partners exchange knowledge in talking or documenting the agreement, e.g., in writing, a poster, a contract, health record, community agreement?
Mediate agreement on a plan	Mediate a plan based on collaborative partnership: What goals, objectives and outcomes will be targeted and how will the underlying occupational justice issues be communicated? What programs or services would have the greatest collective impact to reduce occupational injustice for a group, community, or population? What programs/services are needed and possible – goals, objectives, locations, times, action-based, occupational, participatory approaches? What education on occupational injustice needs to be included to engage the population, public, or government in recognizing occupational injustice as a serious issue? What evaluation and documentation is needed to demonstrate program/service accountability to the population, professionals, and funders? How will the design be participatory and involve engagement in occupations? How participatory (all partners involved equally) is the process of setting goals, objectives and designing the program and its evaluation? How does the program and evaluation plan incorporate qualitative and quantitative methods, e.g., narratives, self-reflection, self-monitoring, peer evaluation, surveys, measures of change What types of documentation will communicate the plan to interested parties? What is the knowledge transfer and mutual knowledge exchange strategy in the plan?

Continued

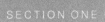

Table 8.3 Critical occupational therapy practice processes, reflexivity and power relations in a participatory occupational justice framework (POJF 2010)—cont'd

Practice Processes	Critical Reflexivity and Attention to Power Relations
Strategize resource finding	Linked with mediating agreement on a plan, find human, financial, space and other resources: Who will advocate for human and financial resources and what are the funding options? What forum, method, database or other documentation will identify potential population, nonprofessional, and professional resources? What government, corporate, or philanthropic financial resources are available? What qualitative, quantitative, and critical analysis methods are available? What education is needed to identify and confirm resources? What are priority occupational performance, spiritual and environmental issues, strengths, resources and challenges for the population or social groups of concern? What enabling processes have been used to support population, community, policy, or other changes? What is occupational therapy's contribution worldwide as a human resource, and what might occupational therapists learn through partnerships with others in enabling occupational justice? How might occupational therapists coordinate our work with efforts by the population, lay persons, governments, businesses, and other professionals? How will all resources be documented and evaluated? How will documentation confirm available resources? What is the knowledge translation and knowledge exchange strategy to let others know about resource opportunities and restrictions?
Support implementation and continuous evaluation of the plan	Integrate professional and partner approaches to achieve the partners' desired results: How are the partners enabling change in occupations through occupational engagement? How are occupations being simulated, for instance in an occupational therapy simulated kitchen, garden or industrial area for adults or a play area for children? How is the translation of simulation learning into real-life supported by professional or non-professional helpers? How does the population collaborate in decision making about strategies for continuous evaluation? How is a 'learning through doing' philosophy explicitly used and understood by all partners? How will the impact of services be monitored throughout from population, professional, management, and other perspectives? What formative evaluation processes and data are feasible and useful? What summative evaluation data display whether or not the goals and objectives in the mediated plan are being met for enabling occupational justice? What qualitative evidence, such as narratives or images, suggests a change in occupational injustice, if any? What quantitative evidence indicates whether change was achieved? What documentation will enable partners, including funders and managers to track progress and points of contention?
Inspire advocacy for sustainability or closure	Inspire advocacy with or for partners to sustain or end the mediated plan and renegotiate or end the professional relationship: How might professionals inspire advocacy with and for the partners? What decisions would guide advocacy for sustainability or closure? What is the perception of success and lessons learned for each partner? What empowerment strategies might professionals inspire to positively conclude professional involvement and end the professional relationship? What conditions might warrant termination or renegotiation of professional involvement? What will be the documented legacy of the referral, contract or project? What will be visible and traceable beyond professional records and in professional records? How will the occupational justice service involving occupational therapy be known by others? What will be the documented legacy of the referral, contract or project, and how would sustainability or closure be documented? What knowledge translation or knowledge exchange strategies would communicate plans for sustainability or closure with targeted audiences?

posters, brochures, YouTube postings, websites, theatre, music, visual arts, and other arts-based media. One could raise attention to population experiences of occupational injustice by inviting narratives and posting blogs on Facebook, MSN, or other social networking sites, or news about injustice on Twitter exchanges and email, where people can discuss their experiences and possibilities for change.

Although practice processes in the POJF 2010 may seem familiar to many occupational therapists, a critical occupational therapy practice would diverge from general occupational therapy, as described at the beginning of the chapter, by critical reflexivity to challenge practice and systems where there is a gap between the vision of enabling occupational justice and the everyday practices, protocols, standards, policies, laws or funding that govern practice.

Raise consciousness of occupational injustice

A foundational process toward enabling occupational justice is to raise awareness of occupational injustice as a concern for social inclusion in everyday life. The aims, issues of power and actions to address occupational injustice and the absence of occupational rights are about *enablement of different participation* in economic and social occupations regardless of ability, age, gender, race, sexual orientation, social class, or other difference. Critical questions to enable consciousness raising might be (Table 8.3): Is a particular community or population inequitably excluded from participating in typical occupations? What forms of consciousness raising are culturally appropriate? What forms of early collaboration will include those with diverse perspectives in raising consciousness of occupational injustice? How is social exclusion experienced? Does the population experience exclusion as alienation, hopelessness, or meaningless in what they are expected to do, or is the experience of life so imbalanced that the population is overoccupied with too much to do or underoccupied with too little to do? Does the population experience exclusion through prolonged occupational deprivation because of isolation or poverty? Is a population marginalized without access, for instance, to participate in civic, leisure, employment, or other occupations? Is the population persistently and historically dependent on others in daily life occupations, such as disabled persons and seniors? Or is there a conscious

occupational segregation, possibly for economic and political reasons – meaning that some community members participate in the occupations they choose and define as meaningful or useful, while others in the same geographic, social, cultural, and political context are politically or legally restricted from such opportunities? Who dominates community occupations and who is not present or is sitting on the sidelines in community occupations? What communities have bountiful resources to enable everyone to participate to their potential, and what communities struggle to provide shelter and basic living structures?

Professionals with little time and without a mandate for community- or population-based practice might reflect on their professional values, beliefs, and visions of justice, and begin naming the tensions and gaps they experience in trying to stay true to their ideals to make a difference in people's everyday lives. A critical practice would generate relentless optimism with those involved about the possibility of an occupationally just world, and employ enablement skills to consult with, educate and engage everyone as appropriate to be alert to collaborative negotiation; enablement would advocate to focus on adapting or changing the environment (context), and coordinate with others to target occupational outcomes and to change unjust structures that regulate what people do.

Questions for professionals might be, for instance, about the occupational rights to play safely and learn for all children, the occupational rights to engage in meaningful employment and civic life for all adults including disabled or chronically ill adults, or the occupational rights to make choices and experience autonomy and balance in leisure, employment, and community participation for older people. Professionals can start to enable occupational justice by actively listening to the individuals and groups with whom they work, and meet with representatives of populations to listen to narratives of everyday life. In some situations, professionals may supplement their experience by scanning websites that provide population data on employment, housing, leisure, child development, or retirement opportunities.

Professionals with a planning or research mandate might investigate social indicators or contextual forces that appear to cause occupational injustice. To analyze occupational injustice in collaboration with partners, one would combine micro, meso, and macro data on occupational participation. Micro data (measurements, stories, documents) on individual or group occupational performance can be used with meso data on community, family, or friendship (reports, stories, etc.), and with macro data (often statistical tables, policies, laws, regulations, etc.) on cultural, social, geographic, economic, political or other conditions.

One might collaborate with partners on a community needs assessment, or an environmental scan of employment (by ability, age, or gender and type of employment), or an analysis of housing/homelessness, education, gender, health services, social or community services. The analysis could examine the economic infrastructure, such as the availability of small loans programs to start a business or to address poverty and marginalization. It is important to analyze population-based data both for population-based practice and as a background for considering individual or family client-specific issues. To fully understand whether or not these data signal injustice, one would expand quantitative and qualitative data collection, for instance to gather narratives about participation in occupations. We caution readers that it is important to determine boundaries to delimit the amount of data to be synthesized in examining social indicators.

One imperative in raising consciousness is to record what is known about a community or population experiences of occupational injustice. Naming and documenting issues with reference to occupational injustice may be appropriate in some settings and require translation in others. Ways of naming occupational injustice are evolving along with the theory of occupational justice and the naming of occupational rights (Table 8.4). Individual occupational injustice issues may be named occupational alienation, deprivation, marginalization, or imbalance. However, occupational injustice is essentially a population issue resulting from structures that routinely produce these experiences. Beyond these four examples, one might consider naming other issues of occupational injustices, such as occupational discrimination, occupational isolation, or occupational victimization or violence. Professionals would engage in critical reflexivity with populations to consider culturally appropriate ways of naming and documenting occupational injustice.

Documentation would be done with a knowledge transfer or mutual knowledge exchange strategy in mind, particularly using language to clearly explain occupation, enabling, and justice to those outside occupational therapy. One can ask: Do professional records alert others about occupational injustice?

Table 8.4 Naming and documenting occupational injustice

Individual occupational	Population-based occupational
Alienation	Alienation
Confusion	Apartheid
Deprivation	Deprivation
Disengagement	Discrimination
Disorientation	Displacement
Dysfunction	Exclusion
Disruption	Imbalance
Dissatisfaction	Isolation
Exclusion	Oppression
Imbalance	Marginalization
Inability/incapacity	Victimization/violence
Isolation	Other?
Loss or recovery	
Underdevelopment	
Other?	

Have narratives or images of occupational injustice been documented in the creative and performing arts – plays, posters, paintings, sculpture, poetry, novels? Whiteford illustrates the process of her own and others' consciousness raising about occupational injustice by gathering multiple forms of data about HIV/AIDS and Grandmothers Against AIDS and Poverty (GAPA) in South Africa (Box 8.1).

Engage collaboratively with partners

Engaging collaboratively with partners may be to respond to a request, referral, contract offer or other arrangement, or to initiate a partnership. Collaborative enablement means that professionals may be neither the primary leaders nor the dominant force in forming a partnership. Key to negotiating engagement with partners is naming concerns to make a difference beyond the level of the individual. Also key in engaging collaboratively with partners is a mutual process of

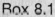

Box 8.1

Collaborating with partners to raise consciousness and analyze occupational injustices: grandmothers against poverty and AIDS partnering, facilitating, and handing over

Whiteford: The first time I went to South Africa I heard a group of women speak so movingly and powerfully that I wanted to find out more about them and their story: this was the Grandmothers Against AIDS and Poverty (GAPA). What I found out in a subsequent visit where I was privileged to meet and interview some of the founding members in the town of Khayelitsha outside of Cape Town South Africa, was that it is a story of transformation. It is also a story illustrative of critical occupational therapy.

South Africa is a country devastated by the HIV AIDS epidemic. Statistically it is the region most affected in the world with an estimated 22.5 million people being infected and, in 2007 alone, 1.7 million people were newly infected (UNAIDS 2007). This is compounded by the fact that 80% of people don't know they are HIV positive; in sub-Saharan Africa only 12% of men and 10% of women have been tested and collected the results of their tests (WHO 2001). One of the particularly tragic outcomes of the HIV/AIDS epidemic has been the number of children orphaned each year. According to WHO's formal definition, an AIDS orphan is one who has had either a mother or both parents die from AIDS before they turn 15 – estimates are that globally the number will reach 41 million by 2010 and 90% are currently in sub-Saharan Africa (WHO 2001). Women, as the major caregivers, particularly carry the burden of this devastating phenomenon which has both economic and social impacts.

GAPA's story is set against this backdrop of hardship and alienation and relative to the HIV/AIDS orphans scenario. Founded in 2001 by Alicia Mdaka in conjunction with occupational therapist Katherine Broderick and a number of other grandmothers, GAPA was established as a response to the impoverishment and burden experienced by the grandmothers in caring for their grandchildren and the stigma of having had their children die from HIV/AIDS. They created a small business through which craft items made by the women were sold, thus providing a means of income generation and addressing the double structural injustices of poverty and stigmatization directly through grass roots action. In this respect, occupational therapist Katherine Broderick worked actively and directly to mobilize resources, to facilitate skills development including everything from small business skills to communication and negotiation and educational skills. She worked in **partnership with the women**, using a number of enablement processes including advocacy, group facilitation, and lobbying to assist the women grow, develop and take ownership of the organization. She, as I understand it, purposefully kept herself out of the growing attention to and profiling of GAPA in the media nationally and internationally, which culminated in several members being invited to speak at international conferences – a transformation of status of real and lasting significance.

GAPA, however, is not just a story of income generation possibilities, it is also a site of participatory citizenship at work in that it has also constituted a supportive space for the women: many have faced prejudice and social stigma because of their connection to HIV/AIDS and it is estimated that to date, more than 900 grandmothers have been involved in the project. The women have developed a community garden, growing and preparing nutritious food, provided HIV/AIDS education sessions and free condoms, and provided childcare and after-school care facilities to support other mothers in the town. They run a number of shops and service a number of contracts – when I was there, the women explained that they were making teddy bears for a Norwegian design company. Over time, Katherine Broderick tailored her input and reduced her influence on the directions and development of GAPA and there is now a business manager, Vivienne, and an independent governance structure inclusive of a board. GAPA is a vibrant, sustainable organization making a real difference in the face of injustice and disadvantage at many levels.

---

critical reflexivity to uncover commonalities and differences in the values, beliefs, assumptions, and frameworks through which partners understand justice and injustice. Professional frames of reference, such as occupational therapists' biomechanical, psychosocial, neurodevelopment, cognitive-perceptual, and other professional frames of reference, would need to be integrated with the frameworks of beliefs and values of indigenous populations and other partners, always asking how frameworks would make occupational injustice issues explicit.

Documentation of mutually agreed terms of the referral, contract, or partnership is essential to ensure clarity and understanding. Although documentation would need to be done by professionals in their practice documents, a point of departure for the POJF 2010 and critical occupational therapy is that all participating partners, not just professionals, would be engaged in documentation using their own methods in their own records. Public forms of documentation noted in the 'Highlights of the POJF 2010' above include websites, theatre, music, and visual arts as well as dialogues using the many communication tools available in the twenty-first century.

Occupational therapists might facilitate engagement with partners by asking open-ended questions (see Table 8.3), such as: What population or community is of central concern, and what issues have sparked a link with occupational therapy? How ready are all partners to participate, and how resilient do they hope to be for the process, notably how ready and resilient are occupational therapists? What conflicting and congruent beliefs, values, cultural, and power issues need attention? What education, mediation, or negotiations will actively show respect for the worth, dignity, and rights of all? How will the designated client and other partners participate, e.g., by verbal interaction, written documents, third-party reports, nonverbal expression in photographs and other objects, talking circles, focus groups? Is there a knowledge translation or knowledge exchange strategy to communicate with the partners and to tell others about the partnership and the focus on occupational injustice?

Mediate agreement on a plan

Sound program design is based on setting broad goals as well as specific behavioral objectives that can be evaluated qualitatively, quantitatively, or both. To mediate a plan based on consciousness raising and collaborative partnership, critically reflexive questions might start with (see Table 8.3): What goals, objectives and outcomes will be targeted and how will the underlying occupational justice issues be communicated? What programs or services would have the greatest, collective impact to reduce occupational injustice for a community or population? What programs or services are needed and possible – goals, objectives, locations, times, action-based, occupational, participatory approaches? What education on occupational injustices needs to be included to engage the population, public or government in recognizing occupational injustice as a serious issue? What evaluation and documentation is needed to demonstrate program or service accountability to the population, professionals, and funders? How will the design be participatory and involve engagement in occupations? How participatory (all partners involved equally) is the process of setting goals, objectives and designing the program and its evaluation? How does the program and evaluation plan incorporate qualitative and quantitative methods,

e.g., narratives, self-reflection, self-monitoring, peer evaluation, surveys, measures of change. What are the documentation and knowledge translation and exchange strategies to ensure that the plan is accessible and known by all who have or need to have an interest in it?

The plan would be documented in writing or through other visual media as appropriate. Ideally plans would be documented in multiple forms for knowledge exchange with diverse audiences. The plan presented to a community or population may be written in multiple languages, or presented using culturally understood images whereas the same plan might be sent to funders and managers in a highly professionalized format. One version of a documented plan may highlight a few key points for the public, whereas another version might include data charts, population stories of injustice, and an integrated model for service delivery.

To develop evidence-based programs, the partners would consider diverse forms of qualitative, critical (structural), and quantitative evidence. Attention to occupational justice issues may arouse interest if the proposal is action-based for 'learning through doing' by involving people as participants and active agents in addressing the injustice they experience. Look, for example, at the interest aroused by Simo-Algado et al (1997, 2002) who engaged child survivors of the war in Kosovo in healing processes using creative occupations, such as doing puppetry and becoming street clowns and artists. Population proposals may succeed best if goals, objectives and concepts relate not only to practical matters in daily life, but to the cultural, aesthetic and spiritual concerns of the community.

If a program or service already exists, the partners could examine how the program actually addresses occupational injustice. One enabling strategy could be to survey participants and ask what outcomes they believe would make the most difference in gaining equitable opportunity and resources for them to participate to their potential in society. Or one could visit and observe them to determine and document their occupational possibilities and barriers. To address occupational injustice, managers could examine, critique, and reformulate the data that are required or useful to demonstrate program accountability. To guide continuing education, professionals could examine their knowledge, skills, and competence to work using an occupational justice framework. Townsend illustrates the process of mediating agreement on a plan with partners in a primary health care community health centre (Box 8.2).

Box 8.2

Mediating agreement on plans in a small urban, resource-challenged community health center

Townsend: Planning is a common professional process, but mediating agreement by multiple partners on plans to address occupational injustice requires special attention to partners' diverse values, beliefs, and assumptions about what will be most helpful. One recent project has been with a resource-challenged, small urban community within a medium-sized city. Individual occupational performance assessments have been done with a sample of persons identified as patients/clients of a community health center. Using the COPM, pre- and postprogramming assessments have documented perceptions of change in identified occupational performance issues, such as 'need to improve lifeskills for living in the community after incarceration' and 'want to take off weight and get more involved in the community' to reverse the negative health effects of obesity. These individual issues are also population issues, exacerbated by social conditions. For example, incarceration utilizes occupational deprivation as a form of punishment. Restorative justice supports the rehabilitation of offenders as a principle, yet professional rehabilitation efforts are severely restrained by concerns for safety that limit access to knives, internet searching, and other life skills experiences. The individual COPM scores are like canaries in a mine. We are alerted by working with individuals that incarceration systems may need to protect the public, but in doing so they may perpetuate the lack of life skills of those who run afoul of the law. The community center has a partnership with the university occupational therapy program to plan, implement and evaluate a primary healthcare, occupation-based program to address inequities in occupational transitions and other occupational issues. Global economics, racism, poverty, and cultural divergence with larger communities in the area are all social determinants of occupational participation. The analysis of occupational injustice supports the community health team to make injustice explicit beyond the physical, mental, and psychological challenges that are on record for the individuals who refer themselves or are referred to the center. One challenge is to find ways to document an analysis of injustice in everyday life that the whole team recognizes. With occupational therapy students and the staff of the community health center, we have designed an occupational therapy service to address the occupational injustices which were assessed in partnership with occupational therapy and the collaborative health team at the community health center. Mediation of an agreement on the plan is a partnership with key leaders of the center, and with a potential funding source that is interested in community outreach. To reach agreement, we are emphasizing the win-win-win-win situation for all – for residents of the community, for the funder to establish community outreach where it matters, for the centre to include occupational therapy in the collaborative community health team, and for students at the university to learn about primary healthcare occupational therapy in a real-life setting.

Strategize resource finding

Resources are such an important force for enabling occupational justice that strategizing to find resources is distinguished as a process on its own in the POJF 2010. Managing funded programs and seeking funds for new programs is not easy in a climate of competition for resources. Nevertheless, occupational therapists who work with population representatives create a powerful partnership for generating innovation and human, financial, space and other resources.

As illustrated in Table 8.3, this process involves asking critically reflexive questions such as: Who will advocate for human and financial resources and what are the funding options? What forum, method, database or other documentation will identify potential population, nonprofessional, and professional resources? What government, corporate or philanthropic financial resources are available? What are the strengths and challenges in current resources? Additionally, one might ask: What qualitative, quantitative, and critical analysis methods are available and respected for analyzing and confirming resources? What are priority occupational performance, spiritual and environmental issues, strengths, resources and challenges for the population or social groups of concern? What enabling processes have been used to support population, community, policy or other changes?

Using the example of occupational therapy as a worldwide human resource (see Table 8.3), occupational therapists may also self-consciously reflect on the following: What is occupational therapy's contribution worldwide as a human resource, and what might occupational therapists learn through partnerships with others in enabling occupational justice? How might we coordinate our work with efforts to advance justice by a population, lay persons, governments, businesses, and other professionals?

Table 8.5 Occupational therapist members of national occupational therapy associations*

Country	OTHR	Country	OTHR	Country	OTHR	Country	OTHR
Argentina	230	France	870	Luxembourg	153	Russia	38
Australia	4674	Georgia	NA	Macau	NA	Singapore	396
Austria	1408	Germany	11812	Malaysia	143	Slovenia	50
Bangladesh	76	Greece	139	Malta	54	South Africa	1155
Belgium	944	Hong Kong	244	Mauritius	8	Spain	560
Bermuda	20	Iceland	233	Mexico	20	Sri Lanka	86
Brazil	260	India	2548	Namibia	NA	Sweden	9466
Canada	7490	Indonesia	100	the Netherlands	3403	Switzerland	1821
Caribbean	25	Iran	100	New Zealand	973	Taiwan, ROC	900
Chile	250	Ireland	312	Nigeria	NA	Tanzania	38
Columbia	300	Israel	850	Norway	3211	Thailand	200
Cyprus	26	Italy	773	Pakistan	34	Uganda	48
Czech Rep.	265	Japan	35 946	Palestine	NA	UK	28 018
Denmark	6490	Jordan	140	Panama, Rep	50	USA	37 740
Estonia	50	Kenya	300	Peru	NA	Venezuela	980
Finland	1948	Korea	1453	Philippines	178	Zimbabwe	10
		Republic of Latvia	100	Portugal	50		

*WFOT Database (2008). Presented are numbers of members of the national occupational therapy associations where WFOT recognizes that occupational therapy education programs meet WFOT minimum educational standards (email correspondence with the WFOT Executive 25 August 2009).
OTHR, occupational therapy human resources (WFOT 2008).

Table 8.5 provides 2008 WFOT data on the growing world supply of occupational therapists. Data gathered by WFOT in 2005–06 for the Occupational Therapy Human Resources Project (WFOT 2008) indicate that access to occupational therapy is highest in Denmark (114 per 100 000) followed by Sweden (104), Iceland (59), Israel (58), Belgium (53), and Australia (50). Resource-rich countries such as Canada (30) and the United States (29) appear to have invested less to date in funding access to occupational therapy services. Denmark's seven occupational therapy programs educate only about 400 new graduates per year, while Canada's 12 educational programs (soon to be 15 with three new Francophone programs in Quebec) graduate around 600 new occupational therapists per year. Australia's seven programs graduate around 700 occupational therapists, and the 149 programs in the US graduate about 5000 occupational therapists. These data suggest that there is a crisis in access to occupational therapy in most countries, and that the retention of practitioners who are nationally recognized as occupational therapists appears to be a major challenge. One hears about crises in access to professions such as medicine, nursing, and pharmacy, yet a crisis to access occupational therapy is monumental despite variations worldwide. Of course population ratios need to be considered in relation to other factors, such as the presence or absence of related services that diminish or expand the need for occupational therapy, or the social, health, and educational systems that determine how a society organizes support networks for those with everyday occupational challenges.

Occupational therapy practitioners may feel that there are overwhelming challenges for enabling occupational justice. Nevertheless, in strategizing to find human resources, this profession might look inward to consider how to improve access to occupational therapists, and particularly to retain graduates who have been educated to make occupational justice explicit. With awareness that occupational therapy faces challenges to build this human resource, the POJF 2010 profiles strategies to mobilize a small, largely female force to make a difference: tapping our tremendous potential for raising consciousness about occupational injustice, engaging collaboratively with partners, mediating agreement on plans, strategizing resource finding, supporting implementation and continuous evaluation of plans, and inspiring advocacy around the sustainability or closure of programs and services.

Support implementation and continuous evaluation

Processes to implement and evaluate occupational therapy services have been described extensively in occupational therapy literature, particularly for individualized programs. We emphasize in the POJF 2010 four important markers associated with enabling the implementation and continuous evaluation of occupational justice plans: occupation is the process of engaging partners in implementing change and evaluating it, and occupation is the targeted outcome of implementation; partners including the designated persons or populations participate in all planning, implementation and evaluation decision making; openness to critique and revise the plan are markers of critical reflexivity in continuous evaluation; and, a strong focus is on evaluating the effects of implementation on changing the environment.

The essence of this process for professionals is to support the integration of professional and partner approaches to achieve the partners' desired results as agreed in the plan. A critically reflective, participatory approach would raise questions (see Table 8.3) such as: How are the partners enabling change in occupations through occupational engagement? How are occupations being simulated, for instance

in an occupational therapy simulated kitchen, garden or industrial area for adults or a play area for children? How is the translation of simulation learning into real life supported by professional or non-professional helpers? How does the population collaborate in decision making about strategies for continuous evaluation? How is a 'learning through doing' philosophy explicitly used and understood by all partners? How will the impact of services be monitored throughout from population, professional, management, and other perspectives?

Continuous evaluation throughout implementation means that evaluation is not a single, discrete process. Nor is conclusion a final, isolated act. Monitoring and evaluation are central to the process of conducting and concluding the partnership. Examples of questions (see Table 8.3) are: What formative evaluation processes and data are feasible and useful? What summative evaluation data display whether or not the goals and objectives in the mediated plan are being met for enabling occupational justice? What qualitative evidence, such as narratives or images, suggests a change in occupational injustice, if any? What quantitative evidence indicates whether change was achieved through implementation of the plan?

Documentation is particularly important for formative and summative evaluation. Formative evaluation with critical reflexivity could track narratives of progress; record challenges and approaches to resolve them; document positive and negative experiences; post revised directions for the plan; and analyze the power dynamics and resources associated with each of the six processes. Summative evaluation with critical reflexivity might challenge survey, narrative or other data. Summative evaluation of outcomes in enabling occupational justice may focus on recording narratives of change (or lack of change); critiquing changes in processes or the context for decision making; or measuring change in participation in occupations that have been targeted in raising consciousness of social exclusion.

Documentation, as in all processes, would be in culturally appropriate forms that may range from professional records to visual images and the use of videos or internet blogs. Partners and others could track progress, milestones, or points of contention. Knowledge translation and knowledge exchange would be a constant process of distributing current news, updates, and data in reports, brochures, posters, websites, Facebook updates, or television interviews. Ideally, there would be diverse knowledge translation strategies in professional and lay language and in multiple formats that are culturally accessible.

Inspire advocacy for sustainability or closure

The process of inspiring advocacy for sustainability or closure is future oriented and visionary, and also critically reflexive. The professional responsibility is to inspire advocacy with or for partners to sustain or end the mediated plan, and to renegotiate or end the professional relationship. Central to the POJF 2010 is the notion that professionals may be catalysts to enable occupational justice and advance occupational rights, although by definition of the funding and mandates for professionals, professional services are a temporary stimulus. In fact, Hammell (2008) reminds us that occupational therapists might consider making occupational rights our signature focus, since occupational therapists are not currently indispensable or always helpful.

Inspire and advocate are combined here as key enablement skills through which professionals would seek to enable others to advocate for their own needs. Inspiring advocacy effectively would, as always, require critical reflexivity of the dangers of ineffective enablement, as highlighted in discussing occupational therapy epistemology above. In inspiring advocacy, professional knowledge translation and exchange would be in partnership with others. Possibly closure would reflect that specific goals and objectives were reached and the program and professionals are no longer needed. Or closure may reflect ongoing consciousness raising and a realization that alternate approaches may be more effective. Critiques of assumptions underlying the three pillars of knowledge (see Fig. 8.1), suggested earlier in this chapter, are necessary to challenge and develop what we think, say and do about occupation, enabling, and justice (Hammell 2009). Funding, professional mandates, and partner perceptions of helpfulness will be factors in deciding whether the partnership may be renewed or extended with or without professionals. Ending the professional relationship is complex to pay attention to emotional ties including dependency, and to address partners' expectations of the professional legacy of involvement. Inspiring advocacy with funding agents to support the partners after professional involvement may be a major factor in sustainability or closure.

Questions to inspire advocacy for sustainability or closure might be (see Table 8.3): How might professionals inspire advocacy with and for the partners? What decisions would guide advocacy for sustainability or closure? What is the perception of success and lessons learned for each partner? What empowerment strategies might professionals inspire to positively conclude professional involvement and end the professional relationship? What conditions might warrant termination or renegotiation of professional involvement?

Professionals will want to attend carefully to their own responsibilities and the expectations of others by asking: What will be the documented legacy of the referral, contract or project? What will be visible and traceable beyond professional records and in professional records? How will the occupational justice service involving occupational therapy be known by others and will the legacy be that of a helpful profession? What public forms of documentation will provide knowledge translation and knowledge exchange opportunities?

Reflections and conclusions

The POJF 2010 is a conceptual tool to guide critical reflexivity around six, nonlinear, interrelated, participatory occupational justice processes for thoughtful utilization and experimentation, not as techniques. One key point in the discussion has been a persistent focus on addressing occupational issues through engagement in occupations. A second key point in the proposed collaborative, enabling processes has been a commitment to make population inequities explicit, work in participatory partnerships with attention to power relations, and focus enablement on changing environment structures, particularly policies and other governance. Our questions arise from a participatory framework which includes community members and population representatives. The third key point has been to name empowerment, social inclusion and participatory citizenship as the ultimate and desirable occupational justice outcomes and as part of longer-term social transformational processes when professionals and partners unite to address occupational injustice.

Although analyses of occupational injustice will differ across the globe, our focus is on injustice that results in social exclusion where some populations are restricted inequitably in their opportunities, resources, privileges, and rights for occupational engagement. The focus is on a justice of difference that takes diversity into account. We hope that readers are motivated to refer to the discussion and questions around the six processes and to adopt what we have described here in its nascent form as critical occupational therapy. Using the POJF 2010 will require different ways of thinking and acting from typical occupational therapy or other professional practice. As occupational therapists, we have written this chapter because we believe that an evolution in occupational therapy to make occupational justice explicit in partnership with others is timely as well as morally and ethically defensible.

Acknowledgment

Our gratitude is extended to Dr Helene Polatajko, co-primary author of Canada's 2007 practice guidelines for occupational therapists: *Enabling Occupation II: Advancing an Occupational Therapy Vision of Health, Well-Being and Justice Through Occupation*, and primary author of the Canadian Practice Process Framework 2007 in those guidelines (Townsend & Polatajko 2007). Dr Polatajko provided comments on a draft of the description and visual format of Figure 8.2, the Participatory Occupational Justice Framework 2010. We would also like to acknowledge Dr Anne Kinsella for her important contribution on this section on epistemic reflexivity in this chapter.

References

Aronson J: Conflicting images of older people receiving care: Challenges for reflexive practice and research. In Neysmith SM, editor: *Critical Issues for Future Social Work Practice with Aging Persons*, New York, 1999, Columbia University Press, pp 47–69.

Baily R, Brake M: *Radical Social Work*, New York, 1975, Pantheon Press.

Bourdieu P, Wacquant L: *An Invitation to Reflexive Sociology*, Chicago, 1992, The University of Chicago Press.

Bourdieu P, Johnson R: *Practical Reason: On the Theory of Action*, Oxford, UK, 1998, Polity Press.

Byrne C: Facilitating empowerment groups: Dismantling professional boundaries, *Issues Ment Health Nurs* 20:55–71, 1999.

Canadian Association of Occupational Therapists: *Occupational Therapy Guidelines for Client-Centred Practice*, Toronto, 1991, CAOT Publications ACE.

Canadian Association of Occupational Therapists: *Occupational Therapy Guidelines for Client-Centred Mental Health Practice*, Toronto, 1993, CAOT Publications ACE.

Canadian Association of Occupational Therapists: *Enabling Occupation: An Occupational Perspective*, Toronto, 1998, CAOT Publications ACE.

Deegan P: Recovery and empowerment for people with psychiatric disabilities, *Soc Work Health Care* 25:11–24, 1997.

Denton MA, Kemp CL, French S, et al: Reflexive planning for later life, *Can J Aging* (Suppl 1):S71–S82, 2004.

Freire P: *Pedagogy of the Oppressed*, Harmondsworth, 1972, Penguin.

Habermas J: *The Philosophical Discourse of Modernity. Twelve lectures* (Lawrence F, translator), Cambridge, MA, 1995, MIT Press.

Hammell KW: Reflections on … well-being and occupational rights, *Can J Occup Ther* 75:61–64, 2008.

Hammell KW: Sacred texts: A sceptical exploration of the assumptions underpinning theories of occupation, *Can J Occup Ther* 76:6–13, 2009.

Iwama M: The issue is – toward culturally relevant epistemologies in occupational therapy, *Am J Occup Ther* 57:582–588, 2003.

Iwama M: Occupation as a cross-cultural construct. In Whiteford G, Clair Wright-St V, editors: *Occupation and Practice in Context*, Marickville, NSW, 2005, Churchill Livingstone.

Jarman J: What is occupation: Interdisciplinary perspectives on defining and classifying human activity. In Christiansen C, Townsend EA, editors: *An Introduction to Occupation: The Art and Science of Living*, ed 2, Upper Saddle River, NJ, 2010, Prentice Hall Publishing, pp 81–99.

Kinsella A, Whiteford G: Knowledge generation and utilisation in occupational therapy: Towards epistemic reflexivity, *Australian*

Occupational Therapy Journal 56:249–258, 2009.

Kronenberg F, Simo Algado S, Pollard N: *Occupational Therapy Without Borders. Learning from the Spirit of Survivors*, Edinburgh, 2005, Elsevier/Churchill Livingstone.

Kuhn TS: *The Structure of Scientific Revolutions*, Chicago, 1989, University of Chicago Press.

Law M, Baum CM, Baptiste S, editors: *Occupation-based Practice: Fostering Performance and Participation*, Thorofare, NJ, 2002, Slack, Inc.

Polatajko HJ: Muriel driver memorial lecture: naming and framing occupational therapy. A lecture dedicated to the life of Nancy B, *Can J Occup Ther* 59:189–200, 1992.

Polatajko HJ: National perspective – the evolution of our occupational perspective. The journey from diversion through therapeutic use to enablement, *Can J Occup Ther* 68:203–207, 2001.

Rolfe G: Postmodernism for healthcare workers in 13 easy steps, *Nurse Educ Today* 21:38–47, 2001.

Sandywell B: *Reflexivity and the Crisis of Western Reason: Logological Investigations*, London, 1996, Routledge.

Simo-Algado S, Gregori JMR, Egan M: Spirituality in a refugee camp, *Can J Occup Ther* 64:138–145, 1997.

Simo-Algado S, Mehta N, Kronenberg F, et al: Occupational therapy intervention with children survivors, *Can J Occup Ther* 69:205–217, 2002.

Stadnyk R, Townsend EA, Wilcock AA: Occupational justice. In Christiansen C, Townsend EA, editors: *An Introduction to Occupation: The Art and Science of Living*, ed 2, Upper Saddle River, NJ, 2010, Prentice Hall Publishing, pp 329–358.

Townsend EA: Power and justice in enabling occupation, *Can J Occup Ther* 70:74–87, 2003a.

Townsend EA: *Occupational justice: ethical, moral and civic principles for an inclusive world.* Paper presented at Annual meeting of European Network of Occupational Therapy Educators, Prague, Czech Republic, 2003b. Online. Available at: http://www.enothe.hva.nl/meet/ac03/acc03-text03.doc. Accessed March 23, 2008.

Townsend EA, Landry JE: Enabling participation in occupations. In Christiansen C, Baum C, editors: *Occupational Therapy: Overcoming Human Performance Deficits*, ed 3, Thorofare, NJ, 2004, Slack, Inc.

Townsend EA, Polatajko HJ: *Enabling occupation II: Advancing an occupational therapy visio for health, well-being and justice through occupation*, Ottawa, 2007, CAOT Publications ACE.

Townsend EA, Wilcock AA: Occupational justice and client-centred practice: A dialogue-in-progress, *Can J Occup Ther* 71:75–87, 2004.

Townsend EA, Ripley D, Langille L: Professional tensions in client-centred practice, *Am J Occup Ther* 57:17–28, 2003.

Townsend EA, Beagan B, Kumas-Tan Z, et al: Enabling: Occupational therapy's core competency. In Townsend EA, Polatajko HJ, editors: *Enabling Occupation II:*

Advancing an Occupational Therapy Vision of Health, Well-Being and Justice Through Occupation, Ottawa, 2007a, CAOT Publications ACE, pp 87–133.

Townsend EA, Coburn L, Letts L, et al: Enabling social change. In Townsend EA, Polatajko HJ, editors: *Enabling Occupation II: Advancing an Occupational Therapy Vision of Health, Well-Being and Justice Through Occupation*, Ottawa, 2007b, CAOT Publications ACE, p 153171.

Townsend EA, Trentham B, Clark J, et al: Enabling individual change. In Townsend EA, Polatajko HJ, editors: *Enabling Occupation II: Advancing an Occupational Therapy Vision of Health, Well-Being and Justice Through Occupation*, Ottawa, 2007c, CAOT Publications ACE, pp 135–151.

United Nations Development Program (2007). UN Development Program in S. Africa 2007–2010. Retrieved Feb 26, 2008 from http://www.undp.org.za.

Whiteford G, Wilcock A: Centralising occupation in occupational therapy curricula: Imperative of the new millennium, *Occup Ther Int* 8:81–85, 2001.

Whiteford G, Wright St.-Clair V: *Occupation and Practice in Context*, Marackville, NSW, 2005, Churchill Livingstone.

Wilcock AA: *An Occupational Perspective on Health*, ed 2, Thorofare, NJ, 2006, Slack, Inc.

Wilcock AA, Townsend E: Occupational justice: Occupational terminology interactive dialogue, *Journal of Occupational Science* 7:84–86, 2000.

Wilcock AA, Townsend EA: Occupational justice. In Crepeau E, Cohn E, Schell B, editors: *Willard and Spackman's Occupational Therapy*, ed 11, Baltimore, MD,

2009, Lippincott Williams & Wilkins, pp 192–199.

Wilding C, Whiteford G: Language, identity and representation: Occupation and occupational therapy in acute settings, *Australian Occupational Therapy Journal* 55:180–187, 2007a.

Wilding C, Whiteford G: Occupation and occupational therapy: Knowledge paradigms and everyday practice, *Australian Occupational Therapy Journal* 54:185–193, 2007b.

World Federation of Occupational Therapists: *Occupational Therapy Human Resources Project*, 2008. Online. Available at: http://www.wfot.org/office_files/WFOT%20HR%20Project%20and%20PPS%20web.pdf. Accessed August 25, 2009.

World Federation of Occupational Therapists: *Position Statement on Human Rights*, 2006. Online. Available at: http://www.wfot.org/office_files/Human%20Rights%20Position%20Statement%20Final%20NLH.pdf. Accessed July 27, 2009.

World Health Organization: *International Classification of Functioning, Disability and Health (ICF)*, Geneva, 2001, World Health Organization. Online. Available at: http://www.wfot.org/office_files/Human%20Rights%20Position%20Statement%20Final%20NLH.pdf. Accessed July 27, 2009.

Yerxa EJ: Some implications of occupational therapy's history for its epistemology, values, and relation to medicine, *Am J Occup Ther* 46:79–83, 1992.

Yerxa EJ, Clark F, Frank G, et al: An introduction to occupational science, a foundation for occupational therapy in the 21st century. In Johnson JA, Yerxa EJ, editors: *Occupational science: The foundation for new models of practice*, New York, 1990, The Haworth Press, pp 1–17.

Situated meaning: a matter of cultural safety, inclusion, and occupational therapy

9

Michael K. Iwama   Nicole A. Thomson   Rona M. Macdonald

OVERVIEW

In this chapter we use vignettes to examine how occupational therapy practice, knowledge, and theory are culturally 'situated', and potentially culturally unsafe when taken across boundaries of meaning. Culture is defined broadly and taken beyond its familiar and usual consideration as an embodied, static attribute of individuals (such as in the common forms of race and ethnicity), and is understood as 'shared spheres of experience and ascription of meaning to objects and phenomena in the world' (Iwama 2007, p. 184). Some dominant features of occupational therapy models developed in the Western world are briefly examined to illuminate how culture is implicit in the fundamental structure of these ideas, instead of culture's usual location as a secondary consideration or afterthought in occupational therapy practices. Occupational therapists are challenged to look inward into what constructs their own individual collections of 'normal' and also probe the cultural boundaries of occupational therapy. Only when this is achieved can we truly contemplate a more relevant, inclusive, safe and effective practice – where we practice occupational therapy equitably across varying contexts of shared experience.

An occupational therapist from the North brings her expertise to living in a developing nation in the South.[1]

DAY ONE

Dear Diary

Arrived at the airport today. It is hot and chaotic here in the tropics, but miracles, I still have my luggage! Met with the group and took vans to compound, our luggage piled up top. It all looks so different here, very different from my own city. The streets are filthy, garbage everywhere, cars with no doors, the roads falling apart, huge holes, unbelievable chaos. These people have it hard! Thank God I don't have to live here. Buildings in shambles, street vendors with no shoes hawking food. Shacks on small pieces of land, like debris, welded together, skinny stray dogs lying in the crazy heat or wandering around. Children on the streets in the day, staring at the van and at us, some wearing uniforms – the wealthy ones probably, and some not. Everybody carrying things, women with things on their head, men carrying heavy long poles on their shoulders.

I feel *white* here, I don't *fit* here. Overwhelmed by the heat, the sounds, the rubber burning smells, and garbage everywhere. What will the clinic and the orphanage be like? What will the kids be like that I have come here to help? I hope I will know what to do, how to help? I worry that I have so little experience to draw from but want to do my bit to help these unfortunate people ...

Introduction

When we decide to take *our* occupational therapy across cultural borders, we often do so confidently with the belief that what we offer is right, equitable, and beneficial for all of our clients. After all, what could possibly be wrong with our *just* mandate of enabling, empowering, and enhancing occupation and participation in daily life activities that have meaning? However, the question the authors of this chapter would like to ask is 'meaning for whom?'

One of the fundamental ideas suggested in this chapter is that the meaning, forms, and purposes of occupational therapy are located or 'situated' within particular and culturally specific spheres of shared experience. When those spheres of experience are translocated into different cultural settings, could the resulting cross-cultural tensions result in practice that is culturally unsafe and exclusionary? By doing so, we raise the notion that our forms, purposes, and meanings of occupational therapy are located or 'situated' in particular spheres of shared experience that may differ greatly from clients abiding in a different cultural reality. The occurrences of such cross-cultural tensions raise fundamental concerns about cultural safety (Ramsden 1990), and possible inclusionary and exclusionary practices of occupational therapy.

For the purposes of this chapter, we will define culture to mean: 'shared spheres of experience and the ascription of meaning to objects and phenomena in the world' (Iwama 2007, p. 184). Occupational therapists, for example, who have acquired and shared a common set of experiences, a specialized language, similar patterns of professional behavior, etc., may define wellbeing and the concept of occupation in a different way from how people and cultural groups might have learned to make sense of the same concepts. If occupational therapists accept a pluralistic way of defining culture, then the question of whether the cultural norms and imperatives of (their) occupational therapy and (of its) therapists are congruent with and safe for their clients' cultures must be raised. Along with the spheres of shared experiences and worldviews held by therapists, the occupational therapies that are taken across sociocultural borders also embody the social and cultural contexts from which they emerged and may not necessarily resonate with and be relevant to other people and their uniquely different contexts of daily living. The results of such dissonances between worldviews can be difficult – even unsafe, for both client and therapist. Instead of enabling, helping, emancipating, empowering, and supporting, an occupational therapy out of sync with others' worldviews and day-to-day realities may end up disabling, limiting, constraining, and even disempowering them.

This word of caution is not necessarily directed only to practitioners of occupational therapy but also to occupational therapy researchers, educators, students, scholars, theorists, and occupational scientists. What is found (For what we find) worthy of investigating, knowing, and explaining, also results in the casting onto others (casts) a certain view of reality based in one particular sphere of shared experience. This what is referred to as we refer to as 'situated meanings'; how these meanings are exercised in any occupational therapeutic situation (even in your own local practices) can be culturally unsafe for clients and exclude many people.

In the foreign therapist's Day one diary entry above, the abrupt collision of cultural realities, or dissonance in 'shared spheres of experience', is apparent and sets the tone for a potential awakening for the well-intentioned occupational therapist. Many such well-meaning health professionals who embark on similar journeys that cross cultural boundaries complete volunteer or work contracts, have remarkable experiences, and return to their familiar and comfortable contexts of work and living with mixed and unsettled thoughts and feelings. In some cases, therapists' outlook on culture, occupational therapy and related issues of equity, and the provisioning of culturally responsive occupational therapy has been extraordinarily upset.

As the chapter unfolds, the reader will be challenged to consider how such experiences of taking occupational therapy across borders and the comprehension of 'differences' or abnormalities are actually apparent and at play in our very own familiar spheres or contexts of daily living. The universality and uniformity with which we come to regard our local practices and clients can be largely elusive. They tend to exist as 'normal' because that's the way we have learnt it in our own familiar spheres of shared experiences – in home life, at school, within our social circles, through the media, etc. Those of us who abide in the rational-oriented Western world have also learned to locate *difference* – or what we find to be remarkable and 'abnormal' as abiding outside of our own selves, embodied in a distinct other and in the external environment. 'It all looks so different here', says our diary writer. Different from what she is used to; different to the familiar contexts of *normal*.

If our diary writer had grown up in these very streets of an impoverished town in a developing country, with the shared experience of daily life there becoming familiar and 'normal', and without having experienced any different spheres of experience elsewhere, would he or she necessarily see it as 'different'? Would there still be the disconcerting feeling of being in an unfamiliar and abnormal environment? Such questions can but lead to the asking of a weightier professionally significant question:

'Are there diverse worldviews that differ from our own familiar and proper ways of viewing and making sense of reality?'

Social constructionism and worldviews

If we follow a social constructionist (Burr 1995, Gergen 1999) view of knowledge – that human beings socially construct and make sense of their realities, and that such constructions of reality will vary between people, then the notion that different world-views exist is fundamental. For example, a therapist, who has been acculturated and trained in the scientific tradition, may see childhood physical impairment as a congenital condition while the child's parents might explain the same condition or phenomena of interest as a penalty for social transgressions committed by their ancestors. The former view is explained through the power of measurable observation (from *valid* instruments) while the latter is credited to faith in an unseen, immeasurable, spiritual element or deity. Which version of truth is *more* 'valid' and trustworthy? It depends on whose situated standards are being employed as the arbiter of validity and truth.

Are these diverse worldviews attributed to biology, whereby our understandings are 'hard-wired' within us, or are they acquired? Or are they artifacts of everything that a person has acquired and experienced since birth; that our experiences since the earliest days have informed or populated a kind of lens through which we view the world and make sense of it? The authors are inclined to believe the latter, and that acquired lenses – or *spheres of shared experiences* – are the templates or filters through which the world is viewed and made sense of. And that sense of the world that exists within and without is uniquely configured. Every person possesses their own particular view and interpretation of the meaning of it all, and no one person's lenses are exactly like another's. These 'cultural' lenses also inform how you make judgments and decisions in daily life. They enable you to determine whether an object or phenomenon you encounter is: safe or unsafe, good or bad, morally right or wrong, beautiful or unsightly, etc. or some variation on a continuum. 'One person's treasure is another's trash', 'Beauty is in the eyes of the beholder' are common adages in the Western world that illustrate the uniqueness and varying feature of our lenses or views of the world and our situations within it.

What patterns or spheres of shared experience have you acquired over your lifetime? How have your occupational therapy education and experiences added to your views of the world? And how do your spheres of experience impact on your interpretation and appreciation for your client's issues of day-to-day living? How do these reference points affect your understanding and provision of 'client-centered' occupational therapy? When we take our selves and our occupational therapy across borders, we essentially take our 'lenses' with us. The lenses can for the most part remain invisible, exempt from any critical scrutiny, particularly if we have been acculturated into an objectivist worldview that regards reality as existing out there, outside of our selves. Reality, including objects, other people and their patterns of daily life and occupations need only be uncovered, described, and measured. In such instances, one's own acquired sociocultural norms also tend to escape critical evaluation. After all, one's own normal view is assumed to be universally shared by all humankind, therefore not a threat to the validity of one's own judgment of the other.

Ironically, this pattern of 'objective' views of the world which still dominate the ways of thinking and knowing in the northern or Western industrialized countries, are not that divergent from the rationales that supported past colonial attitudes and conquests. The moral need to subjugate and cultivate the 'primitive' other to meet the requirements and norms of the dominant society was often the impetus and rationale employed to justify conquest. Under the guise of beneficence, and emancipation, an enormous structural imbalance of power was cast onto the other, privileging, empowering and advantaging the dominant culture while under-privileging, disadvantaging, and disempowering the other. Often the 'other' was cast into vulnerable and disadvantageous or culturally unsafe circumstances.

Similar imbalances of power inherent in the structure and procedures of occupational therapy processes continue to jeopardize attempts to configure occupational therapy as a client-centered practice. Occupational therapies may never be considered truly client-centered unless the power structures imbedded in the client–occupational therapist relationship, and in the structure of our instruments and therapeutic procedures, are better revealed, critically considered, and replaced by alternative procedures that transfer the power of ownership of the therapeutic process to a more level playing field – one that further privileges and empowers the client.

Where one locates or situates these matters of differences and meanings of everyday life experience holds important implications for how occupational therapists carry out their work across borders in meaningful and equitable ways. Are the differences we perceive located in the *other* person, or are such perceived differences actually located within one's own set of acquired ideas about what is normal and right? Every encounter with clients who come to the therapeutic relationship carrying spheres of experiences that differ significantly from those of the therapist and of the institutions of practice are subject to the basic requirements of inclusion, relevance, and safety of occupational therapy. This is the fundamental challenge that culture and diversity represent to the practice, theory, and knowledge systems of occupational therapy. More than the need to cultivate our clients to reach a certain unfamiliar standard of occupational performance that we bring to them, is there a need for us to cultivate our own perspectives with our clients' views experience and explanations of their day-to-day realities?

We now follow the continuing narrative of an occupational therapist from the North, as she takes her enabling skills and (good) intentions to help across cultural boundaries of meaning into *other* clients' contexts of daily living. How such acts of caring and enablement, given with good intentions, are received and judged may depend on where the standards of valuing and meaning are *situated*.

DAY 2

Dear Diary
    Was driven with the rest of rehabilitation team for almost an hour through the city, to get to the orphanage. From the front, it looked like a mansion. Guards opened the gates to let us in. Around the back was where the children spent their day. They lay on cots, some actually chained and strapped to bed frames at the centre of the yard, in full sun, in the scorching heat. Some children were repeatedly hitting themselves, others were banging on their beds. Our job today was to teach the care-givers and rehab aides (who earn next to nothing) in the orphanage why rehabilitation is important, and the basic information about ADLs [activities of daily living], positioning, feeding, and swallowing. They seemed to listen and were interested and receptive to the ideas and asked questions through the interpreter. But it looks like we've got our work cut out for us – these people need things to be repeated over and over – the material is so easy ... WHY DON'T THEY UNDERSTAND???

Cultural safety

Practice is not the only area of concern that can reflect the culture (spheres of shared experience) of its origin. For many occupational therapists and their clients, who fall outside mainstream Western cultural norms, theory, and models that have also risen out of another culture, filled with tacit standards and ideals for what is considered 'normal' and good can be problematic. When these models with their largely hidden norms and standards are taken from their original cultural contexts and then foisted onto people who abide in differing cultural contexts, the consequences can be disempowering and unfair. Like imported practices and approaches that are out of sync with the local context, they can also be regarded to be culturally *unsafe* by the *other*.

Nurse and health scholars from Aotearoa (Maori term for New Zealand) in the last two decades have impressed upon the world the importance of *cultural safety* (Jungerson 1992, Ramsden 1990), a framework by which power relationships between health professionals and the people they serve are critically considered. The present impact of historical, social, and political processes on minority health disparities in and beyond the Aotearoa context hold important implications for equity wherever health issues of a particular group are being described, mediated and evaluated by other people and their unfamiliar standards. The idea of cultural safety is pertinent to occupational therapists when taking their ideas and processes into new cultural domains – especially when the transfer involves applying models to individuals and collectives who have not fully acculturated into mainstream Western society. Often the recipients are in disadvantaged positions and are thus vulnerable to being discriminated against by standards and norms representing a different cultural context. Further, they may lack the experience and means to critically examine the veracity, utility, and *safety* of the material being imposed upon them.

The cultural safety of occupational therapy and its theory

There are also relevant issues of cultural safety at the interface between theory construction and theory application. Theories and models are often developed in academic settings. These products can be far removed from the very people, situated in diverse, dynamic and changing practice contexts, for which these theoretical materials and models are universally given. When we ask where the ideas have come from, on what realities these materials and ideas have been based, and who has participated in the production of such knowledge, we gain valuable insight into the cultural features of a profession's knowledge and theory, and challenges to its *universal* appropriateness and safety for its diverse clientele.

If culture, as it is defined and used in this chapter can mean 'spheres of shared experience and the ascription of meaning to objects and phenomena in the world', then even the profession of occupational therapy itself can be considered a culture. Occupational therapy possesses in its world: a shared specialized language, tacit rules of conduct in carrying out its activities, established social practices that follow a pattern that help to identify its members from other professionals, and certain institutional conditions of knowledge production (Smith 2000) that help to legitimize its discourse. Occupational therapy researchers, educators, and practitioners alike can be observed engaging in organized systems that abide in such shared spheres of experience. When such organized systems are narrowly developed within a particularly dominant cultural grouping, then one has to question the universality and utility of those systems for those who are located outside of its norms. Critical examination of occupational therapy theory will reveal that our existing conceptual models are culturally situated and that their specificity can often exclude both clients and therapists who abide in cultural contexts that diverge from the norm.

DAYS FIVE AND SIX

Dear Diary

What am I doing here? Why don't these people understand what autism is? They ask me why the kids hit themselves, and so I explained a bit about autistic tendencies and sensory deprivation. I explained this several times but they didn't seem to get it.

I asked them through the interpreter 'Why is this boy tied up?' and they say because that is just the way he is, he is crazy. But if they see him as crazy and that is just the way he is, THEN just where does rehab fit in? What is the point of being here? I try to explain to them, to emphasise that these children are occupational beings. They need to have occupations to have a sense of well-being. To be independent, to be autonomous, at least to have CHOICE is important.

This is impossible; I am supposed to do 65 initial assessments in 3 hours. An assembly line of children

lined up, passed from therapist to therapist: nurse, to physiotherapy, to me (as if I had something to offer them!) and then on to the 'speech path' who listens to their chests. Where do I begin here? These assessments I have brought with me don't fit. What is occupation here? What does occupation mean here? And how can I get an understanding of that from them?

And my precious OT models seem to have pieces missing from them. They don't seem to make sense here?

Occupational therapy conceptual models, particularly those that aspire to explain human occupation and its qualities, have Western worldviews embedded within them. Some dominant features of occupational therapy models developed in the Western world are briefly examined here to illuminate how culture is implicit in the fundamental structure of these ideas, instead of culture's usual location as a secondary consideration or afterthought in occupational therapy practices.

If we first examine diagrams depicting established occupational therapy models, we may notice that the concept of the individual self is prominent and commands the central focus of concern. Often the self is situated centrally and construed to be a distinct entity, rationally separated from a distinct environment. Occupation – the phenomenon that often functions as the connector or bridge between the self or person and environment is often defined as another distinct entity. The nature of this depiction of human action and intent is often explained metaphorically (Lakoff & Johnson 1980) in some form of rational description. Diagrams with boxes containing distinct concepts tied together by arrows that explain the principles of relationships between them like a machine or dynamic 'system'. Emphases are placed on individual action and ability, as required to act (and even control) the surrounding environment, with degree of independence and autonomy being important benchmarks of achievement. Situating the self in the central position of concern also creates a temporal emphasis on the future (instead of on the here and now). The central self is empowered to determine his or her future, as if one's own future was primarily dependent on one's own volition. This ideal represents a hallmark of 'best practice' in occupational therapy in the developed world. In the Western world, goals and objectives become important if not imperative foci for occupational therapy (Iwama 2006).

Many of these culturally bound features are not readily noticed or viewed as remarkable to readers who abide in a similar cultural context from which these models emerged. Many of the features of 'normal' remain unremarkable and even invisible. When viewed through lenses that are informed by differing contexts of day-to-day experiences, these same 'normal' features become 'abnormal', remarkable, and clearly visible. A single parent mother trying to survive and raise her children in the inner city of a North American country, under conditions of abject poverty may clearly see white, middle-class, able-ist features or biases to these models. It may be difficult for this person to relate to the narratives of 'doing, being and becoming' (Wilcock 1998) and self-actualization when she is struggling daily – trying to cope with the real demands for safety, nutrition, and shelter for her family. Many concepts of the models may be incomprehensible, as if they arrived from another cultural context, or someone else's reality.

When occupational therapists attempt to apply their models to view and interpret the daily life and occupational circumstances of *other* clients, some problems may arise. The template may not fit well and lead to biased interpretations of the other's ethos and realities of life. Failure of the *other* to fit the conceptual patterns of normal, which are implicit in the model, can lead to unreliable and invalid descriptions and comprehension of the other's reality. At worst, the other can be judged, described and explained in pejorative terms. Instead of a growing interest to understand greater context and complexity around why the other's behaviors or cultural patterns appear so remarkably different (and discomforting) and defy the structure of our theory and expectations, the tendency may be to judge the other as wrong and in need of educating. Some of those judgments can even take on a moral or ethical (our own morals and ethics, of course) tenor, casting the other into subordinate positions in need of *cultivation*.

The emphases on cultivating the other to meet our requirements, rather than on the need to cultivate our selves to appreciate better what the other's requirements might be, remains a challenging, if not problematic, pattern confronting conventional occupational therapy theory and practice.

Empowering the other

What might be indeed irrelevant to the recipient, may be welcomed and sought with open arms because the goods carry the hope for advancement, (if it comes from the West, it must be better!) and the hope of progress and improvement. In the similar way with which occupational therapy students might take on a particular venerated theorist's work with intention to do *proper* and *correct* occupational therapy, health professionals located across *other* cultural boundaries may actually demand to receive the latest Western theory, knowledge and practice forms, no matter how irrelevant (and culturally unsafe) to their context of meanings they may appear to be. Those who are fearful of being left behind the global economy and state of technology may actually put out the welcome mat and not necessarily see it as intrusive. Some may indeed benefit but the parallels to colonialism from past times cannot be ignored. There is always the danger of bringing in 'our' culture and thereby standards of behavior and meanings that can disrupt people's way of life. In the local cultural context, we may actually be modeling and nurturing behaviors that will disadvantage people in their societies. In this way, occupational therapy can oppress rather than empower, encumber rather than emancipate, and disable rather than restore (Abberley 1995).

One solution for culturally safer approaches in occupational therapy is to encourage clients and colleagues to be involved in the therapeutic process from planning, assessing, to treating and evaluating. Culture – when defined as spheres of shared experiences, transcends geographic differences as well as individual embodiments such as race and ethnicity, and acknowledges that such challenges of different meanings and contexts of shared experience exist in our very own locations of occupational therapy practice. The culturally responsive occupational therapist may need to exert some effort to extend this power-sharing option to the client group.

Ideally the concepts that comprise these models of occupational therapy should be in the same language of the client. The structure or principles by which the concepts are tied together should also agree with cultural norms and local worldviews. For example, models that put the individual in the middle of the universe as an autonomous and independent agent may be difficult to comprehend by those who view the relationship of the individual to the environs as being more transactional and not necessarily central and discretely defined (Iwama 2006).

THREE MONTHS LATER

Back in my city in the North, reading through diary and reflecting further.

It all seems unreal now looking back. I went armed with facts and figures about the place, thinking this was going to help, but it didn't. There was so much going on there that I didn't understand, but what I was trying to do there didn't seem to work. I wonder if there was much more going on within me than what I perceived was going on out there. What was it that I was bringing into that situation; a whole bunch of expectations and assumptions?

I saw what I understood as children with a disability. The caregivers there saw, what? I have no real idea how they viewed these children. I assumed that I was there to provide them education, to bring them into right understanding, to bring them up to speed, more than just the right language, the whole ideas behind them, and what rehabilitation is and what it can do. All of this from MY perspective, MY professional and cultural perspective. I didn't know I carried a cultural perspective. Yet there was no fit. Here I am, another privileged White person coming to this country that has had generations of White people arriving and taking over, and I tell them what things are, explain the diagnoses, the ways of managing the functional limitations, what to do about it, how to make things 'better'. My ideas about independence, occupation, occupational therapy, autonomy and choice, they seemed to be so right, just, universal, but now I am not so sure.

I had no idea that my way of thinking about the world was so different from others, I thought I was right and they were wrong, and now? What 'good' did I do, really? In fact, maybe I did harm? Was I just a medical tourist imposing my 'right' way of looking on them; at the time they seemed keen to want to learn the 'right' way. I didn't really understand what I was getting into, I didn't know enough about different ways of knowing in the world, and how different cultures see things differently.

If I went again, I would think about things differently, do things differently. I would want to be more conscious of what values and attitudes I bring with me, and to look at those models and assessments very carefully to see what assumptions could be hidden in them. I would want to listen more carefully, and ask a lot more questions. Try to understand more and to pick up on those moments when something was being revealed that I didn't understand, to follow that and try to learn a bit about it. I would want to learn more about what occupations were important to people and try to understand what meaning they held.

As we contemplate taking occupational therapy into the lives of people living in other locations and contexts, we should re-dedicate ourselves to allow the insiders of client groups to understand and dictate the terms by which occupational therapy should be introduced. Occupational therapists are implored to go beyond the requirements of conventional cultural competence and recognize the cultural construction and features of occupational therapy itself. This involves examining all of its situated subsumed philosophies, knowledge, and theory (Iwama 2003). Failure to do so will ensure that occupational therapy will fall far short of its mandate to 'enable people to engage or participate in activities and processes that have value' (Iwama 2007, p. 184). If meaning in occupation is deemed important to members of this profession, then the issue of culture should be of primary concern.

In this chapter we have attempted to illuminate how knowledge and theory in addition to practice are culturally 'situated' and potentially culturally unsafe when taken across boundaries of meaning. When culture is redefined in broader terms, expanding it beyond its familiar and usual consideration as an embodied, static attribute of individuals (such as in the common forms of race and ethnicity), into the social realm, it becomes much more useful. These principles of cultural relevance and cultural safety are not limited to when occupational therapy is taken across geographic and political boundaries. Differences in worldviews and spheres of shared experience exist in our very own 'local' places of work and daily living. The vignettes contained in the boxes throughout this chapter are not necessarily only about taking occupational therapy to far away places. With a few minor changes in details, the vignettes might easily apply to our own local contexts of practice.

Occupational therapists are now challenged to look inward into what constructs their own individual collections of 'normal' and also probe the cultural boundaries of occupational therapy. The cultural lenses through which we see and make sense of the world and others can change if we welcome new spheres of shared experience. Only when this is achieved can we truly contemplate a more relevant, inclusive, safe, and effective practice – where we practice occupational therapy equitably across varying contexts of shared experience.

References

Abberley P: Disabling ideology in health and welfare; the case of occupational therapy, *Disability and Society* 10:221–234, 1995.

Burr V: *An introduction to social constructionism*, London, 1995, Routledge.

Gergen KJ: *An invitation to social construction*, Thousand Oaks, 1999, Sage Publications.

Iwama M: The issue is ... toward culturally relevant epistemologies in occupational therapy, *Am J Occup Ther* 57:582–588, 2003.

Iwama M: *The Kawa model; Culturally relevant occupational therapy*, Edinburgh, 2006, Churchill Livingstone-Elsevier Press.

Iwama M: Culture and occupational therapy: meeting the challenge of relevance in a global world, *Occup Ther Int* 4:183–187, 2007.

Jungerson K: Culture, theory and the practice of occupational therapy in New Zealand/Aotearoa, *Am J Occup Ther* 46:745–750, 1992.

Lakoff G, Johnson M: *Metaphors we live by*, Chicago, 1980, University of Chicago Press.

Ramsden I: *Kawa whakaruruhau-cultural safety in nursing education in Aotearoa: report to the Ministry of Education*, Wellington, 1990, Ministry of Education.

Smith MJ: *Culture; reinventing the social sciences*, Buckingham, 2000, Open University Press.

Wilcock A: Reflections on doing, being, and becoming, *Can J Occup Ther* 65:248–256, 1998.

Spirituality in the lives of marginalized children

10

Imelda Burgman

OVERVIEW

The contribution of spirituality to children's resilience, agency, and occupational engagement is a neglected area of occupational therapy knowledge. Marginalized children have had limited opportunities to voice their understanding of themselves, and how they wish to be supported in their lives. This chapter explores spirituality's presence in contributing to the resilience of these children through qualities such as hope, trust, and faith from philosophical, theoretical, and research perspectives. Children's connections to their own dreams and desires, to others, to nature and to meaningful cultural experiences all contribute to giving children a sense of purpose and meaning in an often difficult world. As occupational therapists we need to be mindful of the expression of spirituality in the lives of marginalized children, so we can connect with and assist them in ways that have meaning and power for each of them, in the communities, societies, and world in which they live.

Introduction

> The aim of soul work is not adjustment to accepted norms or to an image of the statistically healthy individual. Rather, the goal is a richly elaborated life, connection to society and nature, woven into the culture of family, nation and globe.
>
> Moore (1992, p. xvii)

Occupational therapy theory (Chapparo & Ranka 1996, Townsend & Polatajko 2007) highlights the need for occupational therapists to include spirituality in their daily practice. The core component of spirituality (Townsend & Polatajko 2007) in the lives of children may be a primary enabler for successful adaptation to the challenges in their lives. Children's ability to use spiritual qualities such as hope, courage, and trust, underlies their potential across all aspects of their lives. Children need access to meaningful occupations in order to connect with their spirituality, finding purpose and therefore meaning in their lives. Spirituality is expressed in the daily cultural activities of children; communicated in their self-care, play, connections with nature, conversations, and participation in educational, religious, and work contexts (Burgman 2005). Marginalized children face disconnection from their community and their spirituality through occupational apartheid (Kronenberg et al 2005), which isolates them from meaningful cultural practices.

Traditional Western developmental theories of childhood position children as unknowing and powerless. These theories place the understanding of childhood and the needs of children within adult narratives that do not enable children to live out their own truths (Alderson 2008). Dominant Western cultural narratives do not support the spirituality and meaningful lived experiences of marginalized children. Children who are valued and supported through alternative narratives of childhood are enabled to express their agency and empowered to realize their potential as contributing members of their communities.

We need to develop our understanding and ability to assist marginalized children to identify and connect with their spiritual qualities, to engage the power of their spirituality in the meaning – making

DOI: 10.1016/B978-0-7020-3103-8.00019-5

of their lives. We also need to assist them in building a sense of connection in their own communities and in the world in which they live, enabling them to draw on the collective power and resilience of those connections. In the cultural and daily rituals and activities of life, marginalized children may find peace and connection to be able to sustain, nurture, and heal their spirits. The spirituality of marginalized children is seen in their resilience to the adversities they face and their continuing engagement in life.

The practice of spirit

> Spirituality is the practice of spirit – the conscious, goal-directed activity which brings spirit and soul into being.
>
> (Kovel 1991, p. 198)

Embodiment of spirituality

In the philosophical and theological works of those who have attempted to define its meaning, spirituality has come to encompass many qualities including; faith, courage, love, trust, hope, belonging, compassion, purpose, joy, awe, wonder, creativity, awareness and transcendence (Dalai Lama 1996, 2001, Hardy 1979, McGrath 1999). The embodiment of spiritual qualities is seen in children's responses to their world through; resilience, agency, self-esteem, playfulness, humor, enthusiasm, curiosity, adaptation, engagement, connection with others, forgiveness, and the experience of meaning (Dalai Lama 2001, Goleman 1997, Moore 1992). For example, the spiritual qualities of belonging, trust and faith (in oneself and others) may be evident (or absent) in the relationships children establish with parents, friends and authority figures (such as teachers, police or the military). The way in which children embody spiritual qualities affects their personal realities, and consequently the wider realities of family, community and society. Children's ability to experience love and belonging through meaningful relationships assists their resilience to experiences of occupational alienation and injustice, where their engagement and self-esteem are challenged (Abelev 2009, Rew et al 2001).

Resilience is the ability to cope with and continue to engage in life despite difficulties (Masten 2001). Resilience encompasses coping and optimism, which are built on a foundation of hope and faith in life's

purpose, and ongoing meaning (Frankl 1959, Friesen 2000). The more tenuous children's beliefs of life's purpose and their ability to find meaning, the more vulnerable children become to the stressors of poverty, trauma, illness and abuse (Coles 1990, Moore 1992). However, children's ability to draw on the courage and power of their spirituality facilitates healing through the positive expression of emotions that in turn influences positive actions (Goleman 1997). For example, the Youth Against War Treaty launched in Australia in 1998 (Youth Action Forum 2008), or children using the internet to speak to each other about child abuse (Youth Noise 2008). The embodiment of the spiritual qualities of love, joy and connection assists in building resilience and self-esteem, while alleviating the impact of emotions such as despair, anger and hopelessness. The expression of humor is an embodiment of joy, and supports a connection with others and coping in times of stress (Clowns without Borders 2009). Psychological and physical health have been intricately linked with a 'healthy' spirituality (Frankl 1959, Moore 1992, Goleman 1997). We need to help children to access and utilise spiritual qualities in their everyday lives, through engagement in occupations that provide meaning and support spiritual healing.

The expression of children's spirituality is influenced by their individual reality and the meaning of their lives (Adams et al 2008, Burgman 2010). Children's ability to express their spirituality and access a global spirituality influences their experience of spiritual inclusiveness, where they can embrace, and be embraced by, the world. This spirituality of inclusiveness is a community spirituality (Townsend 1997) in which each child's uniqueness is honored and supported, and children contribute to the health and strength of their community.

Engagement and wholeness

Children's ability and opportunity to respond to life experiences creates the possibility of engagement or disengagement in life. Persistence in the face of daily struggle and trauma, through hopefulness, promotes engagement and wholeness of a child's identity through integration with their spirituality. Subjugation of a child's uniqueness, through feelings of hopelessness, creates disengagement and a splintering of their identity from their spirituality (Bettelheim 1970, Frankl 1959). Continuing to engage in life's experiences despite difficulties supports the develop-ment of children's cognitive, physical and emotional abilities. Children's openness and willingness to engage supports the development of their identity (Adams et al 2008, Masten 2001) and consequently their spirituality. We can observe children's levels of engagement and disengagement in daily life, through the level of curiosity and motivation invested by children in their play and learning.

In many religions and cultures responses to the traumas of loss, abuse and deprivation can be influ-enced by a profound spiritual belief in the purpose of suffering, supporting a continuing engagement and hopefulness in life (e.g., Ali 2000, Dalai Lama 2001, Mascaro 1962, Napoli 2002, Newlin et al 2002). The ability of children to survive extreme suffering and to continue to hope in spite of overwhelming trag-edy demonstrates a strong connection and ability to draw on their spirituality (Simo-Algado & Burgman 2005). We can support children's hope and engage-ment in life through creating opportunities for the expression of healing emotions, through meaning-ful occupations such as play, artistic expression, or religious rituals.

Connection

The need to belong through connection with others is evident in children's active participation in com-munity experiences (Hanson & Hampton 2000, Rappaport 2000, Simo-Algado & Burgman 2005), such as sport, religious events, and national celebra-tions. Marginalized children, such as homeless children, create a sense of belonging through their membership in the gangs which form their families (see Chapters 22 and 24, Bomfin 2005). In the myr-iad of relationships that children have with others in their lives, at an individual and collective level, connection to others through love and trust creates respect-full and nurturing relationships. The ability to connect with others, for example through friend-ship, provides additional support in times of emo-tional and thus spiritual need, aiding children's resilience to life's challenges and enabling them to respond knowing that their efforts are valued and supported (Fazel & Stein 2002).

Children who feel disconnected experience lone-liness, a sense of rejection, feelings of alienation from others and they are more at risk of depres-sion and suicidal behaviors (Fazel & Stein 2002, Tsey & Every 2000). If we respect children's need for

connection with others then we are respecting the importance of the love of family and friends. The meeting of community, society and culture supports these connections in a spirituality of inclu-siveness (Townsend 1997) in which children are valued. Collective resilience is experienced through supportive relationships with others (Barrow 2007, Waller & Paterson 2002). This resilience aids chil-dren in sustaining themselves in their daily reality, offering courage and hope.

Children seek to express themselves in ways that are accepted and fostered by others, and in turn seek to connect with others in ways that are meaningful. Spiri-tual expression may be through stories, dance, dress, language, play, and simply the way children choose to live their daily lives (Burgman 2010, McEwan & Tsey 2008). Supportive environments and relation-ships enable children to express their spirituality and identities in safety. Being socially excluded, as in the lives of many children living in poverty (Australian Research Alliance for Children and Youth 2008), requires children to draw upon spiritual resources, including hope, courage, faith and trust, to sustain their resilience and engagement with the world.

The limitations and exclusions of occupational injustice may occur through dominant societal, religious or cultural narratives, and will impact on children's ability to sustain themselves without the support of their world. For children experiencing occupational apartheid and/or alienation/injustice/deprivation; including the poor (Australian Research Alliance for Children and Youth 2008), the homeless (Kronenberg 2005), the displaced (Simo-Algado et al 1997), the victims of war (Simo-Algado & Burgman 2005), those with disabilities (Burgman 2010, Tenberken & Kronenberg 2005), and many cultur-ally distinct minorities (Thibeault 2002b), their spirituality may be an important enabler to their ongoing belief in their value and power as individuals (McEwan & Tsey 2008). Children's connection to their own dreams and desires, and continuing to have hope and faith despite living in an unforgiving world, gives purpose and therefore meaning to their lives. This foundation enables them to remain resilient to the stresses and sorrows of their lives.

Spiritual distress

The occupational alienation experienced by mar-ginalized children leads to an exclusion where their spiritual expression is often not seen, heard, understood, or respected in their dominant society. In an effort to survive in a hostile world, vulnerable children who live in situations of occupational apartheid because of political or religious oppression, or ethnic hatred, may have to subjugate their spirit (Bettelheim 1970, Tomas 2008). Spiritual distress is experienced when children are not allowed to express themselves, or their expression is not accepted by others (Coles 1990, Hart 2003). For children who are victims of ongoing conflict such as the children of Palestine (Lanvin 2005) and Iraq, or high levels of urban violence/intra-community conflict (Korbin 2003), spiritual distress may lead to acts of aggression in an effort to be heard. If distress is not given a voice then children may never heal from the trauma they have experienced (Berman 2001, Bettelheim 1974).

The 'language' of marginalized children may not only be different from that of adults, but also from the dominant societal understandings of children. We need to broaden our perception of how spirituality may be expressed. This means asking, listening carefully, watching closely, and respecting and supporting ways of life and meanings different from our own (Burgman 2005, Unruh et al 2002). When this is done successfully, for example, creating a website showcasing the music of marginalized Indigenous Australian children (Heaps Decent 2008), children are released from spiritual distress through understanding and expression. Children creating change together speaks of collective resilience, supported through hope and trust, which is transformed into creative power that can change their lives.

Marginalized children are vulnerable to societal discrimination, environmental dangers, physical illness, and psychological trauma (Lynam et al 2008). These children are not generally perceived as resilient, nor are they perceived as beings of self-agency. In contradiction to the United Nations Convention on the Rights of the Child (United Nations 1989), they are not listened to, protected, or valued on a global scale. Dominant cultural narratives often do not allow children sociopolitical power, and curtail children's freedom to express themselves and to experience a sense of empowerment within their own lives (King 2007, Tomas 2008).

The expressions of children's spirituality are as varied as their lives, and in our relationships with children we need to pay attention to their unique narratives and worldviews. Spirituality is not tied to religious education, or cognitive or emotional development (Coles 1990, Hart 2003). The unique worldviews of children, meanings that encompass the influences of community, society, and culture (their own and the one in which they live) must be respected in helping them to maintain or regain their sense of spiritual strength. We are ethically bound to assist children experiencing marginalization to (re)connect with their spiritual strength, so that they can challenge these experiences and create ones of their making.

The movement of existence

The union of soul and body ... is enacted at every instant in the movement of existence.

Merleau-Ponty (1962, p. 88–89)

Interactions with people, art, music, stories, dance and nature, and the motivation for achieving goals and dreams all manifest children's spirituality in daily life (Adams et al 2008). Coles (1986, 1990, 1992) spent many years interviewing children about their experiences and the meaning of their lives. These children lived in segregated societies, rich and poor neighborhoods, rural and urban landscapes, in war and peace times, and demonstrated the influence of cultural and religious backgrounds. The children's lives were challenged by the changing cultures in which they lived and were nourished by their sense of purpose and opportunities to express themselves. Opportunities for expression gave children emotional and spiritual strength to pursue the meaning of their lives. Expression through art, craft, and nature (e.g., planting a garden, arranging flowers in a vase), and participation in music, dance and stories, are time honored ways in many cultures of exploring and deepening the connection to one's own spirituality, the spirituality of the earth, and a global spirituality (Kronenberg 2005, Newlin et al 2002, McCoy 2008).

The extensive work of Kubler-Ross and her colleagues (1969, 1975, 1981) was instrumental in challenging Western beliefs regarding the understanding and needs of children. Her work presented children's ability to express their philosophical understanding and spiritual connections in the midst of deep suffering through the use of 'non-verbal symbolic language' (1981, p. 19), such as drawing, painting, and play. Kubler-Ross's work opens up a space for adults to remember the language of childhood, which can enable greater respect and engagement with children. Children's use of symbols and nonlanguage-based expression of thoughts and experiences is often forgotten by the world of adults. Their ways of communicating demand the respect of closer attention, if we are to assist children in expressing their spirituality within the meaning of the daily occupations of childhood (Burgman 2005).

The search for meaning and the exploration of understanding of the self, others and the world, are integral to spiritual growth (Frankl 1959, Moore 1992). That there is more to understand and become known, is made explicit through children's need for time away from the world, in order to consider it and reframe it and then to re-enter it. Children need access to a 'space' where they can explore the personal meaning of both positive and negative experiences. This 'space' can enable a much greater healing of a damaged spirit for children exposed to war, poverty, sexual abuse, or simply a lack of caring from the world in which they live. Simo-Algado's work with children in a Kosovo refugee camp (Simo-Algado & Burgman 2005), Kronenberg's (2005) engagement with street children in Guatemala, and Georgian occupational therapy students' experiences with orphans and internally displaced people in Tbilisi (Kapanadze et al 2008), highlight the power of this 'space' to help children reclaim themselves and to find the strength of spirit to continue their lives with hope. Children can find a sense of connection and meaning through opportunities to reflect on their daily lives, be it via daydreaming, play, or the practice of religious faith and its rituals.

Healing spaces

Play

Play as a vehicle for expression and connection to children's spirituality and to the world also provides a space away from the world, for the consideration and reframing of the world. Children engaging in pretend war play in Afghanistan are dealing with the meaning of ongoing trauma in their lives and their emotional reactions to its impact, helping themselves to heal. Children with HIV/AIDS laughing together over a hospital incident (Ragga Mundo 2005) are reframing a difficult experience. Children making toy boats from scraps and floating them in a drain are removing themselves for a time from the harsh realities of their Manila shanty town and reconnecting with their imaginative and joyful spirit. The necessity of play without adult rules, for expression of spirituality outside of the confines of society, is necessary for sustaining children's spirituality and for its growth (Burgman 2005, Moustakas 1959).

Csikszentmihalyi (1975) considered the concept of flow as most evident in children when they are at play, where the self is absorbed within the activity and also forgotten. In play, spirituality can be fully expressed through the self, entering into a state of serenity where the world can unfold (Ackerman 1999). The possibility that this unfolding world can be very different from their daily world gives children respite from their cares and sorrows. Children can be anything or anyone they want to be, can express dreams and desires, and create meaning they can carry with them into their day-to-day world.

We can support children's access to healing and nurturing play experiences through the creation of play spaces. These spaces can be the intimate spaces children share with us, or they can be community spaces (Bettelheim 1974, see Chapter 19). Urban children who are marginalized through poverty, such as children living in caravan (trailer) parks or housing projects, may not have access to dedicated play spaces (Stuart 2007). As occupational therapists, one of our roles is to advocate for play spaces to be made available (Ziviani et al 2008), in which children can express themselves in safety and have opportunities to replenish their spirit.

Cultural rituals

The expression of spirituality and immersion of the self are intrinsic to many cultural rituals. In the cultural rituals of Indigenous Australians and the First Nations people of North America and Canada, communal spirituality supports individual transcendence (Gold 1994, Waller & Patterson 2002). In all cultures, children may create gang rituals to replace the loss of meaningful cultural rituals of transition to a stronger self and immersion in a self that is greater than the power of one. However, as a response to spiritual distress or feelings of spiritual alienation, children may also engage in substance abuse or sexual promiscuity to remove themselves from their reality, in an attempt to find a better one where their sense of aloneness and despair is eased for a time (Bomfin 2005, Choi 2002, Tsey & Every 2000). These ways do not ultimately support the spirit, but can be seen as an attempt to find relief from spiritual distress.

The practice of rituals that reflect inclusiveness of children within their communities, such as the corroborees of Indigenous Australians, support children in learning ways to positively connect; to themselves, their community and the supportive beliefs of their culture. This inclusiveness has been strong in many cultures (McEwan & Tsey 2008, Waller & Patterson 2002), helping children to sustain their spirituality and to contribute to an ongoing communal spirituality, which they can draw on in times of need. Indigenous people who have been displaced and marginalized within their own country, such as Australia, may experience difficulty in maintaining their connection to their cultural rituals. The disconnection then impacts on children's ability to experience the spiritual nourishment of cultural rituals. We can support displaced communities to re-establish cultural practices that will spiritually benefit children and their families, supporting their resilience in times of hardship.

Children who experience ethno-cultural marginalization within the dominant culture, such as Indigenous Australians or the First Nations people of North America, may become emotionally torn between theirs and the dominant culture. Positive and healing connections with their own culture may be set aside in an attempt to be accepted and valued by the dominant culture (Kvernmo & Heyerdahl 2003, McCoy 2008). Children experiencing cultural alienation include those who are displaced, such as refugees, or otherwise marginalized, such as homeless children or children in the juvenile justice system. Alienation and the absence of cultural rituals, places them at risk of emotional vulnerability (Berman 2001). Inclusive spirituality needs to be (re)-created to offer children the opportunity to experience a sense of wider community, and (re)built in a way that is culturally and personally meaningful. The work of Simo-Algado and colleagues with Mayan refugees (1997) and children survivors of war in Kosovo (2005), and Thibeault's work in Sierre Leone with female ex-combatants and child soldiers (2002a), demonstrates rebuilding in meaning-making ways for each community's children/youth.

Daily rituals

The rituals that lend meaning to daily life, such as tending to a garden, caring for animals, or sharing a meal with the family, are meaningful for children in many cultures (Coles 1986, Hanson & Hampton 2000, Thibeault 2002b), speaking as they do to a sustained connection to others and nature. The flow of these daily rituals offers its own peace to sometimes fractured and terrifying lives. Participation in emotionally and spiritually supportive, traditional ways of living and being, in cultures such as those

of Africans, Indigenous Australians, and First Nations people, provides children with connection to the time honored daily rituals of the community as a whole, and with nurturing connections to the land, nature, and the cosmos (McEwan & Tsey 2008, Nyagua & Harris 2008, Waller & Patterson 2002). The importance of emotionally and spiritually supportive rituals lies in their immediate value, and in their contribution to the laying down over time of experiences and perceptions. Their meaning can then empower children to find enriching ways of developing their spirituality and sense of self.

Refugee children often need to reconstruct meaningful daily activities, which foster and heal their spirit (Simo-Algado & Burgman 2005). As a result of being traumatized, displaced, and with an uncertain future, these children are at risk of developing perceptions of the world as only a dangerous and uncaring place. Re-establishing daily rituals that provide a peaceful rhythm and a sense of identity, in the home, at school and in leisure, are vital to replenishing children's spirituality. Addressing occupational justice issues will enable marginalized children to access meaningful daily experiences (Townsend 2003). These meanings will be influenced by cultural preference and supported by practices that provide cultural safety (DeSouza 2008). For example, what has personal meaning and spiritual power for a child in Tibet (Tenberken 2002) may have a different means of expression in the life of a child on the streets of Guatemala (Kronenberg 2005), in the favelas of Brazil (Coles 1986), or in an urban neighborhood in America (Rappaport 2000). What is important is that we listen to children, and that we respect their stories and the meanings they find in their lives (Burgman 2005). If we also honor those meanings through our actions then we will truly be enabling them to access their spirituality.

The making of meaning

Meaninglessness inhibits fullness of life and is therefore equivalent to illness. Meaning makes a great many things endurable – perhaps everything.

Jung (1933, p. 373)

The importance of meaning and meaningful occupation is central to occupational therapy theory, and practice (Hammell 2004). How then, do occupational therapists enable marginalized children to make meaning in their everyday worlds, when their spiritual expression and participation is restricted or denied in all aspects of societies where the injustice of occupational apartheid exists? First, we need to acknowledge our own spiritual values and beliefs, and how they influence our perspectives. Second, we need to reflect on our therapeutic relationships with marginalized children, and what we are striving to achieve within these relationships, i.e., how *we* make meaning in these experiences.

As occupational therapists and as a profession, what do we bring to our relationships with marginalized children? Our values and principles, our professional knowledge and skills, our valuing of our professional knowledge, our beliefs about childhood and wellbeing, our experience with other children, our successes and failures with children and what we have understood of them, and our experiences of life and of having been a child. However, we are also capable of bringing our joy in working with children, our belief in their power and agency, our belief in their potential (and ours), our interest in who they are and what they feel and want. How this knowledge and understanding is woven together within each of us contributes to the creation of who we are as occupational therapists.

Occupational therapists' understanding and intervention approaches are traditionally based on proscribed Western understandings of children's social and emotional needs and resources (Hallet & Prout 2003). If we do not critically reflect on these understandings we are at risk of positioning children as lesser; lesser than our adult selves, and certainly lesser than they are capable of being. If we consider children to be always in need of adult guidance, from the physical to the spiritual aspects of their lives, then we will also develop a relationship with them that positions them as powerless and will perceive them primarily in that role. We can choose to sustain the therapeutic relationship at the professional level defined by the medical and psychological models of childhood, but we would be doing so at a cost to children's spirituality, identity and agency that we may never appreciate. If, however, we choose to see children as knowing themselves far better than we ever will, then we can approach our relationships with them with a greater openness to what may happen and what we will learn (Oaklander 2007). Children bring much to the therapeutic relationship; knowing of their identity, knowing of their self, knowing of their spirituality, knowing of the difficulties and pleasures of their world, and their wishes for what is important to face, to leave, or to consider.

Understanding stories

In order for occupational therapists to gain insight into and address the spiritual beliefs and values held by children and the way spirituality contributes to children's resilience, it is important to understand the stories of their lives (Adams et al 2008, Hart 2003). We must ask for and listen to children's stories, even if these stories are expressed in ways we may find very difficult to accept. As we wish to facilitate change in the lives of children, we need to remain cognizant of the power of children's perceptions and their understandings of themselves in relation to their ability to achieve (Saleebey 2005).

The purpose of facilitating occupational change is to bring positive influences to bear on children's abilities and desires to attempt and pursue new roles and tasks – awakening confidence and spiritual power (Burgman 2010, Moustakas 1973). By listening with interest and respect, and utilizing spiritual qualities ourselves, we demonstrate qualities for children to identify with within themselves. We must become familiar with the language of spiritual distress across cultures, and to understand cultural beliefs embedded in expressions of spirituality (Darnell 2002, Lang 2002, Thibeault 2002b). Our responsibility is to acknowledge and facilitate access to and expression of spirituality in enabling children on their life journey. Thus, we need to understand what spirituality may mean and how it may be expressed in the lives of children surviving marginalization. We need to build cultural *and* spiritual safety into our relations with marginalized children (DeSouza 2008), so that children have spaces in which to express and heal their spirits in ways that are culturally meaningful for them.

To create spaces of safety we need to be aware that the expression of our spirituality and culture may be very different from that of marginalized children. Further, we need to explore our own spirituality and its cultural expression (Collins 2007, Johnston & Mayers 2005, White 2006). The outcome of this acknowledgment and self-exploration is then embedded in our relational awareness, enabling children to experience safety in the expression of their spirituality (Burgman 2010, DeSouza 2008).

We can also support children's safety at organizational and systemic levels. At an organizational level, we can promote recognition of the unique occupational needs of marginalized children, and seek to work with the communities to which these children belong, for example, the remote communities of Australian Indigenous children or the refugee centers of children from Africa (Northern Territory Government 2007, Zwi et al 2007). At a systemic level, we should aim to actively participate in strategic planning to address the occupational apartheid issues facing these children, and work to ensure their voices are heard (Human Rights and Equal Opportunity Commission (Australia) 2004, Tenberken & Kronenberg 2005). By working with marginalized children at all levels of intervention, we will be supporting their spiritual expression through enabling their occupational choices and participation.

Conclusion

The resilience of marginalized children has its foundation in spirituality. In our relationships with marginalized children we must allow their spirituality to reveal itself and not be defined by us. We have an ethical responsibility to meet children at the places of their being, doing and knowing; thus meeting the challenge of the paradigm change that acknowledges and incorporates spirituality in the heart and practice of occupational therapy. The influence of spirituality on resilience directs our attention to the price we ask of children's physical and emotional selves when we do not heed their spiritual needs. Children's spiritual disconnection is manifested in their difficulty in remaining engaged in life, in not seeking opportunities, and lacking the determination to pursue their dreams. The finding of meaning can create hope for things to come, that each ending or loss is also a beginning of the new. If we wish to serve marginalized children, and the families, communities, and societies in which these children live, we must support children's connection to themselves, their communities, nature and the world, in ways that are meaningful and empowering for them.

References

Abelev MS: Advancing out of poverty. Social class worldview and its relation to resilience, *Journal of Adolescent Research* 24:114–141, 2009.

Ackerman D: *Deep Play*, New York, 1999, Vintage.

Adams K, Hyde B, Woolley R: *The Spiritual Dimension of Childhood*, London, 2008, Jessica Kingsley.

Alderson P: *Young Children's Rights*, ed 2, London, 2008, Jessica Kingsley.

Ali AY: *The Holy Qur'an*, Hertfordshire, England, 2000, Wordsworth Editions.

Australian Research Alliance for Children and Youth: *Children's Lived Experience of Poverty: A Review of the Literature*, Sydney, 2008, Author.

Barrow FH: Understanding the findings of resilience-related research for fostering the development of African American adolescents, *Child Adolesc Psychiatr Clin N Am* 16:393–413, 2007.

Berman H: Children and war: current understandings and future directions, *Public Health Nurs* 18:243–252, 2001.

Bettelheim B: *The Informed Heart*, London, 1970, Paladin.

Bettelheim B: *A Home for the Heart*, London, 1974, Thames and Hudson.

Bomfin V: Once a street child, now a citizen of the world. In Kronenberg F, Simó-Algado S, Pollard N, editors: *Occupational Therapy Without Borders. Learning from the Spirit of Survivors*, Edinburgh, 2005, Elsevier/Churchill Livingstone, pp 19–30.

Burgman I: *Reflections on being: spirituality within children's narratives of identity and disability*, Unpublished doctoral dissertation, 2005, University of Sydney.

Burgman I: Enabling children's spirituality in occupational therapy practice. In Rodgers S, editor: *Occupation centred practice with children: a practical guide for occupational therapists*, Sydney, 2010, Blackwell, pp 94–113.

Chapparo C, Ranka J: *Occupational Performance Model (Australia)*. *Monograph 1*, Sydney, 1996, Occupational Performance Network.

Choi H: Understanding adolescent depression in ethnocultural context, *Adv Nurs Sci* 25:71–85, 2002.

Clowns without Borders: 2009, Online. Available at: http://www.clownswithoutborders.net/. Accessed June 12, 2009.

Coles R: *The Moral Life of Children*, New York, 1986, Atlantic Monthly Press.

Coles R: *The Spiritual Life of Children*, Boston, 1990, Houghton Mifflin.

Coles R: *Their Eyes Meeting the World. The drawings and paintings of children*, Boston, 1992, Houghton Mifflin.

Collins M: Spirituality and the shadow: reflection and the therapeutic use of self, *British Journal of Occupational Therapy* 70:88–90, 2007.

Csikszentmihalyi M: *Beyond Boredom and Anxiety*, San Francisco, 1975, Jossey-Bass.

Dalai Lama: *The Good Heart*, Sydney, 1996, Rider.

Dalai Lama: *An Open Heart*, Australia, Sydney, 2001, Hodder Headline.

Darnell R: Occupation is not a cross-cultural universal: some reflections from an ethnographer, *Journal of Occupational Science* 9:5–11, 2002.

DeSouza R: Wellness for all: the possibilities of cultural safety and cultural competence in New Zealand, *Journal of Research in Nursing* 13:125–135, 2008.

Fazel M, Stein A: The mental health of refugee children, *Arch Dis Child* 87:366–370, 2002.

Frankl VE: *Man's Search for Meaning*, London, 1959, Hodder and Stoughton.

Friesen MF: *Spiritual Care for Children Living in Specialized Settings. Breathing underwater*, New York, 2000, Haworth Press.

Gold P: *Navajo and Tibetan Sacred Wisdom. The circle of the spirit*, Rochester, VE, 1994, Inner Traditions International.

Goleman D: Afflictive and nourishing emotions: impacts on health. In Goleman D, editor: *Healing Emotions*, Boston, 1997, Shambala, pp 33–46.

Hallet C, Prout A, editors: *Hearing the Voices of Children: Social Policy for a New Century*, London, 2003, Routledge Farmer.

Hammell KW: Dimensions of meaning in the occupations of daily life, *Can J Occup Ther* 71:296–305, 2004.

Hanson I, Hampton MR: Being Indian: strengths sustaining First Nations Peoples in Saskatchewan residential schools, *Can J Occup Ther* 19:127–142, 2000.

Hardy SA: *The Spiritual Nature of Man. A study of contemporary religious experience*, Oxford, 1979, Clarendon Press.

Hart T: *The Secret Spiritual World of Children*, Maui, Hawaii, 2003, Inner Ocean.

Heaps Decent: 2008, Online. Available at:http://heapsdecent.com/. Accessed December 25, 2008.

Human Rights and Equal Opportunity Commission (Australia): *A Last Resort? National inquiry into children in immigration detention*, Sydney, 2004, Author.

Johnston D, Mayers C: Spirituality: a review of how occupational therapists acknowledge, assess and meet spiritual needs, *British Journal of Occupational Therapy* 68:386–393, 2005.

Jung CG: *Modern Man in Search of a Soul*, London, 1933, Routledge & Kegan Paul.

Kapanadze M, Despotashvili M, Skhirtladze N: Political practice in occupational therapy in Georgia: 'challenging change' through social action. In Pollard N, Sakellariou D, Kronenberg F, editors: *A Political Practice of Occupational Therapy*,

Sydney, 2008, Churchill Livingstone/Elsevier, pp 163–166.

King M: The sociology of childhood as scientific communication: observations from a social systems perspective, *Childhood* 14:193–213, 2007.

Korbin JE: Children, childhoods, and violence, *Annual Review of Anthropology* 32:431–446, 2003.

Kovel J: *History and Spirit*, Boston, 1991, Beacon Press.

Kronenberg F: Occupational therapy with street children. In Kronenberg F, Simó-Algado S, Pollard N, editors: *Occupational therapy without borders: learning from the spirit of survivors*, London, 2005, Elsevier, pp 261–276.

Kronenberg F, Pollard N, Simo-Algado S: Overcoming occupational apartheid. In Kronenberg F, Simó-Algado S, Pollard N, editors: *Occupational Therapy Without Borders: Learning from the Spirit of Survivors*, London, 2005, Elsevier, pp 58–86.

Kubler-Ross E: *On Death and Dying*, London, 1969, Tavistock.

Kubler-Ross E: *Death. The Final Stage of Growth*, Englewood Cliffs, New Jersey, 1975, Prentice-Hall.

Kubler-Ross E: *Living With Death and Dying. How to Communicate with the Terminally Ill*, New York, 1981, Touchstone.

Kvernmo S, Heyerdahl S: Acculturation strategies and ethnic identity as predictors of behavior problems in Arctic minority adolescents, *J Am Acad Child Adolesc Psychiatry* 42:57–65, 2003.

Lang M: Then and now: how being Jewish has influenced my work as a psychotherapist, *Psychotherapy Australia* 8:22–29, 2002.

Lanvin B: Occupation under occupation: days of conflict and curfew in Bethlehem. In Kronenberg F, Simo-Algado S, Pollard N, editors: *Occupational Therapy Without Borders: Learning from the Spirit of Survivors*, London, 2005, Elsevier, pp 40–45.

Lynam MJ, Loock C, Scott L, Khan KB: Culture, health, and inequalities: new paradigms, new practice imperatives, *Journal of Research in Nursing* 13:138–148, 2008.

McCoy BF: *Holding men. Kanyirninpa and the Health of Aboriginal Men*, Canberra, 2008, AIATSIS.

McEwan A, Tsey K: *Empowerment Research Team. The role of spirituality in social and emotional wellbeing initiatives: the Family Wellbeing program at Yarrabah*, Discussion paper no. 7, Darwin, 2008, Cooperative Research Centre for Aboriginal Health.

McGrath AE: *Christian Spirituality*, Oxford, 1999, Blackwell.

Mascaro J: *The Baghavad Gita*, London, 1962, Penguin.

Masten AS: Ordinary magic: resilience processes in development, *Am Psychol* 56:227–238, 2001.

Merleau-Ponty M: *Phenomenology of Perception*, London, 1962, Routledge & Kegan Paul.

Moore T: *Care of the Soul*, New York, 1992, HarperCollins.

Moustakas CE: *Psychotherapy with Children*, New York, 1959, Harper & Row.

Moustakas C, editor: *The Child's Discovery of Himself*, New York, 1973, Jason Aronson.

Napoli M: Holistic health care for Native women: an integrated model, *Am J Public Health* 92:1573–1575, 2002.

Newlin K, Knafl K, Melkus G: African-American spirituality: a concept analysis, *Adv Nurs Sci* 25:57–70, 2002.

Northern Territory Government: *Ampe akelyernemane meke mekarle, 'Little children are sacred'. Summary report of the Northern Territory Board of Inquiry into the protection of Aboriginal children from sexual abuse*, Darwin, Australia, 2007, Author.

Nyagua JQ, Harris AJ: West African refugee health in rural Australia: complex cultural factors that influence mental health, *Rural Remote Health* 8:884, 2008. Online. Available at: http://www.rrh.org.au. Accessed December 25, 2008.

Oaklander V: *Hidden Treasure: a Map to the Child's Inner Self*, London, 2007, Karnac.

Ragga Mundo EL: Unlocking spirituality: play as a health-promoting occupation in the context of HIV/AIDS. In Kronenberg F, Simó-Algado S, Pollard N, editors: *Occupational Therapy Without Borders: Learning from the Spirit of Survivors*, London, 2005, Elsevier, pp 313–325.

Rappaport J: Community narratives: tales of terror and joy, *Am J Community Psychol* 28:1–24, 2000.

Rew L, Taylor-Seehafer M, Thomas NY, et al: Correlates of resilience in homeless adolescents, *J Nurs Scholarsh* 33:33–40, 2001.

Saleebey D: *The Strengths Perspective in Social Work Practice*, ed 4, Boston, 2005, Pearson/Allyn & Bacon.

Simó-Algado S, Burgman I: Occupational therapy intervention with children survivors of war. In Kronenberg F, Simo-Algado S, Pollard N, editors: *Occupational Therapy Without Borders: Learning from the Spirit of Survivors*, London, 2005, Elsevier, pp 245–260.

Simó-Algado S, Gregori JMR, Egan M: Spirituality in a Refugee Camp, *Can J Occup Ther* 64:138–145, 1997.

Stuart G: *Supporting residents of caravan parks. Principles of promising practice*, Newcastle, Australia, 2007, Family Action Centre.

Tenberken S: *My Path Leads to Tibet*, New York, 2002, Arcade.

Tenberken S, Kronenberg P: The right to be blind without being disabled. In Kronenberg F, Simó-Algado S, Pollard N, editors: *Occupational Therapy Without Borders: Learning from the Spirit of Survivors*, London, 2005, Elsevier, pp 31–39.

Thibeault R: Occupation and the rebuilding of civil society: notes from the war zone, *Journal of Occupational Science* 9:38–47, 2002a.

Thibeault R: Fostering healing through occupation: the case of the Canadian Inuit, *Journal of Occupational Science* 9:153–158, 2002b.

Tomas C: Childhood and rights: reflections on the UN Convention on the Rights of the Child, *Childhoods Today* 2, 2008. Online. Available at: http://www.childhoodstoday.org/journal.php. Accessed February 18, 2009.

Townsend E: Inclusiveness: a community dimension of spirituality, *Can J Occup Ther* 64:146–155, 1997.

Townsend E: Reflections on power and justice in enabling occupation, *Can J Occup Ther* 70:74–87, 2003.

Townsend E, Polatajko HJ: *Enabling occupation II: advancing an occupational therapy vision for health, well-being, and justice through occupation*, Ottawa, Ontario, 2007, CAOT.

Tsey K, Every A: Evaluating Aboriginal empowerment programs: the case of Family Wellbeing. *Aust N Z J Public Health* 24:509–514, 2000.

United Nations: *United Nations Convention on the Rights of the Child. United Nations General Assembly (Resolution 44/25)*, New York, 1989, United Nations.

Unruh AM, Versnel J, Kerr N: Spirituality unplugged: a review of commonalities and contentions, and a resolution, *Can J Occup Ther* 69:5–19, 2002.

Waller MA, Patterson S: Natural helping and resilience in a Dine (Navajo) community, *Family and Society* 83:73–84, 2002.

White G: *Talking about Spirituality in Health Care Practice. A Resource for the Multi-professional Team*, London, 2006, Jessica Kingsley.

Youth Action Forum: 2008, Online. Available at: http://www.icbl.org/youth/yaw/history.html. Accessed December 24, 2008.

Youth Noise: 2008, Online. Available at: http://www.youthnoise.com/MyCauseIs/?cause_id=44&a=index. Accessed December 24, 2008.

Ziviani J, Wadley D, Ward H, et al: A place to play: socioeconomic and spatial factors in children's physical activity, *Australian Occupational Therapy Journal* 55:2–11, 2008.

Zwi K, Raman S, Burgner D, et al: Towards better health for refugee children and young people in Australia and New Zealand: The Royal Australasian College of Physicians perspective, *J Paediatr Child Health* 43:522–526, 2007.

The challenge for occupational therapy in Asia: becoming an inclusive, relevant, and progressive profession

11

Kee Hean Lim   R. Lyle Duque

OVERVIEW

Occupational therapy is a relatively young profession in Asia and attempting to capture the status and future of this dynamic and ever-evolving profession in an equally dynamic and diverse region of the world is an enormous task. Asia is home to more than 60% of the world's human population and covers a third of the earth's land area.
It encompasses a multitude of nations, territories, cultures, ethnic groups, languages, and religions. Asia always had and continues to have a significant and crucial role in world economics, politics, social initiatives, trends, and culture.

This chapter has a fourfold objective: to examine historical factors that have shaped the growth and development of occupational therapy in Asia; explore and examine the different social, political and cultural factors that impact occupational therapy education, practice, and research; identify different factors that have the potential to shape the profession's future; and outline some strategies that can help Asian occupational therapists ensure that the profession will remain viable, relevant, progressive, and inclusive in the years to come. To avoid inappropriate generalizations, we have focused on specific cases and examples of innovative and contextually relevant practice, culturally appropriate research, and creative clinical and educational initiatives in the region.

Introduction

Occupational therapy has grown and evolved significantly in the past decades in the Asian region. This is evidenced by the increasing number of countries where occupational therapy is offered or where occupational therapy educational programs have been developed (Lim 2007b). To date, there are 19 national associations of occupational therapy, which are members of the World Federation of Occupational Therapists (WFOT 2004a). This growth and development has been paralleled, and in some instances spurred, by factors such as: the increase in number of persons with disabilities, those at risk from chronic or lifestyle diseases, and victims of armed conflicts; an aging population; and an increase in the incidence of natural disasters (United Nations Economic and Social Commission for Asia and the Pacific (UNESCAP) 2007). Given these scenarios, it is reasonable to assume that occupational therapy faces a promising, albeit challenging, future in this part of the world. It is at a critical stage where its survival is dictated to a great extent by how it navigates the ever-changing social, political, economic, and cultural landscapes in the region.

The impact of occupational therapy's historical roots on its future

An examination of the history of occupational therapy in Asia highlights some historical ties that bind the different countries, including the role of armed conflicts (such as the world wars) in the genesis of the profession; the importation of occupational therapy from Western countries; and the strong link of occupational therapy with medicine. These have and continue to impact the development of the profession in the region.

© 2011, Elsevier Ltd.
DOI: 10.1016/B978-0-7020-3103-8.00020-1

The need for the rehabilitation of those injured in wars and other armed conflicts spurred the development of occupational therapy in many Asian countries. In most cases, it was introduced by practitioners from Western countries. For example, the Americans introduced occupational therapy to the Philippines (Bondoc 2005) and South Korea (Kang & Lee 2003); and the Danish introduced it to Iran (Rassafiani & Zeinali 2007). In Singapore, occupational therapy was first introduced in the 1930s by the British. However, it was only after the Second World War when it became a formal service within the Singaporean hospital system that its popularity increased (Yang et al 2006). The influence of wars and armed conflicts continue to impact the development of occupational therapy in the region and raises issues related to the allocation of healthcare resources, the development of educational programs, and the configuration of occupational therapy services. These issues will be discussed in detail later in the chapter.

With the increasing popularity of and need for occupational therapists in Asia, came the necessity for more practitioners. However, given the absence of any educational program in Asia until 1962, most local practitioners were trained in Western countries such as the United States, United Kingdom, Australia, and New Zealand (Bondoc 2005, Lim 2007b, Rassafinani & Zeinali 2007). These Western-trained practitioners brought back with them philosophies, values, and practice models steeped in Western culture. This consequently has contributed to the very 'Western complexion' of occupational therapy in Asia, pronounced in areas such as practice models utilized (Iwama 2005, Yau 2007), educational curricula (Coronel & Cabatan 2007), and practice patterns and trends (Liu et al 2006).

The development of occupational therapy in Asia, just like in the West (Yerxa 1992), has had strong historical links with medicine (Chan 2007, Yang et al 2006). This strong affiliation with medicine can be seen as the result of the confluence of several factors: the predominantly medical-oriented content of early occupational therapy curricula; the provision of occupational therapy in hospitals in the early years (Bondoc 2005, Kang & Lee 2003); and the 'political necessity' for occupational therapy to align itself with medicine during its infancy (Yerxa 1992). The implications of occupational therapy's historical link with medicine are both profound and pervasive. An examination of occupational therapy provision in several Asian countries, underscores the influence of the medical paradigm on occupational therapy practice and research.

During its infancy in South Korea, occupational therapy had a predominantly biomedical perspective and practice was influenced by scientific reductionism (Kang & Lee 2003). This medical orientation, while still influential, has become less dominant. Occupational therapy in South Korea has recently adopted a more social model of care and treatment, focusing on issues of quality of life, patient involvement, integration, and social inclusion.

Occupational therapists in India are often schooled in medical universities, spending a year acquiring knowledge on anatomy, physiology, and psychology alongside medical students. This initial medical grounding and esteeming of the medical hierarchy may predispose some occupational therapists to adopt roles and functions traditionally associated with more medical or physical forms of practice (Chavan 2007). While knowledge of medicine can serve practitioners, it is important to recognize that 'we need to understand medical thinking without adopting the medical paradigm' (Yerxa 1992, p. 82). Confusing the philosophy and domain of practice of medicine with that of occupational therapy may limit the opportunities for clinicians to exercise choice and implement occupation-based intervention.

Strong historical ties with medicine have also, in some cases, resulted in the encroachment of medical doctors on the professional autonomy of occupational therapists. In countries such as India (Srivastava 2008), China (Zhou 2005) and the Philippines (Duque & de Leon 2006), occupational therapy practice and education are still largely regulated by medical doctors, and practitioners are struggling to differentiate themselves from physiotherapists. If, as Foto (1998) asserted, 'the decisive dimension of professional status is the achievement and maintenance of autonomy', then occupational therapists in many Asian countries are faced with the formidable challenge of asserting their rights to regulate their own education and practice (see Chapter 14).

Sociocultural influences on occupational therapy practice, education, and research

Although it is inappropriate to make generalizations, it is important to recognize that there are certain values, beliefs, traditions and ways of being that are commonly shared by various socio-ethnic groups in Asia. In Asian societies, hierarchical status, collective roles, and responsibilities are highly regarded; and elders and those in authority are highly respected and esteemed (Helman 2007, Kondo 2004, Lim & Iwama 2006). A related concept, 'saving face' – having respect for someone in authority or an elder – equates to avoiding any form of action or comment that may adversely impact 'another's' credibility, status, and public image (Lim 2007b, 2008a).

Members within such hierarchical societies are not encouraged to question, criticize, or challenge the status quo; neither is it acceptable to contemplate alternative points of view apart from those collectively accepted (Helman 2007, Lim 2008a). Indeed, daring to be different, questioning, speaking to the contrary, or challenging the norm is considered highly disrespectful and can lead to the individual and their family being excluded, isolated, and even ostracized (Fujimoto & Iwama 2005, Lim 2007b). Such a situation can make it difficult for occupational therapists in these countries and communities to critique established patterns of practice or question accepted points of view, as voicing any alternative perspectives may be deemed highly disrespectful (Fujimoto & Iwama 2005, Lim 2007b).

Cultural relevance of occupational therapy concepts

The importation of occupational therapy from the West has meant that several occupational therapy theories, frameworks, and models replete with Western values and beliefs have been promoted in Asia with little examination of their applicability to the local context (Iwama 2007, Yau 2007). The popularity of and uncritical acceptance of many Western occupational therapy models by Asian practitioners can be attributed to an underlying mindset that 'West is Best' – probably a legacy of colonial history (Lim 2007b). Duque (2005) has called this *colonial practice* – the uncritical application of theories and practice models borrowed from foreign countries into the realities of people who have their own unique perspectives of truth, value, and reality. Colonial practice has several unwanted consequences on therapist–client interactions in particular and the image of occupational therapy as a humanistic and client-centered profession in general (Duque 2005).

However, in recent years, there has been an increasing awareness of the need for theories (e.g. Duque 2005, Rassafiani & Zeinali, personal communication, 15 May 2007), practice models (e.g. Iwama,

2003, 2005), educational programs (WFOT 2008), and research agenda that are more attuned to local needs. This has been paralleled by an increasing awareness of the need for culturally relevant and culturally safe practice (Iwama 2005, Lim 2008b, Watson 2006, Wittman & Velde 2002, Yang et al 2006). Several authors have pointed out that many of occupational therapy's concepts and values are not congruent with other cultures such as those in Asia (Duque 2005, Iwama 2003, Kinebanian & Stomph 1992, 2009, Whiteford & Wilcock 2000). For example, in Singapore, clients generally do not view achieving independence as a priority (Lim 2007a, Yang et al 2006); what is valued is the concept of interdependence – individuals actively supporting one another (Lim 2008a). Family members often adopt caring roles for the ill or individual with disability, and ensure that their needs and wants are met. Community members have clear roles and societal responsibilities, and are expected to fulfill certain functions and duties in the interest of the wider community (Fujimoto & Iwama 2005, Lim 2008a).

The collective structure and context is reflected in many Asian countries, where a shared, common destiny supports interdependence (Iwama 2003). Individual ambitions are secondary and therefore far less important than achieving a shared collective outcome (Lim & Iwama 2006). The concept of independence, esteemed in the West, is viewed differently in Eastern societies (Kondo 2004, Odawara 2005, 2007, Yau 2007). The desire to be independent may be associated with isolating oneself from one's family and community; consequently, the individual is marginalized and left without support from family and friends (Fujimoto & Iwama 2005, Lim 2008a). This increased appreciation of the distinctiveness of Asian culture and the availability of Eastern ideologies has encouraged Asian occupational therapists to explore the benefits of Eastern and traditional approaches in promoting and restoring health and wellbeing. This has led to the development of interventions that showcase the melding of East and West.

In Hong Kong, for example, the benefits of Tai Chi Chuan and Qi Gong, traditional methods of restoring health, balance, and wellbeing, are being explored. Cheung et al (2007), in an experimental study, examined the benefits of Tai Chi Chuan in promoting cardiovascular and pulmonary function and shoulder range of motion of people with lower limb disability. Results from the study indicated improvements in the intervention group.

Although only improvements in the range of shoulder motion were found to be statistically significant, the study highlighted the cultural and contextual appropriateness of the intervention and the overall psychological, physical, and participatory value of Tai Chi Chuan for the participants.

At the 'Self Help Group for Brain Damaged', a self-help and user-led organization supported by the Hong Kong Society for Rehabilitation (HKSR), occupational therapists teach post-stroke patients basic Qi Gong techniques to facilitate breathing, posture control, channeling of life energy, promotion of limb movement, and stamina. Group members are then encouraged to teach the Qi Gong techniques and skills to other members. The benefits and value of Qi Gong in promoting rehabilitation and recovery is articulated by one of its members: 'I have found these Qi Gong sessions to be very helpful for my stroke condition. Before I started, I could not move or use my left arm, but now I can do much more. I like Qi Gong as it helps me with my breathing, physical movement and I understand how it can help my overall health and well being.' (Self Help Group for Brain Damaged, personal communication 2008). Apart from its physical benefits, the practice of Qi Gong also contributes to the establishment of a community. In their ethnographic study, Bratun & Asaba (2008) found that 'finding calm and a sense of self in the present (being) as well as performing movements, actions, and thoughts (doing) involved in the practice of Qi Gong, contribute to community because it creates venues for communication both within and with others' (p. 82).

An innovative and creative program for children with autism in Chang Mai, Thailand is the 'Elephant Therapy' project. Launched in April 2007, it is a collaboration between the National Elephant Institute (NEI), and the Occupational Therapy Department and Faculty of Associated Medical Sciences at the Chang Mai University. Children who qualify undertake a three-week program of 'elephant therapy'. Through a graded program of exposure, the children are matched with the respective elephants and get involved in feeding and bathing the elephants and eventually riding the elephants. Initial findings from the 'elephant therapy' research project indicates some potential benefits including increased calmness, reduced stress levels, improved concentration, physical strengthening, dexterity, self control, and improvements in social interaction.

One mother commented: 'Before joining the program, my son had difficulty communicating with other people. He didn't trust anyone. He didn't have any friends. He just drew pictures and played with dolls. But at the camp, he played with everybody' (www.asianelephantresearch.com, accessed 6 December 2008). Further research is being carried out to examine the potential benefits of 'elephant therapy' with other client groups and also the ecologic and emotional benefits to the elephants that are part of the project (http://www.thailandqa.com/forum/showthread.php, accessed 6 December 2008).

While the aforementioned interventions are relatively new and need more research to document their effectiveness, they reflect a growing awareness among Asian occupational therapists of the need for culturally safe and culturally relevant practice. More importantly, they highlight the possible paradigm shift occurring where East can be blended with the West.

Education

Occupational therapy education and research in Asia reflect a growing awareness of the need for practice that is attuned to the local and global contexts. Educational curricula and research agendas have become more occupation-based and geared towards international collaboration. All countries need to examine their educational programs to ensure that they comply with the new minimum standards of educational competency of the WFOT (Hocking & Ness 2002), and more crucially ensure that the curriculum they provide is inclusive, relevant, and progressive in meeting the unique requirements of the local context.

However, producing practitioners who critically examine the cultural safety and relevance of their practice requires the nurturing of critical thinkers who are encouraged to question and exchange ideas. The opportunities to engage in educational and cultural exchange is a positive step toward encouraging debate, examining practice, sharing perspectives, challenging trends, and promoting discourse (Lim 2007b).

Cultural immersion

A unique program established to promote and enhance cross-cultural learning among occupational therapy students from Curtin University

(Perth, Australia), Brunel University (London, UK), the Hong Kong Polytechnic University, and the BoAi Children's Rehabilitation Centre (Shanghai), is the Go Global Project. Originally conceived at Curtin University, it provides students, through a process of cultural immersion, the opportunity to deepen their own cultural awareness, enhance their knowledge of service development, and acquire global perspectives of occupational therapy education and service provision (Goddard & Gribble 2006).

Healthcare students including occupational therapists, physiotherapists, and speech and language therapists from Curtin University and occupational therapy students from Brunel University undertake a five-week placement in a children's rehabilitation center in Shanghai, China. Students begin with acquiring basic language skills and undertaking preparatory exercises that promotes examination of their own attitudes, values, and perspectives. Through interaction with children, parents, care providers and health professionals at the BoAi rehabilitation center, local students, health professionals, and families, students are provided the opportunity to share, discuss, develop, and acquire valuable cultural skills and knowledge (see Section 3).

Students also acquire a wider perspective of and deeper insight into how health and social care is provided in different contexts, sociocultural views on therapy and how occupational therapy is culturally perceived and provided in different countries. Additionally, students acquire knowledge about and experience in how nongovernmental organizations (NGOs) work and how educational programs are designed. Through this process of cultural immersion, students who have completed the project indicate that they have gained insight into their own values, beliefs, prejudices, frailties, and developed a better understanding of cultural and social differences. One student who participated in the program describes the gradual development of a new perspective and understanding:

> At first I found it really hard as the difference in attitudes to how children are brought up and the treatment of children in Shanghai seemed totally in conflict with my own values, beliefs, and occupational therapy training. However, as I spend time within this new context and at the BoAi centre, I began to appreciate why things are done differently and that different sociocultural attitudes and priorities have their own value.

Research

The quality of occupational therapy research has improved substantially in Asia over the past decade, with studies becoming more complex (Chan 2007, Wright-St Clair et al 2004, Wong & Li-Tsang 2007), collaborative (Hocking et al 2008), and culturally relevant (Cheung et al 2007). Occupational therapy research in Asia is increasingly reflecting the need for assessments (Chan et al 2006, Tay et al 2007) and interventions (Chung et al 2007) to be more culturally inclusive, relevant, and responsive to the needs of the local context, highlighting the importance of having a new generation of occupational therapists trained and skilled in a range of research approaches and methods that will promote culturally safe and inclusive occupational therapy research.

However, many Asian practitioners still do not engage in research. For instance, Duque (2007) highlighted the difficulty associated with building a research tradition in developing countries such as the Philippines. He cited several reasons for this low priority for research: time constraints; lack of funding, infrastructure and resources; practitioners' lack of research competencies; a general perception of the 'clinician-researcher' divide; brain drain and colonial practice. He proposed a three-pronged strategy to address the problem: development of research interest and competencies among practitioners; provision of infrastructure and resources to support research; and formation of networks and interprofessional collaboration.

Politics, economics, and occupational therapy

The development of occupational therapy in the majority of Asian countries continues to be influenced by strong political agendas, demographic changes, social policy initiatives, and economic resource allocation (Lim 2007a). For example, Jordan, geographically located in an area of continuous political conflict and unrest (the Iraq War, the Palestinian/Israeli war, and the unstable Lebanese situation), is confronted by conflicting health priorities and demands. Questions are raised as to whether limited health resources and funding should be focused on treating refugees from areas of conflict or reserved for the health needs of its own citizens (Al Heresh, personal communication 2008). The political, socio-cultural, and economic debate in deciding resources allocation, treatment priorities, and cost management, is crucial and ultimately influences how occupational therapy is viewed within the Jordanian context. Al Heresh (personal communication 2008) indicated that societal views on disability, the importance of rehabilitation and disagreement with resource allocation for those with refugee status in Jordan has a significant influence on how occupational therapy interventions and resources are prioritized.

The system and source of funding for health services influence which areas of occupational therapy practice are prioritized. In countries such as Japan, Taiwan, Singapore, South Korea, and Malaysia, where there is an increasing proportion of older persons, more investment has flowed into services that support the needs of this specific population. Similarly, resources are also concentrated in socially regarded areas such as stroke and cardiac rehabilitation, community rehabilitation and pediatric services, whilst resources for mental health services are more limited (Lim 2007b, 2008a).

In Japan, where health and social care is paid for through the National Insurance system, the provision of occupational therapy is closely linked with these insurance payments. Occupational therapists within Japan are required to substantiate their practice claims through research in order to secure additional funding. The emphasis is more on quantity-oriented outcomes rather than issues of quality of life and improvement in an individual's experience of their personal recovery (Ishibashi, Survey response: occupational therapy in Japan, unpublished data 2008, Yoshikawa, personal communication, 2008).

In China, where there is little or no state benefit available for health services and citizens pay for health services out of their own pockets, emphasis is placed on rehabilitation (Nara et al 2007, Zhou 2006). Clients and their families are keen on accessing medical or therapy services that facilitate rehabilitation and promote productivity. Returning to work and sustaining employment are sociocultural and economic priorities. Persons with disabilities choose to pay for therapeutic services they perceive will enhance their physical health and facilitate recovery. Therefore, being able to walk independently may be considered more of a priority than

being able to perform personal activities of daily living, such as getting dressed and washed (Chan 2007). This is because being able to walk independently is seen as having a direct link to being productive, gaining employment, and therefore providing financially for the family. The need to be productive is such a societal priority that what may be viewed as repetitive work in the West, such as assembling darts or electrical switches as part of work rehabilitation, is well regarded within such a context.

In many parts of Asia, access to occupational therapy services is limited due to several factors such as the scarcity of practitioners and the prohibitive cost of such services. One program that was initiated in response to this challenge was *Thera-Free*.

THERA-FREE: LIBRENG THERAPY PARA SA PILIPINO (THERA-FREE: FREE THERAPY FOR FILIPINOS)

In the Philippines, the combination of a growing number of persons with disabilities, the unabated migration of therapists, and the poor state of the economy and health care system, has led to the creation of an innovative program called Thera-Free: Libreng Therapy Para sa Pilipino (Thera-Free: Free Therapy for Filipinos) (Duque & de Leon 2006). Thera-Free was conceptualized by alumni (occupational therapists, physiotherapists, and speech and language pathologists) of the College of Allied Medical Professions (CAMP) of the University of the Philippines Manila in 2002. It is a joint program of the CAMP Alumni Association (CAMPAA) and the Therapy Centres' Movement (TCM). The TCM is an association of 13 therapy centers owned and managed by alumni of the CAMP (Thera-Free News 2003).

Thera-Free volunteers (therapists and other allied health professionals such as doctors and nurses) offer free therapy and other health services to communities across the country identified as needing health services (particularly therapy services). Aside from free therapy and medical services, volunteers provide home programs for community members and deliver lectures on topics such as prevention of conditions common in the community (e.g, stroke), identifying people who may benefit from therapy, and strategies for supporting people with disabilities in the community.

The realization of the program's objectives (outlined in Box 11.1) is anchored on three vital components: *knowledge of local culture, needs and resources; sense of volunteerism and social responsibility* among therapists; and *collaboration* between clinicians, academicians and government and NGOs (Duque & de Leon 2006).

Box 11.1

Thera-Free program objectives

1. Provide free, accessible, and quality occupational therapy, physical therapy and speech language pathology services to Filipinos who cannot readily avail such services
2. Increase public awareness regarding the benefits of opportune therapy
3. Increase social awareness and sense of social responsibility among Filipino therapists and strengthen their ties with their immediate communities
4. Establish networks and linkages between therapists and other health professionals, cause-oriented organizations and local community leaders
5. Provide a venue for research

---

when needed, translate these into local languages or dialects. The LGUs and NGOs provide logistical support to the volunteers, including coordinating with the community leaders, providing transportation, food, and if warranted, accommodation for volunteers. So far, 54 Thera-Free sessions have been held in 14 provinces and six cities. Over 1800 therapy sessions and 1200 medical and allied health consultations have been provided by more than 250 therapists and other allied health professionals. All these translate to more than 1.5 million pesos worth of free services.

While the program has achieved a lot during its short existence, several challenges remain in order for it to stay viable and responsive to the needs of the country: fewer volunteers due to brain drain; dwindling support from NGOs and LGUs; lack of political action to have Thera-Free incorporated into local and national health programs; and a lack of manpower to synthesize data that can be used as a resource for program evaluation and policy formulation (Duque & de Leon 2006).

Communities are usually identified through the social networks of the alumni. In some cases, local government units (LGUs) that have heard of the program request the TCM or CAMPAA to hold Thera-Free in their community. Prior to holding Thera-Free in a community, the TCM and CAMPAA conduct an informal needs assessment to gain *knowledge of* the *culture, needs and resources* of the community. Factors such as common health conditions in the community, socioeconomic, political and educational background of the community, language/s spoken, cultural beliefs, and norms and local resources available (e.g., the presence of community health workers, indigenous materials that can be used for therapy) are identified. These are vital in making decisions regarding the choice of volunteers and preparation of educational/training materials (Duque & de Leon 2006).

The majority of volunteers are alumni of the CAMP. As alumni of the University of the Philippines Manila, a state-subsidized university, they are considered *Iskolars ng Bayan* (Scholars of the Nation). As such, these alumni consider themselves indebted to the Filipino people who, through their taxes, have partly paid for their college education. It is this sense of indebtedness that underpins the *sense of volunteerism and social responsibility* (Duque & de Leon 2006). This was eloquently pointed out by one of the volunteers:

> *It was a way for me to give back to the community. I am forever grateful to them and it is always a pleasure to be of service to others and touch their lives.*
>
> (Thera-Free News 2003)

The success of any Thera-Free project hinges on the collaboration of clinicians, academicians and LGUs and NGOs. Clinicians provide therapy services and train members of the local community. Academicians prepare home programs, educational and training materials, and

Challenges for the future: reflection, innovation, political action

The future of occupational therapy in Asia is contingent on its ability to respond to the ever-evolving social, cultural, economic, and political challenges in the region. At a time of seemingly increasing political conflict and worsening ecological and economic crises, it is imperative that Asian occupational therapists become reflective, innovative, and political. More importantly, collaboration among Asian countries is needed. While Asian practitioners have become more cognizant of the need to be more critical of trends they adopt from outside their countries, there is still a continuing need to develop practice models that are attuned to the needs and realities of local contexts (Lim 2007a, Yang et al 2006); develop frameworks for service delivery that are relevant and responsive the distinctive needs of the people served; and develop innovative interventions to respond to the evolving needs of the population (Lim 2007b, 2008a).

The tragic events of the Asian Tsunami in December 2004 and the China earthquake in 2008 highlight the need for practitioners to acquire the skills in the areas of disaster response, trauma assessment, and care and relief management (see Chapter 20). These tragedies served as impetus for occupational therapists in Thailand (Sakornsatian 2007), Indonesia (Santosa et al 2007) and China (Hong Kong

Occupational Therapy Association (HKOTA) 2008) to develop strategies for assisting victims and their families deal with the emotional, psychological, occupational, and physical consequences of the disaster. Practitioners have been involved in physical and psychosocial rehabilitation, curriculum development, community training and rebuilding, occupational/ functional assessment and vocational training (HKOTA 2008, Sakornsatian 2007, Santosa et al 2007, Whitford 2007).

The increase in the occurrence of natural disasters has been attributed to climate change brought about by environmental degradation. Healthcare professionals are beginning to recognize their role in this area (Health Care Without Harm n.d.). However, occupational therapists, despite their work on disaster response, have been slower to involve themselves in ecological issues (see Chapter 26). A possible explanation for this can be gleaned from the statement of a young Filipino occupational therapist involved with an environmental protection group: 'Finding a connection between our profession and environmentalism may be a bit challenging but not impossible' (Ochavo, personal communication, 17 December 2008). Hudson & Aoyama (2008, p. 545) argue that occupational therapists can contribute to environmental conservation in three areas: 'understanding how people negotiate and adjust their daily activities in situations of ecological and social stress; interventions that link the conservation of biodiversity with the conservation of occupations; and a renewed focus on balance in the everyday activities of people in the industrialized world'. This is a practice area that Asian practitioners need explore.

Kronenberg et al (2005) and Pollard et al (2008) asserted that occupational therapists need to become more politically aware and engaged in influencing decision making at all levels on a daily basis. They coined the term pADL (Political Activities of Daily Living), referring to politics as part and parcel of daily human occupation and engagement with others. Political action is needed in several fronts: professional autonomy; advocacy for the people we serve; change that aims to advance peace, social justice and equality; change within the profession to make it more socially responsive, progressive, and inclusive of diverse populations, cultures, and perspectives.

This focus on being more political has had mixed success with occupational therapists. The political engagement of Asian occupational therapists has focused more on gaining professional autonomy (Duque & de Leon 2006; Srivastava 2008) and increasing the public's awareness of the unique contribution the profession can make (Duque & de Leon 2006). However, Asian occupational therapists' political action to advance issues such as human rights and occupational justice in the region has been less pronounced. This lukewarm reception of political action may be attributed to prevailing social norms and a misunderstanding of what politics means. Asian practitioners are faced with the formidable task of balancing the need to function within social structures that have strict norms with being critical of the existing practice, social, political, and educational structures that influence their practice, roles, functions, and responsibilities (Yang et al 2006). They need to start to view the process of objectively critiquing practice and established norms as a positive step towards improving the quality of care and service delivery (Lim 2007b).

Conclusion

Occupational therapy in Asia has made significant progress in the past decades. Its future is contingent upon how it can navigate the ever-changing social, political, economic, and cultural landscapes in the region. Asian occupational therapists have myriads of opportunities to contribute to the development of the profession worldwide through innovations in practice, education, and research. However, this is dependent on their ability to capitalize on the gains they have made thus far; recognize and act on the need to attune practice, education, and research to local and global needs; muster the political will to assert their autonomy and advocate for the people they serve; and work collaboratively towards the achievement of a shared vision for an inclusive, progressive and relevant profession.

Acknowledgment

We would like to acknowledge the contribution of all the occupational therapists who have responded to our inquiries and provided us with valuable resources to help us write this chapter. In particular, we thank Mr Lim Hua Beng for sharing his valuable insights into the development and future of occupational therapy in Asia. Lastly, we hope that we have done the Asian occupational therapy community and profession justice by producing an inclusive and respectful chapter.

References

Bondoc S: Occupational therapy in the Philippines: From founding years to the present, *Philippine Journal of Occupational Therapy* 1:9–22, 2005.

Bratun U, Asaba E: From individual to communal experiences of occupation: Drawing upon Qi Gong practices, *Journal of Occupational Science* 15:80–86, 2008.

Chan S: Occupations and activities: a revisit of occupational therapy's core values in the local context, *Hong Kong Journal of Occupational Therapy* 17:34–36, 2007.

Chan V, Chung J, Packer T: Validity and reliability of the activity card sort – Hong Kong version, *OTJR: Occupation, Participation and Health* 26:152–158, 2006.

Chavan SR: Clinical Rating Scale for Head Control: A Pilot Study, *The Indian Journal of Occupational Therapy* XXXIX:59–64, 2007.

Cheung SY, Tsai E, Fung L, Ng J: Physical benefits of Tai Chi Chuan for individuals with lower limb disabilities, *Occup Ther Int* 14:1–10, 2007.

Chan DYL, Chan CCH, Au DKS: Motor relearning programme for stroke patients: a randomized controlled trial, *Clin Rehabil* 20:1–10, 2006.

Chung JCC, Packer TL, Tay G: *Cross-cultural comparison of the activity participation patterns of older adults in Australia, Hong Kong & Singapore*, Hong Kong, 2007, 4th Asia Pacific Occupational Therapy Congress.

Coronel CMA, Cabatan MC: Curriculum redesign – the University of the Philippines Manila Experience, *Philippine Journal of Occupational Therapy* 3:3–5, 2007.

Duque RL: *A theory of occupation from a Filipino perspective*, Unpublished masters dissertation, Plymouth, 2005, University of Plymouth.

Duque RL: Building a tradition of research in a developing country: Mission impossible? *Philippine Journal of Occupational Therapy* 3:3–6, 2007.

Duque RL, de Leon CI: Issues and perspectives: Occupational therapy in the Philippines: Where have we been and where are we headed? *Philippine Journal of Occupational Therapy* 2:57–67, 2006.

Foto M: The Merlin factor: creating our strategic intent for the future today, *Am J Occup Ther* 52:399–402, 1998.

Fujimoto H, Iwama M: Muffled cries and occupational injustices in Japanese society. In Kronenberg F, Algado SA, Pollard N, editors: *Occupational Therapy Without Borders. Learning from the Spirit of Survivors*, Edinburgh, 2005, Elsevier/Churchill Livingstone, pp 351–360.

Goddard T, Gribble N: *A service learning relationship fostering cultural competency: the cultural immersion of occupational therapy students and reflective practice*, Enhancing Student Learning: 2006 Evaluations and Assessment Conference Refereed Papers, 2006.

Health Care without Harm: *Mission and Goals*. n.d., Online. Available at: http://www.noharm.org/globalsoutheng/aboutUs/missionGoals. Accessed January 2, 2009.

Helman CG: *Culture health and illness*, ed 5, New York, 2007, Oxford University Press.

Hocking C, Ness NE: Introduction to the revised minimum standards for the education of occupational therapists, *WFOT Bulletin* 46:30–33, 2002.

Hocking C, Pierce D, Shordike A, et al: The promise of internationally collaborative research for studying occupation: The example of the older women's food preparation study, *OTJR: Occupation, Participation and Health* 28:180–190, 2008.

Hong Kong Occupational Therapy Association: *ProgressReport on Occupational Therapy Voluntary Work for Earthquake Victims in Sichuan*, 2008, Online. Available at: http://www.hkota.org.hk/ot_development.htm. Accessed October 2, 2008.

Hudson MJ, Aoyama M: Occupational therapy and the current ecological crisis, *British Journal of Occupational Therapy* 71:545–548, 2008.

Iwama MK: The issue is … 'Toward culturally relevant epistemologies in occupational Therapy', *Am J Occup Ther* 57:582–589, 2003.

Iwama M: Situated meaning: an issue of culture, inclusion and occupational therapy. In Kronenberg F, Algado SA,

Pollard N, editors: *Occupational Therapy Without Borders. Learning from the Spirit of Survivors*, Edinburgh, 2005, Elsevier/Churchill Livingstone, pp 127–139.

Iwama M: Culture and occupational therapy: meeting the challenge of relevance in a global world, *Occup Ther Int* 4:183–187, 2007.

Kang D, Lee T: The evolution of occupational therapy profession in Korea, *Asian Journal of Occupational Therapy* 2:3–9, 2003.

Kinebanian A, Stomph M: Cross-cultural occupational therapy: A critical reflection, *Am J Occup Ther* 46:751–757, 1992.

Kinebanian A, Stomph M, editors: *World Federation of Occupational Therapists. Diversity Matters: Guiding Principles on Diversity and Culture*, Forrestfield, Australia, 2009, WFOT.

Kondo T: Cultural tensions in occupational therapy practice: considerations from a Japanese vantage point, *Am J Occup Ther* 58:174–184, 2004.

Kronenberg F, Simo Algado S, Pollard N, editors: *Occupational Therapy Without Borders. Learning from the Spirit of Survivors*, Edinburgh, 2005, Elsevier/Churchill Livingstone.

Lim HB: *Sato Memorial Lecture of Dreams and Aspirations: The Future of Occupational Therapy Through the Eyes of Young Practiontioners*, Hong Kong, 2007a, 4th Asia Pacific Occupational Therapy Congress.

Lim KH: *Conference Symposium: Global Occupational Therapy: Asian Perspectives, Challenges and Contributions*, Hong Kong, 2007b, 4th Asia Pacific Occupational Therapy Congress.

Lim KH: Cultural sensitivity in context. In McKay EA, Craik C, Lim KH, Richards G, editors: *Advancing Occupational Therapy in Mental Health Practice*, Oxford, 2008a, Blackwell Publishing, pp 30–47.

Lim KH: Working in a transcultural context. In Creek J, Lougher L, editors: *Occupational Therapy and Mental Health*, ed 4, in print, Edinburgh, 2008b, Churchill Livingstone, pp 251–274.

Lim KH, Iwama M: Emerging Models – An Asian Perspective: The Kawa (River) Model. In Duncan E, editor: *Hagedorn's Foundations for Practice*, Edinburgh, 2006, Elsevier.

Liu J, Ochavo F, Torres E: Handwriting: Current practice of occupational therapy in Metro Manila, *Philippine Journal of Occupational Therapy* 1:5–14, 2006.

Nara NH, Shinkawa H, Sugihara M: *Beginnings of occupational therapy education in mainland China: Opinions of freshly graduated occupational therapists*, Hong Kong, 2007, 4th Asia Pacific Occupational Therapy Congress.

Odawara E: Cultural competency in occupational therapy: Beyond a cross-cultural view of practice, *Am J Occup Ther* 59:325–334, 2005.

Odawara E: *A Japanese perspective of occupational therapy intervention*, Hong Kong, 2007, 4th Asia Pacific Occupational Therapy Congress.

Pollard N, Sakellariou D, Kronenberg F, editors: *A Political Practice of Occupational Therapy*, Edinburgh, 2008, Elsevier Science.

Rassafiani M, Zeinali R: *Occupational therapy in Iran*, 2007, Online. Available at: http://www.wfot.org.au/documents/History_Occupational_therapy_in_Iran.pdf. Accessed May 18, 2008.

Sakornsatian S: *The experience of Thai occupational therapist in helping the survivors from tsunami disaster*, Hong Kong, 2007, 4th Asia Pacific Occupational Therapy Congress.

Santosa TB, Kuncor B, Buana C: *The roles of occupational therapist in disaster preparedness and response*, Hong Kong, 2007, 4th Asia Pacific Occupational Therapy Congress.

Srivastava A: Editorial, *Indian Journal of Occupational Therapy* 40:1, 2008.

Tay G, Khau LT, Hobman J, et al: *Activity sort card (Singapore Version): Psychometric properties*, Hong Kong, 2007, 4th Asia Pacific Occupational Therapy Congress.

Thera-Free News: Volunteers speak out, p4, 14, January–June, 2003.

United Nations Economic and Social Commission for the Asia and the Pacific: *Statistical Yearbook for Asia and the Pacific 2007*, 2007, Available at: http://unescap.org/stat/data/syb2007/8-Chronic-diseases-and-other-health-risks-syb2007.asp. Accessed May 19, 2008.

Watson RM: Being before doing: The cultural identity (essence) of occupational therapy, *Australian Occupational Therapy Journal* 53:151–158, 2006.

Whiteford GE, Wilcock AA: Cultural relativism: occupation and independence reconsidered, *Can J Occup Ther* 67:314–323, 2000.

Whitford A: *The meaning of occupation for persons affected by the tsunami in Thailand*, Hong Kong, 2007, 4th Asia Pacific Occupational Therapy Congress.

Wittman P, Velde BE: Attaining cultural competence, critical thinking, and intellectual development: a challenge for occupational therapists, *Am J Occup Ther* 56:454–456, 2002.

Wong JKK, Li-Tsang CWP: *Enhancing visual search in people with intellectual disabilities*, Hong Kong, 2007, 4th Asia Pacific Occupational Therapy Congress.

World Federation for Occupational Therapists: *Country Profile*, 2004a, Online. Available at: http://www.wfot.org/countryprofileLinks.asp. Accessed May 11, 2008.

World Federation of Occupational Therapists: *Educational Programs*, 2008, Online. Available at: http://www.wfot.org/schoolLinks.asp. Accessed May 17, 2008.

Wright-St Clair V, Bunrayong W, Vittayakorn S, et al: Offerings: Food traditions of older Thai women at Songkran, *Journal of Occupational Science* 11:115–124, 2004.

Yang S, Shek MP, Tsunaka M, Lim HB: Cultural influences on occupational therapy practice in Singapore: a pilot study, *Occup Ther Int* 13:176–192, 2006.

Yau K S Mathew: Universality and Cultural Specificity in Occupational Therapy Practice: From Hong Kong to Asia. *Hong Kong Journal of Occupational Therapy* 17:60–64, 2007.

Yerxa EJ: Some implications of occupational therapy's history for its epistemology, values, and relation to medicine, *Am J Occup Ther* 46:79–83, 1992.

Zhou DH: *Opportunity of developing occupational therapy in China*, Paper presented at the International Conference in Occupational Therapy, Qingdao, China, 2005.

Zhou DH: Present situation and future development of occupational therapy. In *China 2006 Hong Kong Occupational Therapy in China, Hong Kong Journal of Occupational Therapy*, vol 16, 2006, pp 23–25.

Influencing social challenges through occupational performance

12

Moses N. Ikiugu

OVERVIEW

Occupational therapists' knowledge uniquely equips them to contribute substantially to addressing many social challenges that may be attributed to occupational choices and performance. In this chapter, a framework (Modified Instrumentalism in Occupational Therapy (MIOT)) is presented as a conceptual model that therapists could use to guide empowerment of individuals and groups so that they can alter their occupational choices and performance patterns in an endeavor to address such challenges. A case study is presented to illustrate how the framework may be applied. Occupational therapists can use its guidelines to justify funding of community-based occupational therapy services.

Introduction

The ubiquity of occupation and its link to human wellbeing (Reilly 1962) mandates occupational therapists to contribute their unique knowledge to illuminating many occupation-related social challenges beyond the medical settings. As Wilcock (2006) states: 'Occupational therapists have a valuable contribution to make to the prevention of illness for all people, not just those who are sick and disabled' (p. 275). Many occupational therapy leaders and scholars have started exploring that possibility. Townsend & Wilcock (2004) introduced the construct of *occupational injustice* as a human condition that occupational therapists can help address, separate from the more recognized issue of social injustice. They argued that occupational therapists have a duty to empower those who are affected by occupational deprivation, alienation, disruption, and/or imbalance, enabling them to choose and participate in occupations that are meaningful to them, their families, and communities. Their pioneering conceptual work prompted inquiry by a number of occupational therapy scholars such as Duncan & Watson (2004) and Fourie et al (2004) among others.

Similarly, Werner (2005) argued that occupational therapy should embrace 'the human struggle to build healthier communities – and ultimately to build a civilization – which both celebrate diversity and provide equal opportunities for all' (p. xi). Ikiugu (2008a, b) explored ways in which occupational therapists and occupational scientists could contribute to: building organizations that were healthier for workers; helping resolve pertinent global issues of our time such as poverty, economic inequalities, diseases, environmental damage and subsequent climate change, overpopulation; etc. In this chapter I add to the above endeavors a proposed conceptual framework for guiding empowerment of individuals and communities to enable them to address social challenges through occupational performance. The framework is based on the Instrumentalism in Occupational Therapy (IOT) theoretical conceptual model of practice that was developed by Ikiugu (2004a–c) based on the philosophy of pragmatism and the chaos/complexity/dynamical systems theory (see also Ikiugu 2007, Ikiugu & Anderson 2007). In the rest of the chapter, I will introduce the model. Its application as a conceptual framework for guiding therapists in empowering individuals to address issues of concern to humanity through occupational performance will be discussed. In the discussion, consistent with Kronenberg & Pollard's (2005b) call for more inclusiveness in

© 2010, Elsevier Ltd.
DOI: 10.1016/B978-0-7020-3103-8.00021-3

the profession, individuals with whom occupational therapists collaborate to create change will be referred to as 'partners' rather than 'clients', to emphasize the collaborative approach to addressing challenges of priority to these individuals.

Evolution of the modified instrumentalism in occupational therapy

Instrumentalism in Occupational Therapy was created in response to the conclusion reached by a number of scholars that the philosophical foundation of occupational therapy was American pragmatism (Breines 1986, Cutchin 2004, Ikiugu 2001, Ikiugu & Schultz 2006, Wilcock 1998). Pragmatism is a school of philosophy developed by Charles Sanders Peirce based on the premise that the human mind exists in one of two states: belief or doubt (Peirce 1955). According to Peirce, belief is the preferred state of the mind because doubt creates conflict. Human beings seek to dispel doubt by establishing belief. Once belief is established, action is initiated to produce consequences to confirm its veracity. If the consequences are as expected, it is confirmed. If they are other than expected, a state of doubt ensues and further action is generated to investigate and re-establish belief in order to dispel doubt. Therefore, in Peirce's view, all human inquiry and actions are a way of confirming (or fixing) beliefs. He concluded that belief is a rule for action (all actions emanate from beliefs).

William James (1981) and later John Dewey (1981) elaborated on this idea by suggesting that through beliefs as a basis for action, the mind can be construed as a means of guiding actions that shape the environment. In that sense the mind is a tool like any other that human beings use to shape the environment to make it supportive of their survival (*adaptation* according to Darwin (1985), whose theory of evolution was regarded highly by Peirce and colleagues and which influenced the development of pragmatic philosophy (Buchler 1955, McDermott 1981)). Dewey called the notion of the mind as a tool for adaptation *instrumentalism*. Ikiugu (2004a–c) developed a theoretical conceptual model of practice for occupational therapy by operationalizing the construct of instrumentalism for clinical application. Constructs from chaos/dynamical systems theory that appeared to be more appropriate than Darwin's evolutionism for explaining the complex

phenomenon of occupational performance (Kielhofner 2004, Royeen 2003) were borrowed to develop a theoretical core for the model.

Following are the basic propositions of the model. Consistent with the theoretical propositions of the chaos/dynamical systems theory

1. The occupational human being is conceptualized as a complex, dynamical, adaptive system, interacting with the environment through occupational performance.
2. The system has an occupational life trajectory (a temporal path that it follows) which consists of a repertoire of occupations that constitute a pattern that is self-similar. By self-similarity is meant that a part of the trajectory consists of occupational performance patterns that are similar to those of the entire trajectory spanning a significant period of an individual's life (Bassingthwaighte et al 1994).
3. The trajectory may be adaptive or maladaptive. The therapist's role is to assess a portion of the trajectory, determine its adaptability or maladaptability, and establish an intervention plan to make it more adaptive if indicated.

Ikiugu (2008b) modified the IOT theoretical conceptual model (modified IOT (MIOT)) so that it could be used to help individuals and communities identify potentially maladaptive occupational choices and performance patterns and alter them (for example, walking rather than driving on short trips; as an individual action this may not seem like much, but as a collective action, it may significantly impact global issues such as climate change). Such occupational choices can be seen as steps in building a personal or community legacy, based on occupational performance, and can be applied to a range of social challenges such as poverty, material inequality, diseases, corruption, institutional failures, etc. The intervention process based on guidelines of the MIOT conceptual framework is illustrated in Figure 12.1.

Assessments

As is evident in Figure 12.1, three assessments are used to help identify occupational performance issues and guide the process of addressing them using the MIOT framework as a guide: the Modified Assessment and Intervention Instrument for Instrumentalism in Occupational Therapy (MAIIIOT); the Daily

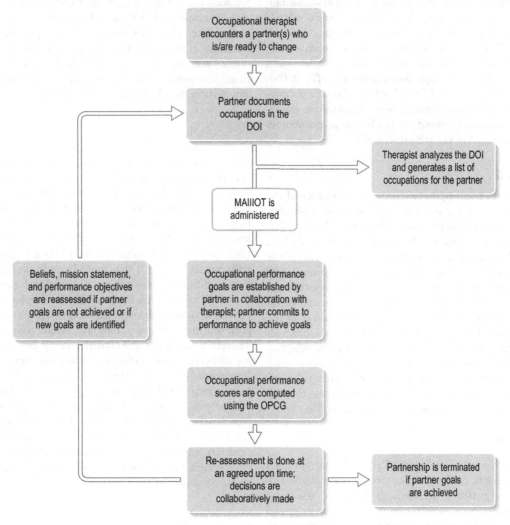

Fig. 12.1 • The Modified Instrumentalism in Occupational Therapy (MIOT) framework. DOI, Daily Occupational Inventory; MAIIIOT, Modified Assessment and Intervention Instrument for Instrumentalism in Occupational Therapy; OPCG, Occupational Performance Calculation Guide.

Occupational Inventory (DOI); and the Occupational performance Calculation Guide (OPCG). The DOI and OPCG are used together, with the DOI as a means of documenting occupations performed within a specified period of time, and the OPCG as a guide for computation of performance scores based on those occupations.

The MAIIIOT

This assessment consists of four parts.

Part I

Partners engage in a visualization exercise in which they imagine what people in their life (family members, friends, colleagues at work/school/other productive activities, community members) would say about them if they were no longer living among them. Based on the imagined statements, a mission statement specifying the partner's desired legacy in the world is created. The statement consists of achievements that would lead to imagined positive statements by people in four areas of the partner's life: family (including intimate partners); sociali-zation (partner's friends and peers); work/school/ other productive occupational colleagues (includ-ing colleagues in occupations such as volunteering, home management, etc. as defined by the American Occupational Therapy Association (AOTA 2008). According to the AOTA, school qualifies as a produc-tive occupation and therefore is categorized as work); and community members (including acquaintances in virtual networks (the internet)).

Part II

Partners choose up to two occupations in each of the four areas of the mission statement, for a possible total of eight occupations, which they believe that if performed consistently and adequately would lead to achievement of the stated mission. In terms of the chaos/dynamical systems theory, establishing a mis-sion statement and choosing occupations that are likely to lead to achievement of the mission intro-duce perturbation to the system and push it in the desired direction away from a stable, steady, but mal-adaptive state. Reorganization into a more adaptive system (Okes 2003), through performance with desired frequency and adequacy of meaningful occu-pations, enables partners to develop patterns that are conducive to achieving their missions in life.

Part III

For each occupation listed in Part II, the partner rates him/herself on four scales: frequency with which the occupation is performed; perceived adequacy of performance; satisfaction with performance; and belief about ability to perform the occupation with desired frequency and adequacy. Each scale is based on four-point Likert-type ratings, and is operationa-lized independently. For example, responses in the frequency scale range from '1 = does not engage in the occupation' to '4 = frequently engages in the occupation.' Responses in the belief scale range from '1 = I do not believe that I am capable of engaging in the occupation' to '4 = I believe I can engage in the occupation adequately and independently' (Ikiugu 2007, p. 410–411).

Part IV

The ratings are aggregated to produce a quantitative score for each scale (for details, see the above cited source). Finally, the partners, in collaboration with the therapist establish short term- and long-term goals

for each occupation whose satisfaction with perfor-mance is rated at less than 4. The goals are designed to facilitate action that would lead to improved per-formance of the occupations in question with the fre-quency and adequacy desired by the partner, leading to achievement of the stated mission. The therapist and partner decide on a time of reassessment.

The DOI

This is an inventory in which the partner documents occupations engaged in for a specific period of time (4, 7, 14 days, etc.) on an hourly basis from 6:00 am through 12:00 midnight. One may notice that occupations performed after midnight are not accounted for. The partner and therapist may decide to document occupations in the 12:00 am through 6:00 pm time cycle if that period would illuminate better the partner's unique occupational perfor-mance patterns. This instrument was developed to provide a window through which the partner's occu-pational life trajectory may be briefly observed. Therefore, it is not deemed necessary to account for all occupations performed at any one time. Just a sample of the occupations is considered adequate for the purpose of analyzing a segment of the trajec-tory to indicate its adaptiveness or maladaptiveness (see Ikiugu & Rosso 2005). The partner completes the DOIs and submits them to the therapist who compiles a list of occupations and the frequency of engagement in each of them before the MAIIIOT assessment is administered.

The OPCG

After the MAIIIOT administration, partners are presented with a list of occupations compiled from the DOIs submitted to the therapist earlier and asked to rank them in order of importance in helping them achieve the missions articulated during part I of the MAIIIOT assessment. Using the OPCG guidelines, the top five ranked occupations are used to calculate a performance score for the partner using the following formula (Ikiugu & Rosso 2005): $P_t = \sum(P_i) = \sum(F \times PI)$, where P_t = total performance score, P_i = performance score associated with each of the five occupations, F = frequency of engagement in the occupation, and PI = performance index accord-ing to the occupation's rank ($PI = 5$ for occupation ranked number 1, 4 for number 2, 3 for number 3, 2 for number 4, and 1 for number 5).

The resultant quantitative score (P_t) is sensitive to change in frequency of performance of valued occupations (valued because they contribute the most to realization of the desired legacy in life). The partner's progress towards established goals can be determined by readministering the assessments at reasonable intervals. From the outcome of reassessment, the partner and therapist collaboratively make a decision regarding whether to terminate the partnership (if established goals have been achieved), or to re-evaluate the partner's beliefs, mission statement, and/or goals.

Internal and external validity of the MIOT assessments

The assessments described above are new and their validity and reliability have not been determined conclusively. Face validity was established through extensive literature review and feedback from at least three colleagues who are well versed with client-centered occupational therapy practice. Pilot validity and reliability studies indicate that the assessments show promise of being valid and reliable measures of occupational performance across a range of partner groups (Ikiugu & Ciaravino 2006, Ikiugu & Rosso 2005, Ikiugu et al 2008). Efforts are being made to conduct more studies with robust samples to reach firm conclusions about the validity and reliability of the assessments. Because the MIOT framework focuses on occupations that are perceived by the partner to be a priority, it does not seek to impose any notion of cultural performance appropriateness and therefore should present no cultural validity problem. The partner makes decisions about the personal mission, occupations to help them achieve it, and acceptable level of performance. The therapist merely facilitates the process.

Application of the MIOT framework

Before discussing the application of the MIOT framework, it is necessary to examine what individual and community empowerment means. For individuals, it refers to facilitation of 'a sense of control over one's life in personality, cognition and motivation' (Koelen & Lindstrom 2005, p. S11). Empowered individuals have an inner sense of control over their lives, and of ability to change the world around them. Community empowerment could be defined as promotion of increased participation of community members in a discourse geared towards creating a better community life and improved social justice (Wallerstein 1992), or occupational justice (see Whiteford & Townsend elsewhere in this book). Given the above definitions, the six propositions on which application of the MIOT framework is based are:

1. People in disadvantaged situations (the disabled, the poor, minorities of all types, and all those who are disenfranchised in any way) often get stuck in unfavorable circumstances not because they are completely powerless, but because they learn to accept their circumstances as inevitable. This phenomenon is referred to as learned helplessness (Kay et al 2000, Meyer 2005, Yale University School of Medicine 2001). Powerlessness is experienced when individuals are placed in situations of oppression for so long that they come to accept their situation as inevitable, and to believe that they can never change things by their own efforts because structural barriers are too formidable to confront. Even when circumstances change and opportunities for self-improvement present themselves, the individuals are unable to take advantage of those opportunities because they do not believe that they can make a difference, or because they have not learned to take advantage of such opportunities. For example, a child who grows up in poverty may not succeed in school even when presented with an opportunity to acquire an education and may drop out of school altogether. Sometimes, this inability to take advantage of opportunities may be due to an internalized sense of inferiority, or a feeling that one is not deserving (a consequence of self-alienation and possible loss of identity as discussed by Fanon (2005) and wa Thiong'o (1997)), followed by possible self-hatred (see wa Thiong'o 1981).

2. The experience of powerlessness often results from abdicating one's power to other people, such as political leaders, administrators, etc., and elevating them while devaluing oneself. This abdication of power is accompanied by habitual ways of thinking, feeling, and acting that are consistent with perception of oneself as lacking in value in comparison to those in positions of power, and as ineffective in the world and therefore powerless (Meyer 2005). One way in which occupational therapists can empower people is by helping them break their habitual way of thinking so that they can act in new ways, and thus exercise their agency in the world.

3. As pointed out by Meyer (2005), complete abdication of one's power is not logical because irrespective of circumstances, people have a certain field of influence, however limited, by virtue of whom they interact with and affects by their actions on a day-to-day basis. It is therefore important that people exercise their agency within their field of influence as individuals and as communities so as to effect change for the better. For example, an economically impoverished parent may commit to attending Town Hall discussions in order to ensure that concerns about educational accessibility for poor children are part of political discourse. Such actions may contribute to policy change for the better in regard to poor families in the community. In my opinion, it is the responsibility of occupational therapists in the community to assist individuals to recognize their own fields of influence so that they can be proactive in changing circumstances within their power for the good of their communities through what Kronenberg & Pollard (2005a) term the political activities of daily living (pADLs).

4. Empowering individuals in the community means in part assisting them to break away from typical self-defeating habits and adopting new, adaptive ways of thinking, feeling, and acting so that they can take back their personal power and exert it within their field of influence. This means that change has to begin from within the individual, a notion that is consistent with the pragmatic principle of beliefs as a rule for action (Peirce 1955). If one modifies beliefs to reflect the thought that their actions could lead to desired consequences, then they are motivated to act in order to achieve those consequences. The MIOT framework aims to guide the partner in addressing issues of priority at the individual level, by changing beliefs about self, other people, and the world. This facilitates change in occupational performance for better adaptation to the environment. Of course, the therapist can only work with partners who are ready to change and to act for the common good. Otherwise, the therapist's role is confined to sensitizing individuals and communities to the need to consider change. Also, I would like to point out that therapists have to go through this transformative change themselves so that they adopt new habits of thinking, feeling, and acting

that are consistent with their own power before they can work with partners effectively.

5. True empowerment comes from self-enlightenment by individuals so that they realize that the most meaningful existence is that characterized by creative actions, love for another person or thing, and a focus on the future and on the welfare of others beyond the self (Frankl 1997). In other words, meaningful existence calls for self-transcendence, and meaningful existence is extremely empowering. The MIOT framework guides the collaborative creation of circumstances favorable to such meaningful existence by focusing on the partner's self-transcendence articulated through a mission statement. The mission promotes competency through creative occupational performance motivated by the love of one's family, friends, colleagues, and community.

6. True community empowerment begins at the grassroots, with what Kronenberg & Pollard (2005a, p. 71) termed 'people-centered self-empowerment'. Therefore, by supporting individuals so that they feel empowered, the occupational therapist ultimately supports the community in which those individuals belong. When people individually act on the basis of missions that are self-transcendent, collectively they can create a better community for everybody. In other words, community empowerment begins with rescuing of individual responsibility (Kronenberg & Pollard 2005b), by shedding light on the fact that individuals are responsible not only for their own existence but also for the world in which they live. It is important to point out that the onus of change is not purely on the individual. Many of the challenges that threaten human wellbeing are global in nature and require systemic solutions (for example, legislation to allocate resources more equitably). Elsewhere in this book, Whiteford and Townsend discuss in depth how such systemic problems can be addressed in order to achieve occupational justice. This chapter highlights the fact that structural barriers notwithstanding, individuals are not pieces in a game of chess to be moved around at will by whatever powers that may be. They have a field of influence through which they can cause change in the desired direction, however limited.

Bearing in mind the above six propositions, in Box 12.1 I illustrate the application of the MIOT framework. (Note: The case of Muita is based on the author's clinical experience but does not describe any specific partner.)

Box 12.1

Application of the MIOT framework: the case of Muita

Muita, is a 23-year-old man from the rural Central Province of Kenya. He graduated from high school with a grade C in the Kenya Certificate of Education (KCE) examination at the age of 18 years. He was the fifth child in an economically poor single-parent family of eight. All his siblings had dropped out of school for various reasons and Muita was his mother's only hope for a better future. She hoped that he would get a good education, attend university, get a job, and support her and his brothers and sisters.

The minimum grade for admission into any of the private universities in Kenya was C+, and a grade B was required for admission into public universities. Therefore, Muita did not meet the minimum requirements. After graduation, he became moody and his behavior erratic. He would stay out all night and not bother to inform his mother when he would be returning home. His mother suspected that he was smoking *bhang* (*Cannabis sativa*, a common mood-altering drug in Kenya). She requested a family friend, who was also an occupational therapist, to talk to Muita and find out what was happening. (This is common practice in the Kikuyu culture where it is expected that elders provide counseling to the young.) When the therapist talked to Muita, he was very negative. He felt that the system was not fair, and he did not think that his mother had done enough to help him succeed. He thought that he deserved to get a college education and that it was society's responsibility to educate him since once he graduated, he would be working for the community.

The therapist pointed out to Muita that it was understandable that he was angry because he thought that his mother and the community had failed him. He asked him to think about what they could do, considering that his grades did not qualify him for admission into college. After reflection, Muita admitted that he was probably partly to blame for his predicament since he had not studied hard enough to pass his exams well. The therapist suggested that he could look at the situation from another perspective. Instead of thinking that his mother and the community had failed him, he could conceptualize education as a privilege, which he could use to serve other people rather than just for his own material comfort. The therapist gave him assignments consisting of literature discussing the role of education in society and the responsibilities of educated people.

Most of the books that Muita read are familiar to Kenyan students: for example, Ngugi wa Thiong'o's *Writers in Politics* (1981) and *Decolonizing the Mind* (1997), as well as Frantz Fanon's (2005) *The Wretched of the Earth*. These sources were meant not only to conscientize him about how Western education might have shaped his identity as a young African man, but also to impress on him his responsibility as one who had been privileged to receive some education in helping fashion out community change

for the good of all those who share in his black African identity. This was part of the belief establishment phase of the MIOT framework. The therapist hoped that Muita would begin identifying issues that would motivate him to change his views so that he could act in a different way (in dynamical systems terminology, a perturbation was introduced).

In a subsequent meeting a week later Muita informed the therapist that through his readings, he had realized that education was about service rather than selfish self-enhancement. He said this motivated him to get an education, but this time for a different reason: to serve society. He agreed that he needed guidance in order to figure out how to act on this awareness. MIOT assessments were administered. Following is the outcome of the assessment.

1. Muita documented occupations in which he engaged for a period of four days (Tuesday through Friday). At the end of the four days, the therapist made a list of all the occupations in which he engaged.

2. Based on part I of the MAIIIOT, Muita articulated the following personal mission statement: I intend to live my life in such a way that when I leave this world, my family, friends, colleagues, and other people in my community will say that I was a wonderful man, who was committed to a life-long fight for equal opportunities and fairness for all people and: cared for my mother, brothers and sisters; and contributed to building a better Kenya for future generations.

The only occupation in which he had engaged in the previous four days that he thought was important for achieving the mission was helping his mother on the farm and in running her small business establishments. He ranked this occupation first in importance. He had engaged in the occupation only once in the four days. His performance score based on the OPCG was: $P_t = \sum P_i = \sum(PI \times F) = 5 \times 1 = 5$. He identified six occupations whose regular performance would lead to achievement of his mission and rated the frequency, adequacy, and satisfaction with performance of each of the occupations, and belief about his ability to perform each of them with desired frequency, and adequacy. The aggregate scores on the 4 MAIIIOT scales were: $X_{11} = 6$, $X_{12} = 6$, $X_{13} = 6$, and $X_{14} = 24$. With the therapist's guidance, Muita established the following four long-term and six short-term goals:

Long-term goals

By the end of six years, I will:
1. Have graduated from a university with a bachelor's degree in business administration
2. Have a job

Continued

Box 12.1

Application of the MIOT framework: the case of Muita—cont'd

3. Be in the process of constructing a nice house for my mom

4. Be engaged in political and volunteer activities to contribute to improvement of the lives of people in my community.

Short-term goals

1. Within six months, I will be back in school and studying hard in preparation for a repeat of the KCE exam.

2. Within two weeks, I will be working on the farm or helping mom with business at least six hours/day, three days/week.

3. Within three weeks, I will have discussed my future career with at least three friends.

4. By the end of one month, I will have located at least three organizations that could sponsor me to study at the university, and identified application procedures to these organizations.

5. Within three weeks, I will be participating in at least one volunteer activity for two hours/week at my church.

6. Within four weeks, I will have read literature and written a paper about the process and effect of Kenyan politics on my community's economic wellbeing.

After four weeks of implementing the intervention plan, all the assessments were administered again. At that time, the five top ranked occupations from his DOI were: searching for a school that would admit him so that he could attend classes and repeat the KCE exam, helping his mother on the farm and in running other small commercial activities, participating in volunteer activities in his church, educating himself about political processes and their effect on his community's economic wellbeing, and searching for organizations that would sponsor him for University studies. His performance score at reassessment (P_{t2}) was calculated as follows:

Occupation (Listed by rank)	Performance Index (PI)	Frequency (F)	P_i
Searching for a high school	5	4	20
Helping mom on the farm and business	4	7	28
Volunteering in the church	3	2	6
Self-education about political processes	2	0	0
Searching for sources of financial support	1	1	1

$$P_{t2} = \sum P_{i2} = \sum (PI_2 \times F_2) = 55$$

Muita's aggregate MAIIOT scores at reassessment were: $X_{21} = 14$, $X_{22} = 17$, $X_{23} = 12$, and $X_{24} = 24$. His performance score therefore changed by 50 points ($P_{t2}-P_{t1} = 55-5 = 50$) and his aggregate MAIIOT scores changed as follows: $X_{21}-X_{11} = 14-6 = 8$, $X_{22}-X_{12} = 17-6 = 11$, and $X_{23}-X_{13} = 12-6 = 6$.

Clearly, a change had occurred in Muita's outlook in life, and this change was reflected in actions as indicated by changed occupational performance patterns. His initiative in tasks such as searching for a school, searching for sources of financial support, etc. indicated that he was becoming empowered. He was developing a sense that he could change circumstances in his life through his own efforts as he performed daily occupations. Eventually, Muita returned to school, repeated the KCE and earned a grade of B–, was admitted to a private university, having secured a scholarship from a church-based organization that supported education of young people from poor families.

Conclusion

This chapter proposed that occupational therapists can contribute their knowledge of human occupation and occupational performance to help illuminate wider societal occupation-related challenges such as global warming. The occupational therapy profession needs to engage in a process of strategically positioning itself to influence such global concerns. This means that it opens itself to exploring how understanding of human occupation can be employed in seeking ways to empower individuals and communities to create change through occupational choices and performance patterns. As the case study illustrates, therapists could use the MIOT theoretical conceptual framework to guide this process of empowering and sensitizing individuals and communities to enable them to influence individual and global events positively through judicious occupational performance.

References

American Occupational Therapy Association: *Occupational Therapy Practice Framework: Domain and Process*, ed 2, Bethesda, MD, 2008, Author.

Bassingthwaighte J, Liebovich L, West B: *Fractal Physiology*, New York, 1994, Oxford University Press.

Breines E: *Origins and Adaptations: a Philosophy of Practice*, Lebanon, NJ, 1986, Geri-Rehab.

Buchler J: *Philosophical Writings of Peirce*, New York, 1955, Dover Publications.

Cutchin MP: Using Deweyan philosophy to rename and reframe Adaptation-to-Environment, *Am J Occup Ther* 58:303–312, 2004.

Darwin C: *The Origin of Species*, New York, 1985, Penguin Books.

Dewey J: From absolutism to experimentalism. In McDermott JJ, editor: *The Philosophy of John Dewey*, Chicago, 1981, Chicago University Press, pp 1–13.

Duncan M, Watson R: Transformation through occupation. A prototype. In Watson R, Swartz L, editors: *Transformation Through Occupation*, London, 2004, Whurr, pp 69–84.

Fanon F: *The Wretched of the Earth*, New York, 2005, Grove/Atlantic.

Fourie M, Galvaan R, Beeton H: The impact of poverty: Potential lost. In Watson R, Swartz L, editors: *Transformation Through Occupation*, London, 2004, Whurr, pp 69–84.

Frankl VE: *Recollections: An Autobiography* (Fabry J, translator), London, 1997, Plenum Publishing House.

Ikiugu MN: The philosophy and culture of occupational therapy, *Dissertation Abstracts International* 62:5678, 2001.

Ikiugu MN: Instrumentalism in occupational therapy: an argument for a pragmatic conceptual model of practice, *International Journal of Psychosocial Rehabilitation* 8:109–117, 2004a.

Ikiugu MN: Instrumentalism in occupational therapy: a theoretical core for the pragmatic conceptual model of practice, *International Journal of Psychosocial Rehabilitation* 8:150–162, 2004b.

Ikiugu MN: Instrumentalism in occupational therapy: guidelines for practice, *International Journal of Psychosocial Rehabilitation* 8:164–177, 2004c.

Ikiugu MN: *Psychosocial Conceptual Practice Models in Occupational Therapy: Building Adaptive Capability*, St. Louis, MO, 2007, Elsevier/Mosby.

Ikiugu MN: A proposed conceptual model of organization development for occupational therapists and occupational scientists, *Occupational Therapy Journal of Research* 28:52–63, 2008a.

Ikiugu MN: *Occupational Science in the Service of Gaia: an essay describing a possible contribution of occupational scientists to the solution of prevailing global problems*, Baltimore, 2008b, Publish America.

Ikiugu MN, Rosso HM: Understanding the occupational human being as a complex, dynamical, adaptive system, *Occupational Therapy in Health Care* 19:43–65, 2005.

Ikiugu MN, Ciaravino EA: Assisting adolescents experiencing emotional and behavioral difficulties (EBD) transition to adulthood, *International Journal of Psychosocial Rehabilitation* 10:57–78, 2006.

Ikiugu MN, Schultz S: An argument for pragmatism as a foundational philosophy of occupational therapy, *Can J Occup Ther* 73:86–97, 2006.

Ikiugu MN, Anderson LM: Cost effectiveness of the Instrumentalism in Occupational Therapy conceptual model as a guide for intervention with adolescents with emotional and behavioral disorders, *International Journal of Behavioral Consultation and Therapy* 3:53–76, 2007.

Ikiugu MN, Anderson A, Manas D: The test-retest reliability of a battery of new occupational performance assessments, *International Journal of Therapy and Rehabilitation* 15:562–571, 2008.

James W: *Pragmatism*, Indianapolis, Cambridge, 1981, Hackett Publishing Company.

Kay J, Tasman A, Lieberman JA: *Psychiatry Behavioral Science and Clinical Essentials: A Companion to Tasman, Kay, Lieberman: Psychiatry*, Philadelphia, 2000, WB Saunders.

Kielhofner G: *Conceptual foundations of occupational therapy*, Philadelphia, 2004, FA Davis.

Koelen MA, Lindstrom B: Making healthy choices easy choices: the role of empowerment, *Eur J Clin Nutr* 59 (Suppl 1):S10–S16, 2005.

Kronenberg F, Pollard N: Introduction: a beginning. In Kronenberg F, Algado SS, Pollard N, editors: *Occupational Therapy Without Borders. Learning from the Spirit of Survivors*, Edinburgh, 2005a, Elsevier/Churchill Livingstone, pp 1–13.

Kronenberg F, Pollard N: Overcoming occupational apartheid: a preliminary exploration of the political nature of occupational therapy. In *Occupational Therapy Without Borders. Learning from the Spirit of Survivors*, Edinburgh, 2005b, Elsevier/Churchill Livingstone, pp 58–86.

McDermott JJ: *The Philosophy of John Dewey*, Chicago, 1981, University of Chicago Press.

Meyer G: Power, powerlessness and chances of productive action: 10 theses, *From Forum* 9:17–23, 2005.

Okes D: Complexity theory simplifies choices, *Quality Progress* 36:35–37, 2003.

Peirce CS: The fixation of belief. In Buchler J, editor: *Philosophical Writings of Peirce*, New York, 1955, Dover Publications, pp 5–22.

Reilly M: Occupational therapy can be one of the great ideas of 20th century medicine, *Am J Occup Ther* 16:1–9, 1962.

Royeen C: The 2003 Eleanor Clarke Slagle lecture – Chaotic occupational therapy: Collective wisdom for a complex profession, *Am J Occup Ther* 57:609–624, 2003.

Townsend E, Wilcock A: Occupational justice and client-centered practice: A dialogue-in-progress, *Can J Occup Ther* 71:75–87, 2004.

Wallerstein N: Powerlessness, empowerment, and health: implications for health promotion programs, *Am J Health Promot* 6:197–205, 1992.

wa Thiong'o N: *Decolonizing the Mind: The Politics of Language in African Literature*, Portsmouth, NH, 1997, Heinemann.

wa Thiong'o N: *Writers in Politics*, London, 1981, Heinemann Educational Books.

Werner D: Foreword I. In Kronenberg F, Algado SS, Pollard N, editors: *Occupational Therapy Without Borders. Learning from the Spirit of Survivors*, Edinburgh, 2005, Elsevier/Churchill Livingstone, pp xi–xii.

Wilcock AA: *An Occupational Perspective of Health*, Thorofare, 1998, Slack.

Wilcock AA: *An Occupational Perspective of Health*, ed 2, Thorofare, NJ, 2006, Slack.

Yale University School of Medicine: *Holistic Health Recovery Program: Client Workbook*, New Haven, Connecticut, 2001. Online. Available at: http://info.med.yale.edu/psych/hhrp.i2001.32. Accessed May 7, 2010.

(Re)habilitation and (re)positioning the powerful expert and the sick person

13

Mershen Pillay

OVERVIEW

The Relationship of Labouring Affinities (RoLA) is presented as a theoretical framework to explain the process of transforming rehabilitation practice. Contextual demands force a shift from traditional deficit based, medical model practices towards socially responsive, collaborative practices – framed broadly as democratic practice. The elements of RoLA viz., communication, thinking, and labor, are offered as theoretical concepts to explain the ways in which practices may be repositioned in the interests of social justice, and may be applied to a wide array of rehabilitation practices.

Introduction

The focus of this chapter is on the transformation of the nature of the clinical relationship between rehabilitation professionals (powerful experts) and people with disabilities ('sick' persons). By transformation of this relationship I mean a radical movement of ideologies, a continuous re-placing of thoughts and actions across all forms of practice: professional higher education, research, and service. This kind of professional transformation is a necessary part of our development. Why?

Rehabilitation practitioners act as powerful arbitrators on behalf of (or with) people living with disabilities. Intrinsic to this arbitration function is the maintenance of an undemocratic relationship between rehabilitation professional and patient. Rehabilitation practitioners have – predominantly – been positioned as experts who decide diagnoses, prognosticate outcomes, design and deliver interventions, report progress, and classify disabilities. Rehabilitation practitioners are undoubtedly regarded as powerfully intertwined with the lives of people living with disabilities, as worthy experts who (re)produce knowledge of disability, decide who deserves state-funded care/equipment, or who are dominantly cited/referenced as authoritative sources on issues of disability. There are progressive practitioners in countries such as Australia, South Africa, the United Kingdom, and the United States who position their work within disability activism. Such practitioners' regard their social and political biographies as dissembled away from being experts toward being, e.g., caring collaborators invited as participants to work alongside disability survivors. Even then how the practitioner and person with disability share power ought to be analyzed. We must 'see' ourselves not only as innocent professionals but as powerful practitioners, people who are politically endowed. In this chapter, I reveal how rehabilitation practice cannot be seen as an apolitical, objective act. Instead, I trouble this notion by presenting an analysis of deeply political professionalization, including professions' engagement with:

- A specialist focus
- A biologic metaphor
- Deficit theories.

In addition, three interrelated processes are presented:

- Dis-othering,
- Essentialism
- Reductionism.

DOI: 10.1016/B978-0-7020-3103-8.00022-5

These processes directly contribute an undemocratic practitioner–client relationship. As this is an undesirable relationship, an alternative ideological framework (promoting democracy) is sought from one of the world's newest democracies: South Africa. An analysis of ideologic positions, from South African policies, is presented as a conceptual resource to inspire democratic practice. Furthermore, a conceptual framework developed out of a practice-focused study (Pillay 2003b) is presented. This framework, (the Relationship of Labouring Affinities (RoLA)) contains non-mainstream notions of 'communication', 'labor', and 'thinking'. These notions are discussed as transformation-potential mechanisms for repositioning the powerful expert and sick person dyad toward a more democratic relationship.

While much of this chapter has been informed by research and/or dialogue regarding professional transformation in audiology and speech pathology (Kathard & Pillay 1993, 1994, 2005, Kathard et al 2007, Pillay 1998, 2001a, b, 2003a, Pillay et al 1997), fundamental intuitions and communiqués may reverberate within occupational therapy and other rehabilitation professions. Indeed, Kronenberg & Pollard's (2005) situating of occupational therapy practice as political in nature robustly harmonized with my own intuitions of audiology and speech-language therapy as a political practice (see Pillay et al 1997). Hence, this chapter may be considered as a reflective talkback to Kronenberg and Pollard for the rehabilitation professions in general.

Rehabilitation processes engaged by powerful experts with sick people

Many new/student rehabilitation practitioners are often asked to 'establish rapport' with their clients/patients, which is intended to create a trusting relationship toward a positive therapeutic and caring end. However, in our effort to care, several processes have become naturalized as common practice. In schools, clinics, homes, hospitals – or in streets – our practices are imbued with ideologies emanating from our birth alongside, and allegiance with, our Brotherhood of Care, the medical fraternity. Across much of the world, therapists working in education/schools, hospitals or in communities are recognized as healthcare practitioners. This seemingly obvious statement needs analyzing when powerful experts

and sick people are considered as political biographies. In uncovering the etiology of the obvious (William 1999), this sick-person trope through the Parsonian tradition, 'reduces the ill person to the patient, and this patient's agency is limited to compliance; the physician becomes the active agent in the illness process . . . [the] expectation of the patient is to return to health, and the physician is to facilitate that return' (Frank 1995, p. 131–132).

This biography is largely due to our alignment with an empirical, medical science and it is no wonder 'Rehabilitation' is ideologically premised on the sick trope. The sick person is ideologically positioned in several ways, viz. via the use of a:

* Specialist focus
* Biologic metaphor
* Deficit theories
* Dis-othering
* Essentialism
* Reductionism.

In considering clinical tools such as case history pro forma, it is possible for rehabilitation professions to identify their specialist foci as being rooted in medicine, psychology, genetics, education, sociology, etc. Across professional rehabilitation higher education programs, it is a truism that courses are prescribed from the medical sciences such as anatomy, physiology, medical pathology, and psychology. Our professional education, practices, and resources represent our specialist focus, which we use to map the foreign space that the patient is. The practitioner (tacitly, explicitly) refers to specialist knowledge to enter the patient's world. Like Christopher Columbus and his kind, the practitioner discovers the patient, occupies their world and colonizes their disabled life.

* The interview.
* The questionnaire.
* The survey.
* The test.
* The asking. The looking. The listening.

Whatever the method, practitioners build biologic images of patients through their medical gaze (Foucault 1976). We actively look at people who cannot walk or talk through medical processes of 'diagnosis', 'treatment', 'patient', and 'pathology'. While we do focus on the tangibility of people's bodies and biologies, illnesses and diseases what is questioned here is the way we have used this reality to enact our roles as powerful experts with the natural chaos of lives.

What's the problem with a focus on the problem? There is a denial of the aesthetic, of intrinsic strengths, functional abilities, possibilities, and of self-perceived resources. The patient is not beautiful or able. The patient is a problem. Sick. Disordered. The patient has a ...

• Handicap ...
• Impairment ...
• Disability ...

... all of which were cornerstone theoretical notions of the International Classification of Impairments Disability and Handicaps (ICIDH) (World Health Organization (WHO) 1980). The WHO has reformulated the classification system into the International Classification of Functioning (ICF) (WHO 1999) so as to 'include positive experiences' (WHO 1999, p. 7). Although ICF authors espoused a social model of disability, they have failed to question the legitimacy of classifying what really is: disfunction (deficit). Even this modern system which may be traced to early nineteenth-century classification systems resonates with well-bottled beliefs that people with disabilities must necessarily be understood as 'imperfect' (Goldstein 1938).

Dis-othering is an adaptation of othering, as used by postcolonial theorists when referring to those who are outside of the politically, culturally, and socially dominant group. How has the practitioner othered the patient? Gayatri Spivak (1985) refers to othering as the seizure and control of the means of interpretation and communication. Othering is made possible via several crucial colonial processes where the colonized other is spoken for, i.e., the colonizer assumes authority (or 'voice') to represent the colonized. Others are necessary to legitimize the existence of those in power. Without others, powerful experts' authority cannot be defined. Othering involves imposing values of the culturally dominant, group (the colonizers) onto their imperial subjects' lives that remanufactured within dichotomies: us & them, men & women, black & white, abled & disabled.

Practitioners begin by, through a medical gaze, highlighting essential characteristics of the disorder done in binary opposition to normative criteria. These criteria, the main subject of study, best represent the cultural capital (Bourdieu 1991), viz.: white, Western, Anglo-Saxon Protestant cultures, developed from predominantly researching/servicing these populations. Criteria are not only established as 'normal' but are done so by rendering other's

experiences lesser, invisible. Pathology, disability, or disorder is defined by measuring others' against the cultural capital's version of normal. Othering is intimately related to our use of deficit theories that, like the African American term (perhaps derived from disrespect) 'disses' people. Hence the term dis-othering: an amalgamation of *dis* and *othering*.

But why do we dis-other? Consider where rehabilitation practitioners may be if we did not focus on pathology. The stutterer, the spinal cord injury, the developmentally delayed child, the autistic – and similar pathological labels help to display a professional reality. Significantly, our disorder focus helps to keep our legitimate space in society. Without it, we may cease to exist (in our present form, anyway).

The practitioner creates the dis-othered patient by engaging essentialist perspectives to define the true, fixed essence of a thing (Thadani 1996). Essentialism has produced knowledge of 'deaf speech', 'the head injured adult' or 'the learning disabled child' among a plethora of essentialized notions. Arguably, essentialist notions are necessary for expert practice. Though, the question remains: Is it ever possible to get at the essence of any person – with or without a disorder. Possible or not, practitioners enter lives armed with conceptual resources belying essentialism: Classification systems, rating scales, coding, assessment tools, and therapy programs – things that define 'good' rehabilitation.

Inherited from the medical fraternity via empiricism is reductionism, which is when 'complex phenomena are partitioned into smaller segments that are then dealt with piecemeal' (Dunbar 1995, p. 19). From even the tiniest level of damaged cochlear hair cells to the grandest notions about emotional-behavioral disorders in autism, we have engaged reductionism. The heuristic-device of methodologic reductionism (Fleck 1935) reduces the complexities of cultural influences (among other notions) to produce scientific facts. And all of this to (ironically) understand the whole. Even such practice innovations, that purport to value people holistically, hobble behind an entrenched practice of reductionism,

Why is this version of science dominant in rehabilitation? Epistemologically, empirical science has long been associated with white, Western cultures (Vidich & Lyman 1998). In this way, empiricism may be regarded as an expression of cultural beliefs regarding the nature of people, relationships, knowledge, and of how knowledge should be created, re-created, seen and re-seen. I do not suggest that empirical science is strictly within white, Western cultures. Of all the types of sciences, an empirical science is valued by those who are politically, socially, and culturally dominant. In our recent history, it is still an empirical science that is served by and best serves the cultural capital, viz.: white, Western cultures. It is possible that ideologic allegiance to those with greater social and political power have seeped into rehabilitation practice. In South Africa, for example, the power triumvirate of race, class, and gender (white, middle-class, male) has influenced how rehabilitation best serves white (English and/ or Afrikaans first language) clientele. At a global level, it is certainly not an occidental accident that cultural capital is matched to the community of rehabilitation practitioners! Practitioners (even when gender is considered) are a product of a society (a world) that has privileged the interests of rich white men, and this power base has predominantly influenced the development of the professions. I do not ascribe to this kind of power and the expert practitioner–sick person relationship this engenders. So, if this is unappealing, what else may we consider for a future state without occupational apartheid?

I have chosen to turn to ideas generated from subjugation and oppression, powerlessness and resistance: South Africa. Being a recent project on humanity, of how we relate to each other; South African policies represent a viable theoretical inspirational source for democratizing relationships engaged by rehabilitation professionals.

Why policies? Why South African policies?

South Africa's policy statements may be positioned as a conceptual resource for our practice. Why? Post-Apartheid, South African policies (1994) contain several democratically aligned beliefs about how we relate to each other as people. The World Bank, the United Nations (UN), and (for my thematic focus) the WHO espouse liberal, democratic ideologies (Storey 2000). Hence, as a political project, South Africa may be synchronized as a world project on humanity inasmuch as there has been an interest on the act of Barack Obama's installation as the first African-American president. South African policy ideologically interacts with globalized notions of

democracy, of social justice, and such-like. These policies may be referred to as ideologic inspirations, reflecting an appreciation of Jansen's (2001) assertion that policy – which may be critiqued as un-implementable – is largely symbolic. Ideologically, current South African policy is inspiring because it enmeshes resistance-politics emanating from organizations such as the African National Congress and the South African Communist Party. It also focuses socialist epistemologies in healthcare, which interact with social models of healthcare from, e.g., the WHO.

There is ideological coherence among most South African policies across health, education, and social welfare – most of which makes direct reference to the South African constitution. Below, I make reference to five *paired* ideologic positions as contained within the South African Constitution and several other documents (for more details, see Pillay 2003b). These ideologies include:

1. Equality and antidiscrimination
2. Human dignity and *uBuntu* (or *umuntu ngumuntu ngabantu*, which, roughly translated from South African cosmology means that 'a person is a person through other persons')
3. Democracy and a law governed society
4. Social justice and equity
5. Transparency and accountability.

These wonderful ideologies represent a revolution away from oppressive practices. However, what does a cursory review of current realities show in 'post' states such as postcolonial Africa, post-independence India, post-occupation Palestine, post-Katrina, New Orleans – and post-apartheid South Africa? For example, in post-apartheid South Africa traditional healthcare facilities (clinics, hospitals) remain inaccessible to large sections of the population. It is a place where in 2006–2007 over 6615 people developed malaria and up to 65 died of this curable illness (Department of Health (DOH) 2008a). Tuberculosis in South Africa is an epidemic growing at 20% per year (DOH 2008a). Acquired immune deficiency syndrome (AIDS) remains one of the top killers of women, men, and their babies (DOH 2008b). It is also where 'the Poors' (Desai 2000) and 30 082 of their children (under 5 years) suffer severe malnutrition (South African Government 2007). Imagine – in the face of these kinds of needs – how could a practitioner seriously negotiate issues of rehabilitation, of walking, or talking with someone who is, for example, dying or hungry?

Of course, I write as an insider, a believer, someone who has considered how my profession could reinvent itself around maxims that promote communication as a fundamental, essential social activity for the quality of anyone's life. So how do we reinvent ourselves, how do we journey to the other side? In response to this question, I offer the RoLA (Pillay 2003b). At this point, the reader is encouraged to reflect on the following questions:

- Consider what label makes you comfortable: 'disability survivor', 'patient', 'sick person' or 'person with disability'. Why don't we call a person with a disability a 'patient' outside of a hospital/medical context?

- Think about responses to the following headlines as you read the rest of this chapter. What is the connection between these statements and this chapter?

  ○ 'Heterosexual man promotes the use of queer activism to empower lesbians'

  ○ 'Deaf Mexican immigrant wants same rights as US citizens to enter university'

  ○ 'Disability rights group reserves 50% of its executive council seats for the non-disabled'

  ○ 'Judge John Richards rules: Husband allowed to stop brain dead wife's tube feeds'

  ○ 'South African Black economic empowerment deals to include white women'

The RoLA: why 'laboring'? why 'affinities'?

'Laboring' positions the notion of work/labor as dynamically transforming. 'Work', alluded to here, is labor for a very specific purpose, i.e., the transformation of professional affinities. 'Affinities' refer to the practitioners' attachment to ideologies that have created them as powerful experts. 'Laboring affinities' is about working with and through professional attachments, collective professional theory, clinical wisdom, expertness and issues of power towards a different practice. Within the RoLA there are three core elements, i.e.:

- Communication
- Thinking
- Labor.

Each of these elements is an idea-filled notion that was generated by colluding with many theoretical perspectives as described below.

Communication and the RoLA

As rehabilitation practitioners, we depend on communication to derive empirical knowledge of patients' experiences. However, in reality the medium of language limits what can be known (Bhaskar 1989) as language (communication) is an inherently fallible system to convey true meanings of patients' experiences. Communication is further compounded by the narrowness of a technologically derived science that encourages use of expert language, such as professional jargon. This empirical/scientific discourse may be used to survey and control our patients in the way we describe their diagnoses, report their progress, and communicate their outcomes. In a more democratic relationship, we ought to work at re-placing surveillance and control (after Foucault 1976) toward a more meaningful, person-centered interaction. Practically, this means attempting to gain insights about the biologic realities of the patient. But, not to stop there. It also means developing ways to access what it means for the patient to experience 'disorder'. And to do this in a way that (contradictorily, simultaneously) acknowledges that we cannot know the patient. Such an epistemological-ontological shift must lead to an examination of the validity of appropriate methodological choices. And this is where qualitative methodologies may offer the practitioner in research, service, and professional higher education viable alternatives to experimental, technologically-oriented methods. In this way, we may (re)construct relational knowings of lives.

Communication as the object, subject, and medium

One of the ways we may consider communication within the practitioner-patient relationship is to think about what constitutes effective communication. We may position communication as autopoietic. Maturana & Varela (1980) refer to autopoiesis as a process within a system that manufactures its elements by engaging these same elements in a recursive fashion. This implies a kind of production network by which these elements themselves are reproduced. Figure 13.1 is a diagrammatic representation of this meaning of communication.

Figure 13.1 illustrates that communication could be reinterpreted and understood in multiple ways as the

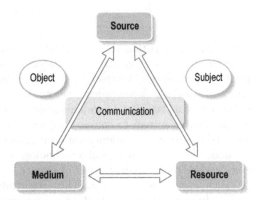

Fig. 13.1 • Communication and the Relationship of Laboring Affinities.

object and the subject. What does this mean? The subject (therapeutic communication) is simultaneously the object of our work toward effective communication. It is also the medium through which practitioners may discover what communication means in complex spaces. When our goal is effective communication we seek to achieve this object by referring to people's communication (the source) as a resource. Their communication becomes the text to develop ideas about rehabilitation goals, methods, and outcomes. Therefore, communication is the fundamental social unit of the practitioner–patient relationship.

Locating a social relationship as a communicative act is not new. In the 1950s, the German philosopher Jurgen Habermas believed that the project of critical theorists (i.e., emancipation) resided in everyday language, in ordinary communication: a belief that led to his theory of communicative action (known as universal pragmatics). Habermas (in Pusey 1987) argued that people (interlocutors) engage issues like truth, justice, intelligibility, and identity.

Communication, as an element within the RoLA, can be used to situate how the powerful expert cannot ever attain total dominance. When we use communication to engage the ordinariness of patients' lives in meaningful ways, we begin to challenge the expertness of experts. We present expert's knowings as delicate shards, remnants of an exploding knowledge in a constantly conflicting world. This kind of communication creates a discursive space for several de-colonization processes. In others' wor(l)ds communication destabilizes power inequalities, moving the RoLA towards a relationship that inscribes things such as conflict, uncertainty – and importantly – moralism as epistemological goals. I shall now turn to the next core element.

Thinking and the RoLA

Thinking can be referred to in many ways. Here, thinking refers to what we think why we think it, how we think when interacting, and *where* we think. Significantly, 'where' refers to social, cultural, political, and related contexts in which thinking occurs. In cognitive psychology the move toward understanding 'where' thinking occurs has resulted in the generation of many new theoretical notions, such as situated cognition or distributed cognition (Salomon 1993). Cognition as a construct may promote a way of thinking about thinking that is not wholly useful because those ascribing to cognitive theories primarily engage the use of a biologic metaphor. This creates a conceptual schism between the way communication and thinking is presented in RoLA. Here, thinking is used to highlight perceptual processes rooted in beliefs, ideologies about people, and the world at large.

Rehabilitation practitioners have meta-theoretically developed an affinity to a thinking centered on certainty. Some realities, such as the biologic bases of hand functioning, bladder control and oral motor movements, may be known. However, we enact practices by closely aligning ourselves with certainty, definite truths, and firm realities. This is inherently in conflict with the realities of an unpredictable world. As illustrated in Figure 13.2, the notion of thinking per se is mediated by uncertainty and certainty. Therefore, thinking (similar to communication, above) is positioned as the source, resource, and medium for addressing the many ways we engage certainty and uncertainty within the RoLA.

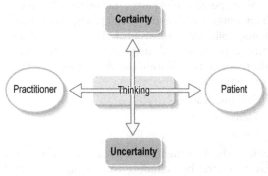

Fig. 13.2 • Thinking and the RoLA (as mediating uncertainty and certainty).

When we initially meet people with disabilities we, or strangers, often seek common ground to reduce uncertainty. This kind of thinking (vis à vis the RoLA) may be understood in relation to Berger & Calabrese's (1975) uncertainty reduction theory. They posited a linear increase in certainty as we attempt to reduce complexity and uncertainty. At times, in professional relationships, we may create closer alliances with either uncertainty or certainty – resulting in ongoing tension. Within the RoLA, it is suggested that practitioners (iteratively) work through this affinity with what is certain towards exploring the usefulness of uncertainties. How may we practically do this?

In extreme situations, e.g., people with disabilities due to terminal illnesses such as multiple drug resistant tuberculosis, and HIV/AIDS, it is possible for the medical, biological nature of the disorder to be certain/known. Thinking within the RoLA requires that we engage a variety of reasonings (thinkings) of and about patients with progressive/terminal illnesses. This may allow multiple communication situations to occur. To explain this, we may consider Babrow's (1995) problematic integration theory for such a purpose. Babrow has argued that people assess probabilities, e.g., 'The patient probably can't retrieve words or ideas from his memory'. Additionally, they evaluate the more/less probable possibilities, e.g., 'An AIDS patient has an unreliable memory'. These assessments of probabilities interact with evaluations, and they often co-occur. In other words, probabilities (or uncertainties) and evaluations affect each other. In this way we integrate forms of certainty (assessment of visual perception) with uncertainty (possibility of a neurologic basis). In engaging certainties with uncertainties we may consider Bradac's (2001) assertion that uncertainty (specifically: probabilities) occurs within frameworks that account for the emotional context of thinking. We should consider how our thinkings about the social, political, and cultural context of our practice may become imbued with emotion. For example, not knowing the reasons for why an adult cannot dress or bathe himself may be perceived as professional insecurity. Hence, we become destabilized as practitioners. This destabilization may perhaps be experienced as ambiguity and confusion. The suggestion is to reposition these emotional thinkings as a useful, positive, constructive resource. But, how could we engage uncertain thinking for positive, perhaps even creative ends?

If we creatively engage uncertainty, then we need to harness our inability to know, to predict, and to engage people living with disabilities. This destabilization is viewed as desirable when we wish to engineer and maintain a meaningful relationship. Neither the person with a disability nor the practitioner may know what effective daily living or effective communication may mean. In such instances, uncertainty may allow our thinking to be filled with ambivalence, to be necessarily ambiguous. This process has potential to admit new ideas, knowledge, and practices; used strategically it can creatively develop uncertainty. Indeed, when we do not know, when we are uncertain – imagine the kind of collusions that may occur between practitioners and people with disabilities.

Labor and the relationship of laboring affinities

Labor has been foregrounded as one of the core elements of the RoLA to emphasize that 'laboring affinities' is essentially a relationship of work. Labor, within RoLA, is charged with transformation (Fig. 13.3). Within a transformatory frame the element of labor has been understood in the following ways.

Labor is positioned relative to Marx's (Marx & Engels 1968) views of labor within capitalism, which is the breeding ground of most professional practitioners. We have developed a core interest in economic gain relative to our market of 'sick people', 'slow learners' who constitute viable capitalistic interests. An extreme perspective may assume that rehabilitation 'patients' are necessary markets without whom we (expert practitioners) could not exist.

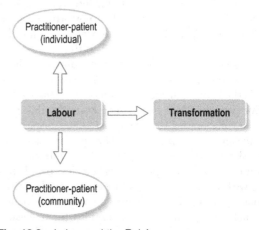

Fig. 13.3 • Labor and the RoLA.

However, a less extreme stance may consider Marx's focus on capitalistic-oriented labor (Engestrom & Miettinen 1999) where labor is seen as a joint, collective activity. Essentially, this means labor in rehabilitation is focused on the solution of a problem, mediated by tools and performed in collaboration with a community of practitioners/other stakeholders like disability rights activists. The structure of our labor, however, is constrained by cultural factors including conventions (rules) and social strata (division of labor) within the healthcare/rehabilitation network. Therefore, we need to be cognizant of that as labor is part of a network of several systems we necessarily have to collaborate. Habermas' (in Pusey 1987) theory of universal pragmatics may further situate the dialogic base of labor, where interlocutors (people) collaborate during interactions, at levels that supersede the individual. Labor is ideologic, as well as a practical endeavor and is the critical element responsible for the production of conceptual and practical/material tools for transformation. In the RoLA (re)formulating the practitioners' relationship with others must engage labor that is in itself conceptually and practically transformative in nature. Practitioners must think and do differently. The production, development and implementation of such tools for thinking and working are in themselves mediated by several processes.

For rehabilitation practitioners, we need to consider how people with disabilities positioned as without agency (or at best as possessing limited agency) can now exercise power/control over the labor within clinics, hospitals, schools, their homes, and their communities. As stated earlier on, labor within a medicalized, deficit tradition has applied an objective science to measure the people's disabilities, separating them from their contexts for intervention. This places the person in a less than powerful position within an expert-driven relationship. Within the RoLA, labor must be shared differently. Such labor-sharing may create multiple understandings of the person with a disability and seek to interact with the very social, cultural, and political forces that have produced him or her. For example, this may mean collaborating to develop 'advocacy' or perhaps 'activism' as conceptual tools. This may be practically translated into the development of organizations to promote advocacy of potentially voiceless people living with disabilities' rights in various social institutions. An example of this may be a social challenge to include sign language/text options for television programs, where the social institution of television

broadcasting (media) is made available relative to the civil rights of nonhearing populations. Elsewhere, we might argue for the valuing of multiple competencies drawing on life experiences and potentialities of people who repeatedly fail in a system which promotes singular ways of knowing, single literacies. In classrooms, for example, we might engage educators and learners on what might be the essence of healthy communication, and the interrelationships between identity, rights, and communication as a significant part of classroom experiences.

Conclusion

The inversion of political ideology in South Africa from an oppressive state to one that aspires for democracy provides the political context for substantive social and cultural change, even transformation, to occur. For South Africa there are many fields of opportunities, especially for ideologic shifts, changes, and/or transformations. However, as we celebrate the fertility of our geopolitical territory; we are also aware that *if* the nature of this ideologic context is *not* nurtured (from 'inside' and from 'outside'), then things such as the Relationship of Labouring Affinities may have an untimely-timely death. We must remain vigilant of the multiple forces which impact on change possibilities. As we celebrate a post-apartheid territory on the inside, we are also a post-colonial territory from the outside. Perhaps it is this perspective that we offer for consideration to others in countries with dissimilar and similar political contexts. Positioning communication, thinking, and labor in a democracy with ideologies driving new practices seeking to free minds comes with a fresh set of threats akin to the repressiveness of apartheid. What are these threats?

In a world of globalizing countries that are soaked in economic concerns, several threats exist in the marketization of policy (and practices) within education and health, foregrounding econometric concerns. This refers practices and rehabilitation outcomes to economic indices, monetary gains or even, as Hammel (2007) has argued, a fiscal related accountability to employers' concerns versus client-centered needs. Specifically, three forces threaten the RoLA: the dominant interests of the private education and health sector; globalization's repressive marketized vision of competence; and interrelated, surging fundamentalist constructions of social, political, cultural, religious, and racial identities.

The complex interaction between these three forces must be understood as yet another dialectic encounter to resist. As it has been with forces such as colonialism, apartheid and the such-like, our practitioner relationships must be considered relative to postcolonialism, neo-liberalism and neo-capitalism. This means that as we encounter these phenomena and work through our laboring affinities we must be able to assess their influence relative to the question of 'Whose interests does our practice serve?'

Acknowledgments

Sandhya Chetty, Ayesha Mohamed for listening, reviewing and editing.

References

Babrow AS: Communication and problematic integration: Milan Kundera's lost letters. The book of laughter and forgetting, *Communication Theory* 2:95–130, 1995.

Berger CR, Calabrese RJ: Some explorations in initial interaction and beyond: toward a developmental theory of interpersonal communication, *Human Communication Research* 16:91–119, 1975.

Bhaskar R: *Reclaiming Reality: a Critical Introduction to Contemporary Philosophy*, London, 1989, Verso.

Bourdieu P: *Language and Symbolic Power*, Cambridge, 1991, Harvard University Press.

Bradac JJ: Theory comparison: uncertainty reduction, problematic integration, uncertainty management and other curious constructs, *J Commun* 51:456–476, 2001.

Department of Health: *Annual Report: the prevalence and distribution of malaria in South Africa 2007*, South Africa, 2008a, DOH.

Department of Health: *Report: the national HIV and syphilis prevalence survey South Africa 2007*, South Africa, 2008b, DOH.

Desai A: *The Poors of Chatsworth*, South Africa, 2000, Madiba.

Dunbar R: *The Trouble with Science*, London, 1995, Faber and Faber.

Engestrom Y, Miettinen R: Introduction. In Engestrom Y, Miettinen R, Punamaki R, editors: *Perspectives on Activity Theory*, Cambridge, 1999, Cambridge University Press.

Fleck L: *Genesis and Development of a Scientific Fact* (Bradley F, Trenn TJ, translator, 1979), Chicago, 1935, University of Chicago Press.

Foucault M: *The Birth of the Clinic: an Archaeology of Medical Perception*, London, 1976, Tavistock.

Frank AW: *The Wounded Storyteller: Body, Illness and Ethics*, Chicago, 1995, Chicago University Press.

Goldstein MA: The otologist and the speech pathologist, *J Speech Disord* 3:231–233, 1938.

Habermas J: cited in Pusey M, editor: *Jurgen Habermas*, England, 1972, Tavistock, 1987.

Hammel KW: Client-centred practice: ethical obligation or professional obfuscation? *British Journal of Occupational Therapy* 70:264–266, 2007.

Jansen JD: Chapter 13: globalisation, markets and the third world university: preliminary notes on the role of the state. In Sayed Y, Jansen JD, editors: *South African Higher Education, Implementing Education Policies: the South African Experience*, Cape Town, 2001, UCT Press.

Kathard H, Pillay M: Educational development and professional transformation: a case study. In *Proceedings of the 9th Annual Conference of the South African Association for Academic Development, 1–3 December*, Cape Town, 1993, University of the Western Cape.

Kathard H, Pillay M: Student assessment: policy and practice in the health sciences. In *Proceedings of the 10th Annual Conference of the South African Association for Academic Development, 30 November to 2 December*, Durban, 1994, University of Natal.

Kathard H, Pillay M: Practice innovations: language practitioners in (South African) classrooms, *International Journal of Learning* 13:9–18, 2005.

Kathard H, Naude E, Pillay M, Ross E: Lead article: improving the relevance of speech-language pathology and audiology research and practice, *S Afr J Commun Disord* 54:5–7, 2007.

Kronenberg F, Pollard N: Overcoming occupational apartheid: a preliminary exploration of the political nature of occupational therapy. In *Occupational Therapy Without Borders. Learning from the Spirit of Survivors*, Edinburgh, 2005, Elsevier/Churchill Livingstone.

Maturana H, Varela FJ: *Autopoiesis and Cognition: the Realization of the Living*, Dordrecht, 1980, Reidel.

Marx K, Engels F: *The German Ideology*, Chicago, 1968, University of Chicago Press.

Pillay M: Developing critical practice: a South African's perspective, *Int J Lang Commun Disord* 33:84–89, 1998.

Pillay M: Do you speak practice-ese? A discourse of practice for sharing communication, *Int J Lang Commun Disord* 36:351–356, 2001a.

Pillay M: Uncertainty in health professional education: a critical discourse?. In *Proceedings of the Cultures of Learning Conference, 19–22 April*, England, 2001b, University of Bristol.

Pillay M: Cross cultural practice: what is it really about? *Folia Phoniatr Logop* 55:293–299, 2003a.

Pillay M: *(Re)Positioning the powerful expert and the sick person: the case of communication pathology*, Doctoral dissertation, Durban, South Africa, 2003b, University of Durban-Westville.

Pillay M, Kathard H, Samuel MA: The curriculum of practice: a conceptual framework for practice with a Black

African first language clientele, *S Afr J Commun Disord* 44:109–117, 1997.

Salomon G, editor: *Distributed Cognitions: Psychological and Educational Considerations*, Cambridge, 1993, Cambridge University Press.

South African Government: *South Africa. Millenium development goals. Midterm country report, September 2007*, 2007, SA Government Press.

Spivak GC: The Rani of Simur. In Barker F, Hulme P, Iversen M, et al, editors: *Europe and its Others*, Colchester, 1985, University of Essex Press, p 1.

Storey A: The world bank, neo-liberalism, and power: discourse analysis and implications for campaigners, *Development in Practice* 10:361–370, 2000.

Thadani G: *Sakhiyani: Lesbian Desire in Ancient and Modern India*, London, 1996, Cassel.

Vidich AJ, Lyman SM: Chapter 2, Qualitative methods: their history in sociology and anthropology. In Denzin NK, Lincoln YS, editors: *The Landscape of Qualitative Research: Theories and Issues*, Thousand Oaks, CA, 1998, Sage.

William M: *Wittgenstein, Mind and Learning: Toward a Social Conception of Mind*, London, 1999, Routledge.

World Health Organization (WHO): *International Classification of Impairments, Disabilities and Handicaps (ICIDH)*, Geneva, 1980, WHO.

World Health Organization (WHO): *International Classification of Functioning and Disability (ICIDH-2), beta-2 draft*, Geneva, 1999, WHO.

Foucault, power, and professional identities

14

Hazel Mackey

OVERVIEW

The aim of this chapter is to outline some of the key insights of social historian and philosopher, Michel Foucault, which I argue have relevance for a re-reading of the professional identities of occupational therapists. The purpose is to illuminate how occupational therapy identities are constructed and understood and not to define what identity occupational therapists as a group or individuals possess. I frame the chapter within a number of broad questions concerned with the construction of professional identities. Typical questions relating to professional identity based on a Foucaultian perspective are:

- How are the professional identities of occupational therapists constructed within a specific locality?
- How do occupational therapists define and practice their work within relationships of power?

Foucaultian approaches are rooted in a recognition that professional identities are contested and thus open to change rather than pre-determined. In this way, occupational therapy is a dynamic concept, shaped and reshaped over time by competing and often contradictory claims. Such approaches open up fields of possibilities for critical reflection and strategic action.

Introduction

For many years I had no theory to explain the professional identities of occupational therapists. For me, occupational therapy identity lay in a number of deeply felt assumptions, often not recognized as such, that shaped my everyday working life. Most often these beliefs were to do with the proper conduct of occupational therapy relationships and were entangled with issues of status, and a frustration based on some ways of existing in the world, being more legitimate, more rewarded, and heard than others. I took comfort and refuge in the occupational therapy collective, believing that we shared an understanding of our professional world. And then I became involved in redesigning the occupational therapy workforce, in line with the modernization of the National Health Service (NHS) in Britain (Department of Health (DH) 2000, 2002). The introduction of a new grade of support worker, the assistant practitioner who could take on extended roles and do some activities that had traditionally been within the role domain of the state registered occupational therapist, forced me to examine my own boundaries, roles, and relationships (Nancarrow & Mackey 2005). At times, this process led me into conflict with professional members of my own discipline. In my practice I fought to promote a vision of what occupational therapy can and should be, but is this vision based on a professional identity that is shared with other occupational therapists, has it been constructed by my own experiences, or have a combination of forces brought it about?

The importance of the concept of professional identity lies in its relationship to professional knowledge and action. Laying claim to being an occupational therapist can be seen as a device for establishing, defending, explaining, and making sense of one's behavior and career. People use the phrase 'I am an occupational therapist' to make sense of themselves and their actions, to find order and consistency over

DOI: 10.1016/B978-0-7020-3103-8.00023-7

the passage of time, to work out where they stand in relation to others, and to make themselves and their interests visible and included. Occupational therapists work together to construct and sustain their collective identity. In strategic terms, a strong collective identity is an ongoing process which enables the group to recognize and define itself, and which also facilitates successful collective action through a cohesive unit with agreed aims and interests. Central to this theory of professional identity, based on social identity theory (Tajfel 1982), is an essentialized, socialized phenomenon that governs occupational therapy action. Typical questions relating to professional identity based on this understanding include:

• What is occupational therapy identity?
• How may occupational therapists be distinguished from other health and social care workers?

It is assumed that although occupational therapists may work in different contexts and present in different ways, underneath that presentation lies a stable identity. Social identity theory explores the process of 'difference' between the 'in-group' and 'the other'. Put simply, according to social identity theory occupational therapists work at maintaining a positive professional identity by making favorable comparisons with other occupational therapists. The emphasis lies in the social cognitive processes of membership and the way that belonging is both initiated and sustained. Irvine & Graham (1994) identify four reasons why the identity of occupational therapists is an important issue for the profession to examine. They argue that for occupational therapy to be defined as a profession brings material and symbolic rewards both to individuals and the collective, that a shared identity is important in obtaining recognition from the public, state and other health and social care workers, that a shared identity encourages unity across local, national, and international occupational therapists, and that the notion of the professional occupational therapist as expert can be used to protect professional boundaries.

The concept of the professional project (Etzioni 1969, Friedson 2001, Larson 1977) explains the methods by which a group of workers acts collectively to aspire to full professional status. Although the exact characteristics of a full profession vary from author to author, the traditional view of a profession is as an organized body of experts who have a systematic, theoretical body of knowledge, have elaborate systems of entry level training usually university based, have a regulative code of ethics, are primarily orientated towards community benefit rather than

self-interest, perform tasks characterized by a high degree of autonomy and have a well-developed sense of community, usually within the form of a national/international association (Greenwood 1957, Parsons 1968). Occupational therapy has strived to acquire the characteristics of a profession (Wilcock 2002). Attempts to create a strong professional identity have been made through changes in the education curriculum, identifying conceptual foundations, producing profession specific models, developing a strong research base and growing networks of practitioners (Illot & White 2001, Kielhofner 1997, Mountain 1997, Wilcock 2001, Yerxa 1998). The result has been the emergence of a rhetoric of generalized certainty about 'the occupational therapist'. Consequently notions of professional identity have traditionally involved continuums of practices and roles that preorder professional identity into an orderly and settled story.

However, this view of professional identity assumes that the goals of individual occupational therapists are wholly consistent with those of the professional bodies, and fails to recognize the active role played by individual occupational therapists in shaping their own professional identity. The portrayal of occupational therapists as a single univocal entity leaves little scope for the consideration of individual difference or the diverse settings in which occupational therapists operate. Watson (2006), in her address to the World Congress of Occupational Therapists, argues that occupational therapists have failed to understand that while they share a common professional foundation, that practice cannot assume uniformity given the cultural uniqueness of different contexts. She calls for the 'doing' of occupational therapy to be diversified across the globe with cultural identity determining what occupational therapists do and practice.

The aim of this chapter is to outline some of the key insights of social historian and philosopher, Michel Foucault, which I argue have relevance for a re-reading of the professional identities of occupational therapists. The purpose is to illuminate how occupational therapy identities are constructed and understood and not to define what identity occupational therapists as a group or as individuals possess. Typical questions relating to professional identity based on a Foucaultian perspective are:

• How are the professional identities of occupational therapists constructed within a specific locality?
• How do occupational therapists define and practice their work within relationships of power?

Foucault: an introduction

Michel Foucault (1926–1984) has been one of the most influential thinkers of recent times and his vast reach extends across many disciplines. He wrote on the history of mental illness, medical practices, the penal system, and sexuality in Western culture. These topics overlap and interlink with the field of occupational therapy and, consequently, his writings are intriguing and relevant to our profession.

Concepts from existing theories act as the lenses through which we read situations. The use of theory is a reflective process. In the perpetual intercourse between ideas about the social world and data collected about it, theories work in two ways. First, the use of theory informs interpretation in a way that allows confirmation, refinement, or contestation of existing beliefs, values, and arguments. Second, theories guide the selection and interpretation of evidence. This is a dynamic use of theory as opposed to the imposition of a definitive structure, and can lead to a much greater understanding of the many dimensions of complex social circumstances. As Foucault argues:

> The role for theory today seems to me to be just this: not to formulate the global systematic theory which holds everything in place but to analyze the specificity of mechanisms of power, to locate the connections and extensions, to build little by little a strategic knowledge.
>
> Foucault (1980, p. 83)

Foucault's work is skeptical of claims of universal truth on the grounds that such totalizing theories are reductionistic and exclusionary, privileging some agendas while excluding or marginalizing others. His aim is to highlight the extent to which there are multiple and conflicting views of the world, some having more power and dominance than others. Language does not simply describe or reflect, but actually creates meaning and understanding, and the self is assumed to be a product of social interaction. In this light, Foucault intended his writing to be used as a 'tool box' by those struggling with and for social transformation. The metaphor of the toolbox may be used in an unsettling, troubling way that maximizes the potential for providing alternative insights into questions of knowledge, truth, and power. As Foucault suggests:

> All my books ... are little tool boxes .... If people want to open them, to use this sentence or that idea as a screwdriver, or spanner to short circuit, discredit or smash systems of power, including eventually those from which my books have emerged ... so much the better.
>
> Foucault (1979, p. 115)

Foucault's compositions offer informed enlightenment on the beliefs that guide professional behaviors and relationships and how they acquire power. His work attempts to defamiliarize present practice and categories in order to make them seem less self-evident and necessary. Consequently, his work is often considered complex and divergent. In a discussion on politics, Foucault explains his desire to see the issue of identity as perpetually unsettled:

> The problem is precisely, to decide if it is actually suitable to place oneself within a 'we' in order to assert the principles one recognises and the values one accepts; or if it is not, rather, necessary to make the future formulation of a 'we' possible by elaborating the question. Because it seems to me that the 'we' must not be previous to the question; it can only be the result –and necessarily temporarily result – of the question as it is posed in the, new terms in which one formulates it'
>
> Foucault (1997, p. 114–115)

By being skeptical of definitive answers, and contesting the taken for granted assumptions which underpin much of our everyday customs, Foucault's work offers a possibility of re-envisioning occupational therapy practices. For Foucault, the notion of a fixed and unified professional identity is difficult to accept (Mackey 2007). He stresses that identity is neither predetermined nor consistent but is constructed within and by the relationships which make up our societies. Occupational therapists understanding of their own identities change as they are enacted and performed within the hospital, clinic, home, or other workplaces. These interpretations may vary from situation to situation as the events and the stakes people have in these events change. We all have many potential individual and collective identities. At the level of collective identity, occupational therapy identities are constructed in the multiple intersections of experiences of the symbols, languages, and practices available within the sociohistorical context of the occupational therapy world. However, there is no neat separation of personal, professional, and political identities as occupational therapists are also created within their belonging (or lack of) to the positions within the various class, racial, gender, sexual orientation, economic, and other groups of society. As such there is a certain artificiality in dealing with occupational therapy identities in isolation.

To illustrate the implication of Foucaultian thought for occupational therapists, I will explore the narratives of Keith (pseudonym). They arise from my own work in progress towards a Doctor of Philosophy degree that investigated the impact of policy-directed workforce redesign in the NHS on the professional identities of occupational therapists. The empirical research was conducted over a 12-month period (April 2006–March 2007), across five NHS organizations in England. There were 13 participants. Over a period of 12 months, I interviewed Keith three times. The main focus of the interviews was on the way in which Keith experienced himself and constructed his identity as an occupational therapist. The interviews followed a semi-structured format, and were geared towards encouraging Keith to express himself in narrative terms, elaborating on issues of importance to his own working life and policies within the UK, yet they can be considered on a global scale as local variants of professional experience. The examples used are brief and by no means exhaustive of the discourses or subject positions within Keith's narratives, and were selected because of their relevance to this chapter. I look at specific incidents when Keith is negotiating the tensions between the public definitions of 'professionalism' with personally held values, attitudes, and beliefs about what constitutes 'being' an occupational therapist. However, according to Foucault, narrators are not free to tell what they like. Instead narrative identity is multi-voiced consisting of the dynamic interplay between available subject positions within dominant discourses. Stories 'are nevertheless, not something that the individual invents by himself. They are patterns that he finds in his culture and which are proposed, suggested and imposed on him by his culture, his society and his social group' (Foucault 1988, p. 11).

As such, they are based on Keith's local experiences and are the products of specific times, places and people. At the time of the first interview Keith had been qualified as an occupational therapist for five years. For two years he worked as a community occupational therapist where his main role involved assessing local residents who had a long-term physical condition, and if necessary, supplying them with suitable equipment to help with daily living activities. He then moved into the area of mental health.

The relations of discourse, knowledge, and power

For Foucault, one of the most significant forces shaping our experiences is discourse. Discourses are languages, representations and practices which

are available in a historically specific context, and which shape our understanding of ourselves and our abilities to differentiate the truth from a falsehood, the beneficial from the dangerous, the right from the wrong (Donaher et al 2000).

We not only use discourses to explain our values, feelings and actions to others, we use them to explain things to ourselves. Discourses consist of a set of common assumptions. They do not identify objects, rather they create and constitute them, thus framing the way in which people understand and respond. There are a number of discourses which occupational therapists draw on to describe and position themselves. For example 'occupational therapy is an allied health profession' (Cusick & Lannin 2005) or 'occupational therapy is a misunderstood profession' (Harries & Caan 1994, McAvoy 1994).

The status and dominance of a discourse is a product of power relations. Dominant discourses are produced as part of powerful cultures and can be considered as regimes of truth that determine what counts as important, relevant 'true' knowledge at any one specific historical point.

> Each society has its regime of truth, its 'general politics' of truth: that is, the types of discourse which it accepts and makes function as true; the mechanisms and instances which enable one to distinguish false and true statements, the means by which each is sanctioned; the techniques and procedures accorded value in the acquisition of truth; the status of those who are charged with saying what counts as true.
>
> Foucault (1984, p. 51–75)

In this way, the need for occupational therapy is created by occupational therapy itself through an emerging knowledge of occupational behavior gained through a pervading gaze which monitors the behavior of individuals and populations. The significance of occupation and participation, and their emergence as a separate identifiable entity worthy of a special body of knowledge and expertise found in occupational science, arises at a time when the discourses of health, wellbeing, and prevention are becoming dominant. To be guided by Foucault is to look for the roots of knowledge in power relations. Rather than see power in the traditional oppressive sovereign sense, in which power is possessed hierarchically, concentrated in particular places or in the hands of specific individuals, Foucault conceptualizes a capillary form of power. Foucault's concept of power sees a multiplicity of power relationships at work at any one time, considering power to be a mobile and productive network. Power can flow very quickly from one point or area to another, depending on changing alliances and circumstances (Sawicki 1991). Consequently, dominant discourses are under constant challenge. Those groups benefiting from dominant discourses attempt to retain and confirm status by failing to recognize as legitimate, the knowledge within competing discourses.

The normalizing professional discourse: producing the docile therapist

Applying Foucault's concepts it is possible to argue that occupational therapy professional discourses regulate members of the occupational therapy profession by upholding what can be claimed as true expert knowledge. The occupational therapy profession is seen as a micro-society within the larger society. It has its own experts, hierarchies, ranks, and networks, and its own codes of conduct. Such practices require systems of classification which sort out what the occupational therapy professional standards are, who fits the standards and who does not. In this way it is possible to think that the occupational therapy 'profession', which is conceived as representing 'the public interest', is an endeavor aimed at power, status, and keeping control over its own domain (Lukes 2005).

This notion of the normalizing professional discourse is interlaced with Foucault's concept of discipline and surveillance. In order to be accepted into the occupational therapy community, individuals learn how to 'fit' in with the discourse of the profession through becoming familiar with the expertise and knowledge of the profession as found in the likes of books, conference papers, and social interactions with colleagues. The profession lays down rules and procedures to regulate behavior and communications. The term 'discipline' is crucial in understanding the implications of these practices on the individual occupational therapist. The first meaning of discipline is as a verb, an action of regulation, and correction which we perform on other people or ourselves. The second understanding sees 'discipline' as a noun, a body of skills and knowledges that we need to master in order to gain recognition within a particular field. Foucault associates these two understandings of discipline through his concept of power-knowledge. Both concepts of discipline are

concerned with producing docile bodies that can be utilized in work and regulated in terms of time and space.

Within the discourse of professional development involving a reflective search for self-knowledge and self-improvement, the development of professional identity has long been held as a central component of the training of occupational therapy students (Ikiugu & Rosso 2003) and researchers, managers, practitioners, and educationalists have spent much time in examining occupational therapy self-concepts and value systems (Finlay 2000, Kanny 2003). Looking at this process from an alternative viewpoint based on a Foucaultian power/knowledge position it is possible to claim that such education and knowledge is structured not so much to critically inform minds, but rather to preserve minds, to suppress differences, and to mold appropriate professional attitudes and behaviors. In this way, discipline and knowledge creates the occupational therapists and the professional gaze is seen as a form of surveillance which produces normative coercion and may constrain occupational therapists ability to form their own way of working in partially new or different ways (Abberley 1995).

However, normalizing professional surveillance is not something that is simply directed against us by others – it also becomes a way of looking, 'gazing', at our own behaviors. Part of our professional socialization into occupational therapy, influences us to make ourselves the subject of our own disciplinary gaze, and so we constantly monitor ourselves, actions, and feelings in order to gain a sense of self. Occupational therapists who practice this monitoring of themselves against professional standards have become self-policing subjects.

Let's look at an example of this in Keith's narratives.

KEITH'S NARRATIVE

'What am I doing occupational therapy wise, am I an occupational therapist doing this job or is it more about actually ticking the boxes and making sure I see as many people as I am supposed to see, so do I meet the needs of my organisation rather than meet the needs of my clients? And it did start to bring up in me I suppose questions about that particular thing "am I meeting their needs" or a bathing assessment would come along which is kind of standard fare for an OT in the community, whereas "ah, well we will pop out with a bath board and a bath seat, and can you use these?" "Yes I can". There was nothing about quality issues of "well what do you like to do with your bath, what does a bath mean to you, are you the glass of Chardonnay on the side and the book and sink down into the bubbles? Well if you are that doesn't really matter because all we need to do is get on the bath so you can have a wash".'

In this narrative, Keith's identity as an occupational therapist is policed in that he scrutinizes himself for conformity to a core notion of occupational therapy professionalism. Here Keith's role as an occupational therapist in the community is to enable self-care, but Keith monitors himself against the ideology of meaningful activity and finds that his occupational therapy practice has become a technical fix. It is assumed that this kind of technical fix misses out 'quality of life' issues for the service user. However, Keith's definition of 'quality of life' has been created through his experiences within the discourses of occupational therapy. According to Foucault's power/knowledge position, there is no definitive, universal, stable set of characteristics that comprises 'quality of life' as differing discourses impose their own regimes of truths.

Multiple, shifting, and resistive subject positions

I have shown that according to Foucaultian concepts, occupational therapists are not free agents who make their own individual or collective meanings; rather they have their working lives scripted for them by the discourse within social forces and institutions. Often, the occupational therapist is not aware of this process. These discourses construct particular positionings that are available to the occupational therapist to take up. It is important to recognize that occupational therapists have access to many forms of discursive practice and may position themselves differently in relation to a range of discourses. The different subject positions give access to, for example, images, expectations, and practices, and are therefore crucial in the construction of different understandings of the world and our place within it. Each subject position may be inconsistent or contradictory with other subject positions also held by the occupational therapist, thus producing resistance and struggle. In his later work, *Care of the Self*, Foucault (1990) discusses how individuals have the potential to be more than docile bodies. Although our identities may be the effects of power relations, these relations are never seamless but are always

changing. With an understanding of these processes we can choose to respond to or resist these practices, and hence gain a certain amount of freedom. Different subject positions are constructed within a variety of different rhetorical, political, and ideologic operations. The occupational therapist may want career advancement, to attract professional recognition, establish and maintain relationships or engage in meaning making processes. All will create differing subject positions. In this way, the production of occupational therapy identities comes about by the process of classifying, analyzing, and naming ourselves as a certain type of subject. There are several possibilities for occupational therapists to name themselves, although the possibilities are limited to the existing discourses in any given context. For example, occupational therapists may name themselves as, and take up the subject position of 'the autonomous professional', 'the expert in occupation for health', 'the occupational therapist without borders'. These subject positions are not bounded, unique, or consistent, but are enmeshed and produced in relations of power which are shifting, rendering them at one moment powerful and at another moment powerless.

Subject positions are also open to interpretation, as we can see from this example from Keith.

KEITH'S NARRATIVE

'We had the occupational therapy away day and the last half of it was really a lot to do with how the culture was going to change, so we had the Chief Exec's right hand man telling us how he wanted us to challenge everything and social entrepreneur is one of the words that gets bandied around a lot and then we had one of the business managers who came along and they were saying there that when it comes to put the business part together he is more than happy to sort of help people to put business plans together and almost one of those words that was never bandied around in health care before, whether they were using it or not is that's the profit, if they are making a profit out of something and ploughing that profit back in again and then we finished off with the accountant and again, it was that strange sensation of business manager and accountants walking into a National Health Service. But, having said that, I suppose I did come away from it feeling quite positive and quite sort of energized by the way that they had sort of sold it, I did have and still have a few reservations about "will any possible profits actually be, as they should be, ploughed back into it or down the line are we looking at the possibility of nice big bonuses for people who have managed to keep the organization doing what it is supposed to do?" I suppose I am quite cynical in that way, so I didn't actually voice that question but it was hanging around in the back of my mind'.

In this narrative, we can see the discursive construction of occupational therapists as potential business people. This is a relatively new concept for occupational therapists working in the UK's NHS. Keith's use of the terms 'profit', 'business plan', and 'big bonuses' connote a very different picture from the traditional discourse of occupational therapists as public servants, motivated by social values that he is more familiar with. The discourse of occupational therapists as business people looks inwardly at the activities of the healthcare organization, and outward to the market (Foto 1998, Pattison 2006) It is important to note that while Keith recognizes the increasingly dominance of the business discourse, he positions himself in relation to it as the 'cynic'.

Within the interview setting, our shared understanding of this term was that Keith was positioning himself as an autonomous professional and disidentifying with any imposed business ethos. However, by remaining silent he was signifying his ability to work within the business culture and remain in his current organization. In other words, he could act the part without internalizing the beliefs. But the term 'cynic' also has alternative meanings dependent on the discourse used. Another, equally plausible version constructs cynicism as a defense mechanism which acts as a block to the perceived imposition of a set of ideas or actions. In this discourse the cynic actively resists the dominant discourse. The cynic here has the opportunity to leave the organization or to remain but continually voice his skepticism.

We can also tell the story of the 'cynic' from a managerial discourse in which cynicism is a psychological fault that needs to be overcome through leadership and personal development (Flemming & Spicer 2003).

The reflexive ethical self: a field of possibilities

The reflexive ethical self is a strategic term used to describe the individual's active negotiation of the self. The term ethics, from a Foucaultian sense, is linked to the process of self-definition and constraint by which individuals train themselves to be ethical persons, thus permitting,

> Individuals to effect by their own means or with the help of others a certain number of operations on their own bodies and souls, thoughts conduct, and way of being, so as to transform themselves in order to attain a certain state of happiness, purity, wisdom, perfection or immortality.
>
> Foucault (1988, p. 18)

Through the practice of the reflexive ethical self, individuals can choose to respond to or resist the practices of normalization. Such thoughts require the individual to analyze specific assumptions and to question how those assumptions were created. When the individuals attempt to work through these assumptions, they may become aware of the power of discourses. They are then in a position to deconstruct those discourses and to reconstruct aspects of their own identities.

In order to bring this about Foucault examines technologies of the self (Foucault 1988). Technologies of the self are a series of techniques that allow individuals to work on themselves through careful consideration of the self, of experiences, and on the surrounding discourses. These techniques are not something the individuals invent, but are patterns found in the cultures which the individuals can model themselves against and within. This is not a solitary exercise, but a social practice. Rather than existing outside of relations of power and knowledge, the reflexive ethical self is conceptualized as their third dimension (Heikkinen et al 1999). The intention is to allow ourselves to be shaped, co-created within our relationships with others.

By being open to the influence of the 'other', the contradictions, the dilemmas and unintended consequences of our own beliefs and behaviors become apparent. The reflexive ethical self requires the repeated experiences of struggling to overcome these difficulties. By examining our own practice through more critical eyes, it is possible to open it up to reinterpretation. The self conceived in this way allows for agency and creative action. It does not preclude the very real possibility that the self-regulating processes will replicate dominant powerful discourses, but it does show that resistance is possible, and that there are several ways of behaving, and many fields of possibilities. The identity of the occupational therapist, from this perspective, is perceived to be a subject who influences social relationships and events, rather than as a passive observer or object of relations. Hence, the search for professional identity is not driven towards finding an external truth, but is instead enmeshed within 'excavating our own culture in order to open a free space for innovation and creativity' (Foucault 1988, p. 163). The excavation of everyday assumptions and beliefs has a creative force because it makes us aware of what we consider common sense and thereby also 'right', or 'good'. Such awareness increases the ability to recognize and understand systems of power within institutions and discourses. The reflexive ethical self involves individual occupational therapists making choices about behavior. As Keith identifies ...

KEITH'S NARRATIVE

'In the past, they have always sort of looked at the occupational therapists to provide the activity and if that's one kind of change, almost cruel to be kind, we have pulled ourselves bodily away from that, we are not activity co-ordinators, we are there to do specific occupational therapy therapeutic input ... "well what we are going to do is reclaim the occupational therapy crowd and we are actually not going to be the activity co-ordinators anymore, so we are not going to do Bingo on a Monday morning and we are not going to do the crossword anymore, the stuff is there if the nursing staff want to use it or if they have got to – they don't want to use it, great, but we are not going to do it anymore". I can't remember once where somebody actually was saying "well aren't you denying activities, aren't we taking the activity away and if anything making the ward environment worse for people?" How ethical is that?'

In this narrative we can see Keith struggling to overcome a dilemma between two incongruent discourses prevalent in occupational therapy. The first discourse, based on the professional project is based on occupational therapists advancing the professions own social status and persuading others of its expert knowledge by drawing back from engagement in low status activities, and replacing this by the establishment of ring-fenced prestigious, specialized activity. However, being an advocate for the profession in this way has unintended consequences, in this specific context, as it clashes with another important discourse within occupational therapy, that of occupation for health.

From a Foucaultian perspective, I argue that it is in the attempt to overcome the struggles between powerful competing discourses that occupational therapy identities are constructed as each therapist creates the specific, localized, incidents according to the network of personal concerns, values and aspirations against which events are judged and decisions made. In this way, occupational therapy is a dynamic concept, shaped and reshaped over time by competing and often contradictory claims.

Conclusion

Using Foucaultian concepts as a 'tool box' to examine the professional identities of occupational therapists has offered me the opportunity to develop and use a wide range of theoretical resources. Because Foucault's writings see expert, universal truth as just one truth among many, they encourage me to relinquish positions of certainty in favor of detailed, local, and specific knowledges formulated by those concretely involved in the situation. This commitment to a plurality of occupational therapy ways of being means that no one version of occupational therapy is more correct than others. This produces more diverse, fragmented and heterogeneous occupational therapy discourses, with different value systems existing side by side within the profession. This does not necessarily rob occupational therapy of a coherent identity. Instead it acknowledges the creation of localized and specific professional identities, where the self is defined by local meanings and practices alongside a self-defined through a global profession.

References

Abberley P: Disabling ideology in health and welfare – the case of occupational therapy, *Disability and Society* 10:221–232, 1995.

Cusick A, Lannin N: Constructions of allied health. Making considered choices. In Whiteford G, Wright St-Clair V, editors: *Occupation and Practice in Context*, Edinburgh, 2005, Churchill Livingstone, pp 158–178.

Department of Health: *Meeting the Challenge: a strategy for the allied health professions*, London, 2000, HMSO.

Department of Health: *HR in the NHS Plan*, London, 2002, HMSO.

Donaher G, Schirato T, Webb J: *Understanding Foucault*, London, 2000, Sage.

Etzioni A: *The Semi-professions and their Organisations*, New York, 1969, Tree Press.

Finlay L: The OT role: meanings and motives in an uncertain world, *British Journal of Therapy and Rehabilitation* 7:125–129, 2000.

Flemming P, Spicer A: Working at a cynical distance. Implications for power, subjectivity and resistance, *Organisation* 10:157–179, 2003.

Foto M: Competence and the occupational therapy entrepreneur, *Am J Occup Ther* 52:765–769, 1998.

Foucault M: Cited by Patton P, Of power and prisons. In Morris M, Patton P, editors: *Michel Foucault: Power, Truth, Strategy*, Sydney, 1979, Ferral Publications, p 115.

Foucault M: *Michel Foucault, Power/knowledge: Selected Interviews and Other Writings*, Brighton, 1980, Harvester Press.

Foucault M: Truth and power. In Rabinow P, editor: *The Foucault Readers*, New York, 1984, Pantheon, pp 51–75.

Foucault M: Technologies of the self. In: Martin LH, Gutman H, Hulton P, editors: *A seminar with Michel Foucault*, London, 1988, Tavistock.

Foucault M: *The History of Sexuality: the Care of the Self*, vol 3: (Hurley R, translator), 1990, Penguin History Books. London.

Foucault M: In Rabinow P, editor: Essential Works of Michel Foucault. vol 1. *Ethics; Subjectivity and Truth*, New York, 1997, New Press, pp 114–115.

Friedson E: *Professionalism: the Third Logic*, Cambridge, 2001, Polity Press.

Greenwood E: Attributes of a profession, *Soc Work* 2:45–55, 1957.

Harries P, Caan AW: What do psychiatric inpatients and ward staff think about occupational therapy, *British Journal of Occupational Therapy* 57:219–233, 1994.

Heikkinen S, Silvonen J, Simola H: Technologies of the truth: peeling Foucault's triangular onion. Discourse, *Studies in the Cultural Politics of Education* 20:141–157, 1999.

Ikiugu M, Rosso HM: Facilitating professional identity in occupational therapy students, *Occup Ther Int* 10:206–225, 2003.

Illot I, White E: College of occupational therapists research and development strategic vision and action plan, *British Journal of Occupational Therapy* 64:270–277, 2001.

Irvine R, Graham J: Deconstructing the concept of profession. A pre-requisite to carving a niche in a changing world, *Australian Occupational Therapy Journal* 41:9–18, 1994.

Kanny E: Core values and attitudes of occupational therapy practice. In Crepeau EB, Cohn ES, Schell AB, editors: *Willard and Spackman's Occupational Therapy*, ed 10, Philadelphia, 2003, Lippincott, Williams & Wilkins, pp 1005–1007.

Kielhofner G: *Conceptual foundations of occupational therapy*, ed 2, Philadelphia, 1997, FA Davis Company.

Larson MS: *The Rise of Professionalism*, Berkeley, 1977, University of California Press.

Lukes S: *Power: a Radical View*, ed 2, Basingstoke, 2005, Palgrave Macmillan.

Mackey H: Do not ask me to remain the same: Foucault and the professional identities of occupational therapists, *Australian Occupational Therapy Journal* 54:95–102, 2007.

McAvoy E: Occupational who? Never heard of them! An audit of patient awareness of occupational therapists, *British Journal of Occupational Therapy* 55:229–232, 1994.

Mountain GA: A review of the literature in the British, Journal of Occupational Therapy 1989–1996, *British Journal of Occupational Therapy* 60:430–435, 1997.

Nancarrow SA, Mackey H: The introduction and evaluation of an occupational therapy assistant practitioner, *Australian Occupational Therapy Journal* 52:293–301, 2005.

Parsons T: Professions, *International Encyclopaedia of Social Sciences* 12:536–547, 1968.

Pattison M: OT – outstanding talent. An entrepreneurial approach to practice, *Australian Occupational Therapy Journal* 53:166–172, 2006.

Sawicki J: *Disciplining Foucault: Feminism, Power and the Body*, London, 1991, Routledge.

Tajfel H: *Social Identity and Intergroup Relations*, Cambridge, 1982, Cambridge University.

Watson RM: Being before doing. The cultural identity (essence) of occupational therapy, *Australian Occupational Therapy Journal* 53:151–158, 2006.

Wilcock AA: Occupational science: the key to broadening horizons, *British Journal of Occupational Therapy* 64:412–417, 2001.

Wilcock A: Occupation for Health. *A Journey from Prescription to Self Health*, London, 2002, College of Occupational Therapists.

Yerxa EJ: Occupation: The keystone of a curriculum for a self-defined profession, *Am J Occup Ther* 52:365–372, 1998.

Occupational therapists – permanent persuaders in emerging roles?

15

Nick Pollard

OVERVIEW

This chapter considers the potential for occupational therapy as a critical dialog about everyday life from the perspective of some of Gramsci's writing, drawing on a relationship between Wilcock's (1998, 2006) and Hammell's (2004) doing, being, becoming, and belonging, the occupational narratives of worker writing and community publishing, and the analyses of 'everyday life' offered by De Certeau and Lefebvre. The chapter offers an introduction to some of Gramsci's ideas and their relevance for occupational therapists as individuals whose work can be persuading people to make changes in the everyday and ordinary but significant aspects of life.

Introduction

The political philosopher Gramsci (1891–1937) wrote in the 1920s that the professional (then a growing social class of new workers in many sectors, particularly healthcare (Paterson 2002, Wilcock 2002)) has a social transformational role as a 'new intellectual' who has to become an 'active (participator) in practical life, as constructor, organizer, 'permanent persuader', and not just a simple orator' (1971, p. 10). This seems to resonate with the present reassertion of occupational therapy's social commitments, but also presents a challenge, as Gramsci (1971, p. 12) says, the process is difficult, full of contradictions, and through it 'the loyalty of the masses (for example, service users with different cultural perspectives) is sorely tried'. Since service users

might also be among the 'new intellectuals', occupational therapy's professional notions of client-centeredness and negotiated outcomes may well be tested. Gramsci's thought offers a process of critical consciousness and intercultural dialog that may speak to occupational therapy's emerging role and the new partnerships it will obtain as more practitioners engage in non-traditional settings and community development projects in the present changing definitions of the profession (Pollard et al 2005a). Gramsci has been a significant influence in the critique of culture, history, politics, and sociology. His work is applied in the recognition of the value of accommodating debate, difference, and adaptability to different contexts.

Our occupational engagement with the world around us is one of the elements of our human nature: all people can potentially play a transformational role in society. Given the organization of modern society with its many strata ordered to functions such as the maintenance of health or social care, there are many opportunities for individuals to mediate or channel social outcomes. Occupational therapists are members of what Gramsci called 'the political society' or the 'civil society' (1971, p. 12) depending on which sector (state or private) they work for. As 'new intellectuals' they carry out the operations of society such as mediating care processes and assessing entitlements to forms of treatment or state benefits. These functions set them apart from service users since their professional status depends on managing such processes for others. Consequently occupational therapists' social transformational role is limited but can have a critical role, for example generating evidence to raise awareness of conditions and support interventions and collaborations. Occupational therapy is experiencing difficulties in identifying a constituency as boundaries in health and social care are being redrawn. On the other hand, therapists are identifying new areas of work in response to the occupational needs of a culturally diverse society outside the traditional care environment and into the community at large (Christie & Simpson 2008, Friedland et al 2001, Hook & Kenney 2007, Pim & Russel 2008, Thew et al 2008, Wheeler 2008). While, in the name of occupational justice, authors such as Wilcock and Townsend have called for 'a social revolution' (2000, p. 84), Gramsci (1971) suggests that the most a transformation through occupation would produce is social reform in which the underlying class relationships that determine occupational deprivations and occupational injustice remain.

Nonetheless, throughout its history some members of the profession have attempted to reach across concepts such as class, gender, cultural, and racial difference through what Peloquin (2007, see Chapter 7) has called its ethologic beliefs, for example in co-creating lives and personal engagement. The profession has not always been successful in doing so, and has been saddled, perhaps in some countries more than others, with the perception that it is a white, middle class, and predominantly female profession concerned with rather quaint therapeutic activities (Beagan 2007, Pollard & Walsh 2000, Sakellariou & Pollard 2008, Wilcock 2002) overshadowed by its more dominant allies in the healthcare pantheon. Nursing and medicine not only command greater resources for education and research but also the public imagination through their greater contact with the public.

Vernacular and narrative

The vernacular understanding of the hospital experience, the narratives that people tell and expect of each other in competing with their stories of treatment do not often include occupational therapists, yet narrative is a key factor in the spread and the developing awareness of the profession (Detweiler & Peyton 1999, Schwammle 1996). Few occupational therapists surface in the professional literatures of other professions, indeed most health and social care professions plough parallel furrows in the development of their discourses (Peck & Norman 1999), and so the value of occupational therapy is incompletely communicated across disciplines, not through the narratives we tell, but the stories others hear.

It is often not until people meet an occupational therapist that they begin to understand what they do (Craik et al 2001, Thew et al 2008). Practitioners' communicative exchanges are frequently *extra* professional, reaching outside their professional base to the world of the carer or service user and the communities they inhabit. Although they may also belong to the same community, and blend back into it perhaps when they are out of uniform, this is an intercultural exchange: these communities do not use the technical vocabulary of the interdisciplinary process. Wilcock (1998, 2006) and Hammell's (2004) doing, being, becoming and belonging $(d+b^3)$ is expressed in the vernacular languages and practices of daily life. A participatory process of negotiating with communities about their needs entails dealing with a different set of practices and forms of vernacular knowledge that De Certeau (1988) and his colleagues (De Certeau et al 1998) have called 'the practice of everyday life'. Health systems and corporate institutions may be slow to respond or even exclude those with needs that cannot be accommodated in the dominant culture. A recent report into mental health service users needs focussed particularly on the demand for communication in lay language (Lloyd et al 2007). The dissonance or assonance between individual experience and the values of larger social actors such as institutions can be the point at which people recognize the political dimension in their daily occupations (Pollard et al 2008).

Gramsci (1971, p. 34, 323) realized the importance of the vernacular from his interest in linguistics and in folklore. In their everyday interactions professionals share stories with each other, perhaps also with service users, developing a lore or a common folk narrative consciousness, and also an occupational literacy (Pollard 2008, Schwammle 1996). Through my active interest in community publishing and worker writing I have read many examples of how social opportunities shape the occupational narratives of both individuals and communities and are indicated in everyday practices such as the know-how or making-do involved in cooking or hand-wringing washing (Gatehouse 1996, Lawrence & Mace 1992) and often indicate particular preferences or cultural interpretations that express identity (Fair & Barnitt 1999, Lawrence & Mace 1992). These stories contain what De Certeau et al (1998) describe as 'microhistories' of specific and intimate aspects of community knowledge about practices, things and places, of occupational deprivation and occupational opportunities, in accounts which emerge through people's resilience, determination to learn or to communicate their experience for others. The political perception of occupation emerges from the daily experiences of the wider community with whom occupational therapists work (Kronenberg & Pollard 2005a,b, Pollard et al 2008) in relation to these cultural spaces. These experiences are the basis for questioning the status quo, of the direction of occupational therapy's goals of social transformation, or an actor's agency for social change.

Community published literature generally exists in small quantities and is somewhat ephemeral and elusive. Though some of its practices and its occupationally focused content have been discussed in the profession (see Chapter 18), it has understandably not made a wide impact. Such writing is often concerned with a detailed witness account of a life ordered to the needs of the writer rather than the reader and consequently can prove challenging to read, not least because of the frequent and sometimes celebratory use of dialect (Bonfim 2005, Landry 1990, Morley & Worpole 1982, Vincent 1981, Woodin 2005a–c, Worpole 1984). It is the written form of the oral autobiographical narrative all people use in their everyday lives, but have been educated and trained not to respect or value such testimony as much as written and researched evidence with its veneer of objectivity (De Certeau 1988, De Certeau et al 1998, Morley & Worpole 1982). On the other hand, working-class autobiographical narratives (for example Hart et al 2008) are ordered to the needs of a bottom-up perspective rather than a dominant order. This is where their difference from other forms of literature lies (Gramsci 1985, p. 132–133, Not 2003). In Ross's (1984) or Williams' (1984) accounts of railway work, people carry on living their everyday lives despite the events around them or efforts to contain or manage them, developing what De Certeau (1988, p. 28) describes as tactics, such as 'la perruque' (literally 'the wig') in order to get by. This describes the work someone does for themselves while appearing to do the job they are paid to do for their employer, which De Certeau describes as a tactic of appearing to conform. One popular and expert example of such wangling is Hasek's (1974) *Good Soldier Svejk*, who maintains a comfortable life in times of war through what Goffman (1969) has termed 'impression management'.

It is not unknown for occupational therapists to develop these skills in order to get some opportunity or extra activity for service users, but to provide examples would challenge the professional culture: such narratives are only spoken of in Goffman's (1969) backstage areas. The professional culture of occupational therapy is distinct from, and may not always readily admit a working class culture (Beagan 2007, Sakellariou & Pollard 2008). In my classes students have often assumed that the experiences of financial insecurity, unemployment, hard and dangerous work, industrial accident or disability described in workers' autobiographical writing is something from the past. Other students recognize the similarity of these experiences to that of relatives or themselves. Bromley (1988) has described how a dominant middle-class culture has domesticated, contained, and made safe the challenges presented by harsh working realities by presenting them as historical events that have now been resolved. Working-class students or those with disabilities often feel silenced by normalizing pressures, or experience a lack of comprehension from their student peers when they talk about things that arise from differing social backgrounds to those dominant in the academic environment (Abel et al 2008, Beagan 2007).

Contact zones

Pratt (1991), a teacher of community literacy, uses literary texts which talk about marginalized experiences in the classroom to explore different experiences with students who may not share these themselves. She calls this the contact zone, but the contact may be rather less direct in literature. Often the protagonist who provokes the reader's sympathy is actually a middle-class person who has entered the working-class world. Oliver, the famous Dickensian orphan boy, is not really a member of the lumpen proletariat but the child of a fallen middle-class woman. Orwell, though down and out in Paris (1940) and London or on the road to Wigan Pier (1962), is really a gentleman. Despite the sympathy these characters evoke, and the authors' good intentions, there is no real contact zone, the true voice of the working-class remains excluded. Despite the grimness of the story, it is reportage. The audience are separated from uncomfortable truths by the reasonable tone of the author, telling them where to cry or laugh.

Occupation and hegemony

The characters who end up in the hospitals depicted in popular UK and US television programs such as *Casualty*, *Holby City*, or *ER*, are snap-shot stereotypes, plot devices which cannot tell stories written by ordinary people themselves in the space of an episode. Occupational therapists rarely feature in these popular dramas in spite of the human interest stories they could illustrate (Hockenberry 2006). Occupation, expressed through $d+b^3$, underpins all society. Therapists need to actively and effectively command more of the popular discourse to generate greater demand for their skills and interventions.

Occupational therapists can reconsider their position in the power structures that maintain society and form alliances with their users by challenging the limitations that people experience in occupational choice in many aspects of the services they work in (Gramsci 1971, p. 12–13, Pollard 2007). User demand can be among the tactics employed to achieve change (Abel et al 2008, Pollard & Kronenberg 2008, Pollard et al 2005b). Autobiographical material or cultural representations of needs and inequalities can show how lack of occupational choice, lack of things to do, be, or become or belong to reduces self-worth, decreases personal horizons, promotes depression, and slows recovery. Recent reports on what clients want from 'person-centered practice' repeatedly call for flexibility (Dowling et al 2006, Lloyd et al 2007), the capacity for people to enact their own decisions according to their own needs, and say that a one-size fits all approach to healthcare does not work.

My operation

Berne (1964) describes the interpersonal transactions or games people play to obtain status and recognition from each other, such as 'broken skin' which might be better understood as 'my operation'. This is an exchange of stories of treatment processes and the characteristics of the people involved, embellished with gruesome details and advice to potential fellow sufferers. It is popular in care environments due to the lack of other things to do, prompted by the regular stimulus of people receiving further interventions. Six people in a ward bay can maintain a game despite the disruption of players' discharge and admission.

Essentially 'my operation' offers a safe zone for people to learn something of each other through a form of intimacy restricted to 'treatments'. It also involves the exchange of a vernacular knowledge of clinical procedures. Many medical and nursing terms are employed in everyday language and perhaps also misunderstood. One difficulty that can arise is that

things which are misnamed have to be re-explained to the service user – in other words there is often some element of un-learning for them to do. Many occupational therapy procedures remain unknown. Being a smaller profession, the specialized vocabulary occupational therapists use has not become taken up in the popular discourse. Occupational therapists have to explain practices in everyday terms to service users and perhaps other workers in order to negotiate them (Pollard & Sakellariou 2008). However, in order to distinguish the purpose of occupational interventions from 'common sense' they require a specialized vocabulary to talk about everyday occupation in a way that allows it to be objectified and in order to develop theoretical concepts.

Cultural exchange

This kind of boundary between professional and vernacular discourses and forms of knowledge is a point of cultural exchange. Occupational therapists do not share an entirely separate culture from service users, thus it is conceivable that although the allied in allied health professionals refers to medicine, it could also be considered in terms of the service user (Pollard 2007, Pollard & Sakellariou 2008). Occupational therapists and service users meet in care environments or community settings which represent a set of hegemonic institutions, or consenting alliances (Gramsci 1978, p. 443), by which their social positions and professional power are maintained. However, professional power and the material benefits from professional salaries and education are purchased through the power of scrutiny over aspects of their lives given to therapists professional associations as a condition of membership.

Client-centered practice and cultural competency may at first appear to be representations of such an alliance. Both suggest inclusion and fit with the holism underpinning most health professionals practice, particularly in a profession concerned with the powerful formula $d+b^3$. $D+b^3$ is the occupational basis of culture, as might be shown in Gramsci's illustration of the emergence of Italian as a renaissance language through the development of commerce, for which it became a *lingua franca*, just as English became later on (1985, p. 170). Latin had been the language of power, but it became increasingly restricted to describing the functions of the church while the functions of trade and the practices of everyday life required new words. Education in Latin was restricted to privileged classes, but the Italian vernacular (the dialect of Florence) was concerned with a widening variety of $d+b^3$ activities – for example of commerce and the organization of labor – and eventually superseded it even in educated usage.

Because it is concerned with the practices of everyday life the development of an intercultural practice has to incorporate vernacular elements from the occupational forms found in the community. Occupational therapists are in a potentially good position to do this through their concern with what people want or need to do, distinct from other aspects of the treatment process – but struggle for the space in which to do it. Occupational therapists can, as Hammell (2007) has pointed out, be so constrained by the process in which they are contractually immersed and bound to by their employers, that there is little room for a true $d+b^3$ equation to produce negotiated outcomes that extend beyond a minimum.

The ethological principles in occupational therapy's professional philosophy center on artistry and skill (Peloquin 2007). Although practitioners have to take account of risk factors and the need to work within the abilities of the people with whom they engage, they frequently work spontaneously (Breines 2005). If an occupational opportunity is missed it may not arise again. In my work in enduring mental health this was frequently an issue, because the chance to do something might be a rare occasion when a person might demonstrate a hidden capacity. One service user in his fifties rarely took the opportunity to go out and presented as somewhat anhedonistic. However, given the time to show a person round his home town, or go with a group to a pub, he demonstrated the ability to be a raconteur, competent pool player and teller of jokes. He had the vernacular 'gift of the gab', but such flashes of ability happened very infrequently for him. Other colleagues found him difficult to engage, and would be surprised when told this story – he just needed more chances.

Although occupational therapists discuss occupation at length, and listen to numerous accounts of occupations from service users, they have relatively recently considered the significance of the occupations their service users engage in as opposed to finding occupations that translate into assessment or to which service users can be introduced. While it seems to be the effect of limited resources, it may also stem from the utopianism of the arts and craft movement, and perhaps a literal interpretation of the 'purposeful' in occupation. It may also as Hocking (2007) and Wilcock (2002) have suggested,

be a response to demands to prove the medical value of exposure to therapeutic occupations.

Working lives

Those readers who are educators have probably despaired at the perennial dissertation problem of topics concerning some novel occupational form to the profession – music, art, dance, writing, yoga, and so forth. I was also guilty of this with creative writing. My interest stemmed from a long involvement in community publication and worker writing, specifically the writing produced from a UK working-class writing movement (see Chapter 18). One of the first community publications I bought was Centerprise's *Working Lives* (1977). Each of its chapters is written by someone then living in Hackney, East London, with accompanying photographs of them working. The story that sold me the book was that of Mike Christou (1977), a Greek Cypriot who describes what it was like to run what was then my local chip shop. *Working Lives* has some relation to Berger and Mohr's photo-documentaries *A Fortunate Man* (1969), about a country doctor's life, and *A Seventh Man* (1975), concerning Turkish guest workers in West Germany. *Working* (Hart et al 2008), written by members of SEU1199, a service worker's union which includes health employees (see Chapter 18) is this community publishing genre's latest example.

In describing aspects of work and involvement in organizations these narratives are perhaps quite similar to the retired members' oral history project run by the College of Occupational Therapists (Wilcock 2002). These books illustrate the ways that different workers' occupations underpin the local community, to which occupational therapists also belong through a complex of hegemonic alliances connected with their employers, union, and professional membership and other activities. Like these alliances, the culture that is developed from them and through which people feel that they belong to, participate in, and own is also multilayered (Gramsci 1985, p. 205–206, Not 2003). In a community these cultural occupations flow in a synergistic relationship, rather than a series of vacuum-sealed activities. Such books demonstrate aspects of social capital, but also illustrate what can be lost if the exchange social capital is disrupted, or people are excluded from access to it.

As occupational scientists, some occupational therapists are already engaged in exploring and unraveling this kind of information through ethnographic study and anthropology, but community publishers tend to develop these occupational narratives *with* communities, rather than about them. The principle of 'nothing about us, without us' (e.g., SUAG 2001) was something that would certainly apply to the majority of the collectively produced publications of the Federation of Worker Writers and Community Publishers (FWWCP) (see Chapter 18, Pollard et al 2005b, Smart 2005).

Occupational therapists as literature sponsors and permanent persuaders

A common exercise to enable people to generate their own writing begins with a list, the most common everyday use of writing (Heath 1983). The list might concern things a person has experienced on the way to work, or a short walk, and is built up rapidly and progressively from simple words to sentences, paragraphs to a full page of writing. This entry into writing, or into composition (because community publishing need not involve the written word, but can mean composing something in your head and repeating it to an audience), generally begins with everyday occupational objects and occupational forms. As it develops sentences and paragraphs requiring descriptions it involves reflection about purpose and the meaning of doing. In facilitating such activity (for example, in a writing group) an occupational therapist is becoming what Gramsci called a permanent persuader (1971, p. 10), someone who is getting people to think about change (Pollard 2004). Because occupational therapy is about doing, perhaps 'practical persuader' is a better term for this new role, but a similar concept from the field of community literacy is the role of literacy sponsor (Brandt 2001), anyone or any institution which encourages people to develop some aspect of their use of the written word, whether in their reading or in their thinking about the world around them, which enables them to access literature.

As a literacy sponsor, or a practical persuader the occupational therapist is engaging in an intercultural dialog that is not just about reading literature but reading the world (Pollard 2008). Often practitioners encourage people to write about their experiences for therapeutic purposes, but writing can be about the expression of the 'moment' (Lefebvre 2002, p. 341) of doing and the articulation of

belonging (see Chapter 18, Pollard et al 2005b, Smart 2005). Community publication and worker writing is about an often critical testimony to the practical experience of doing rather than a fictional doing (Pollard et al 2005b, Ragon 1986, Vincent 1981). Experiences direct the course of the autobiographical story such writers tell, and testimony is usually the motive. They are often tales of that creative essential aspect of everyday life, learning to make do (De Certeau 1988). They are written with a degree of accuracy because, at least in the details of describing a working life, this accuracy is part of its value; the readership is anticipated as local, potentially able to refute a detail which is out of place. The importance of accuracy is also due to the rapid changes in human occupation over the last 170 years (Vincent 1981). People have felt the need to record their experiences because their early life was so different from that being lived by their grandchildren.

The pace of social change has been such that it has often been difficult for working people to organize themselves systematically to represent their culture (Foner 2002, Lefebvre 2005, O'Rourke 2005, Tait 2005). Much of it has simply been obliterated by progress. The FWWCP emphasized facilitating the representation of culture by aiming to be as inclusive as possible. As community 'publishers' they interpreted 'publication' to include many forms of dissemination – performance and even dance. A real problem of vernacular culture – a predominantly oral culture, a folk knowledge, is that it is ephemeral and can appear insignificant (Morley & Worpole 1982). This was appreciated by the middle-class folklorists and folk song collectors, who attempted to record disappearing oral traditions (Lloyd 1969), but it also stimulated a range of working-class people to record their experiences, the way of life they knew, and the culture that went with it (Vincent 1981). The difficulty faced by numerous early nineteenth century working-class writers has been that of appropriation by those with more power, access to education, often professionals who assumed authorship of their working-class tutee's work, or else turned them out like performing monkeys who had learned how to phrase themselves rather quaintly in proper English grammar and use some Latin tags (Landry 1990, Vincent 1981). Other writers struggle to represent their experience authentically in terms defined by the sacred conventions of bourgeois literature (Not 2003). The problem of the power differential remains though the problems express themselves in different ways.

While occupational therapists need to produce generalizable information and to be able to compare information about occupations in unitary forms, using standard assessment tools, the creative element of occupation, the vernacular form of expressions, are not to be easily rendered in the predetermined categories offered by assessment tools. Instead they are to be discovered in everyday occupations, in forms which are articulated by the communities we work with. In his work with Guatemalan Mayan refugees, Algado (see Algado & Cardona 2005) used different forms of cultural engagement to get different generations to work together. Youths exchanged information about the health effects associated with alcohol for the knowledge older community members had of Mayan traditions. Petridou et al's (2005) description of theatre work with psychiatric clients in Greece, Kapandaze et al's (2008) description of the work of Georgian occupational therapists with street children, McNulty's (2008) work with local mental health clients in Lincolnshire setting up their own arts organizations, and the Voices Talk, Hands Write group of people with learning difficulties in Grimsby (Pollard et al 2005b) are further examples (see also Chapter 21). In all of these the participants clearly began to set their occupational agendas, whether adapting the dialog of the plays they were to perform back in their own villages in makeshift stages, or perhaps in working a rapport of trust with the occupational therapists and contributing their own poetry and writing to a photography project, or contributing to the range of arts activities in their own communities. It is in these everyday occupational actions that the small p of politics, the fulcrum of a process of conscientization can be found (Kronenberg & Pollard 2005a, Pollard et al 2008). This doesn't necessarily require an occupational therapy perception; many community organizations, some run by people with disabilities and cognitive issues, are just getting on and doing political or consciousness raising work.

Occupational therapists have a particular dilemma in this intercultural representation since though they work with people with experiences of disability and/or disabling conditions they often do not have this experience themselves. As 'new intellectuals', practitioners have gone through processes of education and acculturation that remove them from vernacular cultures and instill critical perspectives, which distance and objectify the community around them in ways that reflect the dominant cultural view. As therapists they have to make bridges and develop rapport in order to facilitate and enable, but the critical dialog they use to describe the occupational environment is a little removed from it and so less able to accommodate essentially human aspects of it (Lefebvre 2005). Two problems arise from this: once their analyses of the everyday are translated back into everyday terms, they are recognized by service users and other colleagues as expressions of 'common sense' but the translation loses the critical perspective. This difficulty of representation of the everyday is central to the difficulty the profession has in getting the fundamental importance of occupation heard above the medical tumult. The other is that occupational therapy's professional position renders the translation in narrower, 'middle class', and perhaps Western dominant terms with the consequence that the 'common sense' lacks value in the experience of the service user (Iwama 2006, Lefebvre 2005).

Occupational therapy has itself been described as having an oral culture because it is centered in 'doing' (Detweiler & Peyton 1999, Schwammle 1996). The survival of many vernacular and folkloric practices is largely to do with their utility, perhaps in binding communities together and maintaining their identity, and perhaps also because they are fun, but health*care* is not easily connected to the health benefits of frivolity. The ephemeral and mundane issues of everyday life are not as dramatic as the defibrillators and flashing lights or the diagnosis of the doctor leaving the quietened sick room of popular cultural depictions of health dramas.

New intellectual

Science has to isolate something from ordinary life in order to present it as a science, but this process removes the aspect of life examined under its lens from its context (De Certeau 1988, Lefebvre 1991). To make a study of the practice of everyday life is, in effect, to make it other, to create a paradox where the subject becomes an object and loses its point. Working with occupation appears to be 'so ordinary that anyone could do it' (and everyone is, by virtue of $d+b^3$) and so its effect on health and wellbeing is not really seen as important as the other more obviously technical interventions involving medicine, surgery, and regular monitoring with sophisticated equipment and processes.

One of the strategies out of this impasse has been a demand for research, but the reality has been that it is very challenging to get the research published where it will be read by non-occupational therapists and facilitate alliances with those with the power to implement it. There is the student's dissertation problem of where to start and what to concentrate on given the enormous range of human occupations we might research as treatment media. A further difficulty identified by Lefebvre (2005) and De Certeau (1988) in the representation of culture is the range of choice offered by the media available to us. Such is the range of production that while there is perhaps less onus to do things ourselves and more incentive to buy something prepackaged, the immense range of personal choices available make it increasingly difficult to find common ground with others in the community around us. In the 'developed' world, occupation may be becoming less significant than the consumer (De Certeau prefers 'user') or 'lifestyle' choices that we make and the vernaculars we use as a result. At the economically poorer end of the social spectrum it becomes increasingly difficult to catch up with the plethora of choices.

Being a 'practical persuader' as I proposed earlier enables you to consider how to be a 'new intellectual' in challenging times. Occupational therapy is a bit of a mission, and being a professional requires a commitment. Occupational therapists' role is about 'doing stuff' in a way that enables people to balance their lives. Therapists must, above all, show that they are human, rather than commitment junkies, or damage the alliances that keep them human.

The profession retains its inspirational attraction for me through the attention my colleagues in occupational therapy (and nursing and social work) have paid to developing purposeful activities that are fun and stimulating with service users. As Breines (2005) collection of creative anecdotes demonstrates, occupational therapy is far more than a set of clinical treatment objectives, it is often about learning to enjoy life. In recent times resources have been cut back, and many of the spontaneous things we organized – barbecues, walks, sports activities, and so on are often regarded as presenting risks before they can be considered as opportunities, assessments which are often not so prioritized in the practice of everyday life.

A discrepancy between occupational therapists' vision of change and their ability to implement it was partly due to the fact that most of their clients are referred to them by doctors or else have to pay for the services that they offer. A challenge occupational therapists continually face is that the ordinary and everyday things that people want to do and enjoy in order to feel themselves, $d+b^3$, require a level of occupational justice that is a significant challenge for many to obtain. Yet occupation is natural, part of human nature and vernacular experience. Occupational therapists' challenge as 'new intellectuals' is persuading those around us of the value of the ordinary, the vernacular wisdom that arises from the everyday. To do this therapists need to empower themselves and those they work with in demonstrating the value of that knowledge, by the spontaneous and natural use of what is going on around us. Human beings are naturally constructors, organizers of their environments, they are naturally disposed to lives of action, and actions which are often accommodations, adaptations, or wangles. Gramsci is often thought of as a rather difficult, obscure theorist, but he can remind us that change is not an abstract process, it is something that is resourced by the natural skills and abilities that people already possess.

References

Abel B, Clarke M, Parks S: The transatlantic fed: from individual stories of disability to collective action. In Pollard N, Sakellariou D, Kronenberg F, editors: *Political Practice in Occupational Therapy*, Edinburgh, 2008, Elsevier Science, pp 175–181.

Algado SS, Cardona C: The return of the corn men: an intervention project with a Mayan community of guatemalan retornos. In Kronenberg F, Simo Algado S, Pollard N, editors: *Occupational Therapy Without Border: Learning from the Spirit of Survivors*, Edinburgh, 2005, Elsevier/Churchill Livingstone, pp 347–362.

Beagan BL: Experiences of social class: learning from occupational therapy students, *Can J Occup Ther* 74:125–133, 2007.

Berger J, Mohr J: *A Fortunate Man. The Story of a Country Doctor*, Harmondsworth, 1969, Penguin.

Berger J, Mohr J: *A Seventh Man. The Story of a Migrant Worker in Europe*, Harmondsworth, 1975, Pelican.

Berne E: *The Games People Play*, Harmondsworth, 1964, Penguin.

Bonfim V: Once a street child, now a citizen of the world. In Kronenberg F, Simo Algado S, Pollard N, editors: *Occupational Therapy Without Borders: Learning from the Spirit of Survivors*, Edinburgh, 2005, Elsevier/Churchill Livingstone, pp 19–30.

Brandt D: *Literacy in American lives*, New York, 2001, Cambridge University Press.

Breines EB: *Occupational Therapy Activities for Practice and Teaching*, London, 2005, Whurr.

Bromley R: *Lost Narratives, Popular Fictions, Politics and Recent History*, London, 1988, Routledge.

Centerprise Trust: *Working Lives: People's Autobiography of Hackney: 1945–1977*, (vol 2), Hackney, 1977, Centerprise.

Christie D, Simpson B: Self-directed support and personalisation: a new horizon for OT? *Occupational Therapy News* 16:34–35, 2008.

Christou M: Fish and chip man. In Centerprise Trust , editor: *Working Lives: People's Autobiography of Hackney: 1945–1977*, vol 2, Hackney, 1977, Centerprise, pp 158–165.

Craik C, Gissane C, Douthwaite J, Philp E: Factors influencing the career choice of first-year occupational therapy students, *British Journal of Occupational Therapy* 64:114–120, 2001.

De Certeau M: *The Practice of Everyday Life* (Rendall S, translator), Berkley, 1988, University of California.

De Certeau M, Giard L, Mayol P: *The Practice of Everyday Life, Living and Cooking* (Tomasik T, traslator), (vol 2), Minneapolis, 1998, University of Minnesota.

Detweiler J, Peyton C: Defining occupations: a chronotopic study of narrative genres in a health discipline's emergence, *Written Communication* 16:412–468, 1999.

Dowling S, Manthorpe J, Cowley S: *Person-centred planning in social care. A scoping review*, York, 2006, Joseph Rowntree Foundation: Online. Available at: www.jrf.org.uk/bookshop/ebooks/9781859354803.pdf. Accessed November 6, 2008.

Fair A, Barnitt R: Making a cup of tea as part of a culturally sensitive service, *British Journal of Occupational Therapy* 62:199–205, 1999.

Foner M: *Not for Bread Alone*, New York, 2002, Cornell University Press.

Friedland J, Polatajko H, Gage M: Expanding the boundaries of occupational therapy practice through student field-work experiences: description of a provisionally-funded community funded community development project, *Can J Occup Ther* 68:301–307, 2001.

Gatehouse: *Our Experience. Women from Somalia, Tanzania, Bangladesh and Pakistan Write About Their Lives*, Manchester, 1996, Gatehouse.

Goffman E: *The Presentation of Self in Everyday Life*, Harmondsworth, 1969, Penguin.

Gramsci A: *Selections from the Prison Notebooks* (Hoare Q, translator and Nowell-Smith G, editor), London, 1971, Lawrence and Wishart.

Gramsci A: *Selections from political writings 1921–1926* (Hoare Q, translator, editor), London, 1978, Lawrence and Wishart.

Gramsci A: *Selections from Cultural Writings* (Forgacs D, Nowell-Smith G, editors, Boelhower W, translator). London, 1985, Lawrence and Wishart.

Hammell KW: Dimensions in meaning in the occupations of everyday life, *Can J Occup Ther* 71:296–305, 2004.

Hammell KW: Client-centred practice: ethical obligation or professional obfuscation? *British Journal of Occupational Therapy* 70:264–266, 2007.

Hart G, Mangino ME, Murphy Z, Talierco AM, editors: *Working. An Anthology of Writing and Photography*, Syracuse, 2008, New City Community Press and Syracuse University Press.

Hasek J: *The good soldier Svejk and his fortunes in the world war* (Parrott C, translator), Harmondsworth, 1974, Penguin.

Heath SB: *Ways With Words. Language, Life and Work in Communities and Classrooms*, Cambridge, 1983, Cambridge University Press.

Hockenberry J: *Keynote address*, American Occupational Therapy Association (AOTA) Annual Conference ang Expo, North Carolina, April, 2006. Charlotte.

Hocking C: The romance of occupational therapy. In Creek J, Lawson Porter A, editors: *Contemporary Issues in Occupational Therapy*, Chichester, 2007, Wiley, pp 23–40.

Hook A, Kenney C: Evaluating role emerging placements, *Occupational Therapy News* 15:25, 2007.

Iwama M: *The Kawa model; culturally relevant occupational therapy*, Edinburgh, 2006, Churchill Livingstone/Elsevier.

Kapandaze M, Despotashvili M, Skhirtladze N: Political practice in occupational therapy in Georgia. In Pollard N, Sakellariou D,

Kronenberg F, editors: *Political Practice in Occupational Therapy*, Edinburgh, 2008, Elsevier Science, pp 163–169.

Kronenberg F, Pollard N: Overcoming occupational apartheid, a preliminary exploration of the political nature of occupational therapy. In Kronenberg F, Simo Algado S, Pollard N, editors: *Occupational Therapy Without Border: Learning from the Spirit of Survivors*, Edinburgh, 2005a, Elsevier/Churchill Livingstone, pp 58–86.

Kronenberg F, Pollard N: Introduction, a beginning. In Kronenberg F, Simo Algado S, Pollard N, editors: *Occupational Therapy Without Border: Learning from the Spirit of Survivors*, Edinburgh, 2005b, Elsevier/Churchill Livingstone, pp 1–13.

Landry D: *The Muses of Resistance*, Cambridge, 1990, Cambridge University Press.

Lawrence J, Mace J: *Remembering in Groups. Ideas from Reminiscence and Literacy Work*, Colchester, 1992, Oral History Society.

Lefebvre H: *Critique of Everyday Life* (vol 1, Moore J, translator), London, 1991, Verso.

Lefebvre H: *Critique of Everyday Life, Foundations for a Sociology of the Everyday* (Moore J, translator), (vol 2), London, 2002, Verso.

Lefebvre H: *Critique of Everyday Life, From Modernity to Modernism* (Elliot G, translator), (vol 3), London, 2005, Verso.

Lloyd AL: *Folk Song in England*, London, 1969, Panther.

Lloyd M, Carson A, Bleakley C: *Exploring the needs of service users involved in planning and delivering mental health services and education*, Wrexham North Wales, 2007, North East Wales Institute of Higher Education. Online. Available at: www.health.heacademy.ac.uk/projects/miniprojects/mlloyd_finalreport. Accessed November 6, 2008.

McNulty C: The Sleaford MACA Group. In Pollard N, Sakellariou D, Kronenberg F, editors: *Political Practice in Occupational Therapy*, Edinburgh, 2008, Elsevier Science, pp 171–174.

Morley D, Worpole K, editors: *The Republic of Letters*, London, 1982, Comedia.

Not A: Parler 'peuple', du peuple ou au people. In Not A, Radwan J, editors:

Autour d'Henry Poulaille et de la Litterature Proletarienne, Aix-en- Provence, 2003, Publications de l'Universite de Provence, pp 17–24.

O'Rourke R: *Creative Writing, Education Culture and Community*, Leicester, 2005, NIACE.

Orwell G: *Down and Out in Paris and London*, Harmondsworth, 1940, Penguin.

Orwell G: *On the Road to Wigan Pier*, Harmondsworth, 1962, Penguin.

Paterson CF: A short history of occupational therapy in psychiatry. In Creek J, editor: *Occupational therapy in mental health*, Edinburgh, 2002, Churchill Livingstone, pp 3–14.

Peck E, Norman IJ: Working together in adult community mental health services: Exploring inter-professional role relations, *Journal of Mental Health* 8:231–242, 1999.

Peloquin SM: *History Matters. TOG (A Coruna)*, 2007. Online. Available at: http://www.revistatog.com/pdfs/editorial2.pdf. Accessed November 6, 2008.

Petridou D, Pouliopolou M, Kiriakoulis A, et al: Expanding occupational therapy intervention through the theatre and film, *Mental Health OT* 10:99–101, 2005.

Pim L, Russel B: Small steps equal big changes, *Occupational Therapy News* 16:26–27, 2008.

Pollard N: Notes towards an approach for the therapeutic use of creative writing in occupational therapy. In Sampson F, editor: *Creative Writing in Health and Social Care*, London, 2004, Jessica Kingsley, pp 189–206.

Pollard N: Recovering the alliance, *British Journal of Occupational Therapy* 70:459, 2007.

Pollard N: When Adam delf and Eve span: occupational literacy and democracy. In Pollard N, Sakellariou D, Kronenberg F, editors: *Political Practice in Occupational Therapy*, Edinburgh, 2008, Elsevier Science, pp 39–51.

Pollard N, Walsh S: Occupational therapy, gender and mental health: an inclusive perspective? *British Journal of Occupational Therapy* 63:425–431, 2000.

Pollard N, Kronenberg F: Working with people on the margins. In Creek J,

Lougher L, editors: *Occupational Therapy in Mental Health*, ed 4, Oxford, 2008, Elsevier Science, pp 557–577.

Pollard N, Sakellariou D: Facing the challenge: a compass for navigating the heteroglossic context. In Pollard N, Sakellariou D, Kronenberg F, editors: *Political Practice in Occupational Therapy*, Edinburgh, 2008, Elsevier Science, pp 237–244.

Pollard N, Alsop A, Kronenberg F: Reconceptualising occupational therapy, *British Journal of Occupational Therapy* 68:524–526, 2005a.

Pollard N, Smart P: Talk Voices, Write Hands: Voices talk and hands write. In Kronenberg F, Simo Algado S, Pollard N, editors: *Occupational Therapy Without Border: Learning from the Spirit of Survivors*, Edinburgh, 2005b, Elsevier/Churchill Livingstone, pp 287–301.

Pollard N, Talk Voices, Write Hands: Voices Talk, Hands Write. In Crepeau E, Cohn E, Boyt Schell B, editors: *Willard and Spackman's Occupational Therapy*, ed 11. Philadelphia, 2008, Lippincott Williams & Wilkins, pp 139–145.

Pratt ML: The art of the contact zone, *Profession* 91:33–40, 1991.

Ragon M: *Histoire de la Litterature Proletariene de Langue Francaise*, Paris, 1986, Albin Michel.

Ross E: *Tales of the Rails*, Bristol, 1984, Bristol Broadsides.

Sakellariou D, Pollard N: Three sites of conflict and co-operation: class, gender and sexuality. In Pollard N, Sakellariou D, Kronenberg F, editors: *Political Practice in Occupational Therapy*, Edinburgh, 2008, Elsevier Science, pp 69–89.

Schwammle D: Reflections on . . . are you listening? The oral tradition of occupational therapy, *Can J Occup Ther* 63:62–66, 1996.

Service Users Advisory Group: *Nothing About Us Without Us. Department of Health*, London, 2001. Online. Available at: http://www.publications.doh.gov.uk/learningdisabilities/access/nothingabout/index.htm. Accessed November 6, 2008.

Smart P: A beginner writer is not a beginner thinker. In Kronenberg F,

Simo Algado S, Pollard N, editors: *Occupational Therapy Without Borders: Learning from the Spirit of Survivors*, Edinburgh, 2005, Elsevier/Churchill Livingstone, pp 46–53.

Tait V: *Poor Workers' Unions: Rebuilding Labor from Below*, Cambridge MA, 2005, South End Press.

Thew M, Hargreaves A, Cronin-Davis J: An evaluation of a role-emerging practice placement model for a full cohort of occupational therapy students, *British Journal of Occupational Therapy* 71:348–353, 2008.

Vincent D: *Bread. Knowledge and Freedom, a Study of Nineteenth-Century Working Class Autobiography*, London, 1981, Europa Publications.

Wheeler H: Breaking into new areas of practice, *Occupational Therapy News* 16:28, 2008.

Wilcock AA: Doing, being, becoming, *Can J Occup Ther* 65:248–257, 1998.

Wilcock AA: *Occupation Through Health, a Journey from Prescription to Self Health*, (vol 2), London, 2002, British Association and College of Occupational Therapists.

Wilcock AA: *An Occupational Perspective Of Health*, Thorofare NJ, 2006, Slack.

Wilcock A, Townsend E: Occupational terminology interactive dialogue. Occupational justice, *Journal of Occupational Science* 7:84–86, 2000.

Williams A: *Life in a Railway Factory*, Gloucester, [1915] 1984, Alan Sutton.

Woodin T: Building culture from the bottom up: the educational origins of the Federation of Worker Writers and Community Publishers, *History of Education* 34:345–363, 2005a.

Woodin T: More writing than welding: learning in worker writer groups, *History of Education* 34:561–578, 2005b.

Woodin T: Muddying the Waters: changes in class and identity in a working class cultural organization, *Sociology* 39:1001–1018, 2005c.

Worpole K: *Reading by Numbers: Contemporary Publishing and Popular Fiction*, London, 1984, Comedia.

Section 2

Practices without borders

Rebuilding lives and societies through occupation in post-conflict areas and highly marginalized settings

16

Rachel Thibeault

OVERVIEW

This chapter sums up lessons learned while working collaboratively with people living with leprosy or HIV/AIDS and survivors of war, torture, and landmines. It offers an overview of the main occupation-based modalities used with these populations through the course of their recovery, from trauma to full social reinsertion. Not an exhaustive list of possibilities, this chapter is meant as an illustration of a process. At the conceptual level, the content is anchored in community-based rehabilitation (CBR) and community development tenets and in the Paris Principles, the definitive document on the treatment of children associated with armed forces or armed groups. At the grassroots level, it reports participatory action research findings from Burkina Faso, Ethiopia, Laos, Lebanon, Mali, Nicaragua, Sierra Leone, and Zambia, gathered between 1993 and 2008, the result of community decision making informed by the principles of human rights, social inclusion, sustainable livelihoods, service integration, and the rebuilding of civil society.

FREETOWN, SIERRA LEONE 2000

The nearly severed hand, still attached by a single, tenuous tendon, dangles from the wrist and dances around the girl's waist. The crudely cauterized wound is charred and flakes of burnt skin flutter on the bloodied stump. Beads of sweat glisten on her face, around unfocused eyes. She arrived at the camp earlier this evening. From Kenema. When asked, she only vaguely recalls the gang rape and the botched amputation, as if it all happened to someone else or many years ago. She can't remember when or where it took place, or who was there. A common occurrence in Sierra Leone's civil war, where memory can be a liability.

The group leader, a strongly built local woman, reaches for scissors and with a snapping sound cuts the remaining tendon. Holding the dead hand with infinite care, she puts her arm around the girl's shoulders and says softly: 'Tomorrow morning, with your remaining hand, you will go fetch water for the other girls in your barrack.'

For a Western-trained occupational therapist, these words resonated with disbelief. How can anyone ask anything of a young woman so wounded? Couldn't the girl be left alone to find some peace after the horror she had just experienced? The group leader saw my unease and took me aside. 'Do not judge my decision by your own cultural standards. Here, in Sierra Leone, there is one path to healing: finding your place within your community. And this means contributing as soon as possible to collective wellbeing.'

Months later, while discussing significant moments in their recovery, the girl victims of war all agreed that rebuilding their individual identity through securing a meaningful role in their community had been the most pivotal step. The performing of useful and valued tasks had steered them away from drug abuse and suicide. It had saved them from despair and provided them with renewed dignity.

This event led to an irony: an occupational therapist learning essential lessons about occupation from caregivers without any formal training who had spontaneously turned to it for the treatment and reintegration of a highly marginalized group. Over the years, similar learning has taken place with a wide variety of populations, from people living with leprosy or HIV/AIDS to survivors of war, torture, and landmines. Each time, new insights were gained and new possibilities arose from generously shared local knowledge and wisdom.

© 2011, Elsevier Ltd.
DOI: 10.1016/B978-0-7020-3103-8.00025-0

This chapter attempts to sum up lessons learned and offers an overview of the main occupation-based modalities used with these populations through the course of their recovery, from trauma to full social reinsertion. It is not meant as an exhaustive list of possibilities but rather as an illustration of a process. At the conceptual level, the content is anchored in community-based rehabilitation (CBR) and community development tenets and in the Paris Principles, the definitive document on the treatment of children associated with armed forces or armed groups (UN 2007). At the grassroots level, it reports participatory action research findings from Burkina Faso, Ethiopia, Laos, Lebanon, Mali, Nicaragua, Sierra Leone, and Zambia gathered between 1993 and 2008, the result of community decision making informed by the principles of human rights, social inclusion, sustainable livelihoods, service integration, and the rebuilding of civil society.

An occupational continuum, from individual trauma to collective rebuilding of civil society

Occupation-based modalities constitute the golden thread for cross-cultural intervention. Transcending language, they can span the whole continuum, from trauma to social reintegration and the eventual rebuilding of civil society, while creating a space where meaning and healing can be given tangible shape.

The taxonomy used below to classify occupations may surprise as it does not stem from any recognized model. To remain congruent with a phenomenological approach, the selected terms have been coined by the participants themselves and express, in their words, the features they considered key. For them, occupation referred to employment and was mostly used in an income-generating context. Semantically, they overwhelmingly preferred words such as activity, task, duty, routine, work, responsibility, behavior, and action to render the idea of engaging with their inner or outer world. Their choices prevailed.

Also, the observations cut across a realm of different groups with different needs. An elderly woman living with leprosy will not face the same obstacles as a young landmine survivor, and the reader should keep in mind that not all vulnerable communities will undertake an identical process. To a large degree,

the level of stigma seemed to determine the breadth of occupational needs, the most stigmatized requiring the most support. A ranking of sorts arose over time, based not on formal research, but derived from anonymous nominal group exercises and semi-structured interviews with users of community healthcare services in Zambia, Ethiopia, Sierra Leone, and Nicaragua. Clearly, people living with leprosy appeared more ostracized than people living with mental illness, who in turn were more marginalized than people living with AIDS or child soldiers. Torture victims and landmine survivors, on the other hand, faced less prejudice. Because of their many differences, not all groups require the same range of interventions described in this chapter. A case in point: people with leprosy often strongly oppose social integration, deeming it will only bring them greater rejection and suffering. Such a community requires intensive intervention in terms of income generation but minimal involvement for external social networking. They choose to remain isolated, removed from society, a decision that is anathema to most rehabilitation workers and goes so much against the grain that it challenges our adherence to the principle of client-centeredness.

Some occupations associated with the acute treatment phase

Physical trauma occurring in a conflict area

Following physical trauma usually caused by bullets, landmines or machetes, immediate medical needs must be attended. Emergency care (cauterizing, anesthetizing, disinfecting, bandaging, etc.) obviously supersede any other intervention. Only after stabilization is achieved will we occupational therapists take into consideration issues of stump preparation, orthotics, adaptations, and other occupational therapy modalities. These are not always carried in a smooth, logical sequence and must rely on the resources at hand. Not infrequently, the occupational therapist will have to settle for temporary adaptations that will quickly become obsolete once prosthetics become available. Typical of a conflict area are the acute shortage of supplies, difficult delivery to the work site, poor craftsmanship, and arduous follow-up. Adaptability, both on the part of the client and the therapist, is key.

Psychological trauma occurring in a conflict area

Experience has shown that the treatment of psychological trauma need not be postponed until physical healing has begun. In fact, simultaneous psychological and physical care seems to yield the best overall outcomes. Without treatment of post-traumatic shock, learning abilities are seriously impaired, a phenomenon that impedes recovery. If landmine survivors remain too traumatized to process what is said and cannot grasp their own treatment plan, this lack of understanding can translate into fear and disengagement. Since in its immediate, acute phase, post-traumatic shock disorder (PTSD) presents with marked psychomotor changes, hypervigilance, disorganization, and dissociative elements (Kay et al 2000), survivors often react with fright or avoidance. In some cases, hallucinations and paranoia will also be part of the clinical profile and extra care must be taken to create a safe therapeutic space. From an occupational therapy perspective, in the contexts depicted above, six occupational categories have been shown to foster centering, meaning, connectedness, and healing.

1. *Caring duties*: In many non-Western cultures, the collective identity outshines the individual one and contributing to one's community is a sine qua non condition for healing and recovery. In the Sierra Leone conflict and post-conflict eras, survivors of rape and amputation were quickly asked to put their residual abilities in the service of their new-found community. Caring for the elderly and the orphans appeared the preferred choices of those survivors whose hypervigilance had receded and whose social skills had re-emerged fairly intact. For those still in the throes of acute PTSD, more solitary but still meaningful occupations like fetching wood or water, or doing the laundry, brought some sense of peace and usefulness.

2. *Social-status chores*: With some subgroups among war survivors, the issue of dignity poses itself acutely. For example, for those child soldiers who have killed and tortured their relatives, regaining self-respect might seem utopian. To rebuild a dignified identity, matching the severity of committed atrocities with tasks of high social value has proved effective. Caring for the blind elderly carries with it a sense of responsibility, maturity and trust that few other occupations have. When, under careful supervision, the children who have perpetrated the worst crimes are trusted with important duties, their self-perception radically shifts, along with that of others. Their occupational status grants them a second chance to assert themselves in a post-conflict world. These children are often resistant to any occupation associated with play: having lived as soldiers for years, they see such activities as demeaning. They have trained as leaders and often find their new identities in peaceful leadership roles.

3. *Trust-inducing, modeling activities*: In the atmosphere of suspiciousness surrounding any large-scale conflict, trust becomes both a rare commodity and a necessary therapeutic goal. For war survivors, finding oneself in simple social situations like going to the market, attending church, or watching a local soccer game may represent an overwhelming challenge. Several abductions, rapes, and mutilations have taken place in those seemingly harmless contexts and the memories are still vivid. Yet, normal social life must resume. Mentors, carefully selected survivors who have completed the rehabilitation process and can offer a strong, reassuring presence, thus lead newcomers in the re-learning of basic social skills. Together, they set up small booths at the market to sell ground nuts, eggs, or vegetables. Or they go as a safe group to attend church or watch the game. Over time, desensitization occurs and normal patterns of interactions resurface. The programs rest on no clear therapeutic talking sessions, but rather on therapeutic collective interventions woven in the occupational fabric of daily life. Conversations about trauma do take place on the way to the market or at the river, but in a non-stigmatizing environment and with a survivor who can guide without contempt while providing a role model.

4. *Grounding routines*: When the ghosts of PTSD reappear, war survivors express a need for rhythmic, soothing occupations that bring them back to their immediate physical reality in a gentle yet inescapable way. Grinding maize with traditional tools, running, praying, singing all meet that purpose. In a process that could be likened to meditation (Ricard 2008), regular daily practice seems to lead to greater, deeper wellbeing. Spiritual aspects are addressed and survivors are offered the physical means (transportation, books, tapes, visits from religious figures, etc.) to connect more readily with their sources of spiritual solace.

5. *Tasks for belonging*: Fitting back into society and feeling genuinely part of it constitutes the most difficult step for most war survivors and other vulnerable groups. Stigma remains hauntingly present and the sense of connectedness at the core of all mental health becomes elusive. To recreate meaningful webs, survivors often favor collective occupations that can be practiced with minimal initial interaction. Sifting grain with other women at the hammer mill, weaving cotton side by side, fixing the nets when the boats come to shore: these occupations require some contact but little speech. They allow survivors to grow familiar with their environment and control their own reintegration process, gauging when it is comfortable for them to speak or not. A ground rule is established from the start: the meeting place is to be a safe, sacred space, where no pressure is applied and where respect prevails.

6. *Prevocational skills*: When the fear of socializing has been conquered and community ties are being restored, the desire for financial autonomy usually takes hold. Survivors reach a point where they wish to explore their vocational potential. Interviews are carried around each survivor's history, tastes, abilities, values, and dreams. Occupations are then found to expose survivors to situations similar to what has been identified in the interview. If there is a good fit, prevocational training starts, a series of sequential occupations leading to the desired profile.

Some occupations associated with the rehabilitation treatment phase

Once the acuteness of trauma has subsided through the effect of time and the use of appropriate occupations, efforts are geared towards greater integration, beyond the immediate environment, and enhanced performance in all spheres.

7. *Activities of daily living*: Although survivors re-engage early on in their daily routines, schedules at this stage become more demanding and expectations increase. The occupational schedule includes elements from self-care, productivity, and leisure in a way that mimics

more closely the regimen their context and culture will dictate in the long run. That balance is defined collaboratively with the survivor, local mentors acting as cultural brokers, and the program leaders.

8. *Prosthetic*: This includes orthotic fitting, training, and rehabilitation. At this stage, stumps and wounds have healed and the physical rehabilitation process can unfold.

9. *Formal social skills training*: Those survivors who have been heavily traumatized or lacked normal socialization, such as children abducted in early childhood, can elect to take part in formal social skills training. However, research has shown (Bayer et al 2007, Derluyn et al 2004) that living within the community as soon as possible after trauma or demobilization constitutes the best path to recovery. Social skills programs do not match the strong normalizing impact of community inclusiveness. Discrete support systems assisting vulnerable people living within their community appear the best current option.

10. *Schooling*: Especially for women and girls whose access to education is more curtailed, schooling becomes imperative if full social reinsertion is to be pursued. From a social justice perspective, one must pay attention not only to education, but also to the type of education made available to girls. Major gaps exist in opportunities for male and female students within some school systems. In her study of girls' schooling in Sierra Leone, Sharkey (2008) has observed that pedagogical activities such as reading, active learning, and interacting with the teacher are out of bounds for many girls and replaced with systematic debasement. While boys can engage in regular schooling, girls are routinely beaten, flogged, humiliated, or reduced to staring blankly at their desk or the wall. At puberty, some parents also choose to remove their daughters from school because of the prevalence of rape by male teachers. The discrepancy in the treatment of male and female pupils poses the uncomfortable problem of gender-based violence condoned by a key social institution.

11. *Participation in community projects*: Prior to re-entering a full social life, at the close of the formal rehabilitation phase, survivors often still struggle to find their place in their community. Occupational opportunities must then be seized to help shift perceptions of people with

disabilities from burdens to contributing citizens. Brokering a role for survivors in collective occupations such as the organization of a local festival or religious event can make a significant difference in terms of ongoing inclusiveness. Very different from cheap labor, these occupations embody the epitome of citizen participation with an inherent sense of competence and social recognition. Securing even a small part in that larger play helps shape a new, positive identity for vulnerable groups.

Some occupations associated with the social reinsertion phase

In itself, for survivors to acquire skills and competencies is not sufficient to guarantee successful reintegration as it addresses only one half of the equation: their half. The other half, societal attitudes, also needs to be taken into account. In order to render the host settings more accepting of people with disabilities, several steps are required.

12. *Community mobilization through occupation and nonoccupation-based interventions*: CBR has been a source of community mobilization activities from its inception in the early 1980s. Disability-sensitization workshops aimed at entire communities that include simulation games for children and adults, talking circles, and joint leisure activities such as dancing or singing have been successful in decreasing stigma. Leadership training for people with disabilities is also critical in that it produces local advocates who in turn can organize their own group and affirm their presence within the larger social context.

13. *Religious, cultural rituals*: In many cultures, adulthood and kinship are recognized through formal channels. Among those channels are rites of passage that allow for clear public endorsement of individual inclusiveness or exclusiveness. The extent to which people with disabilities are integrated in these traditional events largely determines the level of ulterior community participation. Moreover, in post-conflict areas, other rituals might also modulate the community's response: forgiveness or spiritual cleansing rituals performed by perpetrators can also facilitate their reinsertion.

14. *Microfinance programs*: Financial independence represents one of the most powerful tools for the emancipation of the oppressed. Without it, they are maintained in subservient roles and stripped of their rightful status of adult and citizen. Occupational therapists display a remarkably suitable professional profile to accompany people with disabilities in a microfinance process. Our core values of empowerment, enablement, and social justice blend in well with the underlying principles of microfinance as described by Nobel laureate Mohammad Yunus (Yunus 2003). To a shared philosophy, we add among other assets a holistic perspective, a client-centered approach, skills in activity analysis, counseling, and problem-solving. We focus on needs and abilities, in context, and assist people with disabilities in achieving the difficult balance between the meaningful and the feasible. Without a set agenda, we also recognize those for whom a micro-enterprise is not the answer and seek other, more appropriate solutions (Mersland 2005).

15. *Mentoring*: Long-term success in the reintegration of marginalized groups rests first and foremost on changing societal attitudes relative to difference, disability, and gender equity. The process would thus be incomplete without an initial reflection on power relations within the group itself. Once internal and external power differentials have been identified and acknowledged, strategies can be elaborated to attenuate them and mentors are assigned to the most vulnerable individuals. Mentoring usually goes beyond verbal advice and, at the outset, takes the form of 'doing with' until the vulnerable members can manage on their own with more sporadic support.

Some occupations associated with the rebuilding of civil society

The theme of resource and power redistribution colors most occupations associated with the rebuilding of civil society. These in fact could be labeled 'occupations for a new social order' as they attempt to redress power abuses within a given society. The main issues tackled here are:

16. *Promotion of gender equity*: After a conflict, during which women are often victimized through rape and brutality and pushed into

sudden, forced autonomy, with men away at the front, simply drifting back into the old ways becomes unthinkable. Women want to seize this transition, however sad, to rebuild their world on more equitable grounds. War has awakened them to both their vulnerability and their strength and they are aware of new, fairer avenues. This shift takes roots through social activism, organized political lobbying, and the securing of financial means. Again, microfinance and other forms of income-generating occupations give women the key to a brighter, more peaceable future. In all endeavors involving women, prior to launching new initiatives, a formal analysis of their occupational burden is carried to prevent exploitation and burnout.

17. *Promotion of children's rights*: Inseparable from women's rights are children's rights. The issue is especially pressing for the AIDS orphans estimated to be about 20 million by 2010 (UNAIDS 2008). To protect them, lobbying strategies and legal action are often required to enforce the UN Convention on the rights of children. And while the fight for their basic rights unfolds, these children face harsh occupational realities: as young heads of family, they are expected to provide for their younger siblings and, for lack of other opportunities, often opt for subsistence living, begging, petty theft, and prostitution. Unable to attend school, they find themselves in dead-end occupations that trap them into a downward spiral. As with women, some occupational balance needs to be struck between income- and non income-generating occupations (work versus school and leisure) and attention must be given to the types of occupations suitable for children. In upcoming programs, mentorship and networking will be explored to redistribute the children's responsibilities across a broader base.

18. *Promotion of the rights of visibly vulnerable people*: People living with leprosy, HIV/AIDS, or other stigmatizing conditions undergo the same process women and children do with the added difference that they have to overcome greater social resistance. Debate can be fierce around the topic of disclosing or not one's condition, but activists tend to agree that only through some disclosure can equity be achieved. With this group as well, lobbying and income-generating occupations provide a way out of poverty and

isolation and can be used to overturn stigma. Experience has shown that successful entrepreneurs with disabilities who choose to hire some employees without disabilities exert considerable influence on existing perceptions. From second-class citizens, people with disabilities turn into employers, engines of development in their community. In all cases, one should avoid creating a ghetto of people with disabilities, even a prosperous one. If wealth gets concentrated too conspicuously in the hands of a few vulnerable people, they become a perfect target for widespread resentment and backlash.

19. *The breaking down of social and political barriers*: In post-conflict areas, building bridges between ex-opposing factions is a long-standing objective. Social and emotional scars take years to recede and animosity may remain palpable for generations. *Truth and reconciliation* commissions usually offer part of the answer through dialog and verbal conflict resolution techniques. However, when atrocities have been committed and emotions are still raw, these prove difficult to implement. In Sierra Leone and Nicaragua, occupation has been used as such a bridge between ex-enemies. In the first case, because tension ran too high for dialog, victims and perpetrators were assigned to common 'collective reconstructive occupations' but with significant distance between them and substantial external supervision. At each end of the site where a school or a clinic would be rebuilt, each group focused on its respective tasks. Over time, the distance would lessen and the tasks would become more interactive. Since the rebuilding of communities represented a goal shared by all, the imposed proximity seemed more tolerable and eventually yielded some limited communication. These modest beginnings constituted the first building blocks on which deeper, more meaningful resolution could ultimately occur. In Leon, Nicaragua, the rapprochement between ex-enemies was facilitated through microfinance. For example, loans were granted to fishing teams composed of ex-Contras and ex-Sandinistas. To feed their families, the ex-combatants had to transcend their political differences and learn to work collaboratively with the other side. This project has grown into a myriad of smaller projects that now bring prosperity to a much wider area.

Concluding thoughts

The examples cited above are but a few among many of how occupation can contribute to the rebuilding of lives and societies. They demonstrate that successful intervention in conflict or post-conflict areas or with highly marginalized groups can be tailored on an occupational framework. Occupation travels well across cultures, and so do meaning and social justice: a true *lingua franca*. However, the evidence presented here is still too fragmentary, too anecdotal and further research is sorely needed. But despite its limitations, it highlights nonetheless potential avenues for enquiry and the enablement of vulnerable populations.

Postscript

PONELOYA, NICARAGUA, 2007

It's sunset and, sitting together at an outdoors café, Guillermo and Santiago enjoy a cold beer. A most banal scene, one would think, if it were not for the extraordinary circumstances surrounding it. First, Santiago is an upper-limb double amputee who, with his two hooks, deftly flips the beer caps, passes one bottle to Guillermo and starts sipping from his, sighing with pleasure. During the civil war, Santiago, an ex-Sandinista fighter, was captured and tortured by the Contra army. After days in solitary confinement, he was brought to a clearing where his hands were tied together, and a grenade slipped and detonated between his palms. Both arms were blown off their sockets. But his dexterity, although remarkable, is not what makes the scene so unusual. No, tonight the two men celebrate their village rising from the dead, an accomplishment that seemed utterly impossible five years

ago. They reminisce and joke about all the changes and Guillermo, shaking with laughter, loudly bangs his artificial leg against the loose metal railing. He lost his right leg to a landmine. When he was a Contra.

The small town of Poneloya had always been a resort town for the rich folks from neighboring Leon, but beyond the fancy haciendas, the local fishermen lived in poverty and conflict, trying to cope with the wounds left by the war. Scars were everywhere: in the disabled ex-soldiers, the crumbling healthcare and education systems, the chronic unemployment, and the fights still breaking out between ex-enemies. Poneloya had turned into the social equivalent of a Dr Jekyll and Mr Hyde: it was both a popular tourist attraction and a bleak community in need of healing.

It all started out with a challenge: to offer joint rehabilitation services to the ex-enemies. Individual progress could only be achieved through the sharing of resources and programs, despite the enduring tension. Once function had been restored and income generation became pressing, microfinance schemes were designed that demanded even closer collaboration. Money was lent to teams composed of ex-Contras and ex-Sandinistas, whose financial survival depended on their will to work together. Mistrust gradually gave way to solidarity and, in time, the community founded a fishing cooperative. With the support of biologists, they ensured their practices were sustainable and learned how to protect their environment. The women, included as full-fledged participants, insisted that part of the profit be reinvested into a clinic and a school.

Business flourished and allowed the most visionary members to give shape to their vision: the rehabilitation of the mangrove, an endangered coastal ecosystem vital for the reproduction of land and marine species and for the protection of crops during hurricane season. The fishermen reclaimed a swath of land and reintroduced clams, an indigenous and lucrative species that had vanished through overfishing a generation ago. Their efforts slowly revived the mangrove: birds and fish came back, plants thrived, and a small ecotourism cooperative is about to be launched. The breeze in Poneloya now carries new sounds and scents, including hope.

References

Bayer C, Klasen F, Hubertus A: Association of Trauma and PTSD Symptoms with openness to reconciliation and feelings of revenge among former Ugandan and Congolese child soldiers, *Journal Amer Med Ass* 298(5):555–559, 2009.

Derluyn I, Broekaert E, Schuyten G, De Temmerman E: Post-traumatic stress in former Ugandan child soldiers, *Lancet* 363:861–863, 2004.

Kay J, Tasman A, Lieberman JA: *Psychiatry: Behavioral Science and Clinical Essentials*, Philadelphia, 2000, WB Saunders.

Mersland R: *Microcredit for self-employed disabled persons in developing countries*, 2005, Unpublished Online. Available at:http://www.un.org/children/conflict/_documents/parisprinciples/ParisPrinciples_EN.pdf. Accessed July 6, 2009.

Ricard M: *L'art de la maditation*, 2008, NIL Paris.

Sharkey D: *Education, violence and resilience in war-affected girls in Sierra Leone: An ecological approach*, 2008, Unpublished dissertation Faculty of Education, University of Ottawa, Ottawa, Canada.

UNAIDS: *Executive summary of 2008 Report on the global AIDS epidemic*, 2008. Online. Available at: http://data.unaids.org/pub/GlobalReport/2008/JC1511_GR08_ExecutiveSummary_en.pdf. Accessed July 6, 2009.

United Nations 2007. The Paris Principles. The principles and guidelines on children associated with armed forces or armed groups. http://www.un.org/children/conflict_documents/parisprinciples/ParisPrinciples_EN.pdf.

Yunus M: *Banker to the Poor*, New York, 2003, Public Affairs.

The CETRAM community: building links for social change

Daniela Alburquerque   Pedro Chana   CETRAM Community

Introduction

Chile is located in the extreme south of the Americas. In most Latin American countries inequality is an inevitable consequence of the political and economic climate. On one end of the scale the highest income group, which represents no more than 5% of the population, consumes an extraordinarily high proportion of the region's resources and opportunities, while on the other end, groups with the lowest incomes are unable to satisfy even their most basic needs (Rosembluth 2005).

The economics of the health system reflects the same inequality with a lack of democratic accountability in the distribution of services and resources. In rehabilitation, ENDISC 2004 (first national study on disability in Chile) has identified that of more than 2 million disabled Chileans (12.9% of the population) only 134 000 gain access to rehabilitation, i.e. 6.5% of all disabled persons (Fondo Nacional de la Discapacidad 2005).

In this context nongovernmental organizations (NGOs) (including CETRAM) and groups of disabled persons are created seeking cooperative action to try to obtain benefits not offered by the state, such as the purchase of medicines and access to rehabilitation that is not provided efficiently by any of the existing health systems and to quality of life of its beneficiaries which is the result of the impoverishment implicit in being disabled in Chile.

CETRAM was jointly created in 2001 by health professionals and groups of users (Fundación Distonía and Agrupación de Amigos de Parkinson) (Fundacion Distonia 2008) to develop treatment programs for people with chronic debilitating diseases. The

OVERVIEW

In this chapter we share the social and community experience of CETRAM (Centre for Movement Disorders), a nongovernmental organization in Santiago, Chile, South America, which has addressed the health-disease concept by going beyond the conventional biomedical approach. Chile is a country with extreme inequalities in access to treatment and rehabilitation programs, with vulnerable populations such as adults who are physically disabled by chronic and progressive disease particularly at a disadvantage. In this context, occupational therapy has emerged as a tool for change, by creating awareness of issues in a way that focuses not so much on the disease itself, but on the social conditions that nurture the problem, and – consequently – helping to develop the strategies necessary to produce changes in local practices. CETRAM's practices focus on interdisciplinary work based on social understanding of the problem of health, and interventions directed toward the family and community by the health team, thereby strengthening leaders of disabled persons and generating political and social interest in change. Occupational therapy has been the articulating crux between the contributions of different professionals, users, family and the community, generating a joint understanding of the problem and favoring team work to achieve both individual and collective objectives. We hope that our experience is able to show the impact of occupational therapy on the change of paradigm in understanding health and how it is a key player in the generation of profound social change.

© 2011, Elsevier Ltd.
DOI: 10.1016/B978-0-7020-3103-8.00026-2

main strategy, as agreed by all the stakeholders, adopted a quality of life approach to minimize the effects of the disease. Consequently, the Centro de Trastornos del Movimiento (CETRAM) has became a reflection of the prevailing biomedical approach.

Today, we call our centre 'Comunidad Cetram'. We decided to keep the name CETRAM as a symbol that paradoxically highlights the fact that the disease alone is not the only health problem suffered by people. Underlying each diagnosis is a complex reality produced by the disabling experience.

Comunidad Cetram is a group of actors from different areas, people with functional diversity, relatives, professionals, artists, and an expanding network of social, educational, and health organizations. We believe in a different social health concept, based on the search for wellbeing, not only through the absence of disease, but also through the right of every person to have a good quality of life and to be recognized as a vital part of society. We stand against inequality that entails lack of opportunities, poverty, and discrimination.

Working from this perspective, our interventions aim for an understanding of an individual's health situation in a specific historical and social context which includes the illness. Thus programs to re-establish health involve not only drug therapy or functionalist therapeutic strategies, but also educational, social, analytical, and political elements, right from the very first time a person consults the doctor.

Here we present the way in which we have overcome the reductionist vision of health, which is prevalent in traditional healthcare practices in Chile, and how occupational therapy – with its social and community perspective – has facilitated this change through the use of four intervention methodologies: Joint Care, the Situational Approach, community leaders, and Colectivo Habilitar. These methodologies aim toward social change, 'a movement for the permanent re-creation of collective existence' (Montero 2004) – toward the freedom to be different.

Joint care, encountering collective histories

Those people opposed to small reforms will never be among the ranks of men betting on transcendental changes.

Mahatma Gandhi

Social change, a shared dream that drives the practices of Comunidad Cetram, is a complex process that, in our vision, implies a paradigm change. Kuhn says that paradigm changes are 'immeasurable' since they are not evolutionary processes but scientific revolutions in substance and form, lacking the continuity between the before and after (Pérez 1998).

We call for a global change (Pérez 1998), for a break in paradigms, resulting from understanding reality from a social perspective. That in order to achieve health, we need to recognize that it is the historical, social, political, and economic conditions that produce the health problem in the first place. However, we believe this change should be slow and carefully thought through, because it generates important individual and collective processes, such as the elimination of the supposed 'power' of health professionals or the different 'casts' of professionals, something that has existed for many years and gives individuals a strong sense of security. Thus, we introduce social and health actors to this understanding through the seduction of new ways to collectively construct realities, which helps them recognize that in essence the social paradigm is participatory, as is the construction of reality.

The first stage in Comunidad CETRAM's proposed way to produce changes is Joint Care. Joint Care refers to a collective space constructed by at least two members of the work team. They work with the client and their companions to create a dialog that explores their life history. Through this collective action Joint Care identifies how the existing situation (which may or may not be an illness) impacts the client's wellbeing, by focusing on what the client identifies in their contexts. It takes into account individual and social needs as well as the problems posed by unmet needs. The objective is not to deny the person's subjective experience of illness, but to broaden their perspective and understand the social factors that produce the disability experience given that condition, which we describe positively as a health situation (Vidal 1990).

The Joint Care process has three steps:

1. Interdisciplinary team: Joint Care requires coordinated teamworking based on the principles of interdisciplinary work. At this point it is important to differentiate between the various concepts regarding teamworking. We understand a multidisciplinary team as a group of professionals who contribute their specific knowledge to the understanding of a health

situation, with practice segmented or divided into isolated elements. This type of organization assumes power-based and hierarchichal relations between professionals. The main limitation of this type of approach is the difficulty in integrating knowledge with the understanding of the problem. Traditionally, and in order to segment work, efforts have been made to reduce knowledge to specific aspects. An interdisciplinary team is defined as 'the coming together and cooperation of two or more disciplines, where each one contributes his/her own conceptual schemes, ways of defining problems and research methods' (Inglott 1999). Joint Care is provided by a team that shares knowledge and experiences in a horizontal dialog. In this sense, occupational therapy has been fundamental to the establishment of common criteria to facilitate communication between professionals, such as the prioritization of problems related to quality of life, occupational performance, psychosocial wellbeing and social inclusion, among other goals. Different professionals find tools in their own disciplines to contribute to this process. However, if the reality of the situation is understood based on a social or critical paradigm, teamwork must follow transdisciplinary practice, in which the different actors are all contributing within the same paradigm. It is an alliance whereby 'different theoretical approaches are able to come together harmoniously around certain methodological assumptions through which intervention procedures and techniques are established. These can be developed by any profession or participant (in this case neurologist, physiotherapist, occupational therapist, speech therapist, psychologist, relatives, users and more) that intervenes in the process without contradicting their own viewpoints' (Inglott 1999). At present, CETRAM works through interdisciplinary teams with the expectation of strengthening transdisciplinary experience within the center, which will be subsequently systematically organized and disseminated.

2. Historical narrative: The interdisciplinary team facilitates the sharing of life histories. The tool used is the interview, understood as a conversation with a predetermined purpose and mutual agreement between the interviewer and interviewee. This reciprocal agreement consists in the recognition of verbal and non-verbal cues

that become meaningful depending on the culture, values, and sense attributed to them by the different actors participating in the dialog (Binngham & Moore 1960). The interview aims to reveal the key elements of the problem by taking a socio-historical perspective that values both the person with whom the intervention is being planned and the intervener as part of the same dimension (i.e. intervener–intervened). Such dimensions are being continuously constructed and deconstructed in a dynamic process, in constant movement (Montero 2000). For example, on the one hand, on socially configuring the role of the doctor, the role of the patient is also configured since the latter is the passive recipient of the control exercised by the other. On the other hand, faced with a horizontal dialog, both the intervener and the intervened contribute to the identification of the problem and solution strategies, in a joint and meaningful discourse. In this dialectical relationship, and depending on the situation, the professional may be the person intervened and the 'patient' may become the intervener. Thus, the word 'intervention' is not linked to power structures, but to the context that produces it.

3. Determination of the problem and solution strategies: Understanding of problems is the basis for future intervention. Priorities are determined by the intervener-intervened relationship that has been developed and that jointly identifies how a wellbeing process could be facilitated. This could include one of the vulnerable areas touched on by the intervened, e.g.: 'What bothers me most is when people look at me when I walk'; 'I lost my job because my colleagues don't think I could be useful'; 'My family doesn't understand that I can't move quicker'.

These key problems can be approached in two ways: an analysis of the problems aimed at improvement of the functional performance, reflecting an approach focused only on the individual, physical person; or a strategy that places the intervention closer to the actions collective that would enable social change (Table 17.1).

According to the above, new practices are needed to respond to both ways of approaching the problem. The professional training of all the team members means the team already possesses technical tools for individual intervention. To address the problem

Table 17.1 Determination of the problem and solution strategies. Forms of reasoning.

Difficulties faced	Problem from the individual viewpoint/ actions taken	Problem from the social viewpoint/ actions taken
'What bothers me most is when people look at me when I walk'	Impact of the illness on self-esteem and movement problem/individual intervention, psychology, physiotherapy	A stigma exists because of being 'different'; a sense of discrimination/education in a social context
'I lost my job because my colleagues don't think I can be useful'	Loss of work skills/occupational therapy intervention	Functionalist and productive perspective in the construction of the subject/social perceptions of rights, nonexclusion
'My family doesn't understand that I can't move quicker'	Family is unaware of the effects of the illness/ caregiver education	No consideration of the family in the construction of health-illness/Participatory education about health

from a social perspective, three collective experiences are developed. They are described below as 'practices without borders' and are discussed in order of increasing complexity of action and change produced: the Situational Approach, community leaders, and Colectivo Habilitar. The barriers to overcome are poverty, social deprivation, inequality, and the absence of a collective voice that is recognized in the exercise of their rights.

Situational Approach: interdisciplinary practice in a real context

We all know something. We all ignore something. That is why we always learn.

(Paulo Freire 2009)

The Situational Approach is an exercise that consists of addressing the problem through interventions delivered by the health team at a community level. The subject of the intervention in this case is the community where the problem is being nurtured. The community is understood as a dynamic, historical and culturally constructed and developed social group, in a state of constant transformation, where interrelationships between its members generate a sense of belonging and identity, as well as a capacity to organize the group as a social unit with the potential to develop and use resources for its purposes (Montero 2006).

This Situational Approach aims to strengthen individuals and groups so that they may make transformations to improve their quality of life and access to goods and services within their society.

AN EXAMPLE

Background: A family with conservative and traditional values, consisting of a husband and wife with five adult daughters, where the father (Andrés) has been the breadwinner. Andrés is a man who made great efforts to overcome the poverty and exclusion of his childhood to become a self-employed entrepreneur who could proudly boast that he has provided education for all his daughters. Today, his health situation (Parkinson's disease) prevents him from working and his only source of income is the State disability benefit, which is insufficient for his daily expenses. Andrés' wife and daughters must take charge of the family business and the organization of routine activities, of the finances and responsibilities that Andrés used to handle, thus reducing his participation in family life. They perceive a breakdown in his role as a man and provider.

For Andrés, the problem is his loss of identity both in his community and vis-à-vis the women of his family – as a result of his disability. They have been able to undertake the tasks he did, and although they maintain a relationship of respect and affection with him as father and husband, they feel ashamed in front of their community, and try to isolate Andrés or lie about his disability.

The interdisciplinary team includes three women and a man. Andrés refuses to receive attention from women in general, mentioning his annoyance about the dependency and care he requires. The man in the group is a neurologist. He establishes the link between the patient and the team for planning the intervention and is able to conduct a discourse about Andrés' history and present painful experience.

The rest of the team engages with the women in a joint project that will address management of Andrés' movement, cognitive, and emotional problems. Gender differences are analyzed together with how a balance could be established between their performance as entrepreneurs and Andrés' participation in vocational decision making, recognizing his residual skills as a means of being accepted by others in his environment. Interventions with Andrés' community are again made through the women of the family, who have now acquired knowledge through participatory education and can talk to their peers about gender differences and their roles in life.

In the above example, the roles of the team are determined as a function of the problem in a socio-historical context (Montero 2000). The physician conducts the interview to understand the life history as a result of a link established on the basis of gender. At the same time, physiotherapy and occupational therapy intervene on the basis of the health problem and facilitate a health education process led by the caregivers.

Community work is based on collective work (interdisciplinary and transdisciplinary), seeking to enhance the strengths and actions of the community, towards a better quality of life. Thus, the Situational Approach is the first step to the real context of the state of health of the subject. Continuing in this same line of work are the next stages in the approach: harnessing community leaders and Colectivo Habilitar.

Community leaders: strengthening grassroots

Culture is not the exclusive attribute of the bourgeoisie. The so-called 'ignorant' are cultured men and women who have been denied the right to express themselves and are thus subjected to living in a 'culture of silence' (Freire 2001).

A group of community leaders was formed in response to the need for organized participation on a collective basis. The group collaborates with Comunidad CETRAM through the practice of Joint Care and Situational Approach, and represents the interest of their peers and generates commitment within their community to overcome problems related to the social-health situations they experience (Montero 2006).

Traditionally, ways to generate the participation of subjects have focused on the development of their competencies, training, and employment, functional rehabilitation and recreation, but without appearing to resolve the main problems. The concept of empowerment, an Anglo-Saxon word adopted into the Spanish healthcare terminology, has various origins. For the purposes of this chapter we will use Rappaport's (1984) definition that refers to 'a process of acquiring that capacity to command and control'. Empowerment would have 2 components: 1) Individual capacity to determinate one's own life and 2) The possibility for democratic participation in the life of one's community through social structures. These actions of empowerment reinforce individualism.

Unlike what has just been described, our practice is based on the concept of strengthening, understood as: the 'process through which the members of a community (i.e. as an organized group, rather than an individual process) jointly develop capacities and resources to control their life situation acting in a committed, conscious and critical manner to transform their environment in accordance with their needs and aspirations, and transforming themselves in the process' (Montero 2006).

AN EXAMPLE

Chilean Social Security provides partial reimbursement for expensive medicines, such as botulinum toxin, which is used for the treatment of people with dystonia. Initially, the work of Comunidad CETRAM focused on the empowerment of individuals in regard to their access rights to health, counseling them to request state subsidies from various government institutions. This partial solution lacked continuity and people became dispirited due to the bureaucratic barriers posed by the system. Individuals' anxieties about obtaining their medicines became a sort of social pathology. When community leaders recognized these difficulties, and entered into a dialog with Chile's health authorities, organized through their Fundación Distonía (Fundacion Distonia 2008), they showed that the need for continuous treatment was exercising their fundamental rights, and demanded a state response. The dialog was accompanied by demonstrations in the streets, creating awareness in the community about this situation, through the media and education during the actual demonstration. Finally, the authorities responded by creating a national access programme to botulinum toxin, which is strictly supervised by the community leaders of the Fundación and supported by the professional team at CETRAM. This is an example of strengthening.

Community leaders are representatives of the center in several government and social networks. They meet weekly to generate collective actions. At the beginning, they emerged as promoters of health and education related to the experience of disability. Today, they have expanded their practice to include creation of local self-help groups, represent the community in radio programs and in the media, as well as development of public policies at a local level to facilitate access to social-health programs near people's homes.

We have discussed the practices of CETRAM and the theoretical-practical contribution of occupational therapy during the change process. The last practice without borders represents an action that intends to make every citizen a participant, where the benefit is for all, to the extent that we construct a society that is fairer and more comprehensive: Colectivo Habilitar.

Colectivo Habilitar: 'dreaming about the right to be'

At the beginning the voice became a scream. And the scream became a banner. And the banner became a collective dance. And the dance became a march. And the march became a multitude.

(Ramis 2005)

Colectivo Habilitar is a group comprising students of health professions, primarily occupational therapy, people with functional diversity, relatives, workers, artists, and all those who feel compelled to create a space that evidences the dynamics of exclusion in our society, and that results in many citizens labeled as 'different' simply because they fail to meet an esthetic, functional, or productive assumption (Rueda 2007).

The vision, collectively constructed, states the following:

'Habilitar is a collective, an action and an end in itself. It emerges from the paradox that we are equally different and that such diversity enriches us all.

We intend to generate a space that will enable us to freely express how different we are and minimise experiences of exclusion, in favour of a more just society, with equal rights and opportunities ... promoting scope for discussion about social inclusion, respect for diversity, recognition and social conscience; and raising the voice that summons us by means of art, creativity and non-violence. Habilitar is no longer a utopia, but a space for the construction of justice ... Habilitar will struggle for that freedom to be.'

(Colectivo Habilitar 2008)

The exercise of this collective begins with the evaluation of contextual factors that limit accessibility to less mobile people. Guided by a trainee occupational therapist, who has also been a wheelchair user for more than 10 years, we evaluate accessible routes in key areas of the Chilean capital. The intervention response is not concerned with better mobility training for wheelchairs users, but with the public denunciation of architectural barriers to the state authorities who are responsible for them, according to the legislation regarding accessibility presently in force in Chile.

Over the course of developing their activities, members have stretched the definition of intervention beyond architectural barriers and expanding it to a concern with social exclusion in any of its forms, such as the stigma of mental health, discrimination on the basis of gender or social class, etc. In order to face up to these processes, community work has been put forward through strengthening, Since most possibilities to implement practical and more profound changes are only feasible with the participation of the community, we need to release the forces present in the community. This is an aspect that is not often mentioned in social policies promoted by the state (Rozas 2003).

The collective continues its exercise through education and awareness-raising actions in contexts that could determine exclusion dynamics and those highly frequented by many people, such as educational institutions, streets, cyberspace. The strategies draw on the wisdom and talents of members of the collective. Today, we use art, dance and music as means of expression and denunciation. One example is the experience of November 2008. Colectivo Habilitar took over the streets in downtown Santiago, and by means of gypsy music and circus acts attracted the attention of passers-by, of the press and the radio, to conduct a face-to-face educational process under the motto 'we are all equally different'. This demonstration was about the right of access to the urban public transport system.

The same intervention was made in a traditional health institution and actions are planned in schools, universities and public places. When we refer to political processes of struggle and social change, the needs of social actors are contained within social movements, defined as collective actions with certain stability over time and a given level of organization, geared towards change or conservation of society or of some other sphere of interest. The idea of social movement tends to vary between two theoretical extremes. One is the vision of collective action that responds to specific stresses or contradictions and that is aimed at resolving that specific contradiction; the other is the vision of social movement as a carrier of a sense of history and incarnation and a fundamental agent of social change (Garreton 2001). Colectivo Habilitar focuses on this last assertion. Nonviolent demonstrations are just part of the tasks that this group has undertaken based on a profound belief that even the smallest steps take us further along the path to progress.

Conclusion

We have reviewed a growing process of practices that is laying strong foundations for social change. Beginning with the first encounter, that is, the result of the diagnosis of a person's health situation from a social historical perspective, through Joint Care, an intervention process is generated through community work where the interdisciplinary team conducts the Situational Approach. Community leaders enhance the reach of the practices, making disabled people the most important actors of change. Finally, Habilitar is the last stage in the process that leads to collective strengthening toward a change in values and prejudices about any type of social exclusion, without abandoning the needs of the individual patient, yet moving closer to the desired social change.

Occupational therapy appears as a key facilitator for these practices, its occupational perspective(s) of and approach(es) to promoting experiences of (social) health and wellbeing both with regards to disabled people, and also with the work team, sharing an inclusive and respectful vision of differences, looking at how a persons' problems are situated in the context of their history.

They are small things, they don't end poverty, they don't make us overcome underdevelopment, they don't socialize the media, and they don't expropriate Ali Baba's caves. But maybe they unleash the happiness of doing and translate that into actions. At the end of the day, acting upon reality and changing it, even if a little bit, is the only way to prove that reality can be transformed.

Eduardo Galeano

Acknowledgements

Each step in this history belongs to us all. To the man or woman who approaches CETRAM with the hope of change, and along that path who understands that it is the responsibility of us all. To work colleagues who have no limits in their devotion to this struggle for a better society. To our families that accept our absence in pursuit of a collective dream. To those who suffer, who study and who lead ... to all of them, thank you very much.

References

Binngham W, Moore B: *Cómo Entrevistar*, Madrid, 1960, Ediciones Rialp.

Colectivo Habilitar: 2008, Online. Available at: http://www.habilitar.cl/v2/. Accessed May 17, 2010.

Fondo Nacional de la Discapacidad, editor: *ENDISC-CIF Chile 2004 Primer Estudio Nacional de la Discapacidad en Chile Editorial Fondo*, Santiago de Chile, 2005, Nacional de la Discapacidad.

Freire P, editor: *La Importancia de Leer y el Proceso de Liberación*, Santiago de Chile, 2001, Editorial Siglo XXI, p 14.

Freire P, editor: *Wikipedia, La Enciclopedia Libre*, 2009, Online. Available at: http://es.wikipedia.org/w/index.php?title=Paulo_Freire&oldid=28890565. Accessed May 17, 2010.

Fundaciósn Distonia: 2008, Online. Available at: http://www.distonia.cl/somos.htm. Accessed May 17, 2010.

Garreton M: Cambios sociales, actores y acción colectiva en América latina. In Garreton M, editor: *Editorial División de desarrollo social Naciones Unidas*, Santiago de Chile, 2001, CEPAL.

Granados S, Martínez L, Morales P, et al: Aproximación a la medicina tradicional colombiana. Una mirada al margen de la cultura occidental. Revistas ciencias de la salud, *Universidad de Rosario Bogotá Colombia* 3:98–106, 2005.

Inglott R: La cuestión de la transdisciplinariedad en los equipos de salud mental, *Rev Asoc Esp Neuropsiq* 19:210, 1999.

Montero M: Perspectivas y retos de la psicología de la liberación. In Vazquez Ortega J, editor: *Psicología Social y Liberación en América Latina Editorial Universidad Autónoma Metropolitana*, México, 2000, Iztapalapa Ciudad de.

Montero M: *Cambio Social: Introducción a la Psicología Comunitaria, Desarrollo, Conceptos y Procesos*, Buenos Aires, 2004, Editorial PAIDOS.

Montero M: *Teoría y Práctica de la Psicología Comunitaria la Tensión Entre Comunidad y Sociedad*, Buenos Aires, 2006, Editorial PAIDOS.

Perez C: *Sobre un Concepto Histórico de Ciencia, de la Epistemología Actual a la Dialéctica*, Santiago de Chile, 1998, Editorial LOM.

Ramis A: *Cuando una multitud despierta y avanza Apuntes y Reflexiones sobre el primer foro social Chileno*, Santiago de Chile, 2005, Editorial Aun Creemos en los Sueños.

Rappaport J: Studies in empowerment: Introduction to the issue, *Prev Hum Serv* 3:1, 1984.

Rosembluth M: Políticas sociales y la pobreza moderna. In editor *Magíster en Políticas Sociales y Gestión Local Universidad ARCIS. Políticas sociales de la concertación: una mirada crítica*, Santiago de Chile, 2005, Editorial Arcis.

Rozas G: Política Social y Psicología Comunitaria, *Revista de Psicología* 12:7–9, 2003.

Rueda L: Priorización la perspectiva ocupacional para el abordaje de la Discapacidad en Chile en Estudios de Bioética Social. In *Prioridades es Salud y salud intercultural CIEB, Universidad de Chile, Centro Colaborador en Bioética OMS Primera edición*, In Santiago de Chile, 2007, Editorial Universidad de Chile.

Vidal M: Daño Psicológico y represión política: un modelo de manipulación integral. In *CINTRAS Centro de salud mental y derechos humanos serie monografías N° 6*, Santiago de Chile, 1990, Editorial CINTRAS.

Community publishing: occupational narratives and 'local publics'

Nick Pollard   Stephen Parks

OVERVIEW

Community publishing engages people in developing the means to express and negotiate their own occupational goals, and evaluate outcomes. It can empower people to challenge occupational injustices for themselves. Its outcomes are frequently celebratory narratives of individual and group achievement, enabling people to recognize their own capacities, leading to other social and transformational outcomes both through raising awareness and occupational spin-offs arising from the activities it involves. It has often been used with people whose marginalized situations, arise from their ethnicity, social status, or disabilities (e.g. Hart et al 2008, Lorenzo et al 2002, Ott 2001). This chapter explores how the occupational thread of narrative can be applied to community publishing and gives some practice examples.

Introduction

Occupational therapy, with its concerns in the enabling of people to do, be, become, and belong (Hammell 2004, Wilcock 1999), is very much about the expression of narratives. As professionals we learn to listen to all kinds of stories from the people we work with, to advocate for them and to animate them sufficiently in the interprofessional discourses we engage in to give people the opportunities they want and need for autonomy or for interdependence, rather than dependence, yet frequently these voices and the nuances contained in their experiences are unheard (Hammell 2007, Hammel et al 2007).

When occupational therapy practitioners apply an occupational justice approach to social and occupational needs with specific communities they are concerned with enabling people to identify their needs and ways in which they can work together to resolve issues they experience as a community. The immediacy of these 'local publics' (Long 2007, p. 107) or interaction between individuals, communities, and environmental factors enables them to develop 'emergent narratives' in which people imagine and create new possibilities for themselves (Mattingly 1998, 2000, p. 181). The use of narrative allows free and metaphorical exploration of experience, and lends itself to uncovering nuances that may not be reflected in traditional health and social care environments, the operation of institutional processes or social stigmatization, which operates to silence the voices of those people who are otherwise seen as 'hard to reach' (Dunlap 2007, Goffman 1968, Osgood 2003). In opening the book to people with disabilities or other marginalizing experiences there is a chance that the pages may turn to conflict with dominant cultural taboos over subjects such as sex, behaviors involving risk and disability. Some practitioners who use writing activities with clients have discouraged the expression of these issues instead of working with them (Aubrey 2004, Dowling et al 2006, Lewis 2002, Osgood 2003). Of course, there is the potential for conflict with employing organizations, and legitimate concerns, for example libel, have to be worked through responsibly.

As a phenomenon, community publishing has existed as long as people have had access to print

DOI: 10.1016/B978-0-7020-3103-8.00027-4

and probably throughout that history has been concerned with the dissemination of marginal voices, whether through ballads and broadsides or through the more recent movement which has developed since the 1970s, with groups such as the Federation of Worker Writers and Community Publishers (FWWCP), which represented many such groups between 1976 and 2007, and its re-emergence as the New Fed. This medium has great potential for narrating human occupational diversity, as is clear from just the numerous books concerned with working lives (Bristol Broadsides 1987, 1988, Centerprise 1977, Gatehouse 1997, Hackney WEA & Centerprise 1979, Hart et al 2008). Rooted in human occupation as the very stuff of its content, community publication is a narrative process with many opportunities for occupational spin-off (Rebeiro & Cook 1999) through its embedding in a wide range of supporting activities and enabling people to recognize and celebrate achievements (Griffiths 2007). This is evident from its origins both in the UK as a grassroots medium (Morley & Worpole 1982, Pollard 2004) and the community literacy programs developed in the United States (Goldblatt 2007). One of the key ways in which occupational spin-offs from these practices may be realized is from the concept of the literacy sponsor (Brandt 2001). A literacy sponsor is anyone or any organization that encourages or facilitates other people in developing or enacting their literacy.

In the United Kingdom, where it has been a largely vernacular practice due to its marginal position, developed by people who were justifiably suspicious of institutional appropriation of their aims and have often worked in isolated groups, community publishing has been situated outside both pedagogical and culture norms (Courtman 2000, Morley & Worpole 1982, Pollard 2004, Woodin 2005a,b, 2007). Much of what the movement has produced has been ephemeral, with the groups that made it up changing focus, running out of resources, or people moving on to new emergent narratives. Consequently, like many grassroots activities organized by marginalized groups, it has rarely been written about and objectively described (Tait 2005). Woodin, himself active in the FWWCP for many years, (2005a–c, 2007) describes how the organization's members developed approaches to writing, publishing, and the production of a vernacular literature according to their own needs. While at first the FWWCP had a class-based dimension, it quickly accepted many other groups representing other forms of marginalized experiences – for example 'survivors of mental distress', groups based around ethnic experiences, and adult literacy students.

By the first years of this century, the FWWCP was actively working to bring community publishing experiences to people that might not otherwise have considered the benefits of this kind of activity, an approach which Goldblatt has subsequently called 'knowledge activism' (2007, p. 141). Many of the narratives told in FWWCP publications are about the occupational experiences of ordinary people – a good number of them are autobiographical, describing working lives, domestic detail, and provide a living documentary of social life during the past 70–80 years.

Occupational therapists have often acted as literacy sponsors, engaging clients in writing, developing newsletters and small in-house publications, but with a few exceptions have rarely made explicit use of these practices in literature, despite current emphases in client-centered practice (e.g. DeSouza et al 2005, Griffiths 2007, Schmid 2005a). The profession needs to use its strengths to elicit occupational narratives with the communities it engages, perhaps it still has to reconceptualize creative activities as valuable in their own right, for psychological wellbeing instead of as a psychotherapeutic tool (Reynolds 2005, Thompson & Blair 1998). In mental health, psychoanalytic theory became discredited in favor of cognitive and psychosocial approaches during the 1980s and 1990s, while a culture of positivism has proved a barrier to clinical research on arts activities (Reynolds 2005, Thompson & Blair 1998). As a result, writing groups along with other arts activities were increasingly run by support workers and volunteers, often without reference to other theoretical perspectives (Thompson & Blair 1998). This weakness combines with a lack of diversity in the professional personnel base to present a difficulty in engaging with other cultures (Awaad 2003, Iwama 2006) across social class (Beagan 2007) and gender (Pollard & Walsh 2000, Sakellariou & Pollard 2008), and stands in the way of knowledge activism. However, the necessary theoretical apparatus exists in the profession's links with occupational science and anthropology, its use of narrative expression to elicit occupational history and communicate practices, and the relationship between these aspects of the profession and those of literature in appreciating practice (Detweiler & Peyton 1999, Frank & Zemke 2008, Mattingly 1998, 2000).

How can occupational therapists and literacy sponsors facilitate narratives of doing, being, becoming, and belonging? How can these narratives be celebrated?

Community publishing generally takes the form of the production of materials in print for a specific audience based on geographic location or perhaps a cultural identity. Community publications take a number of genres and writing forms, including poetry anthologies, oral and community histories, novels, short story collections, photographic records, blogs, and social networking websites. They are often autobiographical, combining personal experience and local interest.

Therapists often report that when individuals and communities begin to discuss their experiences the occupational dimension arises because the dialog is located in the processes of doing, being, becoming, and belonging, the expression of which forms narratives (Breines 2005, Schmid 2005b). For many years migrant communities have produced recipe books as a means of asserting their own cultural identity and sharing it with their new neighbors through the explaining of the personal and social significance of foods and associated customs. Recipes are a rich source of occupational narratives.

Many community publications are the products of adult education or the Workers' Educational Association, political or union activity. Others have been edited through a group critical process within organizations such as local publishing cooperatives, which emerged from the counter-cultural organizations of the late 1960s and 1970s (Morley & Worpole 1982, Woodin 2005a). One influence in their development was the application of a Freirean approach to literacy, the use of reflection about ordinary experiences for consciousness raising and what Freire called 'conscientisation' (Freire 1972).

This literature often represents a distinct vernacular and often critical account of human occupation. This connects with the strong narrative elements in occupational therapy's professional discourse (Detweiler & Peyton 1999, Molineux & Rickard 2003, Schwammle 1996) and holistic conceptions of practice determined by the living experience of the client (Mattingly 1994, Pollard et al 2008a). Some occupational therapists have worked with

clients (DeSouza et al 2005, Lorenzo 2004, Lorenzo et al 2002, Pollard 2007, Pollard et al 2005) to produce service user narratives, expressing the political through a living depiction of everyday occupational experience (Pollard 2004, Pollard et al 2005).

Community publishing engages people in developing the means to express and negotiate occupational goals

In a master's study, Pollard (2001) found that people who engaged in community publishing activities valued not only the writing and publishing but the many occupational spin-offs associated with participation in groups. Subsequent work with people with enduring mental health issues and learning disabilities has shown that these benefits arise from engagement in community publishing activities that afford them opportunities to explore new opportunities such as developing performance skills in association with the launch of a publication, or participation in a wider local arts network in their community (McNulty 2008, Pollard et al 2005, 2008a,b, Pollard & Steele 2002, Ryan & Pollard 2002). Writing and publication not only allows people to communicate directly with an audience and raise critical issues about their needs and environments, but also enable people to celebrate their belonging to a community through participation in events and by the creation of local cultural resources such as books or performances. Community publication is not restricted to print, and sound or visual media may be more suited to the needs of some groups and their potential audiences (Schmid 2005b).

Community publications can themselves be useful in articulating the need for a service or in raising or maintaining the profile of a particular group. As a measure of inclusion, community publications have been used for many years to articulate the perspectives of different marginalized groups and tell their stories alongside or counter to an official or more dominant view. They can provide a concrete outcome that can be presented to funding bodies, they can be a local resource for education or a record of local history, particularly as the narratives they contain are often narratives that are not heard elsewhere. The Grimsby group Voices Talk, Hands Write have been included in the discussion of how and where to present their work. They see it as important that other people with learning difficulties have the opportunity to experience the enjoyment and occupational opportunities they have, and recognize that none of this is possible unless they both develop their own group and agree that others can hear about it (Pollard 2007 Pollard et al 2005, 2008b).

Practice examples

DONCASTER DUMFRIES EXCHANGE

A group of enduring mental health clients from Doncaster's Assertive Outreach and Community Rehabilitation services visited Dumfries for a residential course on Scots Literature, funded by the Learning Skills Council (Pollard & Steele 2002, Ryan & Pollard 2002). The weekend was led by Dumfries and Galloway Survivors, people who themselves had had mental health experiences and performed their own work, talked about their writing activities, and brought their skills into the course, for example dramatizing the experience of a medieval reivers' (raiders in the allegiance of feuding Anglo-Scots border families) raid in a ruined castle.

Some participants continued the exchange by attending a residential course in writing with the Dumfries and Galloway group at Northern College, an adult education facility near Doncaster. The group wrote and performed their own poetry to an unknown audience over the course of a couple of days – something none of the service users had done before. A further course in Scots history was organized in Dumfries the following year. Again, the importance of writing up the events for professional publications was demonstrated in that distribution of copies of the articles to health and education managers helped to create a favorable climate in the local public of the healthcare trust, and secure further funding for the facilitation of a second course.

NO RESTRAINTS: AN ANTHOLOGY OF DISABILITY CULTURE

During a period of one year, Gil Ott of Liberty Resources, a disability rights organization in Philadelphia, Pennsylvania, USA, sponsored a collective effort to collect/sponsor writing and artwork being created by the disability community in the city. As Ott wrote, 'It is this active self-identification which transforms a benign social category into a political and cultural force, a community (2001, p. 9).' Meeting monthly, representatives from community writing/art groups, non-profit organizations, and health programs created an anthology which blended personal expressions of identity with materials developed for political campaigns for collective rights. Published by New City Community Press, the book gained wide use in university classrooms as well as disability rights centers. Ott won a 'Mayor's Award' for his work as well.

MUSIC AND CREATIVE ACTIVITIES

The Music And Creative Activities organization, based in Sleaford, United Kingdom, is a self-constituted user-led arts organization staging its own events in the town and producing a local anthology of poetry and art work (McNulty 2008). A day conference with workshops and performances at a local arts centre in 2007 attracted 200 people, practitioners, carers, service users, and arts workers. These events generate numerous occupational activities at every level from making refreshments to organizing performance spaces and publicity. Their significance is that people are able to enjoy participation in them and gain social capital; enjoyment is often a considerable achievement for people with enduring mental health conditions. While outcomes can be simply put: 'I can sing and play guitar', not many people take up instruments in mid-life after a chronic mental illness.

VOICES TALK, HANDS WRITE

A writing and publishing project with people with learning difficulties attending a day service in the center of Grimsby, Yorkshire, United Kingdom, was set up in 2003 (Pollard 2007, Pollard et al 2005, 2008b). A key element of the experience was the participation of people with learning difficulties and other disabilities from Pecket Well College (now Pecket Learning Community, see Chapter 2). This showed the other participants that they, too, could be enabled to take on leading roles, such as acting as 'writing hands' to facilitate others who could not do this themselves, and to think about their own occupational potential. This group became Voices Talk, Hands Write, a self-constituted community publishing group which published an anthology, *Voices Talk, Hands Write* in 2004. This was given a showcase launch at Grimsby Town Hall with the Lady Mayoress and press in attendance. Such events are important in raising the self-esteem of the participants, demonstrating their achievements to the rest of the community in which they live and generating their own means for social capital with their own local public.

Facilitated by several volunteers from a local writing group and support workers from the day centre, the group continued to meet and published a second anthology, *Our Own Work in a Little Book*, in 2006. Voices Talk, Hands Write wants its work to be known to others so that others can benefit from similar opportunities. Sharing its experiences in academic publications gains further recognition for the group and helps to maintain commitments to providing further resources for its sustainability.

THE TRANSATLANTIC FED

An internet exchange was established between students of undergraduate and adult education classes at Syracuse University's Writing and Rhetoric programs in the United States and United Kingdom-based writers from community publishing and writing workshops (Abel et al 2008). Although not an occupational therapy activity, it demonstrates the kind of approach that could be accessed through adult education for people with disabilities. Abel et al (2008) discuss how the discussion of experiences of disability in this and a series of linked encounters resulting from the internet exchange led to the production of an educational manifesto that argued:

1. Education should teach a global humanity (not the humanities) based on an alternative sense of history and where cooperative values and restorative justice are primary
2. Education should take place in a safe environment free from traditional social/economic biases with self-respect for each other as individuals as well as members of different classes, heritages, and sexualities
3. All educators must move from subconsciously teaching students to be a Westernized version of 'them' to teaching the essential equality among all individuals and cultures
4. The conceptual equality taught to students must also be manifested in equal funding and equal access to well-maintained school facilities.
5. To base an educational system on any other values (than these) accepts a fundamental inequity in society and acceptance that now all human potential will be fulfilled.

As a result of the manifesto, additional programs and resources were committed to similar work, including developing a class that would support a long-time disability rights activist completing a memoir of his activism in Syracuse.

WORKING: AN ANTHOLOGY OF WRITING AND PHOTOGRAPHY/ UNSEENAMERICA

Unseenamerica (http://www.myspace.com/unseenamericanys) is sponsored by Bread and Roses/1199C SEIU, a union that represents service workers in the hotel and healthcare industries. The project creates local union photography groups and provides them with cameras to record their working lives. In 2003, *Unseenamerica* partnered with the Writing Program at Syracuse University to add a writing component to the program. During the three-year period in which the project existed, healthcare workers at a local psychiatric hospital were able to create narratives about how writing, when used in terms of patient care, allowed for a broader range of interpretations about patient actions and potential treatments. The results of this project were published in *Working*, a book designed to be used in labor education programs and university writing/labor studies classrooms. In addition, the photography produced from the project was displayed in numerous galleries and local organizations, as well as nationally at the United States Capitol, Washington DC. The *Unseenamerica* as a whole is represented in a book of the same title.

Currently, the Syracuse component of the project has moved to helping hotel workers record how the stresses of their jobs affect their mental health. A publication is expected to follow.

Crossing boundaries/ negotiating practice

As represented in the above examples, community publishing can serve as a means to negotiate the power differential between therapist, the client, and the communities they live in. Each of the above projects works to create a structure where a collective sensibility defines, develops, and executes a particular project. Within such a dynamic, the work of the therapist as primary recorder of a person's experience and primary negotiator of how that experience is deployed for greater individual or collective independence is set within a larger self-defined communal effort. In such a context, the therapist's skills are not excluded but brought into dialog with an emerging self-generated set of goals – goals whose implementation is cast as a set of responsibilities and skills that must be learned by the entire group. For instance, rather than the therapist creating the process by which particular narratives are developed and recorded, the entire group defines the structure and process of how personal narratives are generated. Instead of the therapist managing the creation of meeting spaces, conference schedules, and publication materials, the work is distributed throughout the entire group according to each person's ability to learn/take on such work.

Through such a process, the therapist is able to both witness and participate in the development of a reflective process of defining individual and communal goals. That is, the weekly process of writing and peer critiquing each others work is more than a means to improve literacy skills – although this was certainly an attribute of projects such as Syracuse's *Working* and the FWWCP/Syracuse University 'Transfed' project. Rather, the very process of deciding what language best represents an individual's experience to a larger audience is a means of creating a collective identity – as was the case in projects such as Voices Talk, Hands Write and *No Restraints*. And within this dynamic, the therapist skills in areas such as securing institutional resources or understanding how the 'professional public' will hear such work becomes a valuable, but not dominant, framework through which to organize the work of the writing/publishing group.

Ultimately, then, the very nature of 'community' publications is to embed the development of occupational skills (literacy and organizational) into a larger effort to expand where those skills can be practiced within the larger culture. To make this clear, it might be useful to briefly invoke DeCerteau's (2002) distinction between a tactic and a strategy. DeCerteau argues that a tactic is an intervention that creates a small disruption or alteration in the dominant social structures. An example might be the ways in which patients construct their particular personal narratives to alter how a particular program provides services to them, perhaps because these stories help to engage health workers with the person being treated. A strategy, however, is an attempt to create a new communal space that can demand institutional change at a macro-level – a fundamental change in society. DeCerteau's notions of 'tactics' and 'strategy' correspond with Van Der Eijk's (2001) 'influence' and 'power,' respectively, in the 'means' at the disposal of social actors to develop their interests in conflict or cooperation situations (see also Kronenberg & Pollard 2005, Pollard et al 2008a). By creating a process through which individuals can construct their own publications, stating their self-defined communal goals, community publishing can facilitate the movement from individual tactics to collective strategies – as was the case with the Doncaster Dumfries Exchange, *No Restraints*, and the Transfed projects. The question of how therapeutic practice can act in the service of political rights moves from a marginal to a central aspect of the work.

To return to our earlier discussion of Paulo Freire, a community publishing framework moves the dynamic of therapist/patient beyond a 'banking concept of education' where 'the teacher acts and the students have the illusion of acting through the teacher' or 'the teacher confuses the authority of knowledge with his or her own professional authority, which she or he sets in opposition to the freedom of the students (2002, p. 261)'. Instead, a 'problem-posing' process of learning is put in place where dialog and common exploration help to frame both the individual and communities sense of education and place within the larger world. And while crossing the boundaries that separate professional/non-professionals, accepted knowledge from emergent knowledge, will require everyone involved to reflect on their role in such a process, it is this very process that will lead each toward a process of doing, being, becoming, and belonging to both politically responsive and progressive communities.

Conclusion

Community publishing offers many opportunities for people irrespective of their occupational needs to engage with others through their narratives and other forms of creative expression such as performance. Aside from generating print publications it can provide opportunities to stage community events or participate in community festivals, to make links with other community agencies. It is a tool for increasing self-awareness and self-esteem, reduces the invisibility of disability narratives and provides opportunities for people who may be prevented by their care environments to make direct communication with audiences. It is also a political tool that service users can handle and control for themselves in expressing needs, sharing cultures, and celebrating their own occupational stories within their own local publics; and in so doing share the process of arguing for resources with the professional workers who are working alongside them.

References

Abel B, Clarke M, Parks S: The transatlantic fed: from individual stories of disability to collective action. In Pollard N, Sakellariou D, Kronenberg F, editors: *Political Practice in Occupational Therapy*, Edinburgh, 2008, Elsevier Science, pp 175–182.

Aubrey J: The roots and process of social action, *Groupwork* 14:6–23, 2004.

Awaad T: Culture, cultural competency and occupational therapy: a review of the literature, *British Journal of Occupational Therapy* 66:356–362, 2003.

Beagan BL: Experiences of social class: learning from occupational therapy students, *Can J Occup Ther* 74:125–133, 2007.

Brandt D: *Literacy in American lives*, New York, 2001, Cambridge University Press.

Breines E: *Occupational therapy activities for practice and teaching*, London, 2005, Whurr.

Broadsides Bristol: *Bristol Lives*, Bristol, 1987, Bristol Broadsides.

Broadsides Bristol: *More Bristol Lives*, Bristol, 1988, Bristol Broadsides.

Centerprise Trust: *Working Lives: People's Autobiography of Hackney: 1945–1977*, (vol 2), Hackney, 1977, Centerprise.

Courtman S: *Freirean Liberation, cultural transaction and writing from 'The Working Class and the Spades'*, The Society for Caribbean Studies Annual Conference Papers, 2000 Online. Available at: http://www.scsonline.freeserve.co.uk/carib.htm. Accessed June 26, 2008.

DeCerteau M: *The Practice of Everyday Life*, Berkley LA, 2002, University of California Press.

DeSouza S, Gould A, Rebeiro-Gruhl KL: And then I lost that life: a shared narrative of four young men with schizophrenia, *British Journal of Occupational Therapy* 68:467–473, 2005.

Detweiler J, Peyton C: Defining occupations: a chronotypic study of narrative genres in a health discipline's emergence, *Written Communication* 16:412–468, 1999.

Dowling S, Manthorpe J, Cowley S: *Person-centered Planning in Social Care: A Scoping Review*, York, 2006, Joseph Rowntree Foundation.

Dunlap L: *Undoing the Silence, Six Tools for Social Change Writing*, Oakland, California, 2007, New Village Press.

Frank G, Zemke R: Occupational therapy foundations for political engagement and social transformation. In Pollard N, Sakellariou D, Kronenberg F, editors: *Political Practice in Occupational Therapy*, Edinburgh, 2008, Elsevier Science, pp 111–136.

Freire P: *The Pedagogy of the Oppressed*, Harmondsworth, 1972, Penguin.

Freire P: The banking concept of education. In Bartholemae D, Petrovsky A, editors: *Ways of Reading: An Anthology for Writers*, New York, 2002, St. Martins Press, pp 258–273.

Gatehouse: *Working Lives, The Experiences of Fifteen Workers, from the 40's to the Present Day*, Manchester, 1997, Gatehouse.

Goldblatt E: *Because We Live Here, Sponsoring Literacy Beyond the College Curriculum*, Creskill, NJ, 2007, Hampton Press.

Goffman E: *Stigma: Notes on the Management of Spoiled Identity*, Pelican, 1968, Harmondsworth.

Griffiths S: The experience of creative activity as a treatment medium, *J Ment Health* 17:49–63, 2007.

Hackney Workers Educational Assocation and Centerprise Trust: *Working Lives, vol 1, 1905–1945*, Hackney, 1979, Hackney WEA & Centerprise.

Hammel J, Magasi S, Heinemann A, Whiteneck G, Bogner J, Rodriguez E: What does participation mean? An insider perspective from people with disabilities, *Disabil Rehabil* 1:16, 2007. Online. Available at: http://dx.doi.org/10.1080/09638280701625534. Accessed June 26, 2008.

Hammell KW: Dimensions of meaning in the occupations of daily life, *Can J Occup Ther* 71:296–305, 2004.

Hammell KW: Client-centred practice: ethical obligation or professional obfuscation? *British Journal of Occupational Therapy* 70:264–266, 2007.

Hart G, Mangino ME, Murphy Z, Taliercio AM, editors: *Working, an Anthology of Writing and Photography*, Syracuse, 2008, Syracuse University Press.

Iwama M: *The Kawa Model: Culturally Relevant Occupational Therapy*, Edinburgh, 2006, Churchill Livingstone/Elsevier.

Kronenberg F, Pollard N: Introduction, a beginning. … In Kronenberg F, Simo Algado S, Pollard N, editors: *Occupational Therapy Without Borders: Learning Through the Spirit of Survivors*, Edinburgh, 2005, Elsevier/Churchill Livingstone, pp 1–13.

Lewis JJ: Signs of protest. In: Ott G, editor: *No Restraints, an Anthology of Disability and Culture in Philadelphia*, Philadelphia, 2002, New City Press, pp 47–57.

Long E: *Community Literacy and the Rhetoric of Local Publics*, West Lafayette, Indiana, 2007, Parlor Press/The WAC Clearing House.

Lorenzo T: Equalizing opportunities for occupational engagement: disabled women's stories. In Watson R, Swartz L, editors: *Transformation Through Occupation*, London, 2004, Whurr, pp 85–102.

Lorenzo T, Sanders L, January M, Mdlokolo P: *On the Road of Hope: Stories by Disabled Women in Khayelitsa*, Cape Town, 2002,

Disabled People South Africa, Zanepilo Disability Project, University of Cape Town.

McNulty C: The Sleaford MACA group. In Pollard N, Sakellariou D, Kronenberg F, editors: *Political Practice of Occupational Therapy*, Edinburgh, 2008, Elsevier Science, pp 171–174.

Mattingly C: Occupational therapy as a two body practice: Body as a machine. In Mattingly C, Fleming M, editors: *Clinical Reasoning: Forms of Inquiry in a Therapeutic Practice*, Philadelphia, 1994, FA Davis, pp 37–63.

Mattingly C: *Healing dramas and clinical plots*, Cambridge, 1998, Cambridge University Press.

Mattingly C: Emergent narratives. In Mattingly C, Garro LC, editors: *Narrative and the Cultural Construction of Illness and Healing*, California, 2000, Berkeley, pp 181–211.

Molineux M, Rickard W: Storied approaches to understanding occupation, *Journal of Occupational Science* 10:52–60, 2003.

Morley D, Worpole K, editors: *The Republic of Letters*, London, 1982, Comedia.

Osgood T: *Never Mind the Quality, Feel the Width! Person Centred Planning Implementation and Developmental Disability Services*, Canterbury, 2003, East Kent Community NHS & Social Partnership Care Trust Available at: http://www.paradigm-uk.org/pdf/Articles/nevermindthequality.pdf. Accessed June 26, 2008.

Ott G, editor: *No Restraints: an Anthology of Disability Culture in Philadelphia*, Philadelphia, 2001, New City Community Press.

Pollard N: Community publishing and rehabilitation, *Federation Magazine* 22:12–15, 2001.

Pollard N: Notes towards an approach for the therapeutic use of creative writing in occupational therapy. In Sampson F, editor: *Creative Writing in Health and Social Care*, London, 2004, Jessica Kingsley, pp 189–206.

Pollard N: Voices Talk, Hands Write: sustaining community publishing with people with learning difficulties, *Groupwork* 17:51–74, 2007.

Pollard N, Walsh S: Occupational therapy, gender and mental health: an inclusive perspective? *British Journal of Occupational Therapy* 63:425–431, 2000.

Pollard N, Steele A: From Doncaster to Dumfries, *OT News* 10:31, 2002.

Pollard N, Smart P: Talk Voices, Write Hands: Voices talk and hands write. In Kronenberg F, Simo Algado S, Pollard N, editors: *Occupational Therapy Without Borders: Learning from the Spirit of Survivors*, Edinburgh, 2005, Elsevier/Churchill Livingstone, pp 287–301.

Pollard N, Sakellariou D, Kronenberg F, editors: *Political Practice Of Occupational Therapy*, Edinburgh, 2008a, Elsevier Science.

Pollard N: Talk Voices, Write Hands: Voices talk, hands write. In Crepeau E, Cohn E, Boyt Schell B, editors: *Willard and Spackman's Occupational Therapy*, ed 11, Philadelphia, 2008b, Lipincott, Williams and Wilkins, pp 139–145.

Rebeiro KL, Cook JV: Opportunity, not prescription: an exploratory study of the experience of occupational engagement, *Can J Occup Ther* 66:176–187, 1999.

Reynolds F: The effects of creativity on physical and psychological well-being: current and new directions for research. In Schmid T, editor: *Promoting Health Through Creativity, for Professionals in Health Arts and Education*, London, 2005, Whurr, pp 112–131.

Ryan H, Pollard N: Poetry on the agenda for Scottish weekend, *Adults Learning* January: 10–11, 2002.

Sakellariou D, Pollard N: Three sites of conflict and co-operation: class, gender and sexuality. In Pollard N, Sakellariou D, Kronenberg F, editors: *Political Practice of Occupational Therapy*, Edinburgh, 2008, Elsevier Science, pp 69–90.

Schmid T: Promoting health through creativity: an introduction. In Schmid T, editor: *Promoting Health Through Creativity, for Professionals in Health Arts and Education*, London, 2005a, Whurr, pp 1–26.

Schmid T: Group projects: experiences and outcomes of creativity. In Schmid T, editor: *Promoting Health Through Creativity, for Professionals in Health Arts and Education*, London, 2005b, Whurr, pp 167–201.

Schwammle D: Are you listening? The oral tradition of occupational therapy, *Can J Occup Ther* 63:62–66, 1996.

Tait V: *Poor workers' unions, rebuilding labor from below*, Cambridge MA, 2005, South End.

Thompson M, Blair SEE: Creative arts in occupational therapy: Ancient history or contemporary practise? *Occup Ther Int* 5:48–64, 1998.

Van der Eijk C: *De Kern Van Politiek*, Amsterdam, 2001, Het Spinhuis.

Wilcock A: Reflections on doing, being and becoming, *Australian Occupational Therapy Journal* 46:1–11, 1999.

Woodin T: Building culture from the bottom up: the educational origins of the Federation of Worker Writers and Community Publishers, *History of Education* 34:345–363, 2005a.

Woodin T: 'More writing than welding': learning in worker writer groups, *History of Education* 34:561–578, 2005b.

Woodin T: Muddying the waters: changes in class and identity in a working class cultural organization, *Sociology* 39:1001–1018, 2005c.

Woodin T: 'Chuck out the teacher': radical pedagogy in the community, *International Journal of Lifelong Education* 26:89–104, 2007.

Enabling play in the context of rapid social change

Elelwani Ramugondo   Althea Barry

OVERVIEW

Intergenerational disconnection brought about by rapid social change often renders adults unable to play a facilitatory role in children's play engagements (Ramugondo 2009). Framing childhood play within the seven rhetorics of play (Sutton-Smith 1997), and providing space for carers to contrast their own childhood experiences against current play possibilities for children seems to strengthen the carers' role of enabling play. This chapter will outline how this process was undertaken with five elderly after-care staff from Grandparents Against Poverty and Aids (GAPA), South Africa. The chapter will demonstrate how in the context of rapidly shifting contextual factors, adults' childhood reminiscence, accompanied by engagement with current realities as well as the interrogation of dominant rhetorics of play, has the potential to revive coherence in a community's childhood play story, which across three generations has become disconnected.

Introduction

Theoretical frameworks on children's play have not yet taken an intergenerational perspective in articulating factors that enable or act as barriers to play. Part of this stems from the fact that the interactional nature of play between adults and their children has never been the focus (Davies 2007). Collective story-making as a process of continuous and shared crafting of unfolding life stories (Kronenberg et al 2009, Shades of Black 2007) has also not been viewed with reference to children's play within families (Ramugondo 2009). When this is acknowledged by

practitioners and used to inform practice, both the adult and the child may benefit in ways that enable meaningful and ongoing participation. Through rapid social change adults often feel alienated from children's play activities (Ramugondo 2009). Technology and the media have introduced new ways of doing and literacies into children's worlds that are not always accessible to adults. This is accompanied by exogenous values which often strip the local context of longstanding traditions. Compounding all these is the seeming lack of opportunity for reflection within families and communities of what this ultimately means to their ongoing collective storymaking (Ramugondo 2009).

Occupations are not usually enactments of conscious intent. Even when individuals or communities at large may be aware that they are not coping as well as they ought to, they may not be able to make the necessary link between their everyday struggles, context, as well as what they do. Dealing with chronic poverty and HIV/AIDS, and the resultant occupational imbalance (Wilcock 2006) of pursuing everyday survival or caring for orphans may also deny individuals time for reflection. Creating reflective spaces for adults to reminisce over their own childhood play seems to be a powerful point from which to start when aiming to address dissonance around children's play activities. As will be portrayed in this chapter, these spaces allow adults to contrast their own childhood activities against current play possibilities, while prompting them to confront the complex nature with which change has occurred. Rapid social change and its consequences in this way becomes an explanation to possible feelings of disorientation or alienation, causes of which may have not been exposed before.

DOI: 10.1016/B978-0-7020-3103-8.00028-6

This kind of practice was piloted with aftercare staff at Grandparents Against Poverty and Aids (GAPA) in Khayelitsha, South Africa. GAPA is situated in peri-urban Khayelitsha, Cape Town, South Africa. GAPA is a project that came about to respond to challenges faced by elderly people in Khayelitsha, whose children died of HIV/AIDS-related illnesses, leaving them to raise the grandchildren. Khayelitsha is a partially informal township on the outskirts of Cape Town, with a population at an estimated 1 000 000 people. Most residents of Khayelitsha are Xhosa-speaking, and have the Eastern Cape as their place of origin, having migrated to Cape Town in search for better employment prospects. Khayelitsha is considered one of the largest townships in South Africa, with one of the highest HIV prevalence rates in South Africa. The majority of the population lives in informal housing, and there are alarming rates of poverty, unemployment, and crime, including sexual violence.

The second author, an occupational therapist working with aftercare staff at GAPA approached the first author as a sounding board on how to develop a programme for the aftercare. Her reflections in her journal during this time indicate that she was challenged in bridging the gap between her own expectations and those of the grandmothers working as aftercare staff.

> Today in the workshop I was concerned that the grandmothers were still asking me for answers of what to do with the children. I want them to develop a programme that empowers them to play with the children even when I am not there.

The second author felt that due to her cultural (white) and educational background and age (young adult), there was a gap between her vision and that of the aftercare staff. She was facing internal conflicts that her 'Western' upbringing and understanding differed from what she assumed to be an African perspective on play. She then invited the first author to work with her and carers in developing a program that the carers could implement themselves. Key to the approach followed by the authors was an appreciation of contextual factors that seemed to explain the carers' apparent 'disconnect' with the aftercare program at GAPA at the time, as well as possible dissonance between the dominant rhetoric of play as progress (Sutton-Smith 1997), and what the carers traditionally valued children's play for.

Rapid social change and its impact on the narrative of childhood play

There was a time when social theorists generally believed in fairly consistent societal practices straddling generations. Gorer, for instance once said, 'societies continue, though their personnel changes' just because it can be assumed that 'the present generation of adults will be replaced in due course by the present generation of children who, as adults, will have habits very similar to their parents' (1950, p. 105–106). It can be assumed that for Gorer, socializing patterns generally remained fairly consistent over time. However, Gorer also recognized that this theory probably did not hold true in societies undergoing radical transformation.

Rapid social change has been defined in many different ways. Some authors have looked at it as it relates to human behavioral patterns, others have considered the time span within which it occurs, and yet others have referred to change within the macro-environment. With regards to human behavioral patterns, many seem to agree that rapid social change is accompanied by an observable alteration in the behavior patterns of the majority of the population in question (Haste 2001, Pridemore 2006, Tan 2002), with modernization or Westernization being central to the new patterns of behavior (Boehnke & Bergs-Winkels 2002, Dasen 2000, Edwards & Whiting 2004, Kyung-Sup 1999). Time is of significance, with rapid social change often seen as occurring in one generation or less (Mathiason 1972), or within a couple of decades (Tan 2002).

South Africa in the 1990s became revered 'as the land of miracles' (Moller 1998, p. 27). Reviled in the past and barred from international participation by many states while under the apartheid regime for 40 years, South Africa was suddenly a shining example of how white minority rule could be abolished without bloodshed – when its entire people for the first time could vote, and a government of national unity was established in 1994. This marked a turning point in South Africa's history, bringing forth elements which have led a number of social scientists to regard the country as going through rapid social change (Finchilescu & Dawes 1998, Glatzer 1998, Moller 1998). South Africa is of specific interest in that its transition in governance did not constitute merely a change in political leadership but a radical shift to 'democracy', and the reinvention of citizenship, national, and cultural identity. With the removal of pass laws that restricted migration into cities, population movements gravitated towards where promises of the 'New South Africa' seemed most attainable, the cities. Migration from rural settings to cities which themselves are in a state of flux due to challenges as well as opportunities characteristic of a new democracy and globalization seems to have set grandmothers at GAPA up for harsh confrontation with rapid social change. They often tell stories of how different their lives were when they lived in the Eastern Cape. A grandmother once told the second author that she no longer looked forward to Christmas as she used to. She reminisced on how white butterflies would herald the coming of the Christmas season in the Eastern Cape, contrasting this with an anticipated sense of danger as crime increases over the festive season in Cape Town.

A collective cultural identity in the context of rapid social change necessitates that parts of past stories within communities are reconstructed in generations that come after. Personal identities and individual narratives are embedded in broader social narratives (McAdams 1993). Memories of multiple past experiences that are maintained are often based on images that are recalled or re-enacted within the social and cultural milieu. As individuals are reminded of stories of themselves from the past, they gain a sense of who they are (Peters 2006), and becoming over time. The stories individuals tend to tell of themselves are also often in relation to that of the group they identify with (Watts 2006), whether it be family, community or nationality. It is in these narratives that individuals gauge and resolve tensions between personal and collective forms of understanding (Mattingly et al 2008).

New insights in sociology point to the undue importance inherently placed on adult guidance with the use of the concept, 'socialization' (Corsaro 2005). This realization has led to the construction of a new concept, 'interpretive reproduction' (p. 4), which emphasizes children's active engagement in social reality. The authors see this move from 'socialization' to 'interpretive reproduction' as a pendulum swing, which unfortunately sacrifices child–adult co-creation of social reality. In the authors' view, the notion of adults in every society being equally powerful, and dominating the course of development for children, is a myth. Some adults are more powerful than others. In rapidly changing societies, and in communities that are not in control of the factors

bringing about the change, adults can in fact, be disempowered. In some instances, children can even be more powerful than adults. They can be the ones with more ready access to technology and Western education, rendering them more knowledgeable than the adult. Hegemonic rhetorics of play, particularly the rhetoric of play as progress, often serve to perpetuate this adult disempowerment as far as children's play is concerned.

Rhetorics of play

In his seminal work, *The Ambiguity of Play*, Brian Sutton-Smith (1997) demonstrated that by giving critical examination to rhetorics that on the surface seem peripheral to the enterprise of play, our understanding of it may be enhanced. By reminding us that those who study play often select one aspect of its many complex elements, for example the body, behavior, thinking, groups or individuals, experience or language, Sutton-Smith effectively unmasked the bias with which many theorists have approached play. Rhetorics developed and maintained thus become means through which play phenomena are viewed through set ideologies and assimilated into pre-existing value systems. Sutton-Smith identified seven rhetorics, namely, progress, imaginary, self, power, identity, fate, and frivolity. Not only did Sutton-Smith expose the manner in which these rhetorics have become embedded within our understanding, values, and explorations of play, and have permeated both scientific and social discourse on play, but revealed how they have also been used by scholars to assert 'their own authority over the kinds of play with which they are concerned' (p. 217). Implying hegemony in scientific discourse is one thing, but Sutton-Smith goes further indicating that at times rhetorics could mask more pervasive cultural systems through which other groups' play forms are denigrated by those who hold power in society. This being said, rhetorics of play are not necessarily bad, nor can they be avoided. They are inherent in any discourse about play.

Through the rhetoric of progress, play, due to adults' primary concern with socialization and maturity, is regarded as subsidiary to the more 'important' process of adaptation or development. The rhetorics of imagination and self as well, have led to the idealization of those forms of play that foreground the individual qualities of the player, with imagination, creativity, and innovation hailed in the former, and freedom in the latter. These two rhetorics, along with the rhetoric of progress, are individualistic in focus, mirroring the departure from a communal approach to living by humans across societies.

While the rhetorics of power, fate and identity appear to have had little impact on how the play of children is viewed and studied, the rhetoric of progress seems to have asserted its hegemony explicitly. Sutton-Smith notes that adults, having bought into play as progress, or an external and relentless pressure on children to develop, they seek to organize children's play, thereby inevitably neglecting, denying, trivializing or suppressing all other ways that children play. The rhetorics that have been particularly overlooked are those of power, and identity, especially in their application to the play of children.

Reminiscing as a starting point to reconnect with the past

The first workshop held with the carers at GAPA was to give them space to reminisce as a collective, over their own childhood play engagements. The process was led by the carers themselves, and was filled with nostalgia and considerable banter. A particular activity that brought about immense laughter was exposing chests to the rainbow, skipping around and singing *Neta mvula* (Come down rain, come down!), while wishing for bigger breasts.

Below are some of the other recollections of play in childhood by the elderly carers:

> We used to take *inkwinhi*, the beetles from the river and put in on our breasts to make the breasts grow, to bite the breasts. Then go to the aloe to heal the bites.

> If it stormed we used to run outside to eat the ice. When it is raining, everyone used to go naked in the rain. The boys and girls together in the rain.

> In hide and seek our cousin used to dodge [evade] us. We would look for him the whole blessed day everywhere. Cousin taught us to make a snake from mud, we would break our leg from running because we thought it was a real one. This [hide-and-seek] is important because you must know how to look for something, use your brain to know the hiding places. You should know that this place is too small for someone to hide, but if you have no reasoning power you will search and search till you being lonely there and others are gone away.

Reclaiming a relevant rhetoric of play: building bridges between past and present

During the second workshop, carers began to contrast their childhood experiences against current play possibilities for children. Framing childhood play within the seven rhetorics of play (Sutton-Smith 1997) introduced a political dimension into the discussions. For example, carers were able to see how the rhetoric of play as progress was imposed on what they traditionally valued play for. How an emphasis on play activities that were directly linked to schooling had led to an undervaluing of activities they grew up with, which professionals often knew very little about.

The rhetorics of play as identity, as well as fate resonated very strongly with what they saw their play engagements to have been about. The rhetoric of play as identity was expressed in traditional Xhosa song and dance, which grandmothers explained was very distinct from any other cultural group in South Africa. Discussions on the rhetoric of fate framed engagements in which 'toying' with fate opens up possibilities for children and touches on issues of hope. Having started out embarrassed by sharing activities such as the one where they exposed breasts to the rainbow with the two authors, grandmothers seemed to find solace in the rhetoric of fate. In addition to exploring 'theoretical explanations' for their childhood activities, they also began to understand how a number of their games fostered development in many ways. In order to facilitate the carers' new understandings of their own childhood engagements into informing their roles as aftercare staff at GAPA, questions that stimulate analysis of their engagements in terms of value, current existence, and possibilities were asked (see Table 19.1).

Impact of the play workshops

The impact that these workshops have had can be seen through daily changes in the way in which carers now approach their roles as aftercare staff. A major shift seems to be the confidence they now have in themselves as carers. Two grandmothers had the following to say about the workshops, 'Children respect us because we know about our childhoods and had a good education'. And, 'It was touching

Table 19.1 Analyses of some of the carers' childhood play forms against current possibilities with children at GAPA aftercare

Play form during the carers' childhoods	Current existence and form	Enabling possibilities
Playing with clay	Yes – buying or making clay	Children can make playdough
Playing in the bush	No (due to urbanization and crime)	Outings to the zoo and Table Mountain; gardening within the GAPA yard
Singing and dancing	Yes – music from television	Aftercare staff to share what they know
Sending wishes (e.g., to the rainbow)	No (the elderly were not able to identify similarities between their own games involving 'toying with fate' and current forms of expression)	Create space for current expression: birthday wishes; 'bet and salute'; contracts e.g., group pledges
Intsomi (folklore)	Yes – incorporated in new school curriculum (pre-primary and grade 1)	Incorporate in GAPA aftercare program

our hearts so we can speak from experience and have motivation.'

The carers have also taken on new roles as teachers to other grandmothers. They are now also involved in monthly workshops to train parenting skills to fellow grandparents left to care for grandchildren in the community. To date they have conducted four workshops, focusing on how to care for a vulnerable child. The feedback they have received from their participants has been encouraging.

The grandmothers have shifted to a space in which they initiate seeking new knowledge to enhance play experiences for children and use their own creativity. Following a bulk donation of toys and educational games to GAPA, grandmothers requested that they be taught how each of the toy or game could be used. Since this request the carers and second author now hold monthly skills-sharing workshops in which each staff member has an opportunity to teach a game or skill to each other. For the first time the second author and the carers are crossing bridges between their different experiences of play. A specific example of this is the sharing that happened around making and using playdough in play. The second author brought her knowledge on making the dough while the carers took authority in determining how it could be used. They related it to their stories of playing with clay during the play workshops, identifying how it could be used to stimulate creativity and knowledge of shapes. As this happened one of the grandmothers suddenly thought of how playdough could be accompanied by *Intsomi* (Xhosa folktales).

Intergenerational play dissonance: an occupational justice issue

The apparent disconnect the grandmothers at GAPA had with the aftercare program before the workshops may constitute occupational alienation (Wilcock 2006). Wilcock defined occupational alienation as 'a sense of isolation, powerlessness, frustration, loss of control, and estrangement from society or self as a result of engagement in occupation that does not satisfy inner needs' (2006, p. 343).

Occupational wellbeing is another concept recently proposed that provides a useful guide to frame the experience of childhood play transformation across generations in relation to health and wellbeing from an occupational perspective. Defined as 'the extent to which the occupations that [people] choose, engage in, and have orchestrated into their occupational lives generate meaning and satisfaction' (Doble & Santha 2008, p. 185), occupational wellbeing highlights people's need for agency in crafting their evolving occupational identities, in a manner that allows for adequate sense-making. Coherence in particular – one of the aspects of occupational wellbeing alongside accomplishment, affirmation, agency, companionship, pleasure, and renewal – implies that as people's occupational identities evolve with time, their occupational experiences should 'generate evidence that confirms who they are and want to become' (p. 187). Doble & Santha (2008) also suggest that individuals attain a sense of coherence when their occupations 'provide them with connections between their pasts, presents, and futures' (p. 187). Continuing childhood play narratives across generations may serve as a vehicle for collective story-making (Ramugondo 2009). This in turn, offers adults in particular, opportunities to straddle their pasts, presents, and futures. Their occupational wellbeing may also depend on the extent to which experiences in the immediate context generate evidence that confirms who the community as a collective is, and want to become.

Given that social institutions play an important role in the devaluing of local knowledge and traditions, an occupational justice approach (Wilcock & Townsend 2000) in occupational therapy practice is required, as part of the redress. Wilcock and Townsend highlight respect for difference, especially in relation to the meanings derived from occupational engagement, as a key element to ensuring occupational justice. This is particularly relevant for occupational therapy in Africa, where constructs that inform practice are often conceptualized elsewhere. With particular focus on children's play, practitioners need to engage with what education, the media and technology brings into children's worlds.

References

Boehnke K, Bergs-Winkels D: Juvenile delinquency under conditions of rapid social change, *Sociological Forum* 17:57–79, 2002.

Cosaro WA: *The Sociology of Childhood (2nd ed)*, Thousand Oaks, 2005, Pine Forge Press.

Dasen PR: Rapid social change and the turmoil of adolescence: A cross-cultural perspective, *International Journal of Group Tensions* 29:17–49, 2000.

Davies B: *Adult family members' perspectives on the play of a young disabled child within the family*, Unpublished master's dissertation, Cape Town, 2007, University of Cape Town.

Doble SE, Santha CJ: Occupational wellbeing: Rethinking occupational therapy outcomes, *Can J Occup Ther* 75:184–190, 2008.

Edwards CP, Whiting BB, editors: *Ngecha: A Kenyan Village in a Time of Rapid Social Change*, Lincoln, Nebraska and London, 2004, University of Nebraska Press.

Finchilescu G, Dawes A: Catapulted into democracy: South African adolescents' sociopolitical orientations following rapid social change, *Journal of Social Issues* 54:563–583, 1998.

Glatzer W: Introduction: Quality of life in countries undergoing rapid social change, *Social Indicators Research* 43:1–2, 1998.

Gorer G: The concept of national character. In Crammer JL, editor: *Science News*, Middlesex, 1950, Penguin, pp 105–122.

Haste H: The new citizenship of youth in rapidly changing nations, *Hum Dev* 44:375–381, 2001.

Kronenberg F, Ramugondo E, Smile L: *Addressing occupational apartheid through ubuntourism in Cape Town*, Paper presented at the 69th Annual Meeting, Society for Applied Anthropology, Santa Fe, New Mexico, 2009, 17–21 March.

Kyung-Sup C: Compressed modernity and its discontents: South Korean society in transition, *Economy and Society* 28:30–55, 1999.

McAdams DP: *Stories We Live By: Personal Myths and the Making of the Self*, New York, 1993, William Morrow.

Mathiason JR: Patterns of powerlessness among urban poor: Toward the use of mass communications for rapid social change, *Studies in Comparative International Development* 7:64–84, 1972.

Mattingly C, Lutkehaus NC, Throop CJ: Bruner's search for meaning: A conversation between psychology and anthropology, *Ethos* 36:1–28, 2008.

Moller V: Quality of life in South Africa: Post-apartheid trends, *Social Indicators Research* 43:27–68, 1998.

Pridemore WA: *Criminological Transition? Change and Stability in Homicide Characteristics During Rapid Social Change*, Washington DC, 2006, American Sociological Association.

Ramugondo EL: *Intergenerational shifts and continuities in children's play within a rural Venda family in the 20th and 21st centuries*, Unpublished PhD dissertation, Cape Town, 2009, University of Cape Town.

Shades of Black: *Shades of Black Works*, 2007, Online. Available at: http://www.shades-of-black.co.za/mission.php. Accessed November 5, 2009.

Sutton-Smith B: *The Ambiguity of Play*, Cambridge, MA, 1997, Harvard University Press.

Tan JE: Living arrangements of never-married Thai women in a time of rapid social change, *Journal of Social Issues in Southeast Asia* 17:24–51, 2002.

Peters KE: Spiritual transformation and healing in light of an evolutionary theology. In Koss-Chioino JD, Hefner P, editors: *Spiritual Transformation and Healing: Anthropological, Theological, Neuroscientific and Clinical Perspectives*, Lanham, 2006, AltaMira Press, pp 134–151.

Watts F: Personal transformation: Perspectives from psychology and Christianity. In Koss-Chioino JD, Hefner P, editors: *Spiritual Transformation and Healing: Anthropological, Theological, Neuroscientific and Clinical Perspectives*, Lanham, 2006, AltaMira Press, pp 152–167.

Wilcock AA: *An Occupational Perspective of Health*, Thorofare, NJ, 2006, Slack.

Wilcock AA, Townsend E: Occupational terminology: interactive dialogue, *Journal of Occupational Science* 7:84–86, 2000.

Natural disasters: challenging occupational therapists

Nancy A. Rushford   Kerry A. Thomas

OVERVIEW

An increase in the scale, frequency, and intensity of disasters affecting communities and environments worldwide is fueling a growing interest and need among occupational therapists to contribute to disaster response, recovery, and preparedness (DRRP). However, little is known both within the profession and the international community about the potential contribution of the profession to DRRP and, in particular, how an occupational perspective can facilitate the recovery of individuals and communities. The challenge for the profession is to develop the capacity of occupational therapists to engage effectively and meaningfully in DRRP, locally and worldwide, in policy and practice domains and across a range of disasters. A first step toward this goal is to begin to consider the impact of disaster from an occupational perspective and draw implications for practice based on the experiences of survivors and practitioners in the field. This chapter aims to illuminate an occupational perspective on disaster and development in relation to natural disasters and inspire practitioners to consider the role of 'occupation' and occupational therapy in this emerging field of practice. It incorporates a composite case analysis to reveal survivor and practitioner experiences and portray key issues. The chapter is divided into two parts: a general overview of disaster response, recovery, and preparedness; and an exploration of the relevance of occupation and occupational therapy to the field.

Often it is the people with the least who are at risk of losing the most.

World Vision Australia

Introduction to disaster response, recovery, and preparedness

JULIMNA'S STORY: IN THE BEGINNING

Holding her young grandson, Julimna wept quietly as she told how the tsunami had swept away her son and two other grandchildren, her home, and all her possessions. At 68 years, a widow with few financial resources and struggling with cataracts and arthritis, she is numbly distraught, 'What am I to do? I have nowhere to go, I don't know where my daughter-in-law is; there is no one to look after us ... My son was a fisherman ... he got us food and some income ... how are we going to live now? ... What is going to happen to my grandson? He needs milk, rice ... I tried to get some rations but got pushed over in the crush ... Someone gave us a few things – a bucket containing a plastic sheet, a candle, and some matches, a mosquito coil, a pot, and a sarong – but even if I got some rice, trying to make a cooking fire is impossible ... '

A natural disaster is not just an earthquake or cyclone; nor is it a wildfire, or drought. It is the experience of devastation resulting from such an event; it is the threat to ongoing survival; it is Julimna's despair following the tsunami. In this sense disaster is both a natural phenomenon and a human one. Illustrated simply, a wildfire may cause a population to flee their homes, but it does not account for how the person in a wheelchair was left behind; it does not account for why some survivors manage the trauma better than others; it does not account for *differences in vulnerability* to the effects of the event.

DOI: 10.1016/B978-0-7020-3103-8.00029-8

Human devastation and economic losses caused by natural disasters has already marked the twenty-first century. In 2006 alone, 426 disasters occurred in 108 countries and affected 143 million people (United Nations Development Program (UNDP) 2009). The majority of those affected are among the world's poorest, many of whom live in hazard-prone areas in less economically developed countries (Yodmani 2009). High population growth and density, migration and unplanned urbanization, environmental degradation, and global climate change (United Nations Environment Program (UNEP) 2009) are contributing to an increase in vulnerability to natural disaster. Consequently, greater levels of material damage, injury, and loss of life are predicted (International Strategy for Disaster Reduction (ISDR) 2004, Office for the Coordination of Humanitarian Affairs (OCHA) 2006). This is compelling for occupational therapists from around the globe to consider the role of occupational therapy in disaster response and recovery and how to respond to the challenge. 'We're desperate to help ... but are not sure how best we can' was a common heartfelt plea from occupational therapists following the 2004 Indian Ocean tsunami.

The ISDR (2009) defines natural disaster as:

A serious disruption of the functioning of a community or a society causing widespread human, material, economic or environmental losses which exceed the ability of the affected community or society to cope using its own resources ... Disaster results from the combination of hazards, conditions of vulnerability and insufficient capacity or measures to reduce the potential negative consequences of a hazardous event.

Natural *hazards* that can cause disaster may be geophysical (earthquakes, tsunamis, and volcanic eruptions), hydro-meteorological (e.g. floods, droughts, landslides and avalanches, heat waves, and wild fires) and biologic (epidemics) (OCHA 2006). Human *vulnerability* to hazards results from a complex interplay of social, political, and economic factors in a given locale (ISDR 2009, Yodmani 2009). Poverty, in particular, increases vulnerability (Yodmani 2009) by limiting people's access to safe and healthy environments (Disease Control Priorities Project 2009) and everyday occupations that sustain life, give it meaning, and enhance coping capacity. Poor people are more likely to occupy hazardous areas such as flood plains, river banks, and steep slopes, and live within communities that have inadequate infrastructure and housing. They often lack livelihood security, have few or no assets, and may not have access to social security, education, or health care (Satterthwaite et al 2009). People with disabilities and the elderly, like Julimna, are often among the poorest of the poor and are even more vulnerable and at risk (Haar 2005, International Disability and Development Consortium (IDDC) 2009). Other factors that influence a population's vulnerability to natural hazards include conflict, environmental degradation, unplanned and unregulated development including settlement in hazardous zones, and poor preparedness (UNEP 2009).

Natural disaster, survival, and health

The relationship between natural disaster and health extends beyond rising incidences of death and disease outbreak, injury, and disability in a disaster affected population. Health is more than simply the absence of disease. According to the Ottawa Charter for Health Promotion (WHO 1986), health encompasses basic prerequisites including peace, shelter, and education, food and income, a stable ecosystem and sustainable resources, social justice and equity. Natural disaster threatens all of these things and in doing so compromises the health and wellbeing of entire disaster-affected populations. Health-related interventions that follow a disastrous event need to be holistic in approach and implemented within the context of the disaster response, recovery, and preparedness (DRRP) cycle; they also need to address the social and political factors influencing health and recovery and build on existing structures, services, and capacities (Disease Control Priorities Project 2009). Activities that comprise the DRRP cycle are described below including specific illustrations of the role of health and health-related interventions.

DRRP cycle: a process of building capacity

Reducing vulnerability, enhancing preparedness, and building capacity to better respond to and recover from disastrous events is a long-term complex process encompassing three main phases: response, recovery, and preparedness. Each phase is interconnected and involves particular goals, activities, and actors, which operate at various levels from individuals and families through to community groups and government and international institutions (Fig. 20.1).

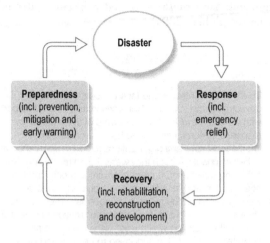

Figure 20.1 • The DRRP cycle.

While the terminology in 'disaster management' varies, what is of fundamental importance is an appreciation that recovery from disaster involves much more than emergency response, rehabilitation, and reconstruction. Increasingly, recovery and future mitigation and preparedness initiatives are being designed and undertaken as an integral aspect of 'sustainable development' (Thomas 2007). Sustainable development involves development that meets the needs of the present without compromising the ability of future generations to meet their own needs (Bruntland 1987); this requires that one see the world as a complex integral system, connecting sociocultural, economic, and ecological wellbeing within wide dimensions of justice, time, and space. Conceiving DRRP within this context represents a conceptual shift from a focus on disaster response toward approaches that reduce vulnerability and increase human and institutional *capacity* to manage hazardous risks and recover from disastrous events (Fig. 20.2).

Building capacity requires coordinated and sustained efforts involving governments, civil society, humanitarian actors (including nongovernmental organizations (NGOs) and donors) and United Nations' bodies (World Health Organization (WHO) 2008). Capacity is the combination of all the available characteristics and resources which improve a community's ability to recognize, assess, and take action to address key issues (ISDR 2009). There are five types of capacity which communities possess: human (e.g. skills and abilities of community members), social (e.g., levels of trust, reciprocity, political influence, social networks, and institutions), financial (e.g., income, credit), physical (e.g., infrastructure,

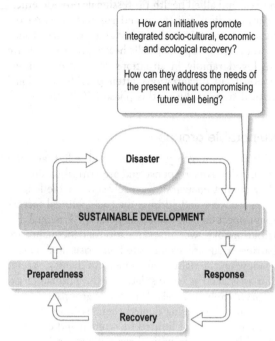

Figure 20.2 • Sustainable development and the DRRP cycle.

public facilities, technology), and environmental (e.g., natural resources, water quality) (Queensland Health 2003). Capacity building in DRRP involves efforts to develop these in ways that will reduce the level of risk or the effects of a disaster. This entails consideration of how hazards, vulnerability, and capacity intersect.

Disaster response: survival and relief

As a disaster unfolds and during its immediate aftermath, the main focus is to coordinate an emergency response and relief program. Survival depends on having access to emergency shelter, food, healthcare, immunization, clean water, and sanitation facilities. As such, the primary goals of disaster response include saving lives, preventing long-term or secondary disabilities, and protecting the public's health. This involves actions such as activating public warning systems and notifying public authorities, mobilizing emergency personnel/equipment and security forces, evacuation, search and rescue, rapid appraisal and assessment, the provision of emergency medical assistance and makeshift shelters, and distribution of relief supplies (Disease Control Priorities Project 2007, Warfield 2009). Locally available doctors, nurses, and allied health professionals provide emergency medical assistance and support to survivors including mental health support. Disease surveillance systems are set up and public health professionals are deployed rapidly in situations of outbreak. International aid organizations often provide additional critical support during this phase (WHO 2008).

Vulnerable groups

Although emergency response and relief are the focus of disaster response and are critical to survival they are not enough in themselves to enable longer-term recovery and address the sociopolitical factors that impact on health and recuperation. Unequal distributions of power, discrimination and inequality are barriers that are exacerbated in crisis and cast a shadow on the right of all persons to dignity, safety, and assistance as encapsulated in the Humanitarian Charter (Sphere 2004). Vulnerable groups are especially at risk of being denied their basic rights, and include but are not limited to, women and children, the elderly, people with chronic illness and disability, and ethnic minorities. Failure to recognize the differing needs of vulnerable groups and the barriers they face in gaining equal access to appropriate services and support can result in further marginalization and denial of vital assistance or information needed to facilitate recovery.

> Julimna and her grandson managed to survive the tsunami with the help of their neighbors who together lifted them to safety on the roof of a local shop. But with limited mobility, difficulty seeing and a small traumatized child to care for, there was no easy way to evacuate Julimna to a temporary emergency shelter a kilometer away. When emergency rations were distributed Julimna, was pushed over in the rush for limited supplies, and she failed to collect basic items for herself and her grandson. A friend from her village helped her to secure some items but they were rendered useless because they did not enable her to cook.

Understanding the needs and strengthening the capacities of affected people and communities is central to effective disaster management and the delivery of effective and equitable programs. This requires the active participation of all groups of people in decision making throughout the DRRP cycle and the processes it entails (assessment, planning, implementation, monitoring and evaluation, and improvement). The protection and promotion of the rights of all people to safety and basic necessities for survival and recovery is a fundamental principle of

humanitarian action as enshrined in the Humanitarian Charter (Sphere 2004).

> ### DISASTER RESPONSE: A PRACTITIONER'S PERSPECTIVE
>
> Initially I felt helpless in the face of such overwhelming devastation and suffering. But working as a 'project officer' with a NGO, I quickly became aware of the emergency response systems established by government and international specialist organizations to coordinate response activities, chaotic though they were. Part of my role involved collecting registration data of survivors and ensuring that age, gender, and assistive devices, including spectacles were included on the forms of all agencies. These data sheets are collated at the disaster coordination centre and provide the basis on which relief plans are made and activated. Although it is supposed to be collected by everyone, data on the aged and people with disability remain especially poor. Knowing the nature and scale of 'special needs' is critical to enabling mobilization, shaping, and coordination of response efforts that address such needs.

Disaster recovery: from rehabilitation and reconstruction to sustainable development

Once the emergency has passed, short-term and long-term 'recovery' activities are initiated with the ultimate goal of rebuilding and strengthening capacity and resilience.

> Prior to the tsunami, Julimna's livelihood was dependent on her son and the strength of the fishing industry within her community. The coping strategies she was able to utilize after the disaster were, in part, a reflection of her community's capacity – the strengths and resources it had available to facilitate recovery, including appropriate healthcare in tandem with access to income – initially through cash grants followed by longer-term income generation activity.

Recovery is a long process of re-building, reconstruction and rehabilitation. In the context of disaster the term 'rehabilitation' refers to the efforts by which the functioning of communities and their environments are restored (WHO 2008). A healthy, functioning ecosystem is as critical to recovery and future development as is the restoration of function for individuals, families, and community groups.

Recovery begins with activities such as building temporary and permanent housing, and re-establishing systems to provide medical and rehabilitative care, counseling services, livelihood support, and income generation (Disease Control Priorities Project 2007, Warfield 2009). During the recovery stage health professionals continue to provide medical care and rehabilitation. They are also involved in planning the redevelopment of health systems and services (WHO 2008). Collaboration and local capacity building should guide recovery efforts, key aspects of which are *participation* of all affected groups and rebuilding of community networks and processes.

Participation engenders culturally and contextually relevant recovery programs. By nurturing community cohesion through participatory processes and tapping into cultural and religious systems, grieving and healing processes are most powerfully facilitated. Research has shown (Thomas 2007, 2008) that where survivors and affected populations are actively engaged in how community recovery programs are developed and implemented, the recovery of individuals is markedly enhanced. In some instances, however, there will be people who may never fully recover from the trauma of their experience, while others may seize the situation to advance their own agendas at the expense of family and/or wider community wellbeing (Box 20.1). Managing participation in a way that respects the rights and needs of all, including how individuals and groups do and do not want to engage at any one time, is an important part of the process.

Disaster preparedness: preventing, mitigating, and preparing for future adversity

Disaster preparedness encompasses prevention, mitigation, and readiness strategies. Prevention and mitigation are aimed at eliminating or reducing the probability of disaster occurring, or reducing the effects of disasters. These include updating vulnerability analyses, building and safety codes, zoning and land use management, preventative healthcare and public education (Asian Disaster Preparedness Centre (ADPC) 2006, Disease Priorities Control Project 2007, Warfield 2009). Preparedness also involves the development of plans to minimize damage and save lives. Efforts are made to establish early warning systems, evacuation plans, and emergency communication systems; identify emergency personnel and establish mutual aid agreements, provide disaster management, training, and public education. Preparedness activities are often informed by previous experiences of disaster, and are primarily focused on building institutional capacity

Box 20.1

The politics of participation

In natural disasters, when law and order is disrupted or the population is anxious to access relief, high levels of tension can endanger affected communities and even humanitarian actors. Tension may be exacerbated in situations of conflict and natural disaster, as occurred for example, in regions of Sri Lanka and in Aceh, Indonesia following the Indian Ocean Tsunami. Engaging with specific groups or recruiting personnel (even inadvertently) who are aligned with certain political factions can lead parties to the conflict, and others, to perceive humanitarian actors as partial. This makes both them and those they are working with potential targets. Ultimately in Aceh the disaster created an opportunity to broker peace and democracy, while in Sri Lanka the conflict significantly hindered ability to distribute relief and progress recovery efforts, with residual effects on already poor, conflict-affected communities. The responsibility lies with humanitarian actors to ensure that their interventions do not increase the security risks to affected populations but rather, reinforces their protection and recovery (Active Learning Network for Accountability and Performance in Humanitarian Action (ALNAP) 2003).

and human resources. As the prevalence and severity of disaster events is predicted to increase, mitigation and preparedness efforts are increasingly being directed toward the building of resilience in the form of social, economic, and environmental capital, as elaborated in the conclusion of Julimna's story.

JULIMNA'S STORY CONCLUDED: FROM SURVIVOR AND DEPENDENT TO EMPOWERED LEADER

'I can't believe how my life has changed!' bubbled Julimna. Two years on from the tsunami, she describes a remarkable process of transformation. 'After I returned to my village I had trouble just surviving day to day. Getting enough money for food and basic provisions was a big problem for me. I felt like a burden – that is, until I joined up with a group of older people like me. There was this local lady, Archana, helping to get us together; I learnt she was from a local NGO that was being supported by an international NGO to help older people affected by the tsunami. Well, the first thing we did was go on a pilgrimage – I never thought I would see that place in my life. It was a spiritual trip, a time to grieve and share losses and fears for the future as old, dependent people; it was two days and we organized a lot of it ourselves with Archana's help. By the time we came back we realized we could help one another a lot more. And that's how our Senior Citizens Association (SCA) was formed.

With help from the two NGOs, our SCA has become an amazing organization. Early on we set-up a revolving micro-credit loan and savings scheme to help older people like myself get a small loan to start a small income-generating business; I started a sweetmeat stall, selling them to the workers. Through the group, I got help in how to manage the money, so I could pay back the loan and also save a few rupees each month. Now I even have a bank account! I am saving to help my grandson's education, and for any emergency in the future, and I can contribute to the household. I now have a role, status, and respect. I'm on the committee of our SCA and have done training in how to get registered and manage an organization. Currently we have 83 members; most pay a small membership fee, and together with a loan we got from the NGO to establish a group enterprise, we are generating income that allows us to provide cash grants to very vulnerable old people and people with disability in our community. Through the SCA, we also work with the NGO to develop a Home Care Volunteers program, that trains volunteers – young-old people are best – to provide simple CBR [community-based rehabilitation] to needy people in the community. And we are working to form a federation of SCAs across the state! All of these things are raising the profile, status, and integration of senior citizens in our society. I never would have imagined this was possible.'

Occupation and occupational therapists: is there a role?

Occupation includes all purposeful human activity and is a fundamental mechanism by which people can influence their health and wellbeing and adapt to change (Wilcock 2006). It provides a means for expression, collaboration, and development on individual and community levels, as revealed in Julimna's story of recovery. Yet, despite its inherent value and transformative potential, the concept of occupation appears to be overlooked in disaster recovery and few occupational therapists are actively involved in the field. A situational analysis conducted by the World Federation of Occupational Therapists (WFOT) following the 2004 Indian Ocean tsunami (Sinclair & Thomas 2005) attributed lack of occupational therapist involvement in South East Asia to a number of factors, including limited awareness of disaster management systems, limited information and data to guide planning for occupational therapy involvement, few opportunities for training and field experience and limited awareness about the potential role of occupational therapists within the profession and with key stakeholders (e.g. coordinating bodies, donors, NGOs).

Occupational therapists often work with people experiencing disability and/or disabling conditions to enhance their abilities and to co-create opportunities to participate in everyday activities either by restoring and maintaining skills, preventing dysfunction or modifying the environment to better support participation (WFOT 2009). Natural disaster is a disabling condition in itself. It creates barriers to the engagement in everyday activities that sustain and give meaning to life. In situations of disaster, livelihoods are destroyed, people are displaced, dislocated, and alienated from their usual activities and roles. Gaining access to occupations of need (for survival) and choice through cohesive and supportive communities and systems is critical to recovery. In order for occupational therapists to respond appropriately to the complexities of practice in the field and play an effective and meaningful role among multiple stakeholders, practitioners must develop basic competencies relevant to humanitarian aid and development and learn to approach DRRP from an 'occupational perspective'. It is through the profession's inherent 'occupational perspective' that the value of occupation-based approaches in contexts of disaster can be further explored and understood and ultimately appreciated and utilized.

An occupational perspective on DRRP

The profession's 'occupational perspective' is based on assumptions that occupation is a basic human need and fundamental human right; it brings meaning to life and has the potential to be therapeutic (Townsend & Polatajko 2007). These assumptions drive the profession's concerns with occupation as the vehicle through which people participate in the social and economic fabric of their communities and influence their health and wellbeing. How such concerns are contextualized in terms of disaster and its impact on individuals and communities is not well understood or articulated within the profession. There is also much to be learned about the role of occupation in recovery, including its therapeutic use and more broadly, its potential to enable just and inclusive disaster response, recovery, and preparedness. Occupational therapy theorists have proposed seven ways in which occupation can mediate the effects of stressful situations and promote health (McColl 2002) which the American Occupational Therapy Association (AOTA) has considered in its formulation of a 'staged model' for occupational therapy's contribution in times of disaster (AOTA 2006). Research is also currently underway that draws on the experiences of survivors and practitioners in contexts of disaster and examines implications for policy, practice, and professional capacity building (Thomas and Rushford (in press)). Initiatives of this nature will help to explore and articulate possible occupational perspectives on DRRP and strengthen occupational therapists' involvement in the field.

A preliminary focus

A preliminary occupational focus on DRRP potentially reveals empowered individuals *and* communities shaping their own destinies through leveraging equitable access to rights and resources, and opportunities to rebuild their lives by participating in self-sustaining, meaningful occupations. In particular, it can be argued that occupation has the potential to help promote inclusive development in disaster contexts where the rights of all persons to dignity, access to humanitarian aid, and assistance and genuine participation in preparedness, recovery, and development activities are fulfilled. Toward this aim, occupation has multiple applications. It can be viewed (and utilized) as:

1. A therapeutic and recovery medium
2. A mechanism through which participation is organized and achieved
3. The primary conduit through which capacity and resilience is built
4. A criterion for evaluating participation and inclusive practice.

Occupation also serves as an external reference point and potentially engenders the mutuality and partnership necessary for community (re)building.

Are occupational therapists prepared for the challenge?

An occupational approach to DRRP would involve identifying and responding to *individuals, communities*, and *populations* from a perspective of social inclusiveness, community participation, and capacity building with 'occupational engagement' and 'enablement of occupation' at the core of an occupational therapy response. This approach necessitates interventions that extend beyond the profession's

markedly 'individual' focus, to address the social, political, and economic factors that influence occupation and recovery more broadly. Although occupation is being reconceptualized in relation to its social, political, and cultural context, and several occupational therapy models exist that recognize the influence of the environment on participation in occupations (Christiansen & Baum 1997, Law et al 1998, Letts et al 2003, Townsend & Polatajko 2007) these developments are not enough in themselves to assist occupational therapists in tackling (from an occupational perspective) the broader environmental barriers influencing disaster-affected contexts and to navigate the sociopolitical realm of disaster.

PERSPECTIVES OF PRACTITIONERS NEW TO THE FIELD ...

I'm not sure what could have prepared me for the culture of humanitarian aid and development in post-disaster contexts – its insularity and competitiveness came to me as a bit of a surprise. When I arrived in Banda Aceh, the streets were lined with the flags of international organizations which gave the impression of 'staking claim'. It struck me that as foreigners we seemed to have a lot of power, and yet due to cultural differences and communication barriers we had no idea of what was really going on within these communities – a sort of 'blind power' so to speak. Where there was mutual respect and collaboration this paradox or tension was manageable. But in situations where the participation of communities was limited, for a variety of reasons, and most of them political, it was detrimental to recovery efforts and most importantly, to the people in those communities.

To achieve inclusive and barrier-free DRRP denotes the provision of opportunities for capacity building in the form of individual and structural empowerment of people, their organizations and networks. Occupational therapists are well versed in capacity building in terms of individual empowerment but are typically less equipped to harness and strengthen community capacity within the complexity of power dynamics and structures that characterize disaster situations. Working in contexts of disaster challenges practitioners to broaden their approach from individuals to communities and in doing so to learn to manage the politics inherent in disaster situations.

A PRACTITIONER'S PERSPECTIVE (CONTINUED)

At the temporary camp, I helped facilitate the establishment of a camp committee comprising authorities and residents. Fighting to have representatives of vulnerable groups on the committee, and ensuring they had a strong voice in how the camp was set up and run was a way of promoting what I now recognize as 'occupational justice'. Enabling survivors to have some control over decisions that affect their lives, however minor or transient, was a powerful factor in trauma management and recovery. Other ways I assisted using my occupational therapy background was to ensure ablution facilities were accessible and provided appropriate privacy and security; and providing basic therapy using CBR principles, including training select residents to undertake simple activities and therapy techniques with others in the camp. As one therapist, I could not possibly meet all the needs on my own. I discovered that providing residents with opportunities for meaningful engagement in a raft of camp activities such as the identification, planning, and management of camp administration activities, play groups for kids, and psychosocial and income-generation training groups, proved effective forms of trauma counseling for many survivors.

New terms, models, frameworks, and discussions are arising in the literature that aim to effect change on a sociopolitical level with populations and communities (Pollard et al 2008b, Sheldon Fisher et al 2008, Kronenberg, Simo Algado & Pollard 2005, Wilcock 2006). The Canadian Practice Process Framework (Craik et al 2007) and the political activities of daily living reasoning tool (pADL) (Pollard et al 2008b) provide a framework and tools through which practitioners can begin to advance notions of occupational justice in complex practice environments that involve multiple stakeholders and interests. Moreover, by actively listening to and reflecting on the stories and experiences of survivors, and practitioners, working in disaster contexts around the globe an occupational perspective can emerge, and give shape to culturally and contextually relevant models to guide practice.

Conclusion

Disaster discriminates; it threatens the health and wellbeing of entire populations, but devastates some lives more than others. People who are poor and (or) marginalized are especially vulnerable. This reality represents a considerable and important challenge to the profession of occupational therapy – a profession that espouses a formidable vision of 'enabling a just and inclusive society so that all people may participate to their potential in the daily occupations of life' (Townsend & Polatajko 2007, p. 2) If the profession is to progress toward this vision it cannot ignore the rising incidences of disaster on a global scale and ever increasing human vulnerability. The particular challenge to the profession is to articulate an occupational perspective on DRRP that is grounded in the realities of the field, and most importantly, the experiences of survivors, from which occupational approaches may be examined, better understood and utilized. DRRP is a long-term and complex process that is increasingly occurring within a framework of sustainable development. Health-related interventions need to be holistic and to build on existing local capacities and nurture community cohesion. Understanding the role of occupation in this process is critical to determining how the knowledge and skills of occupational therapists can be best utilized and capacity strengthened to promote and support ongoing occupational therapy involvement. Context specific research, education and awareness raising, reflective practice, and professional support and networking are all valuable strategies to support occupational therapy involvement and the profession's meaningful contribution to the field. With an increasing number of communities affected by natural disaster around the globe, the time is right for the profession to rise to the challenge.

References

Asian Disaster Preparedness CentreM: *Community-Based Disaster Risk Management. Critical Guidelines*, Bangkok, 2006, Asian Disaster Preparedness Centre.

Active Learning Network for Accountability and Performance in Humanitarian Action: *Participation by Crisis Affected Populations in Humanitarian Action. A Handbook for Practitioners*, 2003, Online. Available at: http://www.alnap.org/

pool/files/gs_handbook.pdf. Accessed.

American Occupational Therapy Association: The role of occupational therapy in disaster preparedness, response, and recovery, *Am J Occup Ther* 60:642–649, 2006.

Bruntland G, editor: *Our Common Future: The World Commission on Environment and Development*, Oxford, 1987, Oxford University Press.

Christiansen C, Baum CM: *Occupational Therapy: Enabling Function and Well-being*, ed 2, Thorofare NJ, 1997, Slack.

Craik J, Davis J, Polatajko H: The Canadian process practice framework. In Townsend E, Polatajko H, editors: *Enabling Occupation II: Advancing an Occupational Therapy Vision for Health, Well-Being, and Justice Through Occupation*, Ottawa, 2007, CAOT Publications ACE, pp 247–272.

Disease Control Priorities Project: *Natural Disasters. Coping with the Health Impact*, 2007, Online. Available at: http://www.dcp2.org/file/121/DCPP-NaturalDisasters.pdf. Accessed January 14, 2009.

Haar A: *Discussion Article. Are People With Disabilities Excluded from Millennium Goals? Dutch Coalition on Disability and Development*, 2005. Online. Available at: http://www.dcdd.nl/?2816. Accessed July 8, 2009.

International Disability and Development Consortium: *Conflict and Emergencies*, 2009, Online. Available at: http://www.iddcconsortium.net/joomla/index.php/conflict-and-emergencies. Accessed July 5, 2009.

International Strategy for Disaster Reduction: *Living With Risk. A Global Review of Disaster Reduction Initiatives*, ed 4, Geneva, 2004, United Nations Publications.

International Strategy for Disaster Reduction: *UNISDR Terminology on Disaster Risk Reduction*, 2009. Online. Available at: http://www.unisdr.org/libraryeng/terminology-%20home@.html. Accessed July 18, 2010.

Kronenberg F, Simo Algado S, Pollard N: *Occupational Therapy Without Borders: Learning from the spirit of survivors*. Edinburgh, 2005, Edinburgh.

Law M, Baptiste S, Carswell A, McColl A, Polatajko H, Pollock N: *The Canadian Occupational Performance Measure*, Ottawa, 1998, CAOT Publications.

McColl MA: Occupation in stressful times, *Am J Occup Ther* 56:350–353, 2002.

OCHA: *The Scale and Impact of Emergencies Across the Globe*, 2006, Office for the Coordination of Humanitarian Affairs. Online. Available at: http://www.globalaging.org/armedconflict/countryreports/general/ocha.htm. Accessed July 19, 2010.

Pollard N, Kronenberg F, Sakellariou D: A political practice of occupational therapy. In Pollard N, Kronenberg F, Sakellariou D, editors: *A Political Practice of Occupational Therapy*, Edinburgh, 2008, Elsevier Science, pp 3–20.

Pollard N, Sakellariou D, Kronenberg F: *A Political Practice of Occupational Therapy*, Edinburgh, 2008, Elsevier Science.

Queensland Health: *Integrating Public Health Practices. A position statement on community capacity development and the social determinants of health for public health services*, 2003, Online. Available at: http://www.health.qld.gov.au/ph/Documents/hpu/20426.pdf. Accessed July 8, 2009.

Satterthwaite D, Dodman D, Hardoy J, et al: *The Heart of the Matter: Underlying Risk Drivers*, 2009, Global assessment report on disaster risk reduction risk and poverty in a changing climate. Chapter 4. Online. Available at: http://www.preventionweb.net/english/hyogo/gar/report/documents/GAR_Chapter_4_2009_eng.pdf. Accessed July 5, 2009.

Sinclair K, Thomas K: *Report of WFOT Post-Tsunami Situational Analysis. The World Federation of Occupational Therapists*, 2005, Online. Available at: http://www.caot.ca/pdfs/WFOTPost-TsunamiSituationalAnalysis.pdf. Accessed July 17, 2008.

Sphere: *Humanitarian Charter and Minimum Standards in Disaster Response, Revised Edition. The Sphere Project*, 2004, Online. Available at: http://www.sphereproject.org/content/view/27/84. Accessed.

Thomas K: *United, We Are Living Again, An Evaluation of the Sri Lanka Tsunami Response Programme*. London, 2007, HelpAge Sri Lanka and HelpAge International.

Thomas K: *Fostering Pioneers. An Evaluation of the Sri Lanka Tsunami Extended Response Programme (ERP)*. Colombo, 2008, HelpAge Sri Lanka and HelpAge International.

Thomas K, Rushford N: *Disaster and Development: An Occupational Perspective*, Edinburgh, in press, Elsevier.

Townsend E, Polatajko H: *Enabling Occupation II: Advancing an Occupational Therapy Vision for Health, Well-Being and Justice Through Occupation*, Ottawa, 2007, CAOT Publications ACE, pp 247–272.

United Nations Development Program: *Crisis Prevention and Recovery*, 2009, Online. Available at: http://www.undp.org/bcpr. Accessed July 5, 2009.

United Nations Environment Program: *State of the Environment and Policy Retrospective: 1972–2002*, 2009, Online. Available at: http:// www.unep.org/geo/geo3/english/pdfs/chapter2-9_disasters.pdf. Accessed July 5, 2009.

Warfield C: *The Disaster Management Cycle*, Online. Available at: http://www.gdrc.org/uem/disasters/1-dm_cycle.html. Accessed July 8, 2009.

WFOT: 2009, Online. Available at: http://www.wfot.org/information.asp. Accessed July 11, 2009.

WHO: *Ottawa Charter for Health Promotion*, 1986, World Health Organization. Online. Available at: http://www.who.int/hpr/NPH/docs/ottawa_charter_hp.pdf. Accessed July 8, 2009.

WHO: *Sustaining Recovery Six Months On. The Role of Health Professionals*, 2008, World Health Organization. Online. Available at: http://www.who.int/hac/crises/international/asia_tsunami/6months/6months/en/index.html. Accessed July 30, 2008.

Wilcock A: *An Occupational Perspective on Health*, ed 2, Thorofare NJ, 2006, Slack.

Yodmani S: *Disaster Risk Management and Vulnerability Reduction: Protecting the Poor*, 2009, Online. Available at: http://www.adpc.net/infores/adpdocuments/PovertyPaper.pdf. Accessed July 5, 2009.

Ubuntourism: engaging divided people in post-apartheid South Africa

Frank Kronenberg   Elelwani Ramugondo

OVERVIEW

Attained in 1994, *post-apartheid* South Africa was meant to evolve into a place that all people who live there could call home. To advance this purpose, the diverse groups of people that make up its population must find ways to meaningfully connect with each other, and possibly engage in *collective story-making*. The Cape Town based initiative ubuntourism came about in response to this challenge. The term is a portmanteau that blends the African humanist ethic of *ubuntu* with the *act of tourism*, the world's largest industry. The conceptualization and practice of ubuntourism are partly inspired and informed by *occupational perspectives* of people's health and wellbeing, which originate in occupational therapy and occupational science. Two experiences are shared: one which gave birth to ubuntourism – a historic intercontinental friendly soccer match between a South African township team and amateur champions from Dublin/Ireland, and one affirming its potential – a unique international occupational justice-gathering in Cape Town. The authors acknowledge that these interactions on their own are not sufficient as evidence to suggest ubuntourism to be an occupational form for social cohesion. It is hoped that further engagements will generate stronger practice-based evidence. This chapter serves to raise debate on the role of collective occupations such as ubuntourism in building and maintaining *working relationships*.

Introduction

The pervasive legacies of apartheid continue to obstruct the unfolding story of democratic South Africa (African Leadership Forum 1991, Hendricks 2002). It seems appropriate therefore to briefly describe this social and political policy of racial segregation and discrimination enforced by a white minority government in South Africa from 1948 to 1994. The term 'apartheid' means '*separateness*' in Afrikaans, which is cognate to the English *apart* and *-hood* (Merriam-Webster 2009). Racial segregation in South Africa began in colonial times. Apartheid as an official policy was introduced following the general election of 1948. New legislation classified inhabitants into racial groups: white, colored (of mixed race), Indian, and Bantu (black African), and residential areas were segregated by means of forced removals (Platzky & Walker 1985). From 1958, blacks were deprived of their citizenship; legally becoming citizens of one of 10 tribally based self-governing homelands or *Bantustans*, four of which became nominally independent states. The state-segregated education, medical care, and other public services, provided black people with services inferior to those for whites (Beinart 1994). Apartheid sparked significant internal resistance, comprising of a series of uprisings and protests that were met with the banning of opposition and imprisoning of anti-apartheid leaders. As unrest spread and became more violent, state organizations responded with increasing repression and state-sponsored violence. International solidarity and liberation movements (whose actions included economic and cultural boycotts) added the mounting opposition during the 1980s, playing a pivotal role in mobilizing international opinion against apartheid and injustices in South Africa and neighboring states (African National Congress (ANC) 1991, Katjavivi 2004). In 1990 President De Klerk began negotiations to

DOI: 10.1016/B978-0-7020-3103-8.00030-4

end apartheid, culminating in multiracial democratic elections in 1994, which were won by the ANC under Nelson Mandela. However, some 14 years later, the vestiges of apartheid still shape South African politics and society (Mbembe 2008).

Former US Ambassador to South Africa James Joseph (2002) indicated that 'society could learn significantly from the South African people about building community and that their emphasis on reconciliation may be at the heart of our search for public values appropriate for a world that is integrating and fragmenting at the same time'. It seems, however, appropriate to also acknowledge that for South Africa – and really any other (emerging) democracy – to become a home for all the people who live in it (South African Government 1996), their historically constructed differences and conditions of unequally lived privileges must be addressed. And just as fighting to bring down the apartheid regime presented a hugely significant purpose that effectively organized and mobilized different groups of people locally and globally (Katjavivi 2004), the building of post-apartheid South Africa may present an equally meaningful challenge. The Cape Town-based initiative **ubuntourism** came about in an attempt to contribute towards this aspiration. It aims to bring about opportunities for divided groups of people – particularly in terms of unequally lived privileges – to meaningfully connect with each other in ways that might trigger collective humane story-making, finding common ground to build on. The conceptualization and practice of **ubun**tourism are partly inspired by the vision of the founders of the occupational therapy profession, which was to share its expertise 'beyond the traditional limits of "therapy" and adopt a perspective that embraces people's occupational needs' (Watson & Swartz 2004, p. 63). The natural progression of this was a realization that it was no longer sufficient to work only with individuals and groups of people, but to take a population approach in pursuing the realization of human potential through what people collectively do every day (Ramugondo 2009, see Chapter 1, p. 9–12).

Situating the unfolding story

It seems relevant to briefly contextualize our personal position related to **ubun**tourism. I (Frank) was born and raised in the Netherlands and after some 20 odd years of traveling, living, and working (education and occupational therapy 'without borders') in different regions of the globe (Middle East, Asia, United States, Central America), in 2004 in Cape Town I met and married Elelwani, a native South African, and found a new home. Borrowing from the Trinidadian author Robert Suresh Roberts, who now has lived in South Africa for over 10 years: 'Home is a notion that has to do with where you feel that what you do matters. And I think that to be part of what South Africa is doing now is something that matters for everyone in the world. It's another way of belonging that has not much to do with the old fashioned idea of roots. I think roots are for plants, not people' (*Conversations on a Sunday Afternoon* 2005). For us, addressing family needs/interests must simultaneously be about helping build up this country. Finding out what contributions we are best positioned to make requires that we activate our occupational consciousness (see Chapter 1, p. 2), and engage in deep and critical learning about what matters to the different groups of people in this local/regional context, as well as how this is influenced by global processes.

After settling in Cape Town in August 2006, being restricted in attaining paid employment due to temporary residence status, I (first author) worked on a pro bono basis for Ishabi (see List of websites, p. 207), a then new community tourism company. It allowed me to learn first-hand about the hegemonic nature of the tourism industry, which is still dominated by operators who were designated as 'white' under apartheid (Witz 2008). The South African government drives a transformation agenda and the growing tourism industry is not excused from this process. Currently, historically disadvantaged populations are at best afforded to provide 'wheels', 'hands' (domestic work, catering, security), 'images', and 'entertainment'. A phenomenon that has picked up since the beginning of the new millennium is so-called township or poverty tourism (Telschow 2003, Passport Day 2009). This kind of tourism allows interested visitors a peek into the environs and lives of township residents, depicting them as places of 'living culture ... political resistance [and] modern life' (Witz 2007 quoting Kurin 1997, p. 273). I have overheard visitors compare their experience to game park safaris, 'instead of watching the wild animals, here you get to look at the poor black people'. Mandated by South Africa's transformation agenda, both local residents in these communities and interested visitors rightfully ask and deserve better and more. That's why we originally conceptualized what we were doing as *transformative tourism*.

Frommer's, the American bestselling travel guides, described Cape Town as 'the oldest city in southern Africa, regularly heralded as one of the most beautiful on earth, thanks to its impressive landscape' (Frommer's 2009). However, it cannot and should not be ignored that this metropolis also continues to reflect the ugly faces of the legacies of apartheid. The first images that may strike visitors' views from airplane or car windows on their arrival to Cape Town are the iconic Table Mountain and a 'sea' of shack dwellings. Very few visitors ever get a chance to meaningfully engage with people who live in the 'downsides' of this tourism hot spot. Many if not most visitors may not be interested, but I (first author) learned that it also relates to a lack of appropriate opportunities for such encounters to come about. Also, residents of local communities do not necessarily welcome a bunch of tourists running around their neighborhood with cameras, unless this represents some negotiated agreement that they can also benefit from. Tourism companies often avoid exposing themselves to unnecessary risks, of which crime perhaps presents the main concern (Ozinsky 2007).

With three South African partners, in 2007 the authors founded Shades of Black Works (SOBW), a Cape Town-based company with a social mission, consisting of three interrelated principles: *strengthening places of origin*, *forging connections*, and *collective story-making* (Box 21.1, see the SOBW website, p. 207). We believe that realizing our mission requires going beyond institutionalized and conventional practices of occupational therapy. **ubun**tourism is our first initiative and the following story gave birth to it.

Experience 1: Intercontinental Friendly Transkei Lions versus Killester United FC

Following up on a friend's recommendation, in August 2007 the first author visited the only township-based museum in the Western Cape, the Lwandle Migrant Labour Museum (LMLM). It is located 'off the beaten track' in Lwandle (Xhosa word for 'sea'), some 40 km outside Cape Town (see List of websites, p. 207). The apartheid government established Lwandle in 1958, with hostel-type accommodation for workers who mainly serviced the nearby fruit and canning industry. Today, Lwandle is

---

Box 21.1

Shades of Black Works: triple social mission

1. **Strengthening places of origin**: Origin here not only refers to geographic location, but also to whatever it is that makes any person ultimately human. A state of mind in this sense can be a place of origin as a starting point for one to feel rooted and fully human. This principle could then be about reaffirming humanness in an individual or a collective.

2. **Forging connections**: Humans have a need as well as an inclination to connect with others. We are basically social animals. It is often superficial factors that create an illusion that we have nothing in common with others in different circumstances. It is only when these superficial factors are stripped that we are reminded of the core within us that essentially makes us the same. Shades of Black plans to use different approaches to remind people across different contexts of this fact.

3. **Collective story-making**: Once people have engaged with each other in any form, they cannot help but be affected by the experience. Their ensuing life stories will more or less be testimony to this meeting point. Shades of Black intends for this collective story-making to be less unconscious. It is in the honoring of the role that others have played in one's life that *Ubuntu* can be realized.

---

a sprawling dynamic township. Most of its inhabitants are Xhosa speaking but it is also diverse, acknowledging that people have multiple identities. The LMLM serves as a memorial to the system of migrant labor, single sex hostels, and the control of black workers through an identity document which under apartheid regulated access to employment and residence in urban areas, the infamous 'dom pas' (pass book) (Witz 2008).

I was welcomed by Lunga Smile, the museum's curator and a local resident. Lunga took me on an informative, engaging story-telling walk through the museum and a visit to the nearby 'Hostel 33', which has been preserved in order 'to sustain a memory of how the system of apartheid had operated' (Witz 2007). At one point Lunga offered a personal reflection of a detail on a displayed photograph which wasn't given any attention in the narratives that accompanied it. It was a poster of a soccer team and he indicated with a wink: 'Historians didn't seem interested in telling us about that story', suggesting that the hostel dwellers' only occupation had been the provision of labor. Lunga told me that he often wondered about what aspirations and dreams they may have held. When he then spoke of his involvement with one of Lwandle's oldest soccer teams, the Transkei (TK) Lions, we discovered a shared passion for soccer. Almost immediately we exchanged some ideas about 'doing something' in relation to the 2010 FIFA World Cup™ in South Africa that could benefit today's TK Lions team. I imagined soccer-crazy visitors from overseas being interested in playing in and against a township team. Although such an experience did not seem to be on offer on the local tourism market, soon after my visit to Lwandle, an established tour operator enquired whether we could organize a friendly soccer match in a township for their client, Killester United FC from Dublin, Ireland.

What seemed like a straightforward request took about six months to get on track. The main challenge constituted establishing working relationships with and between relative strangers. We were curious about why the Irish wanted to play in and against a township team but were unable to ask them directly, given that our client was the tour operator. We arranged for the visitors to act as hosts to a delegation of the TK Lions on the morning after their arrival in Cape Town, at their downtown hotel. This initial encounter extended to lunch feeding into the anticipation of the township visit and soccer match, believed to represent a historic event in South Africa – the first ever international friendly soccer match between a township team and an overseas team (!)

On 5 February 2008, the Irish visitors traveled to Lwandle, where they were warmly received at the museum by Lunga, TK Lions representatives, and a massive number of excited kids. Having anticipated that they would probably appreciate it, the visitors had organized sets of soccer gear to outfit at least three local teams. Lunga's story-telling walk through the museum and part of the surrounding community made a strong impression on the visitors. Some of them were openly emotional and one of them said: 'It's like listening to the stories of my mom and dad and grandparents back in Ireland.' Only then we discovered a significant connection between our visitors and the local community: they shared a similar working-class history. Killester is located in northern Dublin, where *The Commitments* was filmed. One of its protagonist Jimmy Rabbitte's classical lines is 'The Irish are the blacks of Europe. And Dubliners are the blacks of Ireland. And the Northside Dubliners are the blacks of Dublin.' (*The Commitments*1991). From here the players went to the soccer field to prepare for the match. It was preceded by a formal welcome by the local ANC (ruling party) ward councilor, a blessing of the event by a Xhosa praise singer, and a playing of the national anthems. (Actually, we couldn't get hold of the Irish anthem and played an Irish Rugby song instead.) Mainly thanks to word of mouth, local residents flocked to the match in unexpectedly large numbers and the ambiance was fantastic. Local radio and newspaper reporters who were invited also pitched in and conducted interviews with the visiting team and with local attendants. A Cape Town-based Afrikatourism blogger reported: 'the results were magical'; 'working class Irish blokes see reflections of themselves in the faces and places of an African township half a world away'. Here, the report suggested, was 'the possibility to go elsewhere and come back different – kinder, humbler, more connected, more grounded in your own identity because of what you've shared with others' (Ackermann 2008a).

A downtown Irish pub was invited to sponsor soccer balls and in return we ushered the players to enjoy their drinks there. At first it seemed that the Irish amateur champions would walk over the TK Lions, particularly because the latter appeared as teenagers compared with the Irish side. TK Lions, however, only just lost 2–1. After the game, shirts, sportive thanks, and commemoration medals were exchanged. Group pictures, a *braai* (South African barbeque) and drinks (including *mqoboti*, traditional beer) were shared. We had informed various media about this event ahead of time. The international radio station 'Voice of America' and the popular SABC TV show *Morning Live* showed up after the game to record some impressions. These were broadcast the following day, giving positive exposure to both the Lwandle community and the LMLM. An article about the match and overall experience appeared in the *Daily Star*, one of Ireland's main newspapers, which today is on display in the LMLM, not only to commemorate this historic event, but also to inspire future initiatives of this kind (Fig. 21.1).

Here are some testimonies to illustrate how the event impacted locals and visitors:

> A deeply humbling experience; We were reminded not only of our privileged lives in Ireland but also what we may have lost.
>
> Irish visitors

> We live across the N2 [highway] in Somerset West but had never before been to Lwandle. We didn't know that there was a museum here.
>
> Representatives from the local tour operator

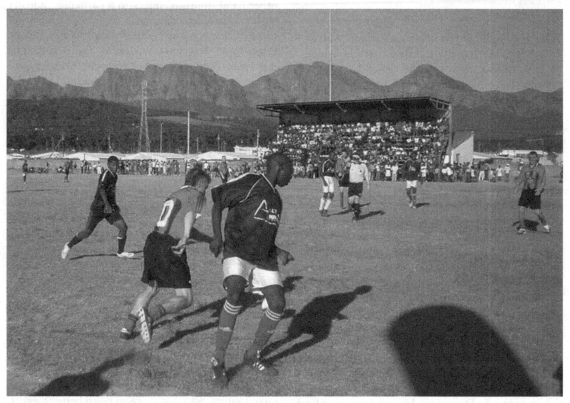

Figure 21.1 • Historical soccer friendly in Lwandle.

The day we went to welcome Killester United at their hotel I was not yet convinced that the team would really play a game with our TK Lions in Lwandle. I mean, it has never happened that a foreign team came to play a match in a former migrant workers community. Top teams like Manchester United and Ajax Amsterdam have been visiting South Africa to play against our famous teams. And, helped by the 6th of February 2008 SABC2 *Morning Live* news broadcast, this event uplifted community interest in the museum.

Lunga Smile – LMLM curator, Lwandle resident, TK Lions supporter

A few weeks after the event I asked a Lwandle teenager what was the highlight for her: 'When the players exchanged their shirts immediately after the match. That moment had the biggest impact on me because I never imagined I'd ever witness something like this. White guys travelling from far requesting to play against our local boys (and paying for it), exchanging sweaty shirts with our boys.' The essence of this response was also echoed by other Lwandle residents who spoke of a 'humanizing experience' and 'restoration of dignity'.

And for us at Shades of Black Works, we had discovered an occupational need and a vision of how to meet it. Negative reactions from the local tourism industry urged us to rebrand 'transformative tourism', as it was correctly perceived as too aligned with the government's transformation agenda, leading to the birth of **ubunt**ourism. This event 'got the ball rolling' . . .

Blending '*ubuntu*' and 'tourism': ubunt**ourism**

The term **ubunt**ourism is a portmanteau that intends to blend the best interpretations and practices of the African humanist ethic of *ubuntu* with the *act of tourism*, the world's largest industry, in everyday contexts of post-apartheid South Africa. Before explaining this concept and practice under construction further, we briefly describe '*ubuntu*' and how we value 'tourism' in order to set out what distinguishes this from other approximations that may not actually be in the same spirit.

Ubuntu

The African philosophy of *ubuntu*, which Watson & Fourie (2004) loosely translated as 'humanness' (p. 20), is associated with the notion that 'persons depend on other persons for the exercise and development of their capacity for self-realization' (Shutte 1993, p. 70). It connects with cultures that Iwama (2005) and Lim (2004) identified as valuing interdependence, social relationships, reciprocity, and belonging. Our increasingly interdependent world that is both integrating and fragmenting at the same time (Joseph 2002) critically needs *ubuntu*. Steve Biko pointed out that what the world can learn from Africa is the focus on humanness and spirituality to complement and possibly replace individualism, which goes with greed (Magadlela 2008). Nobel Prize laureate, Archbishop Desmond Mpilo Tutu often quotes the basic Nguni description of *ubuntu*: '*umuntu ngumuntu ngabantu*', meaning 'I am who I am because of others around me' or 'I am because we are' (Swanson 2007), from which follows that 'to deny the dignity or seek to diminish the humanity of another person is to destroy one's own' (Nussbaum 2003). Akin to the occupational (consciousness) nature of **ubun**tourism, it is useful to also consider the words of Dumisani Magadlela (16 March 2008), a respected South African leadership development facilitator/coach: '*Ubuntu* is best understood experientially, as lived and experienced, and not merely conceptually and as intellectual debate. It's about individual and group behavior and community values, and it is the cultural bedrock from which our common humanity springs ... not just black people, but all of us' (2008). Former president of South Africa Nelson Mandela pointed out that *ubuntu* does allow for people to address themselves as long as this enables the community around them to improve (Morgan & Ojo 2008). For a more critical exploration of *ubuntu* refer to Chapter 1.

Tourism

Tourism is a complex phenomenon. Attempting to define it can be compared to the problems evoked by anthropologists trying to define 'culture' (Wallace 2005) or occupational therapists and scientists attempting to put a definition on 'occupation'. However, in this chapter, on the one hand we value tourism as a 'very particular kind of acting in the world, as real and important in its own right as any other pursuit' (Chambers 2005, p. 43). On the

other hand 'tourism' refers to a particular industry with worldwide occurrence and impact, and of tremendous economic importance (Stronza 2001). Greenwood described tourism as 'the largest scale movement of goods, services, and people that humanity perhaps has ever seen' (1989, p. 171). It also involves face-to-face encounters between people of different cultural backgrounds (Stronza 2001). Lett (1989) credited tourism with bringing about 'the single largest peaceful movement of people across cultural boundaries in the history of the world' (p. 275).

Some, however, argue that tourism has negative effects for local communities (Wallace 2005). Consider for example Reid's definitive assertion that tourism is a dynamic force homogenizing societies and commodifying cultures across the globe (2003). Munt (1994) observed that '[w]hile mass tourism has attracted trenchant criticism as a shallow and degrading experience for Third World host nations and peoples, new tourism practices, such as eco-tourism and sustainable tourism [see List of websites, p. 207], have been viewed benevolently' (p. 50). Mindful of the reported concerns and risks associated with tourism, SOBW embraces a responsible approach to tourism (see Boxes 21.2 and 21.3), 'one in which the act of tourism is clearly recognized' and 'instead of aspiring to be better than mere tourists, why not strive to being better tourists' (Chambers 2005, p. 43), *ubuntourists*, perhaps?

Box 21.2

Responsible tourism: definition

The Cape Town Declaration (2002) defines responsible tourism as tourism which:

1. minimizes negative economic, environmental and social impacts
2. generates greater economic benefits for local people and enhances the wellbeing of host communities
3. improves working conditions and access to the industry
4. involves local people in decisions that affect their lives and life chances
5. makes positive contributions to the conservation of natural and cultural heritage embracing diversity
6. provides more enjoyable experiences for tourists through more meaningful connections with local people, a greater understanding of local cultural, social and environmental issues
7. provides access for physically challenged people
8. is culturally sensitive, encourages respect between tourists and hosts, and builds local pride and confidence.

Box 21.3

ubuntourism: working definition

A participatory form of responsible tourism that is about co-creating unique opportunities for dignified mutually meaningful and beneficial engagements between interested people in local communities and domestic and/or international visitors who are differently situated in terms of lived privileges.

To conceptualize the latter, we find particularly useful Smith's broad interpretation of a tourist as 'someone who is free to (voluntarily) leave his/her place of home in anticipation of experiencing a change' (Smith 1989).

Ubuntourism

The conceptualization and practice of **ubunt**ourism are inspired and informed by concepts such as social and community participation, respect for cultural diversity, human rights, political and economic empowerment and also by *occupational perspectives* of people's wellbeing (Frank & Zemke 2008, Kronenberg & Pollard 2006). The latter is based on the premise that participation in dignified and meaningful occupations of daily life is fundamental to all people's experience of health and wellbeing, as is their basic need and right to food, to belong, and to love (Kronenberg 2009). As indicated earlier, the pervasive legacies of apartheid continue to largely privilege historically advantaged groups in terms of access to dignified and meaningful occupations of daily life in South Africa. The diverse groups of people (ethnically, culturally, languages, religious beliefs) that make up its population by and large continue to live separately. **Ubunt**ourism concerns itself with people who are unequally situated in terms of lived privileges and everyday realities; what they really (want to) know and/or need to know about each other; to what extent they are open to engage with each other, and how? Based on a firm belief in *ubuntu* and the transformative power of every day occupations and sharing stories, **ubunt**ourism – see working definition in Box 21.3 – aims to help activate participants' occupational consciousness (see Chapter 1) of their lived histories and everyday experiences. This holds the potential to contribute to overcoming fear and ignorance, reconciling past and present differences, and finding common ground to engage in *collective story-making* that advances the larger purpose of building post-apartheid South Africa. All this requires participants to develop their capacity to suspend, to 'see their seeing', to see things freshly, stopping their habitual ways of thinking and perceiving (Senge et al 2004).

Smith (1989) describes typical tourism dynamics as hosts–guests interactions, which tend to be asymmetric in terms of power, with guests having the upper hand in determining how any given encounter unfolds. Further, ethnographic accounts have shown that the gaze of tourists can be especially influential in determining how hosts look, behave, and feel (Urry 1990). Generally, hosts are portrayed in these interactions as passive, unable to influence events, as if they themselves were somehow physically locked in the gaze of the tourist. What is missing in these analyses is the possibility that locals can, and often do, play a role in determining what happens in their encounters with tourists (Stronza 2001). A distinctive quality of **ubunt**ourism is that it invites participants to play with the dominant dynamics described here. We call it **ubunt**ourism *ABC–Z*. The letters refer to different engagement possibilities:

A – visitors host locals

B – locals host visitors

C–Z – locals and visitors identify a common purpose and work together to realize it.

A and B follow a (collective) story-telling format, where the hosting party freely shares of/about themselves. C–Z are about collective story-making (see SOBW website, p. 207), and will only come about if the participants express an interest to embark on a joint journey based on the relationship that came about during the A and B encounters. All **ubunt**ourism participants are regarded as 'travel companions' and their roles of hosts and guests are interchangeable, as they are invited to act as both. SOBW acknowledges that this may pose a delicate balancing act between all participants' roles, expectations, and motivations, but we also believe in learning through practicing **ubunt**ourism.

ubuntourism's domestic and international visitors include students/educators/researchers who are interested to learn from and generate contextually relevant knowledge and practices with locals; tourists that seek 'equal playing field' encounters with locals; and special interest groups from the sectors of business, government, and/or civic society.

Although Bockhoven mainly argued a case in point for occupational therapists, his apparent appreciation of everyday occupations as 'a neglected source of community re-humanization' (1972, p. 219) connects with **ubun**tourism's use of these. Everyday occupations of shared interest and/or need serve as a point of departure for bringing people together. The act of tourism is also an example. Visitors to Cape Town want to experience the main tourism sites. It is, however, likely that some of the locals have never had a chance to visit these. Costs may constitute one obstacle, but possibly also internalized perceptions that those sites were 'no-go areas' during apartheid, enforced by the Pass laws (1952), which severely limited the movements of the non-white populace (South African History Organization (SAHO) 2009). This allows visitors to act as hosts to locals, inviting them to accompany them to for example Table Mountain, Robben Island, Cape Point National Park, District Six Museum, or the wine lands. Other examples include the preparation and sharing of food, engaging in conversation, and other social interactions in public or commercial spaces and/or at people's homes. Another possibility is to connect people based on a shared passion, which might be profession or culture oriented (sports, music, dance, expression, etc.) (Ackermann 2008b).

Experience 2: International occupational justice symposium and think tank

The best way to learn about another culture is to meet the professionals in one's own field.

Isaac Stern in From Mao to Mozart(1979)

Although this unique event was not informed by the concept of **ubun**tourism, it does offer a powerful affirmation of its potential as a vehicle for activating occupational consciousness. During 7–10 July 2009, the first ever international occupational science symposium and think tank to be hosted in Africa, took place in Cape Town. Its focus was 'Relevance of an occupational justice perspective in Africa and beyond'. Since 2003, the first author has participated in similar meetings in Europe, Australia, Canada, and the United States. Whereas previous think tanks seemed to have been mainly preoccupied with matters concerning professional and institutional interests, the emphasis of this meeting was on connecting with what matters to people in the local (Cape Town) and regional contexts (Southern Africa) (Conference Management Centre 2009).

Instead of being overly prescriptive and structured, the program's participatory nature and the rather diverse backgrounds of the participants (race, nationality, age, gender, social status, religion, etc.) allowed meaningful engagements with the participants' lived experiences of the very complex and confrontational realities to which the term 'occupational justice' refers. The participants from the local communities were first invited by the community of professionals to take part in the symposium at their 'institutional turf' – the University of Cape Town, followed by the think tank which started with the professionals being welcomed in the (township) communities of Lavender Hill and Khayelitsha, respectively, to engage with people at the programs *Facing-Up* (Galvaan 2004, 2006) and Grandmothers Against Poverty and Aids (GAPA; see List of websites, p. 207, Brodrick 2004; see also Chapters 8 and 19). The fact that diverse voices and genres, representing both popular and professional discourses informed our evolving understanding of bringing about more contextually relevant practices may have constituted a good example of occupational justice in action (see ISOS website report, p. 207).

From an **ubun**tourism perspective, the participants can be viewed to have acted as *ubuntourists*: they were both hosts and guests and they accepted the invitations to leave their familiar physical, mental and/or institutional/professional homes to experience a change, i.e., occupational consciousness, shifting mindsets, etc. This involved risk taking, exposing personal and professional experiences of discomfort with (occupational) injustices, acknowledging 'not knowing', and suspension of habitual ways of thinking and perceiving. Ramose indicated that 'an ubuntu African understanding of justice as balance and harmony demands the restoration of justice by reversing dehumanizing consequences of colonial conquest and by eliminating racism' (2001, p. 1). Within this context, conceptualizing and operationalizing 'occupational justice' ultimately requires people who are unequally situated in terms of lived privileges to first collectively connect with and acknowledge what was and continues to be wrong, before they can plot a way forward to restore justice.

What struck the second author about this event is the extent to which, with our different expertise, mindsets, social positions, and age, no one could be disempowered by the experience. Upset, challenged … absolutely! Often shared conceptually intensive spaces between professionals and communities with whom they work leave community members unable to identify what contribution they have been able to make. This did not happen here, it could not happen. Even though as organizers we hoped for really meaningful shared experiences, we could not guarantee this would happen. I think part of what worked was the fact that individuals from communities we engaged with, through their own power, contributed as they wished to. This included defining terminology in the way they saw fit. An example of this is when GAPA's Executive Director Vivienne Budaza in translating occupational justice to grandmothers in Isixhosa said *'doing well with you'*. As far as empowerment goes, I think very few things beat communities owning the language they use.

Here are some participants' testimonies regarding the question: 'What experience or aspect of the event had the main impact on your unfolding life story?':

> The involvement of communities in what would typically be an 'academic' exercise brought a different dimension to the symposium. Everyone who was there would attest to the fact that when the 'academics' struggled to find answers to very complex issues emanating from discussions about occupational injustice (past and present), the Community Elders from GAPA and Auntie Ellen almost always provided a way forward with the opinions they shared largely because they have lived to experience, with most academics/professionals in the room having experienced to theorize. That surely made the biggest mark for me.
>
> Nick Matyida – UCT lecturer in occupational therapy

> What came out vividly is that, this symposium and think tank marked a new chapter in future of the relationship between the West and the African 'Occupationals' (Occupational Therapists, Occupational Scientists, and Occupational Practitioners). For once the West had a chance to try on the 'big shoes' of occupational injustice that the South dons everyday and even runs on daily. Now transformation is perceptible with the acceptance of apartheid propped white privilege, abandonment of the usual 'cynicism' which characterizes such forums, discarding the culture of individualism hence embracing the true spirit of 'ubuntourism' and the desertion of the black identity that is solely based on the ideology of victim hood. All the above came to be during the symposium and think tank. The Lwandle soccer friendly scenario can be adapted and used in other areas that are bent in uniting the West and the South.
>
> Patrice Malonza – occupational therapist from Botswana

A highlight for me and the grandmothers was interacting with occupational therapists from such diverse backgrounds. Being given the opportunity to tell your story and understand your experience from different perspectives can be incredibly enlightening, particularly when it is facilitated in a manner of shared learning. The honesty and transparency portrayed by participants during the symposium was also amazing. Rich information sharing with regard to our political background and the platform created was a once more wonderful opportunity for reconciliation and healing for a better South Africa.

Vivienne Budaza – Executive Director of GAPA

The journey forward …

> When you're on a journey, and the end keeps getting further and further away, then you realize that the real end is the journey.
>
> Karlfried Graf Dürckheim in Campbell 1988, p. 230

Ubuntourism is still in the early stages of development and its contextual conditions are riddled with challenging contradictions. Although a 2004 government survey data point to increasing levels of social cohesion, in terms of unity, coherence, functionality, and pride among South Africans, this is drawn back by the legacy of inequality, intense migratory trends, rising crime rates related to social conditions and vestiges of racism (PCAS, Social Sector, Presidency 2006). What **ubun**tourism is about doesn't fit the conventional molds of either occupational therapy or tourism, but it attempts to merge a practice of both, that is to be contextually relevant and self-sustainable. For this to happen, firstly, we follow a more collective *ubuntu* African understanding of human occupation – going beyond its traditional and dominant individualistic interpretations and applications (that is, within the discourse and practices of occupational therapy and occupational science) (see Chapter 1). Alternatively, we propose to conceptualize and operationalize 'human occupation' as 'building and maintaining working relationships' (Ramugondo & Kronenberg 2010). Our main role (SOBW) would then be, first, to help build and maintain working relationships with and between divided groups of people (and other relevant stakeholders), whose engagements may result in discovering a shared purpose to be advanced through collective story-making. Second, to allow **ubun**tourism to further develop and to sustain itself, we (SOBW) intend to make it a social enterprise. Simply put, this is a business that trades for social and environmental purposes and its profits are reinvested to sustain and further a mission for positive change

(Bornstein 2007). Examples of social enterprises are the *Big Issue*, Jamie Oliver's restaurant Fifteen and Braille without Borders' International Institute for Social Entrepreneurs (see List of websites, p. 207). Bill Drayton, who has been credited as the 'godfather of social entrepreneurship' (Gergen 2006) captured the spirit – which Jane Addams, early day social innovator and one of the founders of occupational therapy, embodied when she started Hull House in Chicago in 1889 (Schwartz 2009) – that **ubun**tourism attempts to tap into: 'Social entrepreneurs are not content to give a fish or teach how to fish. They will not rest until they have revolutionized the fishing industry.' It requires us to learn about blending value business models that combine a revenue-generating business – to ensure our continued survival and to invest in our aims – with a social-value-generating structure or component – assessing success in terms of the impact **ubun**tourism has on society (Elkington & Hartigan 2008, see also Chapter 1).

Rather than knowing where all this will go, we must trust the journey. **ubun**tourism then can be viewed as a bag of seeds for which we must find the most appropriate soil to plant and grow. Experiences to date taught us that attempting to establish a viable partnership with a particular community, for example Lwandle, proved to be very difficult. Although it is easy to speak of community, this usually has many benign connotations, often its meaning and to whom it refers seems at best unclear and contested at worst (Pollard et al 2008, 2010). A reality check teaches that it is hardly ever homogeneous and within it likely exist multiple groups with conflicting interests. The 2008/2009 xenophobic attacks on township residents from other African countries, such as Zimbabwe and Somalia, in South Africa are but one example of this reality (Consortium for Refugees and Migrants in South Africa (CoRMSA) 2008, Mail & Guardian-online 2009). Hence, without letting go of the intention to connect with and benefit the larger community, the 'soil' in which to plant **ubun**tourism's seeds is 'common ground' (including trust) we have and seek with individuals (friends, colleagues, other interested parties, including organizations) from the various communities that make up the diverse and divided population in and surrounding the Cape Town metropolis. These include but are not limited to Africans, coloreds, Indians, whites of Afrikaner and English descent, foreigners, and also representing different religions (e.g., Muslims, Christians), urban and rural communities, people living with disabilities, organizations, and businesses. Although in this context race continues to be the most obvious dividing factor, we intend to include broad human characteristics that can contribute to the building of this new country, such as religion, (dis)ability, age, gender, class, etc.

In addition, encounters can be documented in a variety of ways to allow these to become part of history in the making, using an approach akin to Brecher's 'history from below', which Terkel said 'enables "ordinary" people, non-academics, to recover their own personal and community's pasts' (Brecher 1997). These documentations would also provide us with means to share and communicate what we are learning and creating with people in other parts of the world.

Although **ubun**tourism originated and developed in the context of Southern Africa, we anticipate that meaningfully engaging divided people around a common purpose will have worldwide relevance and applicability. And we are open to share our learning with interested parties … preferably as *ubuntourists*.

The victory of democracy in South Africa is the common achievement of all humanity.

(Nelson Mandela 1995)

Acknowledgments

The explorative stages that gave birth to **ubun**tourism were made possible with a part of the royalties from the 2005 publication *Occupational Therapy without Borders: Learning from the Spirit of Survivors*. The first author expresses gratitude to fellow editors Salvador Simó Algado and Nick Pollard and to all the contributors and readers who purchased this book.

This chapter presents an adapted version of two papers that were presented at the Society of Applied Anthropology meeting in March 2009 in Santa Fe, New Mexico ('Addressing Occupational Apartheid Through **ubun**tourism in Cape Town') and at the International Occupational Justice Symposium in July 2009 in Cape Town, South Africa ('**ubun**tourism: Engaging with What Matters to People in Context').

References

Ackermann K: *Lwandle Magic: Township Soccer and Tourism*, 2008a. Online Available at: http://afrikatourism. blogspot.com/2008/02/lwandle-magic-township-soccer-and.html Accessed November 18, 2009.

Ackermann K: *Ubuntourism Music Experience in Lwandle*, 2008b. Online Available at: http://afrikatourism. blogspot.com/2008/12/ubuntourism-music-experience-in-lwandle.html. Accessed November 18, 2009.

African Leadership Forum: *The challenges of post apartheid South Africa*, 1991, *Conclusions and papers presented at a conference of the African Leadership Forum, 17 July, Windhoek/Namibia*, Online. Available at: http://www. africaleadership.org/PDFs/ 1991report/The%20Challenges% 20of%20Post-Apartheid%20South% 20Africa.pdf. November 18, 2009.

African National Congress NC: *Historical Documents – Apartheid and the International Community*, 1991. Online Available at: http://www.anc. org.za/ancdocs/history/. Accessed November 18, 2009.

Beinart W: *Twentieth-century South Africa*, Oxford, 1994, Oxford University Press.

Bockhoven JS: Occupational therapy: a neglected source of community re-humanization. In *Moral Treatment in Community Mental Health*, New York, 1972, Springer, p 219.

Bornstein D: *How to Change the World: Social Entrepreneurs and the Power of New Ideas*, Oxford, 2007, Oxford University Press.

Brecher J: *History From Below: How to Uncover and Tell the Story of Your Community, Association, or Union*, (Revised Edition), New Haven, 1997, Commonwork/Advocate Press Online Available at: http://www. stonesoup.coop/historybelow/ historybelow.htm. Accessed November 24, 2009.

Brodrick K: Grandmothers affected by HIV/AIDS: new roles and occupations. In Watson R, Swartz L, editors: *Transformation Through Occupation*, London, 2004, Whurr.

Campbell J: *The Power of Myth with Bill Moyers*, New York, 1988, Doubleday.

Cape Town Declaration: *The Cape Town Conference on Responsible Tourism in Destinations*, 2002. Online Available at: http://www.icrtourism.org/ Capetown.shtml. Accessed November 24, 2009.

Chambers E: Can the anthropology of tourism make us better travelers? In Wallace T, editor: *Tourism and Applied Anthropologists: Linking Theory and Practice*, 2005, Napa Bulletin, p 23.

Conference Management Centre: *Preamble to Occupational Justice Symposium and Think Tank*, 7 July 2009 to 10 July 2009, Cape Town, 2009, University of Cape Town, Online Available at: http://www.uct-cmc.co. za/Conferences/conf-info.asp? Info_ID=168&Conf_ID= 98&Page =Info. Accessed November 25, 2009.

Consortium for Refugees and Migrants in South Africa. Press release: *Xenophobic attacks 'not a crisis'?*, 2008. Press release, 15th May 2008 Online. Available at: http:// 209.85.229.132/search?q=cache: Qo7r0V-Ajv4J:www.cormsa.org.za/ wp-content/uploads/2008/06/ cormsa-press-release-xenophobic-attacks-not-a-crisis.doc+xenophobic +attacks+2008+lwandle&cd= 4&hl=en&ct=clnk. Accessed November 18, 2009.

Elkington J, Hartigan P: *The Power of Unreasonable People: How Social Entrepreneurs Create Markets That Change the World*, Boston, 2008, Harvard Business Press.

Frank G, Zemke R: Occupational therapy foundations for political engagement and social transformation. In Pollard N, Sakellariou D, Kronenberg F, editors: *Political Practice of Occupational Therapy*, Edinburgh, 2008, Elsevier Science.

Frommer's: *Introduction in Cape Town*, 2009. Online. Available at: http:// www.frommers.com/destinations/ capetown/0202010001.html. Accessed November 25, 2009.

Galvaan R: Engaging with youth at risk. In Watson R, Swartz L, editors: *Transformation Through Occupation*, London, 2004, Whurr, pp 186–197.

Galvaan R: Role-emerging settings, service learning and social change. In Lorenzo T, Duncan M, Alsop A, editors: *Practice and Service Learning*

in *Occupational Therapy: Enhancing Potential in Context*, West Sussex, 2006, Whurr, pp 103–117.

Gergen D: *The New Engines of Reform*, 2006. US News and World Report Online Available at: http://www. usnews.com/usnews/biztech/ articles/060220/20gergen.htm. Accessed November 18, 2009.

Greenwood DJ: Culture by the pound: an anthropological perspective on tourism as cultural commoditization. In Smith V, editor: *Hosts and Guests: An Anthropology of Tourism*, Pittsburgh, PA, 1989, University Press, p 171.

Hendricks F: Inter-personal Racism after Apartheid, *CODESRIA Bulletin Nos.* 1 & 2: 2002. Online. Available at: http://www.codesria.org/Links/ Publications/bulletin/ Bulletin1&2_2002_english_.pdf. Accessed November 18, 2009

Iwama MK: Occupation as a cross-cultural construct. In Whiteford LG, Wright-St Clair V, editors: *Occupation and Practice in Context*, Marrickvile, New South Wales, 2005, Elsevier, pp 242–253.

Joseph JA: Public values in a divided world: a mandate for higher education, *Liberal Education* 88: Online Available at: http://www. thefreelibrary.com/Public+ values+in+a+divided+world:+ a+mandate+for+higher+ education.+...-a089022311. Accessed November 18, 2009.

Katjavivi PH: *A tribute to the international anti-apartheid/ solidarity movement*, 2004 Talk delivered at 'A Decade of Freedom' Conference. Durban, South Africa, 10–13 October 2004. Online Available at: http://scnc.ukzn.ac.za/ doc/AAmwebsite/ AAMCONFpapers/Katjavivi,P.doc. Accessed November 18, 2009.

Kronenberg F: *From Apolitical Practice to a Political Practice of Occupational Therapy*, Thieme, Stuttgart, 2009, Ergoscience.

Kronenberg F, Pollard N: Political dimensions of occupation and the roles of occupational therapy. Plenary Address at the 2006 AOTA conference in Charlotte/NC, *Am J Occup Ther* 60:617–625, 2006.

Kurin R: *Reflections of a Cultural Broker: A View from the Smithsonian,* Washington, 1997, Smithsonian Institution Press.

Lerner M: *From Mao to Mozart: Isaac Stern in China. A documentary film about Western culture breaking into China,* United States, 1979.

Lett J: Epilogue. In Smith V, editor: *Hosts and Guests: An Anthropology of Tourism,* Pittsburgh, PA, 1989, University Press, p 275.

Lim KH: Occupational therapy in multi-cultural contexts. Letter to the editor, *British Journal of Occupational Therapy* 67:49–50, 2004.

Magadlela D: Ubuntu: Myth or antidote to today's socio-political and leadership challenges? *ThoughtLeader Blog entry,* 2008, Wednesday, January 9th, 2008. Online Available at: http://www.thoughtleader.co.za/dumisanimagadlela/2008/01/09/ubuntu-myth-or-antidote-to-today%E2%80%99s-socio-political-and-leadership-challenges/. Accessed November 18, 2009.

Mail & Guardian-online: *De Doorns Quiet After Xenophobic Incident,* 2009. Online Available at: http://www.mg.co.za/article/2009-11-18-de-doorns-quiet-after-xenophobic-incident. Accessed November 18, 2009.

Mandela N: *Long walk to freedom – quotes,* 1995. Online Available at: http://refspace.com/users/roadrunner/Long_Walk_to_Freedom. Accessed November 24, 2009.

Matabane K: *Conversations on a Sunday afternoon,* Johannesburg, 2005, Matabane Filmworks Online Available at: http://www.moviesite.co.za/2006/1020/conversations.html. Accessed November 18, 2008.

Mbembe A: *Passages to Freedom: The Politics of Racial Reconciliation in South Africa,* 2008. Online Available at: http://publicculture.dukejournals.org/cgi/reprint/20/1/5.pdf. Accessed November 18, 2009.

Memorable Quotes for The Commitments: 1991, Online Available at:http://www.imdb.com/title/tt0101605/quotes. Accessed November 18, 2009.

Merriam-Webster: *Apartheid,* 2009. Online Available at: http://www.merriam-webster.com/dictionary/Apartheid. Accessed November 18, 2009.

Morgan D, Ojo E: *Women in Africa's development: pushing for progress through entrepreneurship education complimented by on-going coaching sessions – A case study paper.* Presented at The Fifth Pan-Commonwealth Forum on Open Learning 13–17 July , UK, 2008, University of London. Online Available at: http://wikieducator.org/images/3/3f/PCF5_63.pdf. Accessed November 18, 2009.

Munt I: Eco-tourism or ego-tourism? *Race Class* 36:49–60, 1994.

Nussbaum B: African culture and Ubuntu: reflections of a South African in America. World Business Academy rekindling the human spirit in business, *Perspectives* 17: 2003. Online Available at: http://www.barbaranussbaum.com/downloads/perspectives.pdf. Accessed November 18, 2009.

Ozinsky CH: *Township tourism booming in South Africa: Beyond safaris, visitors attracted to the authentic, urban scene,* 2007. Online Available at: http://www.msnbc.msn.com/id/16563904/. Accessed November 18, 2009.

Passport Day: *Poverty Tourism,* 2009. Online Available at: http://www.passportday.com/Poverty_tourism/. Accessed November 18, 2009.

Platzky L, Walker C: *The Surplus People: Forced Removals in South Africa,* Johannesburg, 1985, Raven Press.

Policy Coordination and Advisory Services – Social Sector The Presidency: *A Nation in the making – A discussion document on macro-social trends in South Africa,* 2006. Online Available at: http://www.info.gov.za/otherdocs/2006/socioreport.pdf. Accessed November 18, 2009.

Pollard N, Sakellariou D, Kronenberg F, editors: *Political Practice of Occupational Therapy,* Edinburgh, 2008, Elsevier Science.

Pollard N, Sakellariou D, Kronenberg F: Community development. In Curtin M, Molineux M, Supyk-Mellson J, editors: *Occupational Therapy and Physical Dysfunction,* ed 6, Oxford, 2010, Churchill Livingstone-Elsevier, pp 267–280.

Ramose MB: *An African Understanding on Justice and Race,* 2001. Online Available at: http://them.polylog.org/3/frm-en.htm. Accessed November 18, 2009.

Ramugondo EL: *Intergenerational shifts and continuities in children's play within a rural Venda family in the 20th and 21st centuries,* Unpublished PhD dissertation. Cape Town. 2009, University of Cape Town.

Ramugondo E, Kronenberg F: *Collective occupations: a vehicle for building & maintaining working relationships,* Paper presentation at 15th World Federation of Occupational Therapists Congress. Chile, 2010, Santiago de Chile.

Reid DG: *Tourism, Globalization, and Development: Responsible Tourism Planning,* London, 2003, Pluto Press.

Schwartz KB: Reclaiming our heritage: connecting the founding vision to the centennial vision. Eleanor Clarke Slagle Lecture at the 2006 AOTA conference in Houston/TX, *Am J Occup Ther* 63:681–690, 2009.

Senge P, Scharmer CO, Haworski J, Flowers BS: *Presence. Exploring Profound Change in People, Organizations and Society,* London, 2004, Nicholas Brealey Publishing.

Shutte A: *Philosophy for Africa,* Cape Town, 1993, University of Cape Town Press.

Smith V, editor: *Hosts and Guests: The Anthropology of Tourism,* ed 2, Philadelphia, 1989, University Pennsylvania Press.

South African Government: *Preamble – Constitution of the Republic of South Africa,* 1996. Online Available at: http://www.info.gov.za/documents/constitution/1996/96preamble.htm Accessed November 18, 2009.

South African History Organization: *Pass Laws in South Africa,* 2009. Online Available at:http://www.sahistory.org.za/pages/governance-projects/apartheid-repression/pass-laws.htm Accessed November 25, 2009.

Stronza A: Anthropology of tourism: forging new ground for ecotourism and other alternatives, *Annual Review of Anthropology* 30:261–283, 2001.

Swanson D: Ubuntu: An African contribution to (re)search for/with a 'humble togetherness', *Journal of Contemporary Issues in Education* 2:53–67, 2007. Online Available at: http://ejournals.library.ualberta.ca/index.php/JCIE/article/viewFile/1028/686. Accessed November 18, 2009.

Telschow M: *Townships and the Spirit of Ubuntu,* Cape Town, 2003, Clifton Publications.

Tutu D: *Ubuntu (Philosophy)*, 2008. Online Available at:http://en. wikipedia.org/wiki/Ubuntu_ (philosophy) Accessed November 18, 2009.

Urry J: *The Tourist Gaze: Leisure and Travel in Contemporary Societies*, London, 1990, Sage.

Wallace T: Introduction: tourism, tourists, and anthropologists at work. In Wallace T, editor: *Tourism and Applied Anthropologists: Linking*

Theory and Practice, 2005, Napa Bulletin, p 23.

Watson R, Swartz L, editors: *Transformation through Occupation*, London, 2004, Whurr, p 63.

Watson R, Fourie M: Occupation and occupational therapy. In Watson R, Swartz L, editors: *Transformation through Occupation*, London, 2004, Whurr, p 20.

Witz L: Museums on Cape Town's township tours. In Murray N,

Shepherd N, Hall M, editors: *Desire Lines*, London, 2007, Routledge.

Witz L: *Museums, sustainability and memories of apartheid*, 2008, Leslie Witz, History Department, University of the Western Cape. Talk delivered on the occasion of International Museums Day at the McGregor Museum, Kimberley, 19 May 2008.

Websites

Big Issue: http://www.bigissue.com

Ecotourism: http://www.ecotourism.org/

Fifteen: http://www.fifteen.net

Global Partnership for Sustainable Tourism Criteria: http://www.sustainabletourismcriteria.org/

Grandmothers Against Poverty and Aids: http://www.gapa.org.za

International Centre for Responsible Tourism: http://www.icrtourism.org/

International Institute for Social Entrepreneurs: http://www.braillewithoutborders.org

International Society for Occupational Science: http://isos.nfshost.com/

Ishabi: http://www.ishabi.co.za

Lwandle Migrant Labour Museum: http://www.lwandle.com

Shades of Black Works: http://www.shades-of-black.co.za

Ubuntourism: http://www.ubuntourism.org

Brazilian experiences in social occupational therapy

22

Denise Dias Barros   Maria Isabel Garcez Ghirardi
Roseli Esquerdo Lopes   Sandra Maria Galheigo

OVERVIEW

This chapter seeks to present the basis of social occupational therapy in Brazil. Understanding that theory and practice must be intertwined, feeding each other in a dialogical way, it intends to provide glimpses of practices and the foundations upon which these experiences have been carried out. Occupational therapy in the social field has to take a different stance: it has to put aside the negative aspects which these people have been usually associated with. Thus, it has the tendency to make exclusion visible and seek to value the difference, taking into account the social networks as the axis of the relational support to be strengthened. In order to do that, occupational therapists in the social field have to understand the dynamics of social interchange and learn communication codes and meanings central to each community. Also, it has to consider the social role that human activities play as a means of emancipation and rewriting of life stories, narratives and contexts. Experiences will be presented as representative practical case studies inside boxes, such as street people's political organization, social and cultural activities; youth vulnerability; labor co-ops and community projects.

Introduction

Occupational therapy in Brazil has developed a particular field of knowledge and practice for the last 10 years, which has come to be called social occupational therapy. Those who have been involved with the development of practices and theoretical foundations in this particular field, such as the members of Project Metuia, argue that the so-called 'social field'

asks for a particular reading of social reality and the problems endured by some populations, as it will be presented here (see Chapter 34). Addressing their conditions in research, practice, and teaching requires the use of appropriate methodologies to understand the inner dynamics and organizations of social groups such as urban/rural youth, street people, and specific cultural contexts. This has demanded the development of tools to interpret the connections between personal and social realities, and thus enable innovative occupational therapy practices. It has also called for the engagement into counter-hegemonic activities which may provide alternative paths to appalling life conditions.

This chapter intends to present some of the challenges faced by Brazilian occupational therapy posed by its recent history in dealing with problems that derive from important social issues such as lack of access to social goods and social policies, violence, challenges brought by cultural diversity, the relationship between urban and rural areas, to mention a few. It also explores some theoretical frames which may provide consistency for practice and experiences which may give the theory some substance.

To start, it is necessary to give a brief historical account of the two landmark events, which gave rise to the development of social occupational therapy in Brazil. The first important event was the revision of professional principles, which started at the end of 1970 when social issues were incorporated into occupational therapy curricula. This continued during the 1980s when the academic debate was strengthened. This period of time inaugurated a discussion on the responsibility of the practitioners in the production of social values, and in their engagement on social

DOI: 10.1016/B978-0-7020-3103-8.00031-6

transformation – a demand for a social and politically engaged professional and a claim to commit occupational therapists into the major national move towards the restructuring of the major social policies. The promotion of citizenship became a parameter for an alternative occupational therapy practice and theory (Galheigo 1997, 2003, Lopes 1999). At that time, citizenship became a key concept for the new social movements and policy makers in Brazil (Paoli 1992); a concept understood as the result of a constant social struggle for human rights instead of being considered an expected consequence of the capitalist system or a natural evolution of societies (Marshall & Bottomore 1992). In parallel, there were some questions raised about the usage of the medical and psychological knowledge inasmuch as social problems were usually alienated from their own structurally social and political causes and explained as personal matters. As a consequence, the way social and relational conflicts were addressed as medical problems and the power given to medicine to propose solutions to societies, both were widely challenged.

The second historical landmark development for the emergence of social occupational therapy was the result of continuing confrontation with the contradictions endured by societies such as in Brazil, marked by an intense rise in social inequality. New demands that needed to be addressed were consequently brought about by the growing numbers of people experiencing severe dissolution of familial and social bonds, followed by the weakening of social networks and the insecurity at work, due to social changes in labor relations brought about by the rising of neo-liberalism in the 1990s.

Addressing vulnerability and disaffiliation by open settings approaches

In Brazil the severance of occupational therapy from the biomedical model and the health-disease processes inaugurated a new domain in terms of the production of knowledge and alternative practices after the 1990s. Also, as inequality continues to have an important and deteriorating impact on Brazilian society there is a continuous demand for alternative practices to address the concerns of people living in vulnerable conditions and those experiencing disaffiliation (Castel 1999). The intensity of the social

problems, which appears in various forms, depends on the degree of belonging/not belonging to a family or the degree of communal sociability and the effectiveness of the social support network these people may access (see Chapter 6). Thus the situation when viewed as a whole may indicate a condition of vulnerability or disaffiliation that requires a different type of action.

In this context, work, besides being an economic necessity, is understood as an important medium for articulating relationships, cultural, and social values, and is the principle underlying the organization of work cooperatives for people under the care of occupational therapists in Brazil (Box 22.1).

One of the origins of social occupational therapy in Brazil is connected to the implementation of interventions in community and territorial settings. This open settings context has required different methodologies to attend the specific needs and challenges of a particular setting. One of its most relevant contributions has been the emphasis on collective action and the relations between person, group, community, and society.

Community intervention

The concept of community, as used by Metuia, is related to the sense of belonging and refers to shared identities which take place in social spaces (Santos 1995). Some of Metuia's interventions were designed in specific urban and rural community contexts. Casa Rosa was a two-year youth and women project in a touristic place in Minas Gerais, which was set up in response to a demand by the local women for discussions regarding issues of citizenship involving their young people. In this example of community intervention, Metuia contributed to the organization of the dynamic and the first stages in the establishment of a culture center and a library, both of which are now fully managed by the local association (Vecchia et al 2005). Such community programs are based on the fact that this approach allows more democratic and accountable policy making. Because the community is involved in the decisions, these community programs provide a sense of accomplishment and satisfy real needs and, by doing so, enhance the sense of belonging and solidarity.

However, the ability of a community to engage in participatory action can vary greatly. First, community members may have different and divergent expectations and levels of commitment. Second,

Box 22.1

Occupational therapy, work cooperatives, and the creation of value

In 2002, a group of occupational therapy students at the Universidade de São Paulo (USP), inspired by the debates in their classes, set up a proposal to organize a work cooperative to allow for the exchange of experiences and for the inclusion in the workplace of individuals with various types of disability. This proposal was approved by the Secretaria Estadual do Trabalho (SERT), a board of government appointed experts, which recommended that the program should receive official funding to help implement the work cooperative in São Paulo. The cooperative initially produced handicraft pottery, cloth, and carpets. As a professor at the Occupational Therapy Department at USP, I was invited to beome a technical adviser to this group as the focus of my academic research had been on psychosocial relations in the workplace. I advised the group for two years (2000–2002) on the ways the tenets of occupational therapy might work to shape their practice within the project. The complexities of everyday practices were discussed in their entirety, so as to make it possible to implement means for vulnerable individuals to participate in collective decision-making processes.

A work cooperative is usually a result of an initiative by people who, for different reasons, want to find alternative ways for the production and distribution of market goods. These alternatives posits the cooperation as a starting point for the overcoming of individual differences and it builds on the interdependent character of collective action. Work cooperatives have emerged as a possible way for social inclusion as their power to produce goods and to generate value depends on the very diversity of their members. Having as a starting point the belief that the workplace is a locus for material and affective exchange I have concentrated my social intervention actions for the past two years in a cooperative of artisans, with the aim of enhancing human relations in the workplace and fostering the production of value via the production of market goods. Such cooperative counted, among its members, individuals with different types of handicap. This intervention sought to strengthen collective actions within

the production process so as to break away from everyday relations stigmatized by the idea of handicap. It intended to avoid centering the assessing of the production process on individual performance and to foster collective inter-dependence – not only for the production of goods but also for the daily transformation of the logic of material and affective exchanges. The implementing of an inclusive cooperative of this type was marked by a set of important challenges, once it required a careful reading of market forces as well as a special attention to the human relations within the work cooperative; both potentially tended to replicate forms of social exclusion. Thus with a permanent focus on collective work a series of actions were taken to involve cooperative members in a perception of cooperative work. They were based on an understanding that individual capabilities and limits are an integral part of a collective production process. Mixed groups, which included individuals with different handicaps, with little or no experience as a participant in the labor market, debated extensively the collective norms acting as guidelines for the production and distribution of market goods. That was crucial to counter a logic which focuses on the handicap and which tends to be reinforced by blaming individuals for the difficulties intrinsic to the production process. It is paramount that occupational therapy builds methods of intervention centering on collective work and the production of social value as a means for overcoming social exclusion. Such methods have to take into account the economic values in a highly specialized market so as to be capable of fostering a positive collective perspective which may lead to going beyond tutelage and to producing life autonomy and social production via labor. By being structured as a small business, work cooperatives become highly complex social intervention entities which accept 'the challenge of creating nexuses between what social processes bring as a demand and the scholarly debate occupational therapy has produced on the concept and implications of labor as *mediation*' (Barros et al 2002a).

---

there may be local divisions because of cultural, ethnic, and religious issues, personal interests, and social status. Third, there may be differences in people's access to goods and services and level of participation in the decision making.

To overcome these possible shortcomings, it is important to bear in mind that collective action and community participation are dynamic and in a permanent state of change. The practice of this methodology is based on the principles of nurturing solidarity bonds and good communication networks, both of which are essential for the maintenance of a strong social fabric. However, they demand a

constant problem-solving approach, based on dialog and the negotiation of coexistence, despite diversities and differences. Also, collective action and community participation require a critical view of social reality and an attitude of nonsubmission to oppressive maneuvers, bringing social and political emancipation to the agenda (Freire 1978, 1979a,b).

Collective intervention, as one of the occupational therapy approaches, allows a change of focus from the individual and group approach to something that takes place on collective grounds. When occupational therapists leave behind the traditional therapeutic settings and engage in the organization of folk parties, community radio programs, community fairs, and recycling projects, their action provokes collective community movements, which contribute to the rearrangement of the local social forces and strengthening of the social network.

Territorial intervention

The notion of territorial intervention was adopted by Brazilian occupational therapists following the 1980s Brazilian Movement of Health Reform and the deinstitutionalization of psychiatric institutions, largely influenced by the Italian Democratic Psychiatry movement (Barros 1994, Rotelli et al 1986). The Brazilian Movement of Health Reform led to the creation of a network of local health units, making the public sector responsible for recognizing and resolving health problems in each territory. The Italian Democratic Psychiatry movement understood territory as a field of action of a mental health team, involving the population of a well-defined geographic area. Both views led to the development of an innovative occupational therapy practice based on the principle of territorial responsibility. This involves the acknowledgment of people's needs within a territory and that strategies should be pursued to fulfill them. This also involves the recognition of the person as someone who has rights, knowledge, and aspirations.

Territory, as it is used here, presupposes a geographic space defined historically with social, economic, cultural, and symbolic relations still to be revealed (Oliver & Barros 1999). In this space, different ways of being, dreaming, aspiring, living, and working may take place and different ways of social exchange may be observed. Inasmuch as life chances are believed to determine people's health chances, health interventions should consider people's *life possibilities*, which take into account the ecological and social environment in which people live (Basaglia & Basaglia 1977, Rotelli 1988).

The notion of territory thus implies the fundamental idea of recognizing the other, of accepting otherness. For that to happen, certain conditions need to be established. First, the use of specialized knowledge should be replaced by the use of a plurality of knowledge on social issues. Second, people's actions should be disassociated from the idea that they may be the result of an ill or deviant body or mind, and should be viewed as the result of the mediation of culture, from which nobody can be separated. Third, occupational therapy action should be

moved from the therapeutic setting to the setting of everyday life. Finally, the concept of activity as an individual process should be replaced by the view of activity as historical and cultural processes lived by people or groups.

Box 22.2 is an example of territorial intervention carried out in the city of São Carlos and designed for young people inasmuch as they are the group most exposed to violence in Brazil.

Culture, conflict, *problematization*, dialog, and process

Social inequality has posed most of the problems addressed by social occupational therapy in Brazil. However, recent social changes have brought about the need to recognize the issues of cultural identity and diversity. Both in Brazil and worldwide, practitioners have been presented with new challenges, and have been required to develop new approaches to accommodate the complex and multiple identities that people can adopt in contemporary life. These social demands have raised dilemmas regarding the tolerance of difference and the resolution of conflicts. Individual and collective interventions need to be understood within their contexts and as elements of historical processes which produce personal and social meanings and often call for cultural negotiation.

Social occupational therapy then interacts with two concepts, which transform part of its action: *culture* and *otherness*. Thinking about culture implies interpreting meanings and seeking for the meanings attributed to things and their inter-relationships to determine which are seen as part of a culture and which are seen as different or Other. This is important because differences (personal, cultural, religious, generational, or gender) that cannot be negotiated may generate stereotypes. Culture is the central basis for the actions developed by a non-governmental organization called *Civil Organization of Social Action* (OCAS) (Box 22.3).

The intensification of social conflicts on local and worldwide scale owing to the unequal distribution of wealth and opportunity, has resulted in social antagonism which has led to much misery, migration, and exclusion. Social conflict has been studied from various sociological, anthropological, philosophical, political, and psychological perspectives. Some conflicts

Box 22.2

Poor youth, violence, and citizenship

This account focuses on the results of university projects that problematized ways of confronting violence experienced by adolescents and youths from urban working-class groups in Brazil. Violence has been considered a relevant complex phenomenon by government agencies, media, researchers, and by the general Brazilian society. The vulnerability of these adolescents and youths, manifested by the various violence indicators, has achieved alarming levels in the country, in the light of largely inadequate, fragmented, and inadequate public policies (Lopes et al 2006b). These projects helped to promote and support both a public school work and a territorial action, seeking to setting up collective action for the social development of urban working-class youth. The focus was the Grande Cidade Aracy Region, in São Carlos, a peripheral region of a medium-sized city of 15 200 inhabitants in the interior of the state of São Paulo, which consists of neighborhoods without an infrastructure, and poorly developed public and private service networks. Taking this situation into account, interventions were carried out using an interdisciplinary and multisectoral approach. Examples are given below.

1. **School Violence and Educational Initiatives**: Mobilizing the projects proposed to encourage the political and educational initiatives, training professionals, collecting data and giving support to the school. Also, the aim was to contribute to the participation and effective inclusion of working-class youth in the schools, considering either those attending school classes or the drop-outs.

2. **Urban Violence and Territory**: The projects proposed to carry out interventions with adolescents, youths, and their families on the theme of violence and the opportunities and perspectives of an autonomous life. The idea was that the youth could identify their needs, organizing themselves to demand social changes on a participatory and democratic basis. Discussion groups on violence were also promoted, educational material on the subject was produced and distributed, with training of human resources in the partner social institutions.

3. **Human Rights Violation and Community Organization**: The projects set out to collect data on local forms of violence and the kind of people who were involved. The database was intended to assist in public policy making and to enable professionals working in similar areas to understand, identify, and prevent the violence and its causes. They also set out to promote interventions based around the activities of the local reference youth services in the region of Grande Cidade Aracy, São Carlos, thus seeking to create strategies to answer individual and collective needs, and promoting and strengthening existing public places (public services, youth facilities, places where young people enjoyed going).

Multimedia resources were an important means of engaging in the dialog with young people. Image and sound formed an intermediary resource in workshops, contributing to the enablement of youth to develop self-knowledge and encouraging the process of belonging to a group. Also, this made the youth's approach easier, and contributed to creating bonds with them, which allowed discussion of new life possibilities (Lopes et al 2002). In order to achieve these goals, we emphasize the necessity of maintaining a perspective of youth agency, wherein youths and teenagers play a major role in how to live their own lives. The projects also intended to develop innovative practices in the social field through participative methodologies, which allowed the establishment of partnerships between the professionals and the youths (individually and in groups). By doing so, they also intended to provoke discussion about the social role of the professionals dealing with the contemporary problems of Brazilian society (Barros et al 2002b). The professionals were connected to research projects and undergraduate and graduate learning programs. The sponsorship by the Ministry of Education of a university program designed to support public policies contributed to the development of these five-year-initiatives with resources such as the payment of occupational therapists, scholarships for undergraduate and graduate students who developed fieldwork, materials and equipments (Lopes & Malfitano 2006, Lopes et al 2006a,b, 2008).

---

happen between individuals and groups and others are related to the social, political, and economic organization around them. Despite the structural characteristics of social conflicts, occupational therapy can help address some questions brought about social and cultural contradictions.

Occupational therapy can make use of strategies of conflict resolution through methodologies of social action. This does not mean taking a top-down approach to an occupational therapy program but the use of dialog to reduce and explore the unknown aspects of the person–therapist relationship. Each person, social group, or community needs to talk about how they understand their situation and the potential available to them. Through this process everybody's knowledge is valued. During this process, practitioners need to appraise their own knowledge besides knowing how to overcome diverse social and cultural relations (Barros 2004).

Box 22.3

OCAS and the *Meeting and Culture Point*

OCAS is a social integration project coordinated by a nongovernmental organization created in 2001 (http://blogdaocas.blogspot.com). Its objective is to provide the means of restoring self-esteem for the people who live in the streets by creating the conditions for these individuals to become the subject of their own transformation. The organization accompanies the work of the magazine *OCAS* and seeks partnerships for housing, education, and health services for the members of the project through a cooperative network with public services, journalists, and nongovernmental organizations (Rede Rua, Projeto Metuia, Grupo de Estudos e Trabalhos Psicodramáticos, Homeless World Cup, International Network of Street Papers).

The *Meeting and Culture Point* is a meeting place and a cultural center for people from different regions of Brazil and Latin America and from different social classes, age, gender, and racial groups. It was built by the partnership of OCAS with the University of São Paulo. It has been developed in collaboration with the *OCAS* magazine, and the leaders of the homeless, artists, students, and community members.

In their work with and sharing the daily life of the homeless over the years, Metuia's occupational therapists and students were engaged with different aid organizations and political actions. Due to this involvement, the Metuia became known among the homeless. As a result, the initiatives at the OCAS center that started in 2008, brought together several long-term partnerships.

Anderson, one of the regulars at the Meeting Point and a former partner, is one of the leaders of the 'National Movement of People in Street Condition' (note that not naming the homeless as *street people* is a political decision; street may not be a qualifier of people but of living conditions). Anderson says: 'Because of the issue of struggle, the street people – dwelling, work, health, education, and culture – is one of the actions that you need to recognize … Every time we talk about this, everybody says that the homeless do not want "houses" or education! [They] do want them, you know, at national level, we do want them, but not taxes for the homeless. If a guy has lost his house, how does he feel if we throw him back in a house again? Then he has to live with other people? This is horrible! He first needs to go through the recovery of his citizenship, you know, because later he can come back to build a family, develop ties, you know. You also need work [but] you can't give him a job and lock him up in it. The guy leaves, he wants to run away. He wants freedom. So, you need something little by little, not from one day to another so the guy will have to have a registered job (in the sense that people want to work but they have to be accommodated in working little by little)'.

Other issues are also discussed at the Meeting Point beyond the specific topics of street life, such as prejudice, violence, health, art, music, among others. The activities are always jointly planned by the participants and they happen at OCAS and in other places in the city, such as theaters, movie theaters, events, etc. Besides the group meetings, individual follow-ups are carried out. We try to facilitate new ways of developing participants' individual strengths and promoting their sense of belonging. This needs to be constantly mediated so as not to split up the needs of the individual and the collective.

The notion of activity should also be redefined in order to be a means of emancipation, nurtured by the affective, social, cultural, and political dimensions of persons, groups, and communities. Activities do not hold strict meanings; in fact, multiple meanings are constantly superimposed on each other. They are expressions of identities at the same time as they are creating identities. It is essential that occupational therapists make use of culturally relevant activities. The process of establishing relations and engaging politically with communities requires that therapists get to know their most valued activities and how they are related to their identity-constructs.

Social occupational therapy has adopted some of Paulo Freire's ideas and concepts, namely *process*, as a means of organizing action and addressing social transformation, *consciousness* and *dialog*. For Freire, emancipation comes from the transformation of consciousness and the need, as he puts it, to develop critical consciousness. Thus, the process of becoming conscious goes beyond the level of decision making to the taking of action in a transformative way (Freire 1978, 1979a,b). Therefore, Paulo Freire, like Basaglia & Basaglia (1977), does not disconnect technical action from political action. Occupational therapy may then contribute to the improvement of the quality of life of people who face inequalities, social contradictions, and cultural confrontations. Occupational therapists are invited to provide interventions that are social and culturally coherent, and appropriate to the local context.

Acknowledgments

We would like to thank the people who took part in the projects in various ways, the occupational therapists who directly participated on this project and shared with us these reflections. The Metuia's São

Carlos Branch particularly thanks: Ana Paula Serrata Malfitano, Beatriz Akemi Takeiti, Carla Regina Silva, Patrícia Leme de Oliveira Borba, Patrícia Miola Gorzoni, Sara Caram Sfair, Tatiana Doval Amador and UFSCAR's undergraduate students in Occupational Therapy, Media and Pedagogy; the professionals of the State School 'Dona Aracy Leite Pereira Lopes' and the Pacaembu Social Assistance Reference Center do Pacaembu of the Secretary of Citizenship and Social Assistance of São Carlos; and finally, the young boys and girls of the *Grande Cidade Aracy* in São Carlos/SP – Brazil.

References

Barros DD: *Jardins de Abel: descontrução do Manicômio de Trieste*, São Paulo, 1994, Editora da USP/Lemos Editorial.

Barros DD: Terapia ocupacional social: o caminho se faz ao caminhar, *Revista de Terapia Ocupacional USP* 3:90–97, 2004.

Barros DD, Ghirardi MIG, Lopes RE: Terapia Ocupacional Social, *Revista de Terapia Ocupacional da USP* 13:95–103, 2002a.

Barros DD, Lopes RE, Galheigo SM: Projeto Metuia – terapia ocupacional no campo social, *O Mundo da Saúde* 26:365–369, 2002b.

Basaglia F, asaglia FO: *Los Crímenes de la Paz: Investigación Sobre Los Intelectuales y Los Técnicos Como Servidores de la Opresión*, México, 1977, Siglo XXI.

Castel R: *As Metamorfoses da Questão Social: Uma Crônica do Salário*, ed 2, Petrópolis, 1999, Vozes.

Freire P: *Ação Cultural Para a Liberdade e Outros Escritos*, Rio de Janeiro, 1978, Paz e Terra.

Freire P: *Pedagogia do Oprimido*, ed 7, Rio de Janeiro, 1979a, Paz e Terra.

Freire P: *Educação Como Prática da Liberdade*, ed 9, Rio de Janeiro, 1979b, Paz e Terra.

Galheigo SM: Da adaptação psicossocial à construção do coletivo: a cidadania enquanto eixo, *Revista de Ciências Médicas* 6:105–108, 1997.

Galheigo SM: O social: idas e vindas de um campo de ação em terapia ocupacional. In Pádua E, Magalhães L, editors: *Terapia Ocupacional: Teoria e Prática*, Campinas, 2003, Papirus, pp 29–48.

Lopes RE: *Cidadania, políticas públicas e terapia ocupacional, no contexto das ações de saúde mental e saúde da pessoa portadora de deficiência, no Município de São Paulo*, PhD Thesis. Campinas, 1999, FE-UNICAMP.

Lopes RE, Malfitano APS: Ação social e intersetorialidade: relato de uma experiência na interface entre saúde, educação e cultura, *Interface* 10:505–515, 2006.

Lopes RE, Barros DD, Malfitano APS, Galvani D, Barros GD: O vídeo como elemento comunicativo no trabalho comunitário, *Cadernos de Terapia Ocupacional UFSCar* 10:61–72, 2002.

Lopes RE, Malfitano APS, Borba PLO: O processo de criação de vínculo entre adolescentes em situação de rua e operadores sociais: compartilhar confiança e saberes, *Quaestio (UNISO)* 8:121–131, 2006a.

Lopes RE, Silva CR, Malfitano APS: Adolescência e juventude de grupos populares urbanos no Brasil e as políticas públicas: apontamentos históricos, *Revista HISTEDBR* 23:114–130, 2006b. Online Available at: http://www.histedbr.fae.

unicamp.br/art08_23.pdf. Accessed December 19, 2008.

Lopes RE, Adorno RCF, Malfitano APS, Takeiti BA, Silva CR, Borba PLO: Juventude pobre, violência e cidadania, *Saúde e Sociedade* 17:63–76, 2008.

Marshall TH, Bottomore T: *Citizenship and Social Class*, London, 1992, Pluto Perspectives.

Oliver FC, Barros DD: Reflexionando sobre desinstitucionalización y Terapia Ocupacional, *Materia Prima – Primera Revista Independiente de Terapia Ocupacional en Argentina* 13:17–20, 1999.

Paoli MC: Citizenship, inequalities, democracy and rights, *Social and Legal Studies* 1:143–159, 1992.

Rotelli F: The invented institution, *Per la Salute Mentale/For Mental Health* 1:189–196, 1988.

Rotelli F, De Leonardis O, Mauri D: Deinstitutionalization, another way: The Italian mental health reform, *Health Promot Int* 1:151–165, 1986.

Santos BS: *Pela mão de Alice: o social e o político na pós-modernidade*, São Paulo, 1995, Cortez.

Vecchia T, Barros DD, Sato M: Jovens do bairro da Pedra do Papagaio: notas sobre uma oficina de fotografia – Projeto Casa Rosa, *Revista do Imaginário* 11:335–361, 2005.

From kites to kitchens: collaborative community-based occupational therapy with refugee survivors of torture

23

Mary Black

OVERVIEW

It is overwhelming to imagine the multiple geographic and emotional borders that refugees are forced to navigate and even more impossible to appreciate the experience of refugees who have survived torture. The migratory and resettlement experiences of refugee survivors and the subsequent manifestations of displacement on occupational roles are essential issues that occupational therapists are beginning to address (Davies 2008, Kronenberg & Pollard 2005, Mitchell 2008, Simó-Algado & Cardona 2005, Simó-Algado et al 2002, Smith 2005, Thibeault 2005, Townsend & Whiteford 2005, Whiteford 2004, 2005, Wilson 2008). This chapter will supplement this recent literature, providing an overview of the sociopolitical systems that sustain torture, the consequent traumatic journey and the effects on the emotional and occupational wellbeing of refugee survivors resettling in a new country. Occupational therapy practice in an urban community-based torture treatment program informed by the Canadian Model of Occupational Performance (CMOP) (Law et al 1998, Townsend & Whiteford 2005) will be described. Interventions designed to address isolation, employment barriers, diminished role status, and homesickness will be discussed. The author will also integrate her own experiences of 'crossing borders' that suggest not only lessons learned but also future possibilities for collaboration.

Introduction

Torture. The word is a conversation stopper. It is understandable to want to avoid the unbelievable. As Judith Herman (1992) affirms, in the opening statement of her seminal text *Trauma and Recovery*, 'The ordinary response to atrocities is to banish them from consciousness' (p. 1). Perpetrators deny it. Governments dispute it. Healthcare workers shy away from it. Survivors often underreport it (Amnesty International 2000, Burnett & Peel 2001, Eisenman & Keller 2000, Mehta & O'Dougherty 2008, Mollica 2004). Torture is used systemically and systematically worldwide to silence and break the spirit not only of the individual, but also of the community (Amnesty International 2000).

As a global community, torture affects us all and our challenge is to believe the unbelievable and give voice to the unspeakable. 'Learning how to learn' about the grim reality and profound implications of torture is imperative if we are to provide credible healthcare and aid in preventing further abuses (Fabri 2001, Iacopino 2000, Johnson 2005, Mollica 2004, Patel & Mahtani 2007). But this learning comes about uneasily; there are challenges and possibilities encountered when 'crossing borders' into an unknown practice arena, as the following personal account demonstrates. For though this author felt ill-prepared and anxious, knowing next to nothing of the weighty realities pressing on survivors, she began to 'learn how to learn' through 'doing' as much as through dialog.

Crossing borderlands – kites and Kovler

In 1990, after reading an article by Barbara E. Joe in *OT Week* entitled 'OTs wanted to volunteer with torture survivors', I made a choice that unquestionably changed my worldview. I began volunteering at the

DOI: 10.1016/B978-0-7020-3103-8.00032-8

program described by Ms. Joe, the Marjorie Kovler Center for the Treatment of Survivors of Torture (NCTTP 2006). Currently named Heartland Alliance Marjorie Kovler Center, the program was founded in 1987 to provide therapeutic and social services for survivors of torture who had migrated to Chicago from countries as distant as Cambodia, Afghanistan, and El Salvador. Mario González, a psychologist from Guatemala, introduced me to Kovler, which operated with a staff of three and a large network of volunteers. At the time, Mario, and psychologist Dr. Antonio Martínez, were facilitating a group with Guatemalan adults inspired by the philosophy of the *Madres de Plaza de Mayo* in Argentina. The *madres* of sons and daughters who had been *desparecidos* 'disappeared' and tortured during the 'Dirty War' promoted intolerance of impunity, social transformation through solidarity and acknowledgment of memory (Feitlowitz 1998, Gogol 2002). Mario described comparable political realities experienced by the group and their families whom were among the estimated 200 000 who had fled Guatemala's armed conflict between 1986 and 1990 (Smith 2006). Many, aided by the sanctuary movement, sought refuge in the United States only to face uncertain legal protection; indeed, the asylum approval rate for Guatemalan applicants during this period was only 5% (Barry 1989). These new pressures compounded pre-existing traumas. The families were clearly under stress. While the adult group met, their children congregated in a nearby room and would regularly leave their gathering to check in on their parents. The parents felt their children were masking their own fears so as not to upset them. After one of the teens joined a street gang, parents were fearful others would follow. The parents were requesting assistance for the children and Mario extended an invitation to work with them. I felt totally unequipped. I was only learning about Guatemala and knew next to nothing about torture. What could I possibly do? I had to remind myself that occupational therapists come from a long tradition of 'doers'. I had experience with groups. I knew kids are inherently drawn into play. I knew I liked to play. Despite my anxieties, I felt compelled as Smith (2005) persuaded, to 'feel the fear and do it anyway'.

The first group I attended was held in a home hosting one of the families. I remember feeling nervous. The parents met upstairs and the children were gathered in the basement: sitting around, joking in Spanish and, as Mario had described to me, 'hanging out'. They ranged in age from 6 years to mid teens. There were about a dozen kids. Most of the teenagers spoke English and eventually told me, politely, it was okay to abandon my broken Spanish. Finally I asked, 'What did you like to play in Guatemala? What do you miss?' They responded openly in a mix of Spanish and English, 'Corn, tortillas, climbing trees, grandmas, flying kites, soccer, playing in the dump'. 'The dump?' 'Yes,' they explained, 'Guatemala City has a famous dump'. They casually described the dump and strewn dead bodies on roadsides as easily as they depicted kicking soccer balls. 'What was this indifference?' I wondered.

We ultimately agreed to make kites at the next group. I went to the library and checked out a book on kite making, brought tissue paper, glue, sticks, and string. I arrived with a plan; a plan for a typical American diamond-shaped kite. That, however, was not the kids' plan. Instead they quickly and adeptly began spinning and fastening the sticks in a wheel shape and covering the spine with a patchwork of colored tissue. They mimicked stained glass! They explained they were constructing *barrilettes*, a traditional octagon-shaped kite flown over Guatemalan cemeteries on All Saints Day. The children's were miniature versions of the '*barrilettes gigantes*', which I learned span up to 15 m (40 ft) in Guatemala. They described the kite tradition and the graveyards. Politics were revealed: many did not receive a proper burial. We tried out the kites in the yard and then planned to construct a *barrilette* '*mini-gigante*' for the city kite festival. The group was followed with a big Guatemala dinner. This was the start of a long-standing relationship with the Guatemalan families and the children's group, later named 'Konojel Junam' meaning 'All United' in the language of Maya Quiché.

My tutorial began directly in those initial groups. I did not expect that a seemingly mundane exploration of play and constructing kites could reveal such insight into trauma, cultural traditions, safety, collaboration, and community. Memories of climbing trees, soccer games, and kite flying sandwiched alongside those of corpses and playing in the city dump gave me an initial glimpse of the traumatic becoming 'normalized'. Engaging in a familiar play tradition, such as creating a *barrilette*, affirmed sharing of culture, expertise, and skills. 'Letting go' of my preconceptions allowed for discovery, mutual learning, and creating future possibilities. Trust, and its companion safety, emerged very slowly. In this home, I was the 'other', a guest and graciously, albeit gradually, included in the local community. I found that this cultural borderland, full of complicated assumptions, potential missteps and miscommunications, could also foster common ground (Mattingly 2008).

To appreciate the needs of refugees from an occupational perspective, Whiteford counsels us to 'acknowledge the impacts of the trauma that many refugees have lived through' (2004, p. 187). I learned from the families that survival in Guatemala depended on prolonged hypervigilance and staying quiet. Parents and children witnessed brutalities including bloodshed and rape, countless were *desparecidos*, harassment was constant. I came to understand that the use of intimidation and torture was not random, but had a long well-organized legacy (Guatemalan Commission for Historical Clarification (CEH) 1999). The implementation was dependent on international training and military support, including aid from the United States (Barry 1989, Costello 1997). Tragically the Guatemalan experience is mirrored worldwide. The following section will concentrate on the systemic use of torture and its far-reaching effects on individuals and communities.

Torture and its effects

'Torture knows no borders' (Worden 2006, p. 79). Despite the fact that torture is forbidden and condemned universally, it is practiced in over 150 countries worldwide and this includes nations that are parties to the United Nations Convention against Torture and Other Cruel, Inhuman or Degrading Treatment or Punishment (CAT) (Amnesty International 2000, United Nations 1984, Worden 2006). Routinely used physical and psychological methods include beatings, extended disruption of food and sleep, sensory deprivation, starvation, hanging by the extremities, simulated drowning or 'water-boarding', application of electric shock to sensitive body parts, threatened violence to loved ones, forced observance and/or participation in torture of others, and the sexual humiliation and rape of women and men (Amnesty International 2000, Modvig & Jaranson 2004, Quiroga & Jaranson 2005, Torture Abolition Survivor Support Coalition (TASSC) 2008). Torture is commonly portrayed as necessary for gaining information, to make a person 'talk'. In actuality it creates 'silence'. Torture is used to break the spirit of individuals, to objectify a person into an object to despise. It creates discord in families, perpetuates fear and distrust among communities, and stifles opposition to the 'status quo'. It fuels a cycle of intimidation, and alienation, ultimately corrupting human connections and creating isolation (Johnson 2005, Martínez 1992, Stover & Nightingale 1985).

At the core of this inexpressible torment is loss, to depths beyond what most can comprehend. Because torture falls outside the norm of what humans should ever experience, the symptoms that ensue are generally understood as 'normal reactions to abnormal circumstances' versus pathology (Droždek & Wilson 2004, Simó-Algado & Cardona 2005, Simó-Algado et al 2002, Wenk-Ansohn 2001). Rather, it is the situation of torture that is pathologic, not the suffering. Reactions such as hypervigilance, distrust, or emotional numbing can support survival through these egregious events. The sequelae takes on various forms, but are often manifest as diffuse bodily pain, headaches, sleeplessness, nightmares, poor concentration, flashbacks, intrusive thoughts, shame, guilt, hopelessness, disorientation, and feelings of betrayal. Depression is highly prevalent. Post-traumatic stress disorder (PTSD) though commonly recognized as a helpful explanatory framework, is argued by many as inadequate in capturing the magnitude and complexity of these effects (Quiroga & Jaranson 2005). Most significantly symptoms need to be understood contextually and within the spiritual, cultural, and social traditions of each survivor. As will be discussed next, traumatic experiences are not consigned solely to torture and flight. The post-flight experience of resettlement offers its own set of unanticipated stressors, which can contribute to the persistence of symptoms affecting everyday activities and occupational wellbeing. This extreme journey and the resettlement environments will be outlined, along with the response of torture treatment programs in countries of arrival.

The long and uncertain journey

The chronic repression, flight, and subsequent resettlement elaborated in 'the triple-trauma paradigm' highlights three phases of the protracted experience which include: (i) pre-flight: often years of societal chaos, escalating harassment, fear, and torture; (ii) flight: the escape, negotiating dangerous borders, guarding against further exploitation and violence while in hiding or in refugee camps; and (iii) post-flight: the initial relief of arrival, often followed with overwhelming feelings of loss, isolation, and coping with marginalized status (Center for Victims of Torture (CVT) 2005). The critical reception at the border, during the flight/post-flight period, depends on whether a survivor arrives with the requisite official documents. *Refugees* are granted protective status *before* reaching the host country and arrive with documentation securing entry, though often after years of deprivation in refugee camps. *Asylum seekers* must petition for protection in the new country *once they have arrived*. Escalating restrictions governing global immigration policies put asylum seekers at greater threat for detention at port of entry, thus exponentially increasing risk of retraumatization and severely compromising overall health (Keller et al 2003, Sheikh et al 2008, Silove 2004, Whiteford 2004).

Legal limbo

The United Nations High Commissioner for Refugees (UNHCR) defines a refugee or asylum seeker as a person who 'owing to a well-founded fear of being persecuted for reasons of race, religion, nationality, social group, political opinion, is outside the country of his nationality and is unable, or owing to such fear, is unwilling to avail himself of protection of that country' (UNHCR 1951). The burden of proof to establish 'well-founded fear' is on the asylum applicant. In the United States, asylum seekers have no opportunity for government assistance or permission to work until their asylum case is granted or work authorization is approved. This can take years leaving the survivor totally dependent on others. Meanwhile, families waiting in the home or nearby country rely heavily on remittances from the survivor. Until asylum status is granted and families are reunified, survivors feel as if they are still in flight, living in limbo, often idle, and fearful whether deportation looms. These systemic exclusions and unending uncertainties are the most crushing and unexpected aspects of resettlement (Brady 2008, Davies 2008, Musiyiwa 2006).

Seeking refuge

Migration of traumatized refugee and asylum seekers to industrialized countries escalated in the 1980s. In response, a convergence of human rights and mental health concerns led to the creation of an international network of torture treatment programs (Gorman 2001) that now numbers over 200 programs worldwide (Library of Congress 2007). Founders of the Kovler Center, recognizing that torture systematically silences and disconnects, developed interventions guided by empowerment. A small interdisciplinary staff and large network of clinical and case management volunteers provide therapeutic and social services on-site and in

the community. Since Kovler opened in 1987 the program has worked with more than 1500 survivors of torture from 74 different countries in Africa, Latin America, the Middle East, Asia, and Eastern Europe (Fabri et al 2009). The majority arrive as asylum seekers. While it is recognized that torture will indeed change a life forever, it does not mean it will eternally define it (Woodcock 1995). Many survivors recover their strength and voices, reclaiming the personal spirit and core humanity the torturers sought to destroy. Survivors lobby officials in Washington DC, speak to the media, file civil lawsuits against perpetrators living in the United States, and establish activist and community support organizations. TASSC is one such national group hosting local meetings at Kovler.

This contagious spirit kept me volunteering with Konojel Junam and felt so compelling that in 1995, when it was announced there was a job opening at Kovler, I jumped. It was for a case manager, one of the three staff positions. I knew if I wanted to work as an occupational therapist I would have to help create a position. I quickly found all my energy was devoted to direct service and thus relied on articulating and promoting occupational therapy to our administrator who was able to secure the inclusion in future grant proposals. In 2000, Kovler was awarded funding from the Torture Victims Relief Act (TVRA) (Library of Congress 2007), effectively expanding staff three-fold and this included occupational therapy. An overview of occupational therapy within the context of Kovler concludes the discussion.

Commonplace tasks, uncommon challenges

Experience in case management brought home the extent of environmental segregation and occupational challenges facing survivors, particularly asylum seekers. These new social realities exacerbate survivors' existing stress and trauma by contributing to forced dependency, loss of dignity, diminished self-esteem, and occupational deprivation (Davies 2008, Simó-Algado et al 2002, Smith 2005, Wenk-Ansohn 2004). As described, denying asylum seekers access to necessary social networks and full participation in daily life tasks is deliberate political policy and a shock to most survivors in post flight. It is not that survivors in the United States have migrated to 'resource-poor' environments, quite the contrary; rather they are denied access to the conspicuous resources that surround them. Occupational apartheid confronts the realities of this socially constructed segregation. Not unlike torture, apartheid demonstrates a 'systemic relationship between the phenomenon and the causes' (Kronenberg & Pollard 2005, p. 79). The systems that support the use of torture also maintain occupational apartheid. Both skew the balance of power, segregate and discriminate based on race, religion, nationality, social group, and political opinion. As social phenomena they warrant participatory action and 'a sustained program of collaboration in order to effect social change' (Kronenberg & Pollard 2005, p. 80).

Reconstructing social networks

Konojel Junam taught me how engagement in meaningful occupations can effect social change. The children did indeed make their *'mini-gigante' barrilette* for the city's kite festival embellishing it with a *quetzal* and GUATEMALA in bold letters announcing, in effect, 'We are here!' They began creating handmade badges for an annual Guatemalan rally; the images drawn and underscored with slogans such as *Viven Los Desparecidos*, '500 Years of Oppression', 'Save Guatemalan Art!' The group became an anticipated presence in the community where they used their art, dance, and drama to voice a political message. In less dramatic fashion, though not any less potent, a group of Bosnian women, *Zlatne Ruke* 'Golden Hands', utilized their shared skills to cope with pervasive isolation, depression, and anxiety. Handcrafting over coffee, then later sharing their wares with the local community, they tagged their own personal message on their distinctive knitted creations: 'We are a group of middle aged Bosnian women who arrived to the U.S. with only the clothes on our backs and the skills in our hands ... we hope you enjoy our contribution.' The women, like the children, had something unique to contribute to the larger community that was not there previously, thus positively shaping and expanding their own environments and boundaries.

In developing relevant occupational therapy services at Kovler it became clear that further alternative social realities needed to be developed. While access to basic needs is most primary, concurrently 'the need to re-engage in meaningful occupations, to re-establish familiar routines and to connect with others, is also important' (Whiteford 2004, p. 187). In fact, an evaluation summary of European-based

torture treatment centers indicated that the impact of rehabilitation was greater 'when the therapeutic program includes occupational therapy or other activities designed to *reconstruct a social network* around the patient, which contribute to his/her integration in the host society' (Guillet et al 2005, p. 8).

Assessments – adapting the Canadian Occupational Performance Measure

While reconstructing social networks, it is also important to get to know the individual. At Kovler a modified occupational history is used to help identify what life was like for a survivor before the flight: mapping out in conversation how days were spent, interests, opportunities for education, for work, family roles, community roles. This begins to reveal meaningful occupations, strengths, and interests and is also useful for prevocational and vocational planning, as employment is one of the most pressing demands. In an effort to better capture current or post-flight occupational concerns, the Canadian Occupational Performance Measure (COPM; Law et al 1998) was adapted with the assistance of a University of Illinois occupational therapy student, Ana Blazevic. Each of the categories were reviewed and cross-referenced with domains in the Occupational Therapy Practice Framework (American Occupational Therapy Association (AOTA) 2002). Common challenges cited in literature and from experiences at Kovler were identified and incorporated. The most predominant challenges self-identified by survivors with COPM echo and supplement in the literature (Datson et al 2004, Davies 2008, Mitchell 2008, Simó-Algado & Cardona 2005, Smith 2005, Townsend & Whiteford 2005, Whiteford 2004 & 2005, Wilson 2008). The most compelling are barriers to employment, isolation, and diminished status.

Interventions

Dignified employment is primary. Richard Mollica (2006) in his lifelong career with refugees cites work as 'a psychological life raft, assuring the survivor that he or she is not completely helpless, that not all is lost' (p. 171). Yet many survivors are despondent waiting for work authorization. Keeping the focus on vocational readiness skills, English acquisition, and exploring future educational options helps to build towards a more hopeful future. Once employed, many nuanced situations can manifest particularly when a client senses injustice. Ongoing support to retain jobs is essential, with an appreciation of how past experiences can impact present emotions in everyday environments (Piwowarczyk & Simon 2008). Additionally, assisting with adaptation of existing roles, e.g., as a parent, student, or community leader can help maintain dignity and status. Maximizing the skills and interests survivors identify from home serve as catalysts for current groups: urban farming (including workdays at a rural farm, through Angelic Organics Learning Center), honey production (there is an apiary on the Kovler roof), and an international cooking group. Universal rituals, e.g., preparing and sharing a meal or sowing and nurturing plants promote predictability, anticipation, enjoyment, safety, and belonging (Davies 2008). Martine Songasonga, colleague and TASSC member from Democratic Republic of Congo, likens the sustainability of these groups to a 'clan or a village. Over time there are people who move on and new people arrive but the village is still here' (M Songasonga, personal communication, 2008).

Summary

When I began volunteering at Kovler I did not imagine I would be still involved with this 'village' almost 20 years later. Then there was a paucity of information on occupational therapy working with survivors of torture and indeed, a paucity of conversation on torture itself. Despite feeling initially 'lost' I found work with survivors offers personal connection to the larger world. There is a natural 'goodness of fit' for occupational therapy in the realm of torture treatment though one does not need to work in a treatment program such as Kovler to meet a survivor. The chance of working with a refugee who is a survivor of torture in any practice area is increasing. Future directions in practice depend on keeping informed on torture and its effects, advocating for prevention and expanding our repertoire of contextually relevant interventions, mindfully collaborating with survivors and colleagues. The initial kite making lessons with Konojel Junam would have been lost without collaboration. The subsequent closing contributions eloquently capture the communal spirit of Kovler and what ritual can offer, not surprisingly in the kitchen.

THE KOVLER KITCHEN

The desire for the familiar and for ritual documented by Whiteford (2005) in her work with displaced refugees is echoed at Kovler. For the last four years, approximately every other Friday evening in the Kovler kitchen, we have been taking turns leading preparation of a meal from one's home country (Fig. 23.1). Anthony C Ibeagha, TASSC member from Nigeria, describes the potency a cooking group can hold. 'We've lost something we're always trying to capture. Where do you find it? In the kitchen! When you get in the kitchen we find it in little pieces, in the food, in the conversation. When you smell that particular herb, you can picture the woman in the market who sells it, what she is wearing – you know where she is from. It takes you back to good places, takes you back home. I still own a culture of food that I can share and that people will accept' (A C Ibeagha, personal communication, 2008). Arantza Jauregi, volunteer and creator of delicious Basque stews, elaborates 'Reconnection can happen while knitting or in the kitchen … definitely in the kitchen. It brings back memories of home that are ingrained with identity and culture. When torture relates to ethnicity or a particular culture the intention is to rip away what is value, what is admired, what is loved and cherished and passed on in a community; to uproot everything and make it disappear. For example when I share with you the way I cut and prepare a plantain – with that ritual I am reclaiming value through the experience. I am bringing back memories prior to torture that make me who I am. People from different cultures reciprocate, 'Oh! We do that too in my country, in my village. It is not only what I do but

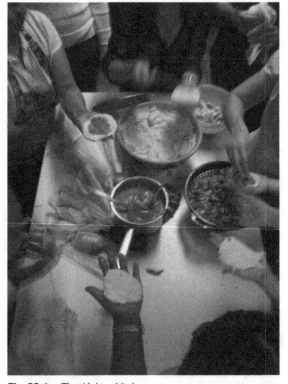

Fig 23.1 • The Kolver kitchen.

what others do too. It no longer is a private experience. In kitchen there are witnesses to my private moment that welcome me and break down the isolation creating a community of acceptance. In the kitchen, not only are we appreciated, but we are excited, because we like each other. In this setting I am telling the torturer, "No!" meaning the torturer did not succeed in destroying the essence and goodness of who I am. Here I am of value and this is shared by others. This means there must be goodness in me!' (A Jauregi, personal communication, 2009). Anthony concurs, 'It is all about acceptance. That is our tradition. In English I can't capture the experience but I can touch the feeling when we're creating, when we're doing. You feel it. It's alive . . . The greatest joys are simple. When we're eating nothing else counts. We're no longer a survivor. We are celebrating family. We are happy.'

Acknowledgments

Recognition and multiple thanks go to Esad Boskailo, Karen Dilfer, Mary Fabri, Anne Flanagan, Mario Gonza'lez, Anthony Ibeagha, Marianne Joyce, Arantza Jauregi, Martine Songasonga, and Mary Beth Tegan for generously sharing their wisdom, guidance and support. Sincere appreciation is extended to Frank Kronenberg, Nick Pollard, and Dikaios Sakellariou for their inspiration, positive direction and patience! To all the survivors, staff, and volunteers who pass through Kovler's doors; for life lessons in maintaining courage, kindling hope and modeling selfless generosity – heartfelt gratitude.

Resources

There is a wealth of information regarding torture, its sequelae and healing that is beyond the scope of this chapter. The following online resources provide comprehensive information, transferable to a multitude of contexts, on rehabilitation, education and advocacy, as well as links to a global directory of torture treatment centers.

International Rehabilitation Council for Torture Victims (IRCT): http://www.irct.org.

Center for Victims of Torture (CVT): http://www.cvt.org.

Medical Foundation for the Care of Victims of Torture: http://www.torturecare.org.uk.

National Consortium of Torture Treatment Programs (NCTTC): http://ncttp.dataweb.com.

Torture Abolition and Survivors Support Coalition International (TASSC): http://www.tassc.org.

The following occupational therapy sites actively support international outreach, networking and capacity building for occupational therapists working in marginalized situations, including those with refugees and asylum seekers.

Occupational Opportunities for Refugees and Asylum Seekers (OOFRAS): http://www.oofras.com.

Occupational Therapy International Outreach Network (OTION): http://www.wfot.com.

References

American Occupational Therapy Association: Occupational therapy practice framework: domain and process, *Am J Occup Ther* 56: 609–639, 2002.

Amnesty International: *Torture Worldwide: An Affront to Human Dignity*, New York, 2000, Amnesty International Publications.

Barry T: *Guatemala: a Country Guide*, Albuquerque, New Mexico, 1989, The Inter-Hemispheric Education Resource Center.

Brady E: The Year of Living Nervously, *The New York Times* CY1, 2008. Online. Available at: http://www.nytimes.com. Accessed December 7, 2008.

Burnett A, Peel M: Asylum seekers and refugees in Britain: the health of survivors of torture and organized violence, *BMJ* 322:606–609, 2001.

Center for Victims of Torture (CVT): 2005, *Healing the Hurt: a Guide for Developing Services for Torture Survivors*, 2005. Online. Available at: http://www.cvt.org/main.php/HealingtheHurt. Accessed April 5, 2008.

Costello P: *Guatemala: Historical Background*, 1997. Online. Available at: http://www.c-r.org/our-work/accord/guatemala/historical-background.php. Accessed July 5, 2008.

Datson S, Hubbard C, McGarrigle J, et al: *Addressing the needs of newly arrived refugees: an occupational therapy perspective*, 2004, OOFRAS: Practice Skills: Occupation Centered Practice. Online. Available at: http://www.oofras.com. Accessed January 19, 2008.

Davies R: Working with refugees and asylum seekers: challenging occupational apartheid. In Pollard N, Sakellariou D, Kronenberg F, editors: *Political Practice of Occupational Therapy*, Edinburgh, 2008, Elsevier Science, pp 183–189.

Drožđek B, Wilson J: Uncovering: trauma-focused treatment techniques with asylum seekers. In Wilson J, Drožđek B, editors: *Broken Spirits:*

The Treatment of Traumatized Asylum Seekers, Refugees, War and Torture Victims, New York, 2004, Bruner-Routledge, pp 243–276.

Eisenman D, Keller A: Survivors of torture in a general medical setting: how often have patients been tortured, and how often is it missed? *West J Med* 172:301–304, 2000.

Fabri M: Reconstructing safety: adjustments to the therapeutic frame in the treatment of survivors of political torture, *Professional Psychology: Research and Practice* 32:452–457, 2001.

Fabri M, Joyce M, Black M, et al: Caring for torture survivors: The Marjorie Kovler Center. In Stout C, editor: *The New Humanitarians: Inspiration, Innovations, and Blueprints for Visionaries*, Westport, Connecticut, 2009, Praeger Publishers, pp 157–187.

Feitlowitz M: *A lexicon of terror: Argentina and the legacies of torture*, New York, 1998, Oxford University Press.

Gogol E: Las madres de plaza de mayo: raising a banner of freedom in Argentina. In Gogol E, editor: *The Concept of Other in Latin American Liberation: Fusing Emancipatory Philosophic Thought and Social Revolt*, Maryland, 2002, Lexington Books, pp 295–306.

Gorman W: Refugee survivors of torture: trauma and treatment, *Professional Psychology: Research and Practice* 32:443–451, 2001.

Guatemalan Commission for Historical Clarification (CEH): *Guatemala: memory of silence–tzinl natabal: report of the commission for historical clarification conclusions and recommendations*, 1999. Online. Available at: http://shr.aaas.org/guatemala/ceh/report/english/toc.html. Accessed July 5, 2008.

Guillet S, Perren-Klingler G, Agger I: *EIDHR (European Initiative for Democracy and Human Rights) Evaluations: Torture Rehabilitation Centres Europe*, 2005. Online. Available at: http://ec.europa.eu/europeaid/where/worldwide/eidhr/documents/evaluations-rehabilitation-torture-europe_en.pdf. Accessed August 9, 2008.

Herman JL: *Trauma and Recovery*, New York, 1992, Basic Books.

Iacopino V: Health professionals cannot be silent witnesses: commentary, *West J Med* 172:304–305, 2000.

Ibeagh A, personal communication, 2008.

Jauregi A, personal communication, 2009.

Johnson D: *Helping Refugee Trauma Survivors in the Primary Care Setting*, Minneapolis, 2005, Center for Victims of Torture. Online. Available at: http://www.cvt.org/file.php?ID=5380. Accessed April 5, 2008.

Keller A, Rosenfeld B, Trinh-Shevrin C, et al: Mental health of detained asylum seekers, *Lancet* 362:1721–1723, 2003.

Kronenberg F, Pollard N: Overcoming occupational apartheid: a preliminary exploration of political nature of occupational therapy. In Kronenberg F, Simó-Algado S, Pollard N, editors: *Occupational Therapy Without Borders: Learning from the Spirit of Survivors*, Edinburgh, 2005, Elsevier/Churchill Livingstone, pp 58–86.

Law M, Baptiste S, Carswell A, et al: *Canadian Occupational Performance Measure*, ed 3, Ottawa, 1998, CAOT Publications, Ontario.

Library of Congress: *Torture Victims Relief Reauthorization Act of 2007*, 2007. Online. Available at: http://www.thomas.gov/cgi-bin/cpquery/T?&report=hr103p1&dbname=110&. Accessed February 6, 2009.

Marti'nez A: The ecology of human development. In Turitz S, Davis P, Heisel J, editors: *Confronting the Heart of Darkness*, Washington DC, 1992, Guatemalan Human Rights Committee/USA, pp 22–25.

Mattingly C: Reading minds and telling tales in a cultural borderland, *Ethos: Journal of the Society for Psychological Anthropology* 36:136154, 2008. Online. Available at: http://www3.interscience.wiley.com/cgi-bin/fulltext/120176437/PDFSTART. December 5, 2009.

Mehta E, O'Dougherty M: *Study: communicating torture and war experiences with primary care providers*, 2008. Online. Available at: http://www.cvt.org/files/pg20/Study_Communicating%20Trauma%20with%20Providers_2006.pdf. Accessed August 9, 2008.

Mitchell A: Reflections on working with south Sudanese refugees in settlement and capacity building in regional Australia. In Pollard N, Sakellariou D, Kronenberg F, editors: *Political Practice of Occupational Therapy*, Edinburgh, 2008, Elsevier Science, pp 197–205.

Modvig J, Jaranson J: A global perspective of torture, political violence, and health. In Wilson J, Drožđek B, editors: *Broken Spirits: The Treatment of Traumatized Asylum Seekers, Refugees, War and Torture Victims*, New York, 2004, Bruner-Routledge, pp 33–52.

Mollica R: Surviving torture, *N Engl J Med* 351:5–7, 2004.

Mollica R: *Healing Invisible Wounds: Paths to Hope and Recovery in a Violent World*, Orlando, 2006, Harcourt Books.

Musiyiwa A: *Refugees, uncertainty and the absence of control: an interview with Claire Smith, occupational and psychological therapist*, 2006, Worldpress.org. Online. Available at: http://www.worldpress.org/Europe/2552.cfm. Accessed January 18, 2008.

National Consortium of Torture Treatment Programs (NCTTP): *Profile: The Marjorie Kovler Center for the Treatment of Survivors of Torture of the Heartland Alliance for Human Needs and Human Rights*, 2006. Online. Available at: http://ncttp.dataweb.com/wsContent/Internal/Tables/wsContent/Profiles/default.view?_mode=details&RowId=23. Accessed January 24, 2008.

Patel N, Mahtani A: The politics of working with refugee survivors of torture, *Psychologist* 20:164–166, 2007.

Piwowarczyk L, Simon C: *Vocational Rehabilitation in Torture Survivors*, 2008, Boston Center for Refugee Health and Human Rights. Online. Available at: http://www.cvt.org/file.php?ID=60350. Accessed October 11, 2008.

Quiroga J, Jaranson J: Politically-motivated torture and its survivors: a desk study review of the literature, *Torture Journal on Rehabilitation of Torture Victims and Prevention of Torture: Thematic Issue* 15:2–3, 2005.

Sheikh M, MacIntyre C, Perera S: Preventive detention: the ethical ground where politics and health meet. Focus on asylum seekers in

Australia, *J Epidemiol Community Health* 62:480–483, 2008.

Silove D: The Global Challenge of Asylum. In Wilson J, Drožđek B, editors: *Broken Spirits: the Treatment of Traumatized Asylum Seekers, Refugees, War and Torture Victims*, New York, 2004, Bruner-Routledge, pp 13–31.

Simó-Algado S, Cardona CE: The return of the corn men: an intervention project with a Mayan community of Guatemalan retornos. In Kronenberg F, Simó-Algado S, Pollard N, editors: *Occupational Therapy Without Borders: Learning from the Spirit of Survivors*, Edinburgh, 2005, Elsevier/Churchill Livingstone, pp 336–350.

Simó-Algado S, Mehta N, Kronenberg F, et al: Occupational therapy intervention with children survivors of war, *Can J Occup Ther* 69:205–217, 2002.

Smith HC: Feel the fear and do it anyway: meeting the needs of refugees and people seeking asylum, *British Journal of Occupational Therapy* 68:474–476, 2005.

Smith J: 2006, Guatemala: economic migrants replace political refugees. In *Migration Information Source*, Online. Available at: http://www.migrationinformation.org/Profiles/display.cfm?ID=392. Accessed July 5, 2008.

Songasanga M, personal communication, 2008.

Stover E, Nightingale E, editors: *The Breaking of Bodies and Minds:* *Torture, Psychiatric Abuse, and the Health Professions*, New York, 1985, WH Freeman.

Thibeault R: Connecting health and social justice: a Lebanese experience. In Kronenberg F, Simó-Algado S, Pollard N, editors: *Occupational Therapy Without Borders: Learning from the Spirit of Survivors*, Edinburgh, 2005, Elsevier/Churchill Livingstone, pp 232–244.

Torture Abolition and Survivors Support Coalition International (TASSC): *About Torture*, 2008. Online. Available at: http://tassc.org/index.php?sn=81. Accessed January 16, 2008.

Townsend E, Whiteford G: A participatory occupational justice framework: population-based processes of practice. In Kronenberg F, Simó-Algado S, Pollard N, editors: *Occupational Therapy Without Borders: Learning from the Spirit of Survivors*, Edinburgh, 2005, Elsevier/Churchill Livingstone, pp 110–126.

United Nations: *Convention against torture and other cruel, inhuman or degrading treatment or punishment, part 1, article 1, paragraph 1, 1984.* Online. Available at: http://www.un.org/documents/ga/res/39/a39r046.htm. Accessed January 16, 2008.

United Nations High Commissioner for Refugees (UNHCR): *Convention and protocol relating to the status of refugees, article 1*, 1951. Online. Available at: http://www.unhcr.org/protect/PROTECTION/ 0b00c2aa10.pdf. Accessed January 5, 2008.

Wenk-Ansohn M: The vestige of pain: psychosomatic disorders among survivors of torture. In Graessner S, Gurris N, Pross C, editors: *At the Side of Torture Survivors: Treating a Terrible Assault on Human Dignity*, Baltimore, 2001, Johns Hopkins University Press, pp 57–69.

Wenk-Ansohn M: Treatment of torture survivors-influences of the exile situation on the course of traumatic process and therapeutic possibilities, *Torture* 17:88–95, 2004.

Whiteford G: Occupational issues of refugees. In Molineux M, editor: *Occupation for Occupational Therapists*, Oxford, 2004, Blackwell Publishing, pp 183–199.

Whiteford G: Understanding the occupational deprivation of refugees: a case study from Kosovo, *Can J Occup Ther* 72:78–88, 2005.

Wilson C: Illustrating occupational needs of refugees. In Pollard N, Sakellariou D, Kronenberg F, editors: *Political Practice of Occupational Therapy*, Edinburgh, 2008, Elsevier Science, pp 191–195.

Woodcock J: Healing rituals with families in exile, *Journal of Family Therapy* 17:397–409, 1995.

Worden M: Torture spoken here: ending global torture. In Roth K, Worden M, Bernstein A, et al, editors: *Torture: Does it Make Us Safer? Is it Ever Ok? A Human Rights Perspective*, New York, 2006, The New Press, pp 79–105.

Argentina: social participation, activities, and courses of action

24

Liliana Paganizzi   Elisabeth Gomez Mengelberg

OVERVIEW

This chapter offers a description of programs that promote creative, social, and inclusive activities, and encourage the social participation and exercise of human rights. Access to education, health, and life in the community become a pillar of an occupational therapy involved in the social context. This goes beyond the traditional work inside asylum organizations and is far from the biomedical approach of the past century. The programs described in this work were developed at a psychiatric hospital and its nearby neighborhoods and public parks. They are especially significant because they reveal the purpose of building and/or recovering a life project with people living in such environments.

Background

Occupational therapy in Argentina developed as a profession in the 1950s. Since then it has followed the changes of the health system together with the different political and social crises undergone in this country. Historically, occupational therapists in Argentina worked with populations who had experienced a breakdown in their social bonds. These exclusions were both a consequence of their physical and mental disabilities and the restrictions operated by psychiatric asylums. In Argentina, more than a million people have some mental pathology and more than 25 000 people are inpatients in hospitals in the largest urban centers (Barrionuevo 2005). Most mental health occupational therapy practice still takes place in psychiatric hospital environments.

In this chapter, we present examples, including two recent programs developed in one of the largest Argentine psychiatric hospitals. The first of these examples describes a program focusing on the families of people having a severe mental disorder. The other example is a report on a community health project developed with women who face difficulties in their daily tasks. Other case examples include professional practices committed to social changes in the population and community experiences addressing the needs of people living in vulnerable situations associated with the increasingly evident phenomenon of urban poverty.

The social situation in Argentina

Around 37 million people live in Argentina. Until the end of the 1990s, 20% of Argentine citizens lived in poverty, while across the Latin American region an average of 40% of the people living in poverty were living in urban areas (CEPAL 2003). In 2001, Argentina went through a political crisis that resulted in the deepest social inequality in the history of the country. While poverty indexes slowly diminished over most of the South American region, the percentage of urban poor people in Argentina increased to 44%. There was also an increase in the number of women breadwinners with principal incomes under the poverty line. Young people between 15 and 24 years who live in cities form the most vulnerable group among others, which include the impoverished women breadwinners. (CEPAL 2007)

According to the International Labor Organization (ILO 2007) around 750 000 teenagers living in cities

© 2011, Elsevier Ltd.
DOI: 10.1016/B978-0-7020-3103-8.00033-X

are neither studying, nor working or looking for jobs. These factors increase urban residential segregation and contribute to stigmatization of poor neighborhoods. This complex panorama is the context for some of the important occupational therapy projects presented in this chapter.

From the hospital to the community

Recovering rights and working with families

Elisabeth Gomez Mengelberg, Occupational Therapist

Workshops in groups

Context

This program was developed at the Dr José Borda Interdisciplinary Psycho Assistance Hospital, which was set up as an asylum at the end of the nineteenth century. In 1999, the Department of External Medical Assistance identified the need of people who had family members with a diagnosis of schizophrenia to receive information about the general features of such illness. They also recognized the need to discuss their relatives' daily lives and to get useful tools to facilitate their relationships.

Group workshops were therefore organized for these relatives. They were initially coordinated by Mrs Blanco, a psychologist, and later, I joined as an occupational therapist. In these workshops, people worked on several aspects such as education, daily life activities, development of social consciousness, rights and obligations; they were also encouraged to mutually help each other. We found that families were unable to deal with their everyday obligations because they lacked knowledge of their rights to the resources and opportunities that would enable them to assume responsibility for the care and maintenance of their family members (Amenta y Otros 2000).

The activity: organization of a nongovernmental organization

Participation

These activities were planned taking into account the real needs of the population with and for whom we worked. The families started to assert their rights by learning how to ask about integral and multidisciplinary healthcare services for their relatives and by participating in the planning and development of programs in mental healthcare. With the notion of defending their citizens' rights and access to social conditions and opportunities which would place them on an equal footing with the rest of the citizens, the suggestion made was that they organize themselves as a non governmental organization (NGO). Some of the essential rights of patients and their relatives in this context are:

1. provision of adequate integral and multidisciplinary healthcare services for people with psychiatric disorders
2. participation of consumers and relatives in the planning and development of programs and mental health services.

With legal assistance provided by a lawyer and workshops coordinated by an occupational therapist, an NGO was established. This activity played a key role in the patients' social vindication. The debates and discussion meetings were intense and members had to learn how to assert their rights, to demystify insanity, to confront and eliminate prejudice. Bylaws were drafted, a board was created, new members were admitted, funds were raised to afford administrative expenses, and a name chosen for the NGO, and *AFAPPE* (association for relatives and friends of people having schizophrenia) was legally created.

Founders' testimonies

This activity was aimed at encouraging emancipation and citizenship. One of the founding members, a 60-year-old woman, is the NGO's secretary. She is the one who ensures board meetings take place, admits new members, and raises funds. Her son is 45 years old and she always remarks that: 'If this workshop had existed when my son became ill, my family and son's quality of life would have been different and we would not have experienced the desperation of visiting several hospitals and doctors without getting emotional support or information beyond the crisis itself', and she adds, 'They taught me how to know about my rights and now I stand up to anyone'.

AFAPPE members have spoken at many congresses addressing the psychosocial problems of patients with schizophrenia. The daughter of one AFFAPPE member says 'Since my mum attends the workshops she really understands me'. AFAPPE's president and his wife stated that the workshop has enabled them to considerably improve their family's quality of life and the relationship with their son.

Difficulties and perspectives

Members and NGO actions

The NGO wanted to open a library, have a television room, and conduct cultural activities and emotional expression and/or labor workshops for people diagnosed with schizophrenia. The organization contacted the city authorities to ask if it could 'borrow' one of the city government buildings to organize a 'clubhouse' facility for this purpose. However, no interview took place and the official answer to the request was negative (Rodríguez Del Barrio Lourdes 1999).

This answer discouraged the NGOs members, who had to support any activity of the NGO with their own time and money. Some members lost their interest in the community tasks and others found it difficult to keep the pace. However, the opportunities for group discussion on the defense and vindication of human rights of people experiencing serious mental disorders have undoubtedly left a mark on them. They have learned to be assertive in their daily lives and recognize that obtaining successful outcomes for the NGO's aims depends mainly on a collectively organized course of action.

'From fears ... to real possibilities': creation of the common spaces program community project management

Adriana M Slaifstein, Occupational Therapist

Context

The community health program developed in La Boca neighborhood in Buenos Aires, in 1999, was organized by the social services of the General Hospital of the neighborhood and the occupational therapy service at Dr José T Borda Hospital. The La Boca neighborhood is a tourist destination and a cultural center known for its special type of dwelling and for its artistic, cultural, and sport activities.

Its population mainly consists of middle, lower-middle, and lower classes, and many of whom are semi-skilled workers or with no education at all, independent contractors, and maids. Most of them are unemployed. Considering their working and housing conditions, it can be concluded that the majority of this population does not have their basic needs satisfied. Local women have a key role in the development of survival strategies concerning food, work, and housing matters. The tasks that women carry out are related to the care of the family group and to household services, generally rendered on an irregular basis. Through developing health prevention and promotion strategies with this community, we identified a local group of women who said that they had difficulties in their daily tasks and personal projects. We suggested their participation in entertainment activities according to their interests, motivations, and needs.

Workshop for women

We started a 'Women's Group Workshop', which was especially set up as a meeting space coordinated by an occupational therapist with the purpose of facilitating the identification of women's personal interests, strengthening social bonds, and determining their own resources through the learning of artistic, creative, and productive techniques implying community action.

Many women participated in this workshop, eager to learn together with members of their community and, at the same time, interested in sharing their own technical knowledge. During the process of learning oil painting technique, they developed an interest in showing what they had learnt. Each woman exhibited her paintings of the neighborhood to families, friends, neighbors, and tourists. The intention was to work on maximizing the autonomous development of their personal skills and attitudes, and the self-management of their current and future personal projects. Despite their initial fears of developing a personal project, it was evident that the group experience offered them the possibility of acquiring new knowledge and skills (OPS, OMS 1986).

A personal testimony

Achievements

In the first preparation phase: 'I don't know, I've never painted before, I was afraid, but with the group at the workshop we experienced, through learning, discovering and creating, how to maximize our potential skills and we were inspired to do that in our neighborhood, La Boca.'

Second phase: Planning and developing their first painting exhibition called 'La Boca Women's Group, neighbors painting their own community'. This exhibition was displayed in the heart of their neighborhood and is a tourist attraction.

Through the workshop, each painting has transformed these women. They have produced goods, works of art shown to the public and put on sale. The exhibition allows them to increase their personal income and, also, it allows the group to financially sustain its activities.

Outcomes of the first painting exhibition

Following discussion of the experience of the first exhibition it was proposed to offer new opportunities for the development of individual potential skills through occupational therapy which in turn would facilitate the development of collective skills.

> We need to learn foreign languages to be able to speak to tourists, learn computing to do our own marketing and learn art history and different drawing and painting techniques.

The schedule for the third stage of the program comprises a year of training according to people's interests and includes: English, computing, drawing and painting, and marketing technique courses. Some of the women have ventured into education and others have resumed education programs that they had previously abandoned.

The planning and development of the second painting exhibition was grounded in this experience and the applied knowledge the group has acquired (Dabas 2001).

Perspectives

Two years on: through their activities, the women have become the main characters of their story: they are more purposeful, less fearful, and more independent. They take an active role and have capitalized on what they have learnt individually, both in the group and in the community.

In neighborhoods

Health, environment and human development

Emma G Cein, Occupational Therapist, Fernando Cacopardo, Architect

Context: occupational therapy fundamentals and role

This project started in 2004, in a Research Group of Environment Emergencies at the Architecture School of Mar del Plata National University (Argentina), in a context of social crisis and increasing urban poverty. We entered into public and private collective bargaining agreements with different organizations related to education, health, and sports. Occupational therapists drew an interdisciplinary and participating working schedule which was mainly aimed at developing human and citizen skills and self-management capacity (Asthon 2000).

The health perspective derives its focus from an interdisciplinary perspective of occupational therapists, social support workers, architects, and psychologists. We are interested in incorporating the environment and the lifestyle as essential aspects of a health policy within a framework that we can call 'quality life improvement'. We present a trial experience in two neighborhoods in the city of Mar del Plata. These are vulnerable communities with shortages of drinking water and accumulated rubbish piled in front of houses. These are often uninhabitable due to poor construction materials, sanitary problems, untidiness due to lack of basic dwelling elements (furniture, cupboards, and closets) and overcrowding. All these issues represented serious obstacles to health.

Course of action

In this precarious local residential setting, it is evident the main cause of many health and human development problems experienced by the children lay in the surrounding environment. We proposed to use a participatory course of action, which modifies such environments by reinforcing people's participation in their daily activities (García & Veyra 2005).

Occupational therapy contributed in the organization and use of the resources that families already have.

Work strategies and results: facilitating home order to create a suitable environment for daily household activities

Different participatory courses of action were planned, which enabled gradual improvements in people's lifestyle. We simultaneously worked three different aspects:

3. **Internal home equipment**: Restoring order to homes by providing furniture is a trigger and promoter of household activities that are now carried out naturally. For example: Sitting down, gathering together, doing homework in a space with a table and chairs; a personal 'space' where individuals can keep their clothes. A sense of belonging is created in an environment where this

is frequently not possible (clothes are shared with all family members and, before, they had belonged to 'strangers' ...).

4. **Adjustments at home for children at risk**: We worked with mothers by giving them simple suggestions on how to modify their living environment thus facilitating children's development and reducing the risk of domestic accidents.

5. **Development of personal skills**: Creation of handcraft (portrait frames, decorative ornaments, simple toys for children) using the papier mache technique (a decorative technique in which pieces of paper are stuck together to create an object). This activity encouraged inter-family cooperative working. The children looked for bottles and concrete bags, and expressed their creativity with elements found while scavenging (papers, cloths, recyclable containers).

Contributions and discussion

This trial experience has allowed extending the horizons of the occupational therapy discipline in Argentina with regard to the problem of the urban poverty.

In the community

Inclusion of teenagers and the overcoming of occupational apartheid

Elisabeth Guadalupe Gaziano, Occupational Therapist

In the city of Santa Fe, province of Santa Fe, Argentina, the 'Coming Back to School' program was implemented in area development centers of the Social Development Ministry in surrounding neighborhoods and illegal shanty towns.

ABOUT TEENAGERS, THEIR FAMILIES, OCCUPATIONS, RIGHTS, AND DEPRIVATION ...

In 2006, 58 teenagers between 14 and 18 years participated in this project. They belonged to families living in chronic poverty and unemployment with a deep breakdown of their basic rights to food, health, education, home, work, and occupational development (Kielhofner 2004). They came from large families, with an average of seven family members each, living together in the same room. Only 18% had regular incomes from employment; 82% of adults received incomes from government aid programs, had temporary

jobs, or scavenged for food. Many teenagers, as well as their parents and/or siblings, had problems with the law and had dropped out of their state-funded education program. The youth and their families experience constant and progressive subjugation of their rights to have a job and a decent education, and we understand this situation to be a form of occupational apartheid (Kronenberg et al 2007).

'Coming Back to School': an opportunity to overcome social exclusion

We worked on access to education as a basic right: we encouraged the teenagers who were school drop-outs to resume their studies and the ones who were still studying to continue despite adverse conditions such as pregnancy, precocious maternity or paternity, delinquency or addictions. To fulfill such purposes, different strategies of support for the teenager and their family were planned and developed (Duschatzky & Corea 2007).

Course of action: collecting information from the available community resources, conducting personal and family interviews, meetings, visits

We did exploratory community work by collecting information from different organizations, by conducting individual and family interviews (to know about interests, occupations, education level); we also visited children's orphanages and schools and coordinated the courses of action with different social players (nongovernmental organizations (NGOs) and other organizations such as penitentiaries, addiction rehabilitation centers, neighborhood community centers, churches, organizations for teenagers, etc.).

With the intention of making teenagers feel part of the program, we had some meetings to think and organize in groups the working method for the year. The team leaders were one occupational therapist and two social workers who were also responsible for implementing other programs involving promotion and social assistance. In these meetings, we worked on:

6. **Personal strengthening**: self-esteem, interests and choices, communication, values, conflict solutions, individual problems, among others.

7. **Community integration**: collecting information from different organizations, visiting occupational workshops and cultural spaces in the area, knowing about resources and neighbors' associations.

8. **Occupational orientation to studies or work**: individual interviews, interest list, analysis of local possibilities, drafting of CVs, attending job interviews, and selection of job opportunities in newspapers and magazine ads, etc.

9. Meetings with families, visits to places in the open air, celebrations, participating in entertainment and cultural shows.

The program provided a monthly economic incentive. To get this benefit students were required to be involved in different educational activities (whether official or not). At the beginning, the economic incentive was the only motive for teenagers to participate in the program but later, they developed a deeper interest in participating, thus giving the activity its true meaning.

Results and conclusions

The contribution of occupational therapy to community programs is important to achieve occupational justice. In our program, 86.2% of the teenagers finished their school year, either by passing in subjects or with some pending (they were not examined at the end of the year in the subject). Two teenagers were in jail and one of them underwent drug rehabilitation treatment. Others did not start formal educational activities, but they attended courses or occupational workshops and went to literacy and special education centers; a proportion, 13.8%, officially dropped out from school (due to pregnancy or delinquency reasons).

We would like to highlight that:

10. the teenagers gained access to new places which had a positive impact on their personal self-esteem

11. occupational participation is a key factor in people's health and quality of life

12. the community, especially in schools and neighbors' associations, acknowledges implementation of the program as a positive action.

13. in the 'Coming Back to School' program, community strategies were implemented towards achieving occupational justice and providing tools and making contributions to face and overcome occupational apartheid.

Daytime Activities Device (DAD) for children and teenagers in a psychosocially vulnerable situation

Julia Benassi, María E Fraile

Context

There were two big floods in Santa Fe, in 2003 and 2006, which increased the already evident poverty in the city. As a result, many children and teenagers

moved to urban areas from their neighborhoods located in the surrounding areas. These teenagers were children who had undergone severe psycho-physical trauma, and they came from families living in an abandoned and marginal situation, under extreme poverty conditions and within a serious breakdown of support social networks. In this psychologically devastating situation, the Childhood Team supported by the Mental Health Management Department was created. The professional team was supported by different areas such as: psychology, occupational therapy, psycho pedagogy, general practice, psychiatry, nursery, legal assistance on minors and family matters, therapeutic assistants, and people working at art workshops.

After the initial experiences, we decided to create the Daytime Activities Device (DAD), which functions in public and community spaces. The population comprised mainly children and teenagers between 8 and 14 years from psychosocially vulnerable contexts in crisis.

Participation

Two participatory approaches were offered to provide assistance and apply preventive measures. The efficacy of this intervention was directly related to the creation of different strategies of inter-organizational cooperation in each case (Paganizzi y Otros 1999).

Daytime Activities Device: A stage of treatment and linking with other community sectors, such as schools, workshops, and sport clubs in order to integrate children in their own places (Paganizzi y Otros 2007).

Working on the urgency of the case and finding alternatives: creating a space

Due to the urgency of the case, we tried to leave a tangible result for people, something that can be seen as a possible project, a period of transition to some better future, something to hope for, something for which each meeting is worthwhile (Winnicott 2003).

In these circumstances, different outcomes became evident in the process of promoting children's creative capacities. The results are real objects produced in a shared process between children. Occupational therapists and many elements of physical, mental, emotional and experimental nature served as raw materials in this process. The creative attitude is the distinguishing feature in a world where everything is a mere repetition. The idea is to allow for a process in which multiple options are possible, thus inviting them to a world of combinations (Da Rocha Medeiros 2003).

Some achievements

We saw some important changes in the children's lives. New community spaces gave some of the children the possibility of a healthier daily life in the different places where they spent their time, such as orphanages, workshops, and schools. At these places, some of which were completely new for most of them, they were treated in a different manner by their peers and they could feel that they were no longer treated as 'criminals' or 'freaks'. On the contrary, they could meet each other within a valuable social experience.

Final comments

The programs discussed in this chapter, at a psychiatric hospital and nearby neighborhoods and public parks, are especially significant because they reveal the purpose of building and/or recovering a life project with people living in such environments.

At workshops, by promoting creative social and inclusive activities, we encourage social participation and exercise of basic citizen rights. Access to education, health, and life in community becomes central to the social context of occupational therapy and goes beyond the traditional work done in institutions and is far removed from the medical intervention-based approach of the past century.

The social and political panorama of Argentina is recovering slowly (CEPAL 2007). As of now, the Argentine government has succeeded in reducing the excessive numbers of urban poor people by providing the population with government aid programs and non labor income.

Perspectives

14. To actively work for creating links between organizations which support social networks and act as a counterbalance to disintegration and social exclusion.

15. To participate in the formulation of social and public health policies that support the development of other intervention mechanisms in order to achieve coordination among the different areas of the society, that is, social development, public health, education, culture and justice.

References

Amenta y Otros: *Tratamiento grupal ambulatorio de pacientes esquizofrénicos y otras psicosis deficitarias. Vertex*, Buenos Aires, 2000, Polemos.

Asthon J: *Las Ciudades Sanas, Una Iniciativa de la Nueva Sanidad*, España, 2000, Generalitat Valenciana.

Barrionuevo H: *Salud Mental y Discapacidad mental en las Obras Sociales Nacionales*, Buenos Aires, 2005, Ministerio de Salud.

CEPAL. Comisión Económica para América Latina y el Caribe: *Panorama social de América Latina 2002–2003*, Naciones Unidas. Available from: www.cepal.org.

CEPAL. Comisión Económica para América Latina y el Caribe: *Panorama social de América Latina 2007*, Naciones Unidas. Available from: www.cepal.org.

Da Rocha Medeiros M: *Terapia Ocupacional. Un Enfoque Epistemológico y Social*, Sao Paulo, Brasil, 2003, EDUFSCAR.

Dabas E: *Red de Redes. Las Prácticas de la Intervención en Redes Sociales*, Buenos Aires, Argentina, 2001, Paidos.

Duschatzky S, Corea C: *Chicos en Banda. Los Caminos de la Subjetividad en el Declive de las Instituciones*, Buenos Aires, Argentina, 2007, Paidos.

García Cein E, Veyra M: *Algunas reflexiones sobre el rol actual del TO en la comunidad*, Argentina, 2005, Mar del Plata Revista Contexto Psicológico 3(12).

ILO. International Labor Organization: *Panorama Social 2007*. Available from: www.oit.org.

Kielhofner G: *Terapia Ocupacional. Modelo de la Ocupación Humana: Teoría y Aplicación*, Argentina, 2004, Panamericana Buenos Aires.

Kronenberg F, Simo Algado S, Pollard N: *Terapia Ocupacional sin Fronteras.*

Aprendiendo del espíritu de supervivientes, Madrid, España, 2007, Panamericana.

Paganizzi y Otros L: *Del Hecho al Dicho*, Argentina, 1999, Buenos Aires, pp 55–64 Psicoterapias Integradas Editores 83–86.

Paganizzi y Otros L: *Terapia Ocupacional Psicosocial. Escenarios clínicos y comunitarios*, Buenos Aires, Argentina, 2007, Polemos.

Rodríguez Del Barrio Lourdes: *Salud Mental y Rehabilitación: La dinámica de diversificación y homogeneización de organizaciones, discursos y prácticas*, 1999, Polemos Buenos Aires. Vertex Revista de Psiquiatría 10(36).

OPS, OMS: *Promoción de la salud: una antología. Carta de Ottawa para la promoción de la salud*, Ottawa, Canadá, Washington DC, 1986, EE UU.

Winnicott D: *Realidad y Juego*, 2003, Gedisa Buenos Aires.

Crossing borders in correctional institutions

Jaime Philip Muñoz   Louise Farnworth
Toby Ballou Hamilton   Sandra Rogers
John A. White   Gina Marie Prioletti

OVERVIEW

The per capita incarceration rate in the United States is at an all time high and worldwide millions of people occupy prisons and jails. In the United States, as in many countries, contemporary criminal justice practices create social consequences that leave individuals, families, and society at large less able to flourish in occupationally just and stable communities. Occupational therapists and occupational scientists are beginning to make crucial connections between occupational engagement and reductions in criminal behavior. This chapter presents a mix of program descriptions and exploratory and outcomes research on the occupational needs of ex-offenders and several occupational enrichment programs designed to address post-release community functioning. These programs use occupation as a means of promoting adaptive behaviors that not only reduce recidivism, but also increase noncriminal social participation. The intent of this chapter is to stimulate readers to consider a range of possibilities for developing occupation-based programming for ex-offenders and to envision creative strategies that infuse criminal justice practices with an occupational justice perspective.

Introduction

A primary function of a nation's criminal justice system is to secure, maintain, or restore social control (Foucault 1975). Criminal justice systems typically include police (constables, gendarmerie, mishtara, etc.) who enforce a nation's laws, courts that interpret and apply laws, and correctional settings (jails, prisons, etc.) that hold those suspected or convicted of breaking laws. Criminal justice systems vary cross-culturally. These systems are more or less adversarial or compassionate, coercive, and/or focused on rehabilitation (Pakes 2004). Violations include writing bad checks (United States), not standing when the King's song is played (Thailand), breaking religious law (Saudi Arabia) or political activism (Myanmar). A nation's rate of incarceration can be influenced by distribution of wealth, political stability, unemployment rates, sentencing practices, the degree to which disrespect for human rights permeates the correctional justice system, or the use of alternatives to incarceration such as restorative justice programs (Pakes 2004).

Worldwide, prison populations have grown exponentially (Tkachuk & Walmsley 2001). In the United States, more than one in every 100 adults is in jail or prison (Bureau of Justice Statistics 2007) and the number of state prisons has nearly doubled in the past 30 years (Lawrence & Travis 2004). Prison overcrowding increases the probability of substandard sanitation and hygiene facilities, limitations in physical and mental healthcare, and reductions in educational, vocational, and community reintegration interventions (Tkachuk & Walmsley 2001). Moreover, prison can be a brutalizing environment where 'prisoners struggle to maintain their self-respect and emotional equilibrium despite omnipresent violence, exploitation, and extortion; despite an utter lack of privacy; stark limitations on family and community contacts; and the paucity of opportunities for education, meaningful work, or other productive, purposeful activities' (Human Rights Watch 2003).

The profile of the typical offender in the United States is a person with a history of poverty, substance

© 2011, Elsevier Ltd.
DOI: 10.1016/B978-0-7020-3103-8.00034-1

abuse, mental illness, and/or learning disability. Offenders often grow up with diminished social statuses, in poorer communities, with less access to quality healthcare and education, and limited political power (Magnani & Wray 2006). They are more likely to drop out of school and less likely to pursue vocational education (Bernstein & Houston 2000). Female offenders often have a history of addiction or mental health issues and poor educational and vocational histories. Many are single mothers of young children whose lives have been disproportionately affected by domestic violence and poverty (Bloom et al 2003). In short, offenders have a complex set of problems and come from marginalized communities. When they are released they return to these same communities they add to the already heavy concentrations of others with incarceration histories (Travis 2005). The challenge of meeting offenders' needs is complicated by social policies that often do little to address underlying contextual issues.

> Incarceration is big business with increasing resources spent to warehouse poor (people) behind bars rather then addressing issues of violence, affordable housing, equal quality education and universal healthcare as a human right or other healthcare resources that would improve daily life in marginalized communities.
>
> (Magnani & Wray 2006, p. 40)

Occupational therapists working with offenders face challenges that exist not only at an individual level, but also within the social, economic, political, and environmental contexts that influence offenders' experiences. Concepts such as occupational imbalance, occupational alienation, and occupational deprivation (Wilcock 2006), occupational restriction and reconciliation (Galvaan 2005), occupational apartheid (Kronenberg et al 2005) and occupational enrichment (Molineux & Whiteford 1999) can deepen practitioners' understandings of how correctional environments limit engagement in occupation, and provide insights for designing individual and environmental interventions to address these limitations.

For example, correctional settings systematically deny an offender's need for meaningful and health promoting occupations (occupational deprivation), yet many United States citizens believe that prison environments should restrict access or deny opportunities for such participation (occupational apartheid). Systematic denial of occupation and the loss of control over basic choices can lead many offenders to devalue themselves and the occupations they do complete (occupational restriction). Daily prison routines can be so highly structured that the ensuing monotony leads offenders to experience daily occupations as meaningless and purposeless (occupational alienation). Constriction of both choice of and opportunities to engage in occupations can negatively influence an offender's health and wellbeing (occupational imbalance) (Table 25.1).

This chapter presents a mix of literature review, program descriptions, and exploratory research with offender populations. The intent is to provide a broad, but introductory survey of occupational therapy programming in correctional systems that have used concepts from the occupational science literature to design interventions for offenders.

Table 25.1 Occupational science concepts applied to incarceration

Occupational alienation	'Sense of isolation, powerlessness, frustration, loss of control, estrangement from society or self as a result of engagement in occupation which does not satisfy inner needs' (Wilcock 1998, p. 257). The need for correctional settings to control inmate behavior inevitably limits occupational choices and creates conditions where the everyday activities of life lack meaning or purpose. Even occupations that are allowed and that once provided pleasure and meaning, such as reading or physical activity, lose meaning when they become the only choice in a mundane routine
Occupational apartheid	'Refers to the segregation of groups of people through the restriction or denial of access to dignified and meaningful participation in occupations of daily life on the basis of race, color, disability, national origin, age, gender, sexual preference, religion, political beliefs, status in society, or other characteristics' (Kronenberg et al 2005, p. 67). This concept challenges practitioners to examine the social, economic, and political conditions that deny or restrict opportunities for occupational and social participation for incarcerated populations (education, immigration, political and health access, etc.)

Continued

Table 25.1 Occupational science concepts applied to incarceration—cont'd

Occupational deprivation	'Deprivation of occupational choice and diversity because of circumstances beyond the control of individuals or communities' (Wilcock 1998, p. 257). Deprivation is distinguished from a disruption in occupational choice because it is a process that occurs over a long period of time (Whiteford 1997). Occupational deprivation is an implicit characteristic of correctional settings, that is, restriction in occupational choice is the standard operating procedure of institutions that confine prisoners
Occupational enrichment	'The deliberate manipulation of environments to facilitate and support engagement in a range of occupations congruent with those that the individual might normally perform' (Molineux & Whiteford 1999, p. 127). Relative to prisoner populations, occupational enrichment would be direct interventions in the social, physical, and cultural environments to specifically address occupational deprivation
Occupational imbalance	'A lack of balance or disproportion of occupation resulting in decreased well-being' (Wilcock 1998, p. 257). In correctional institutions, the environment creates conditions that can significantly limit the opportunity for a person to be involved in a balance of physical, mental, social, and restful occupations
Occupational reconciliation	This concept describes a person's submissive response to stifling environmental conditions. A prisoner's lack of opportunity to develop their potential as a result of loneliness, lack of stimulation, frequent victimization, and limited resources can lead them to 'give way to their circumstances and engage in limited occupations because of their restricted opportunities' (Galvaan 2005, p. 436).
Occupational restriction	This concept, which was originally used to describe a sense of devaluation experienced by domestic workers who were having their occupational choices severely controlled by their employers needs is applicable to the lived experience of prisoners. Occupational restriction leaves a person feeling as if they have no control, no choices, and no options for engaging the environment except as organized and controlled by the correctional institution's needs (Galvaan 2005).

Synthesis of occupational therapy programming in corrections

Few publications offer examples of occupational therapy programming in correctional settings. Most describe programs designed to address the needs of offenders with mental illnesses (Chacksfield & Forshaw 1997, Farnworth et al 1987, Lloyd 1985, 1987a,b) and most do not specifically address the use of outcome measures (O'Connell & Farnworth 2007). This synthesis is the result of repeated searches of the literature between 1991 and 2008 using several databases including CINAHL, OTDBase, and ProQuest. Primary search terms included correctional facilities, forensic, jail, occupational therapy, incarceration, offender, prison, and public offender. Hand searches of the table of contents for publications (1991–2008) in American (*American Journal of Occupational Therapy*), Australian (*Australian Occupational Therapy Journal*), British (*British Journal of Occupational Therapy*) and Canadian (*Canadian Journal of Occupational Therapy*) journals of occupational therapy were also conducted. Two texts with descriptions of correctional programming were also

reviewed (Cara & MacRae 2005, Couldrick & Aldred 2003). Publications that clearly identified the type of correctional setting and specified key elements of the program's structure were included. We emphasized programs that measured program outcomes (Table 25.2).

These programs operated in a variety of settings (e.g., high security state hospitals, community corrections, forensic rehabilitation facilities, etc). The Model of Human Occupation frequently guided program design (Couldrick & Aldred 2003, Eggers et al 2006, Forsyth et al 2005a). Other practice frameworks included the Canadian Model of Occupational Performance (Clarke 2003, Duncan 2004) and the Role Acquisition Model (Schindler 2004, 2005). These models offer specific concepts for considering physical and social environments and tools for outcomes measurement. Collectively, these programs each focused on independent living, self-efficacy, and pro-social skill development, healthy lifestyles, community reintegration, and social participation (see Table 25.2).

Occupational therapists are beginning to make crucial connections between enriched occupational engagement and reductions in criminal behavior that suggest occupation as a means of promoting adaptive behaviors to reduce recidivism, increase public

Table 25.2 Occupational therapy programs in correctional settings

Author	Population	Program elements	Measures
Clarke (2003) USA	Forensic rehabilitation hostel; females	Based on CMOP; work, education, leisure, community reintegration	CMOP
Duncan (2004) South Africa	Prison pre-release program; females	Story-telling, goal setting, journal writing, self-maintenance	CMOP
Forsyth et al (2005a) UK	High security state hospital; males	Based on MOHO; improve engagement in occupation	OCAIRS, OSA, AMPS, ACIS, WRI
Hooper (2008) USA	Community-based transitional housing program; males and females	Based on Life By Design (LBD) learning model: focus on occupation, dismantle prisonization, and support transformation. Focus on: self-efficacy, skill development, healthy lifestyles, wellbeing, social and community participation, self-understanding, employment, housing, recovery, lifestyle change and transformation	COPM (pre and post), used module facilitator feedback, resident feedback, graduation feedback, and follow-up interviews
Snively & Dressler (2005) USA	Community-based; males	Independent living, social support, skill building, group therapy	KELS, unspecified ed. and vocational tools
Duncan (2004) South Africa	Diversion program; First offender youth	Restorative justice program, life skills, academics	None stated
Garner (1995) UK	Regional secure unit	Prevocational, problem solving skills, social skills	None stated
Jones & McColl (1991) Canada	Forensic inpatient service unit	Life skills, pro-social behavior	None stated
Schindler (2005) USA	Maximum security psych unit	Role development, interpersonal skills	None stated

CMOP, Canadian Model of Occupational Performance; MOHO, Model of Human Occupation; OCAIRS, Occupational Circumstances Assessment Interview and Rating Scale; OSA, Occupational Self Assessment; AMPS, ; ACIS, ; WRI, .

safety, and inform public policy relative to criminal and social justice. Three evidence-based approaches to reducing recidivism include education, treatment for mental illness and substance abuse, and jobs with self-sufficiency wages (McKean & Ransford 2004). In the next section, we discuss four programs designed to address occupational performance needs of offenders through programming designed to enrich opportunities for occupational engagement.

The community reintegration project at the Allegheny county jail

In the United States, jails confine persons before or after criminal hearings and sentencing. Most jail inmates are awaiting sentencing, thus jail environments are more fluid and transitory than prisons where inmates are sentenced to terms of more than one year. The Community Reintegration Project (CRP) at the Allegheny County Jail (ACJ) is designed to ameliorate the effects of occupational deprivation by providing opportunities for incarcerated men to develop adaptive patterns for post-release occupational functioning (Eggers et al 2003, 2006).

In the United States, African American males make up less than 7% of the population but account for nearly 40% of the population in correctional facilities (Logan 2008). In Allegheny County in Pennsylvania, approximately a third of the entire population is African American, yet African American males account for nearly three-quarters of the population in the county jail (Center on Race and Social Problems 2007). Men in the CRP are predominately young (70% are between 20 and 40 years), African American

Table 25.3 Community reintegration project – program profile

Correctional context	Occupational profile of program participants	Program elements	Outcome measures
County jail setting in midsize city	Mean age = 34 (range 19–68) 79% report drug use	Program for males Primary outcome is employment	Intake screening (demographics) Chart review (incarceration history)
	76% are single	Group therapy three months pre-release	Occupational Self Assessment (Baron et al 2006)
	72% have children	1:1 follow-up one year post-release 4 domains of program content	Individual reintegration
	66% worked within past year 60% jailed three or more times 48% report 12th grade education 21% report mental health diagnosis	Education and employment Family and support structure Skills for living wellness	Plans (goal documentation)

(72%), single (76%), fathers (72%) with substance abuse histories (79%). Most are incarcerated on non-violent charges such as nonpayment of child support, driving under the influence, or drug possession. Educational and work histories vary, but most men describe limited schooling and sporadic work histories. Typical jobs prior to incarceration include work in construction, and the food and service trades (Table 25.3). These bleak statistics reflect the systemic, externally observable realities of occupational apartheid. The well-documented racial disparities in conviction and incarceration rates in the United States translate into an incredible loss of human capital. If a community is to sustain itself and advocate for socioeconomic viability and civic and cultural development, it needs educated adults, but for every black male who graduates from college there are 100 black males incarcerated (Lanier 2003). The men in the CRP often return to impoverished communities where the other men, and increasingly the women, struggle to overcome the lack of educational and economic opportunities (Magnani & Wray 2006).

The CRP addresses four domains critical to successful community reintegration: employment, family and support structure, wellness, and skills for living and education. The program fosters productive occupational role functioning with an emphasis on finding and keeping employment. The program begins in the jail. Inmates within three months of release attend group and individual sessions emphasizing self-assessment, skill building, and action planning for post-release. Reintegration specialists provide case management services to each participant for a full year post-release. Participants are considered successful in the program if they meet identified domain area goals, find, get, and keep a job, and do not return to jail. The recidivism rate of all inmates in the county jail is 65–70%, while the recidivism rate for men enrolled in the CRP is 34% (Eggers et al 2006).

Despite the significant reduction in recidivism, interviews with men who have not returned to jail one-year post release describe the continuing challenges of establishing a positive pattern of occupational functioning. Person–environment interactions in employment and community contexts present both barriers and opportunities for meaningful participation in occupation.

> It is hard, cause I am right back in it. Cops, drugs, little kids running around, mothers on drugs, no fathers around and public housing. Geographic change wasn't going to help me. I've got to change within myself.
>
> (Participant C)

Successful participants of the program have identified behavioral routines they felt supported reentry such as avoiding people who might influence participation in criminal activities or increasing their pursuit of non-criminal activities.

> People, places and things. You can't go back into the same environment. I can not go to, like my relatives still sell drugs, use drugs. I haven't visited them since I got outta jail. No, people, places and things will get you in trouble.
>
> (Participant F)

These men also describe intrapersonal processes that support their resolve to remain out of jail. These strategies range from finding spiritual meaning in their life circumstances to specific cognitive processes used to consider consequences before acting.

> I see the same faces coming back in. I told myself right then and there, I'm going to be the one (who remains out of jail).
>
> (Participant G)

> I know peoples gonna sit up there and say, Oh I can't find a job, no one will hire me, you can't find this, you can't find that. You got to make your own way.
>
> (Participant F)

Family also plays an integral role in the reentry process. Men in the CRP program often speak of the need and the challenges of (re)-establishing family connectedness, their efforts to manage family roles, and the insights they have gained about the influence of their behavior on their children's' lives.

> I can't keep running in and out [of the kids' lives]. Cause how you think the kids would feel? Oh, there goes dad, he's gone again. It's not good for the kids.
>
> (Participant A)

Successful community reentry is a complex transition for ex-offenders. Men in the CRP program are faced with a variety of personal, familial, and societal and legal barriers to community re-entry. Typical needs included housing, drug counseling, financial assistance, specific tangible support for items such as food and clothing, custody, parenting and legal issues, and transportation. Family, employment, and meaningful participation in occupational roles within their families and neighborhoods each offered meaningful opportunities for participation in the mores of community life.

Washington County Community Corrections

With over 20 000 people incarcerated in Oregon jails and prisons at an average annual cost of $27 000 per prison inmate in 2002 (cited in Crime Victims United n.d.). Oregon spends proportionally more ($684 million) than any other state on corrections (10.9% of its budget) and is one of five states that spend more money on corrections than on higher education. Nearly half the inmates released from Oregon correction facilities recidivate within one year. Primary factors influencing recidivism include criminal attitudes and beliefs, negative peer association, impulsivity, and chemical dependency (Washington County Corrections 2007). Creatively addressing these concerns, Washington County Community Corrections (WCCC) has decreased recidivism to 37%.

The occupational therapy pilot program designed to address the complex problem-set of ex-offenders is a collaborative partnership between WCCC and the School of Occupational Therapy at Pacific University (OT-WCCC). The OT-WCCC program was integrated into the Center's Drug and Alcohol Treatment Program serving men and women in a residential facility. Most services occurring within this setting use a 'teach and talk' format, featuring didactic discussions and verbal reinforcement of key issues or the use of cognitive-behavioral techniques. Program participants earn pass privileges to seek housing and employment.

Prominent offender health concerns include substance abuse, depression and anxiety, vision problems, headaches, obesity, hypertension, poor sleep habits and unprotected sex with multiple partners (Gietzen et al., Pacific University unpublished study 2005); most offenders have poor educational and vocational histories. Occupational deprivation is evident in patterns of performance from the Occupational Self Assessment (Baron et al 2006), including limitations in habituation (lack of satisfying routine, limited role involvement, managing time and responsibilities) and a constraining physical and social environment (e.g., housing, basic self-care resources, and limited social supports).

The OT-WCCC pre-release component added a critical active component compared with programming provided by WCCC staff. Occupational therapy modules address occupational exploration (e.g., cooking, exercise, shopping, leisure) and occupational balance and enrichment (e.g., stress and time management, communication, health and wellness, personal planning) (Hooper 2008). Primary goals are to increase successful reintegration, decrease recidivism, and create conditions that support occupational re-engagement. Plans for the OT-WCC program are to investigate the impact of occupational enrichment on program outcomes, to extend the scope of services in the residential setting, and to follow participants' for 12 months' post-release. Post-release programming will focus on maintenance of healthy occupational routines in the community, and building, through practice, the skills necessary to manage social pressures that accompany regained independence.

Center for Family Success

The Center for Family Success and the School of Occupational Therapy at Pacific University developed a program (CFS-OT) for female offenders. The mission of CFS-OT the Center for Family Success (http://www.childrensjusticealliance.org/projects_cfs.htm) is to improve the wellbeing of children with parents in the criminal justice system. Women offenders experience high rates of poverty, domestic violence, sexual abuse, and drug addiction (Covington 2002, Oregon Department of Corrections 2008). The center serves up to 60 women and their children through parent education, advocacy, coached family time, life skills development, and building positive social networks. The CFS-OT is grounded in an occupational perspective of health (Wilcock 2006) with engagement in healthy work and leisure occupations essential for the personal transformation and community engagement (i.e., working, living in a habitat, shopping, using public services, transportation, and healthcare services) and participation that supports a productive, clean and sober lifestyle (i.e., the absence of substance use and criminal behavior).

The CFS-OT program was designed to examine engagement or lack of engagement, in satisfying and socially acceptable life activities to support sustained employment and housing, and prevent recidivism. Mothering occupations are emphasized, given that 1.8 million minor children nationally have an incarcerated parent, and women typically are the primary caregivers (Bureau of Justice Statistics 2000). Pre-release limitations in healthy occupations, life skills, parenting responsibilities and social support makes the transition to a clean and sober lifestyle particularly difficult for women (Ritchie 2001). Post-release transition to the community often entails returning to the same economically and occupationally impoverished communities where they practiced unhealthy choices (Logan 2008, Ritchie 2001).

The CFS-OT program helps women engage in occupations with their children, while fostering appreciation of parenting, work, and leisure activities, and directly addresses societal attitudes and barriers that are essential for their re-engagement as parents and as community members (Jose-Kampfner 2004). The CFS-OT program challenges women to transfer the skills learned in didactic classes into healthy habits, routines, and roles. Women have the opportunity to create and engage in a healthy lifestyle through the performance of novel and familiar occupations in their local neighborhoods and within the social network they belong to or have access to.

Geena's challenges are typical of women struggling to make a 'new' life in the community post-release (Table 25.4). If any one of the fragile supports of her occupational life fails she may become homeless, jobless, and at greater risk for returning to violent relationships and drug use. Once Geena completed the CFS-OT parenting skills and housing training she earned a certificate that helped her secure housing (provides financial security for the landlord), and she received on-going support to pursue her education. The CFS-OT program provides

---

Table 25.4 Occupational profile for Geena

Occupational profile	24 years old; physically and sexually abused as a child
	Family history: primary and extended family includes alcoholism and drug abuse
	Employment history: held entry-level, minimum-wage jobs
	Accepted state welfare assistance to raise children and maintain a household
	Criminal justice history: convicted of fraud and stealing and sentenced to 24 months in state prison, inclusive of four months in county jail
	Released six months ago and seeing her parole officer
	Regained custody of her children three months ago
Current situation	4- and 6-year-old children with minor developmental delays; two different fathers; Currently three months pregnant; unplanned pregnancy
	History of homelessness, domestic violence by a series of live-in partners, including one of the fathers
	Family not 'close'; one parent is living; little or no contact with grandparents, parent, or siblings

Continued

Table 25.4 Occupational profile for Geena—cont'd

Strengths	Views education as a way to improve her income and occupational status Completed GED in prison; attends apprentice program for medical technology Committed to sober living Completed 500 hours of therapy/classes in prison (substance abuse treatment; abuse, problem solving, and life skills) Attends Alcoholics Anonymous meetings and sees her sponsor several times a week Concerned parent; striving to be more involved and directive Enrolled children in daycare with therapy services; connected to and willing to use services
Challenges	Financially impoverished and receives limited assistance for food Housing: Currently lives in one room transitional housing unit with her two children; common kitchen and bathroom facilities; limited storage for food or capability to make own food; looking for safe, affordable housing, near childcare and apprenticeship program; needs to complete housing training program Daily schedule: 6 am commutes to childcare, drop off children, commutes to apprentice program then back to pick up children; home by 6 pm No established routines for children; unaware of how to monitor and engage children in appropriate activities in the evenings or weekends Family meals consist of inexpensive low-nutritional meals or fast food Social participation: lacks significant social relationships and social supports Affective: fears return to domestic partner would ensure both greater financial security and return to abuse; feels isolated, chaotic, and sad about her situation
Intervention	Center for Family Success: parenting, housing, and childcare classes Occupational therapy: • Practice engaging in healthy occupations • Skill development for meal planning and setting routines for self/children • Find and participate in low cost play opportunities for play for children (swimming pools, playgrounds) • Finding and attending support groups and occupationally relevant interest groups

Geena with opportunities to identify and engage in desired occupations (e.g., making/keeping appointments, preparing a schedule, shopping for healthy food, finding low-budget social activities for her family). In weekly sessions she set goals, received coaching in the grocery store, and got help structuring her children's bedtime routines. Future programming will include life-coaching and support in building and maintaining social support networks.

Oklahoma Halfway House

'Halfway' implies transition from one state to another. Because 95% of offenders return to their communities of origin (Hughes & Wilson 2002), a correctional halfway house provides offenders an opportunity to make a successful transition from prison into personally meaningful community occupations. Successful re-entry requires a balance of physical, mental, and social wellbeing derived through work, household management, leisure, childcare, and other activities that are socially valued and individually meaningful; in short, successful re-entry requires occupational health (Wilcock 2006). Challenges of re-entry including obtaining employment, housing, transportation, healthcare and childcare, while simultaneously resuming management of household and family roles and routines (Hirsch et al. 2002).

The Oklahoma Halfway House (OHH) is a nonprofit organization whose goal is to provide a secure context for residents to assume community-based employment and family reintegration while providing programming to reduce recidivism. Technically, OHH residents are still in custody and are diligently monitored to ensure they are accounted for at all times while they serve out the remainder of their sentences. At the OHH the physical and social environments are designed to communicate a respect for human dignity while also providing both opportunities and expectations for residents to engage in productive patterns of occupation. Residents immediately exchange shirts marked 'inmate' for street clothes. They live in and maintain dorm-like rooms and the only security fence is around the children's playground. Staff do not wake residents in the morning or call them to mealtimes. Residents fill out their own itineraries, take meals provided in local restaurants, and use city buses to search for jobs.

Many residents are first offenders with drug- or property-related crimes. Most residents report a chaotic home life as a child and 73% of the women have a history of childhood physical, sexual, or emotional abuse. At OHH, federal offenders attend employment-focused groups on job preparedness and job placement and receive career development planning. Mandatory evening groups focus on literacy, critical thinking (exploring decision-making processes using logical methods), family reintegration, recovery from physical, sexual, or emotional abuse during childhood or domestic violence, and relapse prevention.

Most face multiple barriers in obtaining and maintaining employment. The majority have inadequate secondary or vocational education, poor functional literacy skills, and are ill-equipped to overcome public stigma and employer attitudes about felony convictions. Many lack work experience and have few marketable job skills. Some residents may have participated in prison work programs, but such programs are often more focused on increasing the profits of companies that employ prison labor than on developing inmates work habits and marketable skills (Logan 2008).

Once eligible for work, residents have 15 days to obtain full-time employment. Some keep their jobs on release from the OHH, while others must find new jobs on relocation. Unemployed residents have daily housekeeping duties and those with the longest sustained employment earn rooms with fewer roommates. Once employed, the OHH staff confirms that residents are at the job site daily. Employed residents contribute 50% of their pay for subsistence, put 20% of their income into savings for re-entry expenses, and pay 10% to cover court fees, fines, and restitution.

Occupational therapy services are a joint project of the OHH and the Program in Occupational Therapy at the University of Oklahoma Health Sciences Center. The program at OHH helps the university to fulfill its mission regarding community service, while providing a setting for student learning. The occupational

therapist screens residents with physical, cognitive, or psychosocial disabilities referred by staff. Referrals include residents with health conditions or injuries that seriously challenge employability. The occupational therapist evaluates and provides individual intervention directed at life skills; employment readiness, acquisition, and maintenance; leisure pursuits; medication routine; and re-entry skills (Table 25.5).

Individual and group interventions at the halfway houses focus on redesigning a life around occupational health. Occupational therapy personnel provide intervention and supervise students in offering groups in life skills, employment, career planning, leisure, and social participation and provide individual intervention. Occupational therapy provides residents with graded in-community support for identified re-entry challenges. Post-release support groups would focus on immediate and long-term re-entry challenges with assistance from certified peer support specialists (former offenders who have successfully reentered the community). The Occupational Performance History Interview II (Kielhofner et al 2004) can be used to examine whether a person's occupational history predicts recidivism and the Occupational Self Assessment (Baron et al 2006) can help describe offenders' patterns of occupational performance problems and goal setting priorities. Post-re-entry outcome measures include recidivism data and indicators of occupational health, such as employment, career development, family reintegration, household management, participation in family and social roles, and community housing.

Future directions and conclusions

'If you do the crime, you do the time' is a phrase referring to the consequences of criminal behavior. However, most are unaware of the degree to which these consequences permeate an ex-offender's community life post release. Ex-offenders face various forms of occupational alienation and deprivation. Property owners legally deny housing to felons and employers toss applications that reflect a history of incarceration. In many states, convicted felons are systematically denied eligibility for food stamps, public assistance, public housing, student loans, drivers' licenses, and even the right to vote (Legal Action Center 2004).

The negative consequences of incarceration on people already marginalized in multiple ways prior

Table 25.5 Oklahoma Halfway House – program profile

Correctional context	Occupational profile of program participants	Program elements	Outcome measures
Not-for-profit halfway house in midsize city	Males = 140 beds	Screening for mental health, substance abuse and literacy	Intake screening for special needs for disability, chronic conditions, and mental health
	Females = 23 beds	Focus on employment in community setting	Chart review
	75 state beds and 88 federal beds	Dorm rooms; no fences	Incarceration history
	10% with disability or chronic health condition	Accountability 24/7	Interview
	11% with mental illness	1:1 occupational therapy intervention to: find/keep employment, build life, leisure, and wellness skills for re-entry	Employment until discharge
	10% dorm rooms; no fences	Occupational therapy student volunteers run group sessions	
	75% of women are survivors of abuse	Master Social Work staff also run group sessions	
	8–12% recidivism rate from facility		

to incarceration are well known. The number of persons in jails, prisons and other correctional settings in industrialized nations continues to grow. The impact of overcrowding increases the likelihood that such environments further jeopardize opportunities for rehabilitation. Nearly two-thirds of offenders return to prison within three years of release. The human and financial costs for society are enormous. This chapter offered concepts such as occupational deprivation, occupational imbalance, and occupational enrichment as conceptual frameworks for understanding the negative impacts of secure settings on the occupational performance patterns of offenders. Such concepts are also useful to frame interventions aimed at maintaining and developing occupational skills and roles that support successful community reentry. The outcomes of such interventions should influence development of policy within correctional settings and change practices within secure settings, as well as the broader sociopolitical arena. However, echoing O'Connell & Farnworth (2007), these concepts require further definition.

This chapter described occupational therapy programs that demonstrate a range of possibilities for developing innovative, occupation-based practices with positive outcomes for offenders. Occupational

therapists and occupational scientists are just beginning to build a coherent body of evidence of occupational therapy practice in corrections. Still, the potential to undertake multi-site, international studies is feasible. Development of academic-practices partnerships will assist this development as noted in the academic-practice partnership in a county jail in the United States that supported the scholarship of practice and modeled evidence gathering through systematic evaluation (Crist et al 2005, Forsyth et al 2005b, Suarez-Balcazar et al 2005). A list serve such as (http://uk.groups.yahoo.com/group/forensic_occupational_therapy/) indicates the possibilities of research support for practitioners, and an international exchange of ideas on occupational therapy focused on corrections. These activities can help support coordination of research endeavors, and dissemination of occupational therapy best practices in corrections. The collaborators for this chapter illustrate that even geographic distances do not hinder such work. A more significant challenge for the occupational therapy profession is to address the underlying social inequities that help to create conditions that lead people to choose occupations which lead to imprisonment and sustain repeated patterns of recidivism.

References

Baron K, Kielhofner G, Iyenger A, Goldhammer V, Wolenski J: *A User's Manual for the Occupational Self-Assessment (Version 2.2)*, Chicago, 2006, Model of Human Occupational Clearinghouse, University of Illinois at Chicago.

Bernstein J, Houston E: *Crime and Work: What Can We Learn From the Low Wage Labor Market?*, Washington, DC, 2000, Economic Policy Institute.

Bloom B, Owen B, Covington S: *Gender-Responsive Strategies: Research Practice, and Guiding Principles for Women Offenders*, Washington, DC, 2003, National Institute of Corrections.

Bureau of Justice Statistics: *Incarcerated Parents and Their Children*, Washington, DC, 2000, U.S. Department of Justice.

Bureau of Justice Statistics: *Prison Statistics: Summary Findings*, Washington, DC, 2007, U.S. Department of Justice, Office of Justice Programs. Online Available at:http://www.ojp.usdoj.gov/bjs/prisons.htm. Accessed June 1, 2008.

Cara L, MacRae A: *Psychosocial Occupational Therapy: A Clinical Practice*, ed 2, Clifton Park, NJ, 2005, Thompson Delmar Learning.

Center on Race and Social Problems: *Pittsburgh's Racial Demographics: Differences and Disparities*, 2007, Center on Race and Social Problems, School of Social Work, University of Pittsburgh. Online Available at: http://www.crsp.pitt.edu/demographics.html. Accessed July 20, 2009.

Chacksfield D, Forshaw D: Occupational therapy and forensic addictive behaviours, *British Journal of Occupational Therapy* 4:381–386, 1997.

Clarke C: Clinical application of the Canadian model of occupational performance in a forensic rehabilitation hostel, *British Journal of Occupational Therapy* 66:171–174, 2003.

Couldrick L, Aldred D: *Forensic Occupational Therapy*, London, 2003, Whurr.

Covington S: A woman's journey home: Challenges for female offenders. Washington, DC 2002. Online

Available at: http://urban.org/publications/410630.html. Accessed February 9, 2009.

Crist P, Muñoz JP, Hansen AMW, Benson J, Provident I: The Practice-scholar program: An academic-practice partnership to promote the scholarship of 'best practices', *Occupational Therapy in Health Care* 19:71–93, 2005.

Duncan M: Occupation in the criminal justice system. In Watson R, Swartz L, editors: *Transformation Through Occupation*, London, 2004, Whurr, pp 129–142.

Eggers M, Sciulli J, Gaguzis K, Muñoz JP: Enrichment through occupation: The Allegheny county jail project, *OT Practice* 26:1–3, 2003.

Eggers M, Muñoz J, Sciulli J, Crist PA: The community reintegration project: occupational therapy at work in a county jail, *Occupational Therapy in Health Care* 20:17–37, 2006.

Farnworth L, Morgan S, Fernando B, et al: Prison based occupational therapy, *Australian Journal of Occupational Therapy* 34:40–46, 1987.

Forsyth K, Duncan E, Summerfield Mann L: Scholarship of practice in the United Kingdom: An occupational therapy service case study, *Occupational Therapy in Health Care* 19:17–29, 2005a.

Forsyth K, Deshpande S, Kielhofner G, et al: *A user's manual for the OCAIRS: The Occupational Circumstances Assessment Interview and Rating Scale (version 4)*, Chicago, 2005b, Model of Human Occupation Clearinghouse.

Foucault M: *Discipline and punish: The birth of the prison*, Sheridan A, translator, 1977, New York, 1975, Pantheon.

Galvaan R: Domestic workers' narratives: Transforming occupational therapy practice. In Kronenberg F, Algado SS, Pollard N, editors: *Occupational Therapy Without Borders: Learning Through the Spirit of Survivors*, Edinburgh, 2005, Elsevier/Churchill Livingstone, pp 429–439.

Garner R: Prevocational training within a secure environment: A programme designed to enable the forensic patient to prepare for mainstream

opportunities, *British Journal of Occupational Therapy* 58:2–6, 1995.

Gietzen, JW, Hough JA, VanAtta J: Prevalence of medical conditions of inmates in a community corrections population. Unpublished manuscript. Pacific University 2005.

Hirsch AE, Dietrich SM, Landau R, et al: *Every Door Closed: Barriers Facing Parents with Criminal Records*, Philadelphia and Washington DC, 2002, Community Legal Services and the Center for Law and Social Policy. Online Available at: http://www.clasp.org/publications/every_door_closed.pdf. Accessed April 4, 2008.

Hooper B: *Occupational science and occupational therapy in correctional institutions: Community Reintegration Project at Dismas House New Mexico*, Paper presented at the American Occupational Therapy Association Annual Conference Long Beach, CA, 2008.

Hughes T, Wilson DJ: *Reentry Trends in the United States*, 2002, Bureau of Justice Statistics. Online Available at: http://www.ojp.usdoj.gov/bjs/pub/pdf/reentry.pdf. Accessed July 12, 2007.

Human Rights Watch: *Ill-equipped: U.S. Prisons and Offenders with Mental Illness*, New York, 2003, NY Human Rights Watch. Online Available at: http://www.hrw.org/reports/2003/usa1003/. Accessed March 14, 2007.

Jones E, McColl M: Development and evaluation of an interactional life skills group for offenders, *Occupational Therapy Journal of Research* 11:80–92, 1991.

Jose-Kampfner C: Mothering from prison: It can be done. In Esdaile SA, Olson JA, editors: *Mothering Occupations: Challenge, Agency and Participation*, Philadelphia, 2004, FA Davis, pp 259–279.

Kielhofner G, Mallinson T, Crawford C, et al: *A User's Manual for the Occupational Performance History Interview (Version 2.1)*, Chicago, 2004, Model of Human Occupational Clearinghouse, University of Illinois at Chicago.

Kronenberg F, Algado SS, Pollard N: *Occupational Therapy Without Borders: Learning Through the Spirit* of Survivors, Edinburgh, 2005, Elsevier/Churchill Livingstone.

Lanier J: The harmful impact of the criminal justice system and war on drugs on the African-American family. In *The State of Black America*, New York, 2003, The National Urban League, pp 169–179.

Lawrence S, Travis J: *The New Landscape of Imprisonment: Mapping America's Prison Expansion*, Washington DC, 2004, The Urban Institute.

Legal Action Center: *After prison: Roadblocks to reentry. A report on state legal barriers facing people with criminal records*, 2004. Online Available at: www.lac.org. Accessed July 22, 2009.

Lloyd C: Evaluation and forensic psychiatric occupational therapy, *British Journal of Occupational Therapy* 48:137–140, 1985.

Lloyd C: The use of film and literature in the treatment of incest offenders, *Can J Occup Ther* 54:173–179, 1987a.

Lloyd C: Sex offender programs: Is there a role of occupational therapy? *Occup Ther Int* 7:55–67, 1987b.

Logan JS: *Good Punishment? Christian Moral Practice and U.S. Imprisonment*, Grand Rapids, MI, 2008, William B Eerdmans Publishing Company.

Magnani L, Wray HL: *Beyond Prisons: A New Interfaith Paradigm for our Failed Prison System*, Minneapolis, MN, 2006, Fortress Press.

McKean L, Ransford C: *Current Strategies for Reducing Recidivism*, Chicago, 2004, Center for Impact Research.

Molineux ML, Whiteford G: Prisons: From occupational deprivation to occupational enrichment, *Journal of Occupational Science* 6:124–130, 1999.

O'Connell M, Farnworth L: Occupational therapy in forensic psychiatry: A review of the literature and a call for a united and international response, *British Journal of Occupational Therapy* 70:184–191, 2007.

Oregon Department of Corrections: *Quick Facts*, Salem, OR, 2008, Oregon Department of Corrections.

Pakes F: *Comparative Social Justice*, Devon, UK, 2004, Willan Publishing.

Ritchie BE: Challenges incarcerated women face as they return to their communities, *Crime and Delinquency* 47:368–389, 2001.

Schindler V: Occupational therapy in forensic psychiatry: Role development and schizophrenia, *Occup Ther Int* 20:3–4, 2004.

Schindler V: Role development: An evidence based intervention for individuals diagnosed with schizophrenia in a forensic facility, *Psychiatr Rehabil J* 28:391–394, 2005.

Snively F, Dressler J: Occupational therapy in the criminal justice system. In Cara L, MacRae A, editors: *Psychosocial Occupational Therapy: A Clinical Practice*, Clifton Park, NJ,

2005, Thompson Delmar Learning, pp 567–590.

Suarez-Balcazar Y, Hammel J, Helfrich C, Thomas JJ, WIlson T, Head-Ball D: A model of university-community partnerships for occupational therapy scholarship and practice, *Occupational Therapy in Health Care* 19:47–70, 2005.

Tkachuk B, Walmsley R: *World Prison Population: Facts, Trends and Solutions*, Helsinki, 2001, The European Institute for Crime Prevention and Control. Online Available at: http://www.vn.fi/om/heuni. Accessed May 4, 2008.

Travis J: *But They All Come Back: Facing the Challenges of Prisoner Reentry*, Washington, DC, 2005, The Urban Institute Press.

Washington County Corrections: *Community Corrections Biennium Plan 2007–2009*, Hillsboro, OR, 2007, Author, Online. Available at: http://www.co.washington.or.us/deptmts/comm_cor/comm_cor.htm. Accessed February 9, 2009.

Whiteford G: Occupational deprivation and incarceration, *Journal of Occupational Science* 4:126–130, 1997.

Wilcock AA: *An Occupational Perspective of Health*, Thorofare, NJ, 1998, SLACK Inc.

Wilcock AA: *An Occupational Perspective of Health*, ed 2, Thorofare, NJ, 2006, SLACK, Inc.

Occupational apartheid and national parks: the Shiretoko World Heritage Site

Mark J. Hudson   Mami Aoyama

OVERVIEW

Protected areas for the conservation of nature are becoming increasingly common around the world. While imagined as places of 'wilderness', these parks usually have long histories of human occupation. In many cases, however, such occupational histories are ignored and the human populations living in protected areas often have their lives and occupations disrupted by the assignment of park status. This chapter discusses problems of occupational apartheid associated with protected areas using the example of the Shiretoko National Park and World Heritage Site in Hokkaido, Japan. We show how ecotourism and religious ceremonies are used by indigenous Ainu people to re-engage with the 'occupationscape' of Shiretoko. It is argued that an occupation-based perspective derived from occupational therapy and occupational science can provide an important contribution to debates over policy regarding human livelihoods and wellbeing in national parks and other protected areas.

Introduction

This chapter argues that an occupation-based perspective derived from occupational therapy and occupational science can provide an important contribution to debates over human activities and wellbeing in national parks and other protected areas. Parks for the conservation of nature began with Yellowstone National Park, established in 1872, but since the 1970s there has been a tremendous growth in the number and size of such protected areas. There are now more than 105 000 terrestrial and marine protected areas across the world, covering over 11% of the land area of our planet (West et al 2006). This expansion of protected areas has been of enormous benefit for the conservation of biodiversity, but has also had far-reaching impacts on the lives and occupations of populations living within or near these protected areas. Negative impacts of protected areas can include: actual displacement of people formerly living in the park, shifts in the control of resources away from local people, alienation from land and sea, and criminalization of traditional land and sea use patterns (West et al 2006). Physical displacement can be associated with landlessness, joblessness (loss of income and means of subsistence), homelessness, social marginalization, food insecurity, loss of access to common property resources, and increased morbidity and mortality (Cernea & Schmidt-Soltau 2003). In some African parks, conservation has become 'militarized' with paramilitary groups employed to prevent poaching and other 'illegal' uses of park resources (Neumann 1998, p. 6–7).

A growing literature has begun to examine the social problems associated with parks and other conservation sites. However, the geographic coverage is uneven and there are still many gaps in our knowledge of how protected area status actually affects particular human groups over the long term (West et al 2006). This chapter attempts to contribute to this literature by providing an occupational perspective on the human use of one protected area in northern Japan. We suggest that an emphasis on occupation is a particularly empowering way to theorize the issues raised here. Occupation can be defined as 'Things that people do to occupy life for intended purposes such as paid work, unpaid work, personal-care, care of others, leisure,

DOI: 10.1016/B978-0-7020-3103-8.00035-3

recreation, or subsistence' (Christiansen & Town-send 2004, p. 279). This simple but powerful concept has considerable relevance for people living in or around protected areas.

Parks, occupation and wilderness

The idea of protected conservation areas has been intimately entwined with the concept of 'wilder-ness'. However, to borrow the title of Catton's (1997) book on Alaskan parks, many protected areas are 'inhabited wildernesses', a term that has an oxy-moronic ring because the wilderness is a place where nature supposedly takes its course *without* human intervention. In this sense, wilderness is the antithe-sis of the human activities that we call occupations; wilderness places are places that should not have his-tories of occupation. As a growing number of studies have shown, however, this is rarely the case. Many national parks have long histories of human occu-pational behavior and this occupational heritage is often what gives the park landscape its scientific or aesthetic value. The grasslands of Yosemite that so enchanted early Euro-American visitors, for exam-ple, were in part created by Native American horti-culture (Keller & Turek 1998, p. 21).

The dichotomy between wilderness and human occupations, or between nature and culture, is one that is particularly associated with the Western tradition. Indigenous and other non-Western groups, in contrast, typically view humans as more closely embedded in nature (e.g., Berkes 2008, Nelson 1969, Roth 2004, Wenzel 2004). The expansion of protected areas and related environmental policies in the past few decades has usually been associated with the importation of Western views of nature and wilderness, views that often lead to the commodification of these spaces with resulting conflicts in many cases. Forced displacement of the inhabitants of protected areas has been the most extreme result of this view of wilderness conservation. Such displacements almost always involve some degree of occupational deprivation even if new jobs and occu-pations become available as part of the conservation project. In some cases, people are displaced from their homelands only to be 'made to reappear in these land-scapes as purveyors of arts and craft, entertainment, and other services required by visitors' (West et al 2006, p. 260). Displacement and occupational deprivation can result in displaced peoples adopting unsustainable hunting practices simply to obtain food (Fabricus &

de Wet 2002). Paradoxically, too large an expansion in opportunities for work in or around protected areas can also lead to negative conservation impacts. The classic example here is the Wolong Nature Reserve in southwest China where a tourist boom enriched local villagers, increasing pressure on timber and other natural resources inside the reserve (Liu et al 2001).

This chapter examines the Shiretoko National Park and World Heritage Site in eastern Hokkaido, Japan, in the context of these issues surrounding the social and occupational impacts of protected areas. We argue that Shiretoko can be seen as an 'occupationscape' – a landscape formed and molded by human occupations. The concept of occupation-scape brings an occupational perspective to landscape studies (Hudson et al 2010). Within landscape research, Marxist and other critical geographers have been especially active in investigating the relation-ships between labor and landscape. Mitchell's (1996) *The Lie of the Land* analyzes the role of migrant workers in California to show how labor can be hidden or erased from perceptions of landscapes. In this chap-ter we want to make a broadly similar argument that the particular histories of, not just labor, but occupa-tions more generally, have been ignored in many national parks in favor of concepts of pristine 'wilder-ness' largely unaffected by human activity. Linking occupation to landscape is, we suggest, one way to re-engage displaced populations with their traditional homelands inside protected areas.

Shiretoko and national parks in Japan

Urban parks modeled on those found in European cities were introduced in Japan in 1873, but the first national parks were not established until 1934 (Katō 2000, p. 44–45). These parks were initially placed under the control of the Home Ministry before being moved to the Ministry of Health and Welfare in 1938. Apart from a spell under American military control after the Second World War, parks remained at Health and Welfare until the formation of the Environmental Agency (now Ministry) in 1971. This administrative history reflects the fact that Japanese national parks were seen primarily as places for recreation and tourism rather than as reserves for wildlife conservation. The law on national parks actually stated that one of the aims of these facilities was to support the health of the nation (Katō 2000, p. 46–49). The concept of national parks in Japan was developed by urban elites who appropriated and 'redesigned rural landscapes to suit their recreational and aesthetic interests' (Mitsuda 1998, p. 153). This history often led to *de facto* accommodation of multiple uses of parks, but not necessarily to an acceptance of the importance of subsistence occupations by park residents.

Shiretoko was made a national park in 1964 and inscribed as a World Heritage Site in 2005. Both national park and World Heritage Site cover the currently uninhabited eastern end of the Shiretoko Peninsula. With a land area of 487 km^2, the World Heritage site is slightly larger than the national park (386 km^2). A 3 km coastal zone with a surface area of 220 km^2 is also included in the World Heritage listing (Nakagawa 2006a). Shiretoko was designated as a World Natural Heritage Site on the basis of criteria (ix) and (x): 'significant on-going ecological and biological processes' and 'significant natural habitats for in-situ conservation of biological diversity' (UNESCO 2005). The Japanese government initially made no attempt to involve Ainu people – the indigenous inhabitants of Hokkaido – in the nomination process (Ono 2007, p. 133). However, the activities of the Sipetru Ainu ecotourism group discussed below were instrumental in the addition of a proposal in the Shiretoko World Heritage management plan to 'study the culture of the Ainu people and the traditional wisdom and skills of the local residents in order to determine the methods to preserve, manage and realize sustainable use of the natural environment' (International Union for Conservation of Nature (IUCN) 2005, p. 31).

Occupations in Shiretoko

The Shiretoko Peninsula has a history of human settlement reaching back at least 8000 years. Figures 26.1 and 26.2 show the numbers of archaeological sites for each period within the World Heritage park and in Shiretoko in general. Over 120 sites are known from Shiretoko, but the real number is probably much higher since little archaeological survey work has been conducted on the peninsula. Around 15% of known archaeological sites belong to the Ainu cultural period (approximately 1200–1869). The name 'Shiretoko' derives from an Ainu word meaning 'the end of the land', a term originally applied to Cape Shiretoko. A map of Shiretoko drawn by Japanese explorer Takeshirō Matsu'ura in the mid-nineteenth century lists Ainu place names for dozens of rivers and streams around the peninsula.

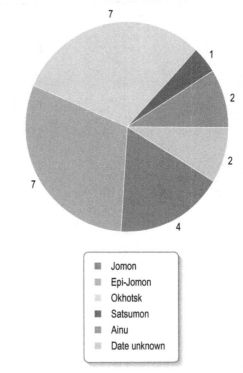

Fig. 26.1 • Numbers of registered archaeological sites by period in the Shiretoko World Heritage area. Data from Shiretoko Museum (2005).

Most of the 8000-year human history of Shiretoko has been based on hunter-gathering. Although agriculture is now an important industry around the base of the Shiretoko Peninsula, farming has never been an important subsistence strategy in the park area. Agricultural migrants from Japan first came to Iwaobetsu in 1914 but conditions were so harsh that they moved out by 1925. Other unsuccessful attempts at agricultural colonization were made in 1937 and 1949–1966, but the last farmers left in 1966 (Nakagawa 2006a). Rather than farming, it was fishing that came to have the most far-reaching influence on Ainu livelihoods in Shiretoko. The Shiretoko Peninsula is characterized by closely linked marine and terrestrial ecosystems (Makino et al 2009). Marine resources have been extensively exploited for thousands of years by Ainu and other cultural groups in Shiretoko and other parts of Hokkaido (Hudson 2004, Okada 1998). From the eighteenth century, however, Japanese colonists established a system of fishing stations in Hokkaido and Sakhalin where Ainu were forced to work as laborers (Howell 1995). In Shiretoko, the Nemuro station on the south side of the peninsula was

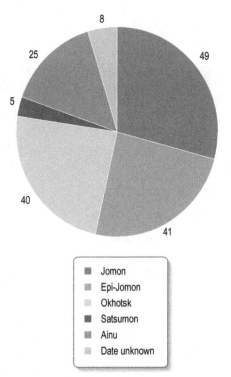

Jomon
Epi-Jomon
Okhotsk
Satsumon
Ainu
Date unknown

Fig. 26.2 • Numbers of registered archaeological sites by period on the Shiretoko peninsula. Data from Shiretoko Museum (2005).

established in 1789 and the Shari station on the north side in 1790 (Nakagawa 2006b, p. 137).

The exploitative working conditions in these fishing stations led to a rapid decline in the Ainu population of Shiretoko. The first mention of Shiretoko in historical documents is in the *Tsugaru Ittōshi* which records that in 1669, about a hundred Ainu men from Cape Shiretoko took part in the Shakushain War between Ainu and Japanese colonists in southern Hokkaido. In 1856, however, Takeshirō Matsu'ura recorded that there were only three Ainu households comprising 10 individuals in the same location (Nakagawa 2006b, p. 136). According to Matsu'ura (2006, p. 37–40), the number of Ainu houses in the Shari station as a whole declined from 316 in 1822 to 173 in 1856. This dramatic decline mirrors that known for Hokkaido as a whole over the same period (cf. Walker 2001, p. 181–182). Almost a century before Shiretoko became a national park, therefore, much of the indigenous Ainu population had already been displaced from the peninsula. Today there are only a handful of Ainu who reside in Shiretoko, all of whom have moved there recently from other parts of Hokkaido.

The history of Ainu people in Shiretoko provides a clear example of occupational apartheid, defined as 'the segregation of groups of people through the restriction or denial of access to dignified and meaningful participation in occupations of daily life' (Kronenberg & Pollard 2005, p. 67). Although this chapter has placed the occupational apartheid experienced by Shiretoko Ainu in the context of forced displacements from national parks, it is of course the case that this displacement occurred long before Shiretoko national park was established in 1964. While the occupational apartheid considered here was thus not a direct result of park conservation policy, it has nevertheless been reproduced in modern Japan by a discourse of wilderness that has ignored Shiretoko's history of Ainu settlement. Since the first tourist boom in 1971, the Japanese public has shown considerable interest in the natural environment of Shiretoko. Property speculation following the departure of the last farming families in the 1960s led to a national trust movement based on the British model in which ordinary people from all over Japan bought plots of land for preservation. Established by the mayor of Shari in 1977, this national trust movement became increasingly involved in green politics on a national scale in the 1980s (Mitsuda 1998). Despite the breadth of the Shiretoko environmental movement throughout Japan, however, it has displayed little interest in the Ainu people who once lived in Shiretoko. Ironically, this has happened despite a general trend in modern Japanese thought 'to incorporate (the Ainu) in the "nature" of Japan, ... to exaggerate their naturalness; in other words to assimilate them into the "nature" of Hokkaido and Nature as a whole' (Berque 1980, p. 129, translation from Hudson 2003, p. 269).

The next part of this chapter briefly considers some ways in which Ainu people have begun to make their voices heard again and to reclaim parts of their Shiretoko heritage. Here we focus on the activities of Sipetru, an Ainu ecotourism group based in Shiretoko, and the associated performance of *kamuy-nomi* rituals by Ainu at archaeological sites in Shiretoko.

Sipetru and *kamuy-nomi*

An acronym of 'Shiretoko Indigenous People Eco Tourism Research Union', Sipetru was formed in 2005 to establish and develop indigenous tourism in Shiretoko. As noted already, lobbying to the IUCN led to the inclusion of statements on the importance of Shiretoko to Ainu people in the World Heritage

Site inscription (Ono 2007, p. 135). Based in the community of Utoro, the northwestern gateway to the World Heritage park, Sipetru has focused mainly on tours to archaeological sites in and around this town. As well as explaining the history of the site and its links with Ainu people, the tour guides perform prayers before and after entering the mountain to climb to the sites. Traditional tea made from the Amur corktree (*Phellodendron amurense*) is served and one guide plays a stringed *tonkori* that he made himself. The Sipetru guides are Ainu men from Sapporo in their twenties to sixties (Ono 2007, p. 137).

Our fieldwork in Shiretoko has developed through a project in community archaeology. In September 2007, the first author participated in a Sipetru tour with other members of this project. This tour lasted about two hours and involved a hike up to the Benzai *chashi* site outside Utoro. *Chashi* were Ainu forts and their strategic location usually makes them good places to view the scenery as well as to learn about Ainu heritage (Fig. 26.3). While on this tour, we discovered another *chashi*, which had not been registered as an archaeological site and, in September 2008, a *kamuy-nomi* ceremony was performed by three Ainu Sipetru guides at this new *chashi* prior to further archaeological work. *Kamuy-nomi* is a general term for prayers or ceremonies held for the deities. These ceremonies are held in a range of contexts and are one aspect of Ainu culture that has proven remarkably resilient (Akino 1999).

Kamuy-nomi have been an important element in Ainu attempts to re-engage with their Shiretoko heritage. Long before the World Heritage inscription, Ainu in Shiretoko 'held religious ceremonies in honor of the forest spirits' to protest logging plans by the national Forest Agency in the mid-1980s (Mitsuda 1998, p. 159). In September 1986, for example, a *kamuy-nomi* was held in Shari by the 'Movement to Stop Shiretoko Logging based on Ainu Spirituality' (Ainu seishin ni yoru Shiretoko tachiki bassai soshi undō no kai) (Yasei Seibutsu Jōhō Center 1988, p. 276). These activities were part of a general revitalization of Ainu ceremonial life that began in the 1980s (Iwasaki-Goodman & Nomoto 2001). The *kamuy-nomi* witnessed by the present authors at Benzai *chashi* in 2008 was led by Kōji Yūki, representative of the Ainu Art Project and a well-known Ainu artist and activist. A simple enclosure was made using fallen tree branches at the centre of the *chashi* platform and a small fire lit. Freshly-shaved willow prayer sticks (*inaw*) were placed against a tree beside this enclosure and Yūki and an Ainu colleague sat cross-legged on the forest floor. Rice wine was sipped and gently sprayed on the earth and on the *inaw* while Yūki spoke to the gods and ancestors, apologizing for having ignored this place in the past.

Occupation, knowledge, and landscape

Indigenous ecotourism and *kamuy-nomi* ceremonies represent small-scale yet significant attempts to re-engage with Ainu occupational heritage in Shiretoko. These activities are occupations related to ritual

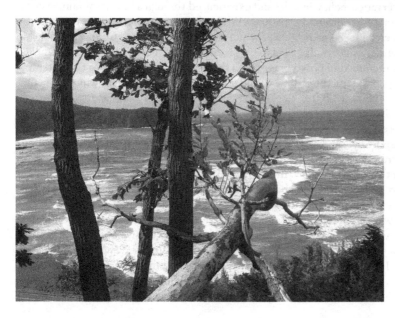

Fig. 26.3 • View of the Sea of Okhotsk from the Benzai *chashi* site.

observances and relationships between people and the environment, yet this should not be construed as evidence that they are somehow unimportant or unrelated to basic livelihood. Through visiting, talking about, and conducting ceremonies on the land, Ainu people begin to re-imagine links with that land and to recapture part of the balance of their ancient occupational heritage in Shiretoko. The use of archaeological sites for ecotours and ceremonies is crucial since these sites provide concrete connections to the past, even though some of the sites used in this respect date to before the Ainu period.

There is already an extensive literature that examines the roles of both spirituality and eco-tourism in indigenous revitalization (e.g. Hinch 2001, Nuttall 2002, Wilson 2003, Wolsko et al 2006). Building on postcolonial writings in indigenous studies such as Smith (1999), occupational therapists and occupational scientists have also begun to use occupational interventions with indigenous peoples (e.g. Frank 2007, Frank et al 2008, Simó Algado & Cardona 2005). Here we want to build on this previous work by briefly examining some further aspects of the significance of occupation for indigenous peoples, particularly in the context of occupational apartheid and injustices in protected areas.

Occupation is important in this context because it forces us to consider how even the most basic daily activities relate to overall wellbeing (see also Blakeney & Marshall 2009). An example here is the separation of 'subsistence' from 'commercial' foraging that has been adopted by many park managers, and indeed many conservationists in general. While conservation policy in some parks has been able to incorporate hunting and gathering for 'subsistence', a commercial element in such activities has usually been regarded as nontraditional and therefore unnecessary in the context of protected areas. A similar dichotomy has structured debates over Aboriginal whaling (Nuttall 2002, p. 101–123). Alaska was one of the first places where broader meanings of 'subsistence' were discussed in the context of national parks. A 1974 report by Yupiktak Bista, a Yup'ik Eskimo NPO, was instrumental 'in redefining subsistence as a cultural rather than an economic issue...'. Subsistence, the report declared, was 'directly related to and affected by everything that is happening within this region in the way of education, land use, economic development, wildlife management and other areas of public policy. Subsistence is really an entire way of life' (Catton 1997, p. 205).

Research over the past few decades has explored the complex ways in which subsistence is embedded into life for many indigenous people. In this context, it makes sense to regard 'subsistence' activities such as hunter-gathering as *occupations* (Hudson & Aoyama 2009). The holistic concept of occupation provides a concrete way of conceptualizing the 'knowledge–practice–belief complex' that we know is so central to livelihoods in many indigenous and traditional societies (cf. Berkes 2008, p. 16–18). In such societies, knowledge is acquired by participating in occupations such as 'moving through the world, living and acting in it, breathing the air, drinking the water, hunting, harvesting, fishing rivers, lakes and the sea, tilling soil, growing crops, and so on' (Nuttall 2002, p. 73). Occupations cannot be separated from the social and physical context in which they are performed.

Landscape and praxis

The concept of 'occupational apartheid' implies a commitment to political engagement (Kronenberg et al 2005, Pollard et al 2009). Such praxis requires working with *communities* (cf. McGuire 2008, p. 231), yet how can we begin this engagement with indigenous people whose communities have been ruptured and displaced by colonialism? In attempting to develop an occupational perspective on this problem, we want to suggest that the concept of 'occupation-scape' (Hudson et al 2010) may be a useful way to think about the links between people, occupations and places in protected areas such as Shiretoko. An occupationscape is a landscape that has been molded by and experienced through a history of human occupations. While the concept of occupationscape can incorporate several approaches to the relationship between landscape and occupation, it nevertheless possesses a deliberately political nature that attempts to consider how the contradictions which structure occupations are reflected in landscape.

While landscape is primarily a spatial concept, the idea of occupationscape also foregrounds the importance of *time* in occupational behavior and assumes that occupations have a cumulative history for both the individual and the group. An occupationscape can be seen as a *palimpsest* of accumulated occupations. Using terminology developed by archaeologist Geoff Bailey (2007), an occupationscape is a 'cumulative palimpsest', in which successive episodes of activity or occupation are superimposed and mixed together and also a 'palimpsest of meaning' in which different occupations acquire different meanings over time. This does not mean that the most recent elements are necessarily the most important. Rather, an occupationscape can work like many so-called 'ethnographic landscapes', which emphasize the 'long and complex relationship between people and land; the idea of people's *unity* with both natural and spiritual environment; [and] the expression of people's ties to landscape primarily through their cultural knowledge' (Krupnik et al 2004, p. 4). The idea of occupationscape adds an occupational element to this perspective by arguing that it is the human performance of occupations that provides the key link between people and the land. Thus, the long history of hunting, gathering, and fishing by Ainu and other indigenous peoples in Shiretoko represent the occupations that, above all, have been responsible for the creation of landscape. The gradual incorporation of these occupations into the capitalist economies of early modern Japan profoundly transformed Ainu livelihoods in Shiretoko and elsewhere (cf. Howell 1995), but landscape remains important because it provides such a concrete link, not just with the land itself, but with the occupations that sanctioned Ainu presence on that land.

Conclusions

This chapter has briefly examined some of the ways in which Ainu people have been able to re-engage with their occupational heritage in the Shiretoko National Park and World Heritage Site. At present this re-engagement has been centered on ritual and ecotourism links with the land. We have argued that because occupation helps (trans)form landscape, such links are a concrete way to begin to negotiate a history of occupational apartheid. Seeing Shiretoko as an 'occupationscape' does not in itself redress occupational apartheid for Ainu displaced from that peninsula, but may be one first step toward that end. Future work must attempt to examine how Ainu people themselves might wish to utilize the idea of 'occupationscape'.

The case study considered here is part of the wider problem of the social impacts of protected areas. There is no easy solution to balancing human needs and biologic conservation. Reed & Merenlender (2008), for example, recently found that even low impact recreational activities such as hiking and mountain biking can upset ecosystems and diminish biodiversity. In the context of a long history of conflict over human presence in protected areas, conservation biology is beginning to emphasize the importance of combining benefits to human livelihoods as well as to nature (Brockington et al 2006). Such thinking can be found in recent fisheries policy in Shiretoko which has stressed community co-management that is 'open to consider a wide range of human needs in the community' (Makino et al 2009, p. 213) – although to our knowledge the role of Ainu people in this co-management has so far been ignored. In this chapter we have argued that a focus on occupation provides both theoretical and practical means to develop policy benefiting both people and nature. Our discussion here has suggested that linking occupation with landscape and with heritage in general is a way to empower groups experiencing occupational apartheid.

Acknowledgments

An earlier version of this paper was presented at the 69th annual meeting of the Society for Applied Anthropology, Santa Fe, New Mexico, USA, March 2009. We thank the editors for their detailed comments on the text. This research was supported by a grant-in-aid from the Ministry of Education, Culture, Sports, Science & Technology, Japan, for the project 'The emergence of indigenous archaeology and cultural resource development in the Shiretoko World Heritage site' (No. 20320121) and by the NEOMAP project of the Research Institute for Humanity and Nature, Kyoto.

References

Akino S: Spirit-sending ceremonies. In Fitzhugh W, Dubreuil C, editors: *Ainu: Spirit of a Northern People*, Washington, DC, 1999, Arctic Studies Center, Smithsonian Institution, pp 248–255.

Bailey G: Time perspectives, palimpsests and the archaeology of time, *J Anthropol Archaeol* 26:198–223, 2007.

Berkes F: *Sacred Ecology*, ed 2, New York, 2008, Routledge.

Berque A: *La Rizière et la Banquise: Colonisation et Changement Culturel à Hokkaïdô*, Paris, 1980, Publications Orientalistes de France.

Blakeney A, Marshall A: Water quality, health, and human occupations, *Am J Occup Ther* 63:46–57, 2009.

Brockington D, Igoe J, Schmidt-Soltau K: Conservation, human rights, and poverty reduction, *Conserv Biol* 20:250–252, 2006.

Catton T: *Inhabited Wilderness: Indians, Eskimos, and National Parks in Alaska*, Albuquerque, 1997, University of New Mexico Press.

SECTION TWO **Practices Without Borders**

Cernea MM, Schmidt-Soltau K: The end of forcible displacements? Conservation must not impoverish people, *Policy Matters (IUCN Commission on Environmental, Economic & Social Policy)* 12:42–51, 2003.

Christiansen CH, Townsend EA: *Introduction to occupation: the art and science of living*, Upper Saddle River, NJ, 2004, Prentice Hall.

Fabricus C, de Wet C: The influence of forced removals and land restitutions on conservation in South Africa. In Chatty D, Colchester M, editors: *Displacement, Forced Settlement and Sustainable Development*, Oxford, 2002, Berghahn, pp 149–163.

Frank G: Collaborating to meet the goals of a native sovereign nation: the Tule River tribal history project. In Field LG, Fox RG, editors: *Anthropology Put to Work*, Oxford, 2007, Berghahn, pp 65–83.

Frank G, Murphy S, Kitching HJ, et al: The Tule River tribal history project: evaluating a California tribal government's collaboration with anthropology and occupational therapy to preserve indigenous history and promote tribal goals, *Hum Organ* 67:430–442, 2008.

Hinch T: Indigenous territories. In Weaver DB, editor: *The Encyclopedia of Indigenous Ecotourism*, Wallingford, 2001, CABI, pp 345–357.

Howell DL: *Capitalism from within: economy, society, and the state in a Japanese fishery*, Berkeley, 1995, University of California Press.

Hudson MJ: Foragers as fetish in modern Japan. In Habu J, Savelle J, Koyama S, Hongo H, editors: *Senri Ethnological Studies 63: Hunter-gatherers of the North Pacific Rim*, Osaka, 2003, National Museum of Ethnology, pp 263–274.

Hudson MJ: The perverse realities of change: world system incorporation and the Okhotsk culture of Hokkaido, *J Anthropol Archaeol* 23:290–308, 2004.

Hudson MJ, Aoyama M: Hunter-gatherers and the behavioural ecology of human occupation, *Can J Occup Ther* 76:48–55, 2009.

Hudson MJ, Aoyama M, Diab MC, Aoyama H: The South Tyrol as occupationscape: occupation, landscape and ethnicity in a European border zone. *Journal of Occupational Science*, 17(4).

International Union for Conservation of Nature: *World heritage nomination IUCN technical evaluation*, Japan, 2009, Shiretoko ID No: 1193 Online Available at: http://unesco.org/archive/advisory_body_evaluation/1193.pdf. Accessed December 16, 2008.

Iwasaki-Goodman M, Nomoto M: Revitalizing the relationship between Ainu and salmon: salmon rituals in the present. In Anderson DG, Ikeya K, editors: *Senri Ethnological Studies 59: Parks, Property, and Power: Managing Hunting Practice and Identity Within State Policy Regimes*, Osaka, 2001, National Museum of Ethnology, pp 27–46.

Katō N: *Nihon no kokuritsu kōen (The National Parks of Japan)*, Tokyo, 2000, Heibonsha.

Keller RH, Turek MF: *American Indians and National Parks*, Tucson, 1998, University of Arizona Press.

Kronenberg F, Pollard N: Overcoming occupational apartheid: a preliminary exploration of the political nature of occupational therapy. In Kronenberg F, Simó Algado S, Pollard N, editors: *Occupational Therapy Without Borders: Learning Through the Spirit of Survivors*, Edinburgh, 2005, Elsevier/Churchill Livingstone, pp 58–86.

Kronenberg F, Simó Algado S, Pollard N, editors: *Occupational Therapy Without Borders: Learning Through the Spirit of Survivors*, Edinburgh, 2005, Elsevier/Churchill Livingstone.

Krupnik I, Mason R, Buggey S: Introduction: landscapes, perspectives, and nations. In Krupnik I, Mason R, Horton T, editors: *Northern Ethnographic Landscapes: Perspectives from Circumpolar Nations*, Washington, DC, 2004, Arctic Studies Center, Smithsonian Institution, pp 1–13.

Liu J, Linderman M, Ouyang J, et al: Ecological degradation in protected areas: the case of Wolong Nature Reserve for giant pandas, *Science* 292:98–101, 2001.

McGuire RH: *Archaeology as political action*, Berkeley, 2008, University of California Press.

Makino M, Matsuda H, Sakurai Y: Expanding fisheries co-management to ecosystem-based management: a case in the Shiretoko World Natural Heritage area, Japan, *Marine Policy* 33:207–214, 2009.

Matsu'ura T: *Shiretoko kikō*, Sapporo, 2006, Hokkaidō Shuppan Kikaku Senta.

Mitchell D: *The Lie of the Land: Migrant Workers and the California Landscape*, Minneapolis, 1996, University of Minnesota Press.

Mitsuda H: National trust and local politics: twenty years of the Shiretoko national trust movement in Japan, 1977–1997, *Journal of the Faculty of Sociology, Bukkyō University* 31:151–167, 1998.

Nakagawa H: Historical view of Shiretoko national park. In McCullough D, Kaji K, Yamanaka M, editors: *Wildlife in Shiretoko and Yellowstone National Parks: Lessons in Wildlife Conservation from two World Heritage Sites*, Shari, 2006a, Shiretoko Nature Foundation, pp 221–224.

Nakagawa H: *Sekai isan Shiretoko ga Wakaru Hon (A Book to Understand Shiretoko World Heritage)*, Tokyo, 2006b, Iwanami.

Nelson R: *Hunters of the Northern Ice*, Chicago, 1969, Aldine.

Neumann RP: *Imposing Wilderness: Struggles Over Livelihood and Nature Preservation in Africa*, Berkeley, 1998, University of California Press.

Nuttall M: *Protecting the Arctic: Indigenous Peoples and Cultural Survival*, Abingdon, 2002, Routledge.

Okada A: Maritime adaptations in Hokkaido, *Arctic Anthropology* 35:340–349, 1998.

Ono Y: *Shizen no Meseeji o Kiku: Shizuka na Daichi Kara no Dengon (Listening to Nature's Message: Messages from the Quiet Land)*, Sapporo, 2007, Hokkaidō Shinbunsha.

Pollard N, Sakellariou D, Kronenberg F, editors: *Political Practice of Occupational Therapy*, Edinburgh, 2009, Elsevier Science.

Reed SE, Merenlender AM: Quiet, nonconsumptive recreation reduces protected area effectiveness, *Conservation Letters* 1:146–154, 2008.

Roth R: On the colonial margins and in the global hotspot: park-people conflicts in highland Thailand, *Asia Pacific Viewpoint* 45:13–32, 2004.

254

Shiretoko Museum: *Data Book Shiretoko 2005*, Shari, 2005, Shiretoko Museum.

Simó Algado S, Cardona CE: The return of the corn men: an intervention project with a Mayan community of Guatemalan *retornos*.
In Kronenberg F, Simó Algado S, Pollard N, editors: *Occupational Therapy Without Borders: Learning Through the Spirit of Survivors*, Edinburgh, 2005, Elsevier/Churchill Livingstone, pp 336–350.

Smith LT: *Decolonizing Methodologies: Research and Indigenous Peoples*, London, 1999, Zed Books.

UNESCO: Shiretoko, 1999: Online Available at: http://whc.unesco.org/en/list/1193. Accessed December 16, 2008.

Walker BL: *The Conquest of Ainu Lands: Ecology and Culture in Japanese Expansion, 1590–1800*, Berkeley, 2001, University of California.

Wenzel GW: From TEK to IQ: Inuit quajimajatuqangit and Inuit cultural ecology, *Arctic Anthropology* 41:238–250, 2004.

West P, Igoe J, Brockington D: Parks and peoples: the social impact of protected areas, *Annual Review of Anthropology* 35:251–277, 2006.

Wolsko C, Lardon C, Hopkins S, et al: Conceptions of wellness among the Yup'ik of the Yukon-Kuskokwim delta: the vitality of social and natural connection, *Ethn Health* 11:345–363, 2006.

Yasei Seibutsu Jōhō Center: *Shiretoko Kara no Shuppatsu: Bassai Mondai no Kyōkun o dō Ikasu ka (Starting from Shiretoko: How Should We Use the Lessons from the Logging Problem?)*, Sapporo, 2006, Kyōdō Bunkasha.

The Kawa (river) model: culturally responsive occupational therapy without borders

27

Michael K. Iwama   Hanif Farhan   Erin Hanrahan
Avital Kaufman   Alison Nelson   Neha Patel

OVERVIEW

The essence of occupational therapy is simple yet potentially powerful: to enable people from all walks of life engage or participate in activities and processes that have value. The forms and meanings of such activities and processes – or what many occupational therapists situated in industrialized countries refer to as 'occupation', will vary from person to person and from context to context. Our clients' occupational narratives – each reflecting a different constellation of shared experiences set in time and space, deserve occupational therapeutic responses that are *culturally safe* and honor diversity. The river metaphor on which the Kawa model is based, is a promising medium for diverse clients to express their daily life narratives. Over the past few years, the Kawa model has steadily spread wherever occupational therapists seek solutions to challenges of diversity and culture (in the broadest sense). A series of short case studies collected from occupational therapists in different parts of the world are presented in this chapter. The cases honor the complexities and challenges of culturally responsive occupational therapy, and offer an alternative to conventional universal approaches when occupational therapy is practiced within and across cultural borders.

Introduction

The essence of occupational therapy is simple yet potentially powerful: to enable people from all walks of life engage or participate in activities and processes that have value (Iwama 2007). The forms and meanings of such activities and processes – or what many Western occupational therapists refer to as 'occupation', will vary from person to person and from context to context. Our clients' occupational narratives – each reflecting a different constellation of shared experiences set in time and space, deserves occupational therapeutic responses that are *culturally safe* (Ramsden 1990) and honor diversity. Many occupational therapists may find this to be elusive if they apply theory in a *colonial* manner, forcing their preferred frameworks and models of occupational therapy onto *other-ed* clients (Iwama 2005a). Clients in such predicaments may find their occupational narratives forced through universal or standardized sets of concepts and principles that were originally constructed on someone else's (unfamiliar) cultural reality.

Culturally responsive (Munoz 2007) occupational therapists practicing across cultural boundaries may eventually discover that they cannot simply bring their usual ways of knowing and practice into *other* sociocultural contexts and assume that these will apply universally and equitably. Despite best intentions, doing so may disadvantage and, in some cases, be disastrous. Some may find, for example, that the largely hidden *Northern* and *Western* sociocultural values around individualism, egocentrism, and able-ism, exercised in mandates for independence, autonomy, personal causation, etc., are problematic, if not disabling. And they may discover that such problems are not isolated to some *other* clients in some *other* places, but that they can actually exist in their own domestic contexts of practice. The challenges to equitable and culturally responsive occupational therapy exist in our very own communities (Iwama 2004) and contexts of daily living as much as they do elsewhere.

The key to culturally responsive and equitable occupational therapy practice without borders lies

DOI: 10.1016/B978-0-7020-3103-8.00036-5

in *cultivating* occupational therapy theory and practice to meet the requirements of diverse clientele in diverse places and time, rather than *cultivating* or forcing the client to meet the requirements of conventional occupational therapy theory and practice (Iwama 2003). In this chapter, applications of the Kawa (river) model demonstrate this therapeutic dynamic of enabling diverse occupational therapy clients to cultivate a comprehensive understanding of their occupational requirements in their occupational therapists. This is achieved through a basic metaphor of nature that uses the image of a river and its parts to translate and enable clients' occupational narrative or the life flow. Clients are empowered to express their occupational lives in the context of their day-to-day realities, in their own words, from their unique cultural orientations. And just as the natural elements of a river flowing, such as water, walls, rocks, and driftwood, cannot be readily separated and viewed in isolation, the client and occupational dimensions of their daily contexts of living are appreciated through the Kawa model in a complex, holistic, and integrated way (Iwama 2006b).

Over the past few years, the Kawa model (Iwama 2005b) has steadily spread wherever occupational therapists seek solutions to challenges of diversity and culture (in the broadest sense). A series of short case studies collected from occupational therapists located across five continents follow. The cases honor the complexities and challenges of culturally responsive occupational therapy, and offer an alternative to conventional universal approaches when occupational therapy is practiced without borders.

A *sungai* (river) flows through rural Malaysia

Hanif Farhan, occupational therapy student, National University of Malaysia (Universiti Kebangsaan Malaysia), Kuala Lumpur, Malaysia

Ms Aini, a 21-year-old Muslim woman of Malay ethnicity, lives in a rural village in northern Malaysia with her elder sister. She was self-admitted to a mental health institution and has been an inpatient for a month. Her psychiatric records revealed that she had previously been institutionalized over 10 times since the age of 13 years due to borderline personality disorder. During previous stays in the hospital,

she was observed to frequently quarrel with other patients. Furthermore, she would also act out from time to time, striking her head against the walls of her room. In order to build therapeutic rapport with Ms Aini and conduct further assessment, the occupational therapist planned to run an art activity during an established weekly group session in the ward.

The sessions

Six patients were selected for the group session. After some warming up and 'icebreaking' activities, the patients were asked to draw a diagram of a river. When possible, patients were encouraged to make the river symbolic for how they thought their life was going – or flowing. First, each component of the *sungai* (river) was briefly described using the simplest manner and language such as *ayer* (water), *batu* (rock), *kayu hanyut* (driftwood), and *dasar sungai* (river bottom). Then, the therapist proceeded to relate those metaphoric components with real-life situations based on the basic phenomena stressed within the Kawa model (Iwama 2006a). The patients were then encouraged to briefly talk about their own drawing while the others were persuaded to ask questions about it. Although she did not talk much, Ms Aini was able to complete her personal illustration of her own river with some rocks embedded within to symbolize her 'dark history' (Fig. 27.1).

After the group therapy session was finished, the occupational therapist decided to carry on with an individual session with Ms Aini. Again, each component of the river was briefly described, but in a more practical approach. During the explanation, the occupational therapist drew a Kawa diagram of a long, flowing river to describe the personal history of the patient in a psychodynamic way. Each significant

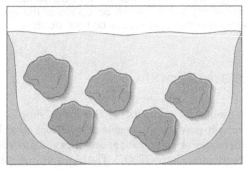

Fig. 27.1 • Ms Aini's personal illustration of her river (rocks symbolize the 'dark histories').

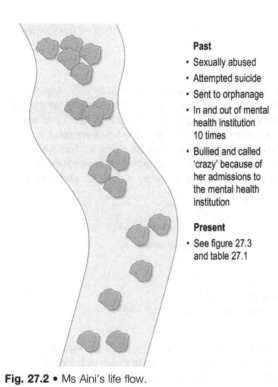

Past

- Sexually abused
- Attempted suicide
- Sent to orphanage
- In and out of mental health institution 10 times
- Bullied and called 'crazy' because of her admissions to the mental health institution

Present

- See figure 27.3 and table 27.1

Fig. 27.2 • Ms Aini's life flow.

life problem Ms Aini had reported was illustrated as obstructions made up of rocks that impeded her life flow. The patient became more talkative and used the word *'batu'* when expressing her major life problems (Fig. 27.2). Finally, the occupational therapist drew another cross-sectional view of the Kawa diagram, particularly focusing on Ms Aini's present life flow (Fig. 27.3, Table 27.1). Collaboratively, the patient and the occupational therapist proceeded to name and ascribe a value to each of the Kawa components.

Conclusion

After the initial assessment using the Kawa model, the occupational therapist and the patient could mutually identify the actual problems and plan for further assessment and intervention. A plan for Ms Aini to focus on – 'here and now' training, psycho-educational support and reality testing using a cognitive-behavioral frame of reference, for example – was made possible by agreeing on outcomes using the Kawa framework. Social and interaction skills training was also suggested by the occupational therapist. As a Muslim, Ms Aini also said she wanted to have spiritual counseling. Her occupational therapist then could suggest that Ms Aini participate in spiritual activities overseen and moderated by the institution's spiritual psychologist.

The Kawa model is not only applicable as a theoretical framework in Malaysian occupational therapy contexts by emphasizing cross-cultural sensitivity, but is also a creative way of determining possible solutions for any occupational condition. The Kawa Model is proving to be a client-friendly framework – a model that makes it easier to achieve the therapeutic relationship.

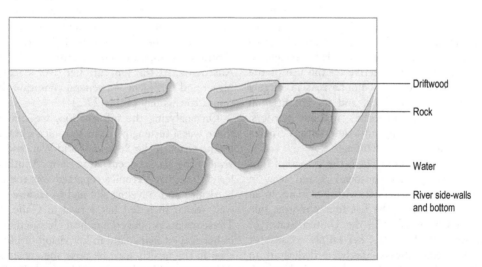

Driftwood

Rock

Water

River side-walls and bottom

Fig. 27.3 • Cross-sectional view of Ms Aini's present Kawa condition.

Table 27.1 Ms Aini's narrative based on the Kawa concepts

Kawa concepts (*bahasa melayu* – English)	Client-centered issues
Batu – rocks	From the early stages of her life, the tragedy of sexual abuse remained the major negative circumstance implicating a major obstruction to Ms Aini's life flow. This, she claims had changed her perceptions about men for the worse. The clinical picture of her mental health condition, borderline personality disorder, represented another large rock. This *batu* is expressed clinically in Ms Aini's case as: unpredictable behavior, self-destructive acts, and hostility – which disturb her normal life. She also reported that when she was within the social community, she carried a stigma of a 'lunatic person' because of her history of numerous admissions to a mental health institution
Dasar sunga i – river bottom and side-walls	Family Patients within the institution Community – including stigma toward people with mental illness
Kayu hanyut – driftwood	Motivation to change Attitude toward men When in crisis, easily gets anxious and depressed Calm when listening to spiritual (religious) counseling 'Hot' temper
Ayer – water	*Ayer* continues to flow through the obstructions along the river. *Kayu hanyut* play important roles in determining the volume of flowing water. The aim of occupational therapy is to facilitate the positive effect of the *kayu hanyut* to change and open the obstruction in a way that *ayer* (Ms Aini's life) will flow to a greater extent

A *folyo* (river) flowing through and beyond Auschwitz

Avital Kaufman, occupational therapist, Santiago, Chile

Veronica, a Jewish woman of Hungarian heritage, currently resides in Santiago, Chile. She is a survivor of Auschwitz and the Holocaust, which resulted in a number of long-term illnesses and daily challenges. Her case provides a perspective on the use of the Kawa model, which originated in East Asia is largely unknown in South America, and its potential in occupational therapy processes without borders. The occupational therapy interview with Veronica took place in her home in Santiago.

Veronica is 77 years old; she is the second of four brothers and sisters. Her husband passed away in 1999 and she lives by herself, with her maid, in an apartment in Santiago. She has four children, one of whom has been living in the United States of America since 1981. Today, her family consists of 23 members. She always has been dedicated to her family and the home. Her hobbies include travel,

movies, and reading. Regarding her medical history, she reports that she has 'general diseases'.

The Kawa model was used as an organizational framework of Veronica's life and occupations. After reflecting on her life, she made a diagram of two rivers. The first one was about her childhood, when she had a happy life in Hungary with her family. It was a *quiet river*, where she could play and share. The second river was about a very difficult stage of her life. In 1944 she and her family were deported to the concentration camps of Nazi, Germany. She went to Auschwitz. At this juncture her river started to get bigger and turbulent – a general condition that continues to this day (Table 27.2).

On analyzing the information, we can see that there was a turning point in Veronica's life, marked by the onset of the Second World War, and her survival of the Nazi concentration camp. Another significant time that Veronica reported was the multiple hardships and traveling she had to endure after the war, which included her arrival in Chile in 1946. These events produced a radical change in her river, in her way of living, and in her vision of life. This is seen in the health area, because she considered her disease states like elements that impede her life flow,

Table 27.2 Veronica's *folyo*

Kawa concept (*Spanish* – English)	Client-centered issues
Rocas – rocks	Veronica does not refer much to the presence of rocks. She describes a quiet river, when her family was fine
Las Paredes del Río – River side-walls	She had few friends. The scattering of her family after the Second World War was a significant factor. A big help is the telephone which allowed her to communicate. Family is important to her; she maintained excellent relationships with family members, and decisions were taken together
Flotante – driftwood	(−) Acquired pathologies affected/limited her performance (+) Her capability to join her family and to solve all the difficulties
El Agua – water	Her life flow is similar to the era in her life when the Second World War began, with highs and lows. Her extraordinary life experiences taught her how to adapt and learn to live. This allowed flow with fewer obstacles
Lagunas – space between obstructions	Occupational therapy can be used to find out how disease affected her life: • Encouragement of the continuity of social activities and the use of alternative ways of communication. • Continuing with supportive family meetings, on important dates, festivities. • Looking for different ways to face health problems, to be able to do things better independently, according to her preferences • Contributing to the continuity of life flow without obstacles, and satisfy personal needs

but she did not talk about them in this way. Veronica's flowing river is representative of her capability to continue, her religious faith, and the support of her family and friends. The most important thing in her life was to be with her family and to see them happy.

Comment

Veronica's narrative allows us to appreciate how the Holocaust experience, which occurred way up-river, not only changed her life course irreversibly, but also gave her the impetus and strength for a better life and hope down-river. She started life again in a new country, had a family, and proceeded through the different stages of her life journey. This included raising her children and taking care of her husband, who had Alzheimer disease.

Given this narrative, would Veronica need occupational therapy intervention? The Kawa model redefines the traditional boundaries of occupational therapy by going beyond medical pathology and function and bringing the client's historical conditions of life and sociocultural context into focus. In Veronica's Kawa narrative we can see certain elements

obstruct her life flow and which may be resolved. We can also think about ways and actions to improve the free flow of her river, such as strengthening family relations. The Kawa framework enables both client and therapist to explore occupational therapy strategies that are relevant and contextually meaningful to the client.

A *nadi* (river) flowing calmly and deeply in Mumbai

Neha Patel, senior second occupational therapist, Willesden Centre for Health and Care, London, UK

This study was conducted in Mumbai, India, as a master's degree dissertation project.

Dr Sharma is a 67-year-old retired medical college lecturer. After the death of his first wife 10 years ago, he remarried and settled with his second wife in Mumbai, India. His second wife was also a lecturer in a medical college in Mumbai. Dr Sharma had two sons and a step-daughter. His children were all married and settled overseas.

Dr Sharma had his first stroke six years ago followed by two strokes within a six-month interval. These resulted in a flexion synergy pattern in his right upper limb and an extension synergy pattern in his right lower limb. He was now walking with one stick under supervision. He had privately employed caregivers to assist him with personal and domestic activities. His wife took care of his meals and his finances (paying bills etc.). He has no speech problems and his cognition was intact.

In the broader study from which this case was drawn, the Kawa model (Lim & Iwama 2006) was used as a framework to assess the effects of sociocultural factors on quality of life of elderly stroke survivors. Two semi-structured interviews were carried out with a one-month interval in between. Perhaps having been a medical professional, Dr Sharma could articulate his health, wellbeing, and quality of life with clarity. Table 27.3 represents his quality of life and life flow in past, present, and future.

Summary

The Kawa model was seen to have an immense potential to explore Dr Sharma's own perception about his illness and issues that affected his quality of life post stroke. Through diagrammatic illustrations, Dr Sharma's occupational status was easily understood by his family members. Moreover, Dr Sharma reported that the Kawa model had helped him to be more aware about viewing his life course and his rehabilitation needs.

In addition to physical and functional factors, the Kawa model framework used as an assessment tool helped the occupational therapist to explore sociocultural factors such as: praying to God, keeping a positive attitude towards life, trying different things of interest, friends and family, support and encouragement, and participation in making clinical decisions.

A contributing factor to a person's health and wellbeing according to Western concepts is 'Becoming' through 'Doing' (Hasselkus 2002). However, one's accountability to one's social relationship is more important in the Indian culture. 'Belonging' rather than 'Doing' becomes an important matter of identity and meaning as described in a collective frame of reference, rather than through an individual-introspective process. In Indian society, where elderly people are not as actively productive, *doing*

Table 27.3 Dr Sharma's occupational therapy assessment results based on the Kawa framework

Kawa concept	Client-centered issues
Rocks	Dependency in his physical activities of daily living (PADLs) due to stroke Strained interpersonal relationship with sons – who are not on talking terms with him His step-daughter's marital problems. He felt 'lost' and 'unhappy' because his wife was unhappy and he could not fulfill his family duties
River side-walls and bottom	His wife was very supportive His strong faith in God and prayers Healthcare professional's care and support in rehabilitation department (occupational therapist, physiotherapist, and other non-clinical staff) The department served as a social network; and he enjoyed talking with his healthcare professional and other patients
Driftwood	(+) His sociable and lively nature (−) His temperament (anger) because the stroke and dependency on everything left him frustrated (−) Difficulty walking without stick (+) His family's finances; owned many properties in Jaipur (a city in India)
Water	Water continued to flow in substantial volume around his stroke and functional consequences, driftwood (see above), and his social physical environment Water was still flowing, but to a lesser extent, through the cracks and gaps bounded by the structures and components in Dr Sharma's river
Cracks and gaps	Potential occupational therapy treatment approaches and points of intervention are in the gaps and channels through which water (life energy) still courses (see Water above) and the specific structures that form the boundaries

is important but may not mean much when separated from the social context in which it occurs and from which meaning is derived. Humans are inseparable from nature, society, and deities (Iwama 2003, Lau et al 2003).

Aborigine *paaka* (river) flowing through urban contexts

Alison Nelson, occupational therapist and doctoral candidate, University of Queensland, Brisbane, Australia

Jacinta is an 11-year-old aboriginal Australian who lives in an urban setting with her aunt and her aunt's partner. Jacinta's older and younger sisters, two younger cousins and an older cousin also live there. Jacinta usually slept on a mattress in the lounge-room as there were not enough bedrooms for all the children. Her mother lived approximately 300 miles away due to her partner's living situation. As a baby, Jacinta was 'given' to her other aunt who was in a same sex relationship and she was raised by this aunt for the first four years of her life. Jacinta had lived with her mother previously and expected she would be living with her again in the near future. Jacinta's mum and aunt were both unemployed. Jacinta was in Year 6 at school.

Application of the Kawa model

River side-walls (environment)

When asked about those aspects of her environment that helped her be active and healthy, Jacinta identified that she had a trampoline in her backyard and that she lived close to a pool and a park. She also noted that she was able to walk to school from her house and played soccer, cricket, and touch football at school, as well as swimming and running.

Rocks (problems)

Jacinta noted that her biggest problem was stress concerning looking after her younger cousins and her younger sister, who has a tendency to get into trouble regularly. Jacinta also identified that eating junk food made it more difficult to be healthy.

Logs (assets and liabilities)

Jacinta generally viewed 'logs' as assets rather than liabilities. For instance, she recognized that having her older cousin help her care for her younger cousins relieved her stress. She also noted that jumping on the trampoline was a major source of stress relief.

Another log was 'junk food'. One way to avoid junk food was when her mother cooked healthy meals for the family. 'Mum when she makes our dinner; she makes healthy salads and everything healthy'.

Fish (relationships) and eels (bad social connections)

It was at this point in the conversation that Jacinta really appeared to 'own' her river. She asked if she could add fish to her river and identified that these could be relationships in her life that helped her (Fig. 27.4). Jacinta identified some family members and friends at school as 'fish' who were able to support her and help her with looking out for her younger sister. Jacinta next added eels to her river stating that these were 'bad connections'. These included other people at school who she felt made the situation with her sister more difficult. Sometimes people whom she felt were 'fish' could also be 'eels'.

Flowers

Next Jacinta drew three flowers in her river to 'represent something that's wonderful in my life'. These appeared to be significant life events that had an overarching quality to her life. The first of these was when she was reunited with her mother at the age of 4. The second 'flower' was when Jacinta was reunited with her sister Nicole.

It seemed that despite the difficulties she had articulated earlier with helping Nicole at school, Jacinta was able to identify the importance of this relationship in her life. This was also true of Jacinta's view of her family, that even though her life was complicated by family, the benefit of having a family was greater.

> The thing that took most of the stress away was just having a family. Just having like my sister and my mum there to help me so yeah.

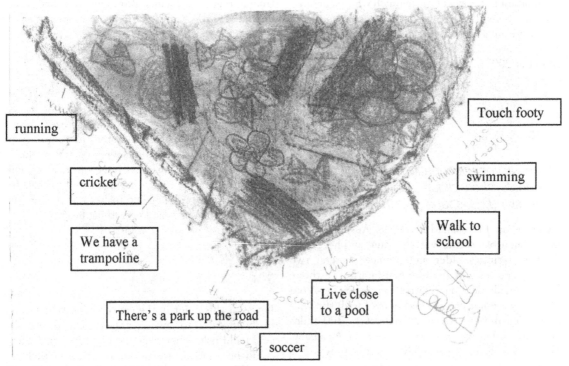

running

cricket

We have a trampoline

There's a park up the road

Touch footy

swimming

Walk to school

Live close to a pool

soccer

Fig. 27.4 • Jacinta's drawing of her river.

Conclusions

Using the Kawa model appeared to enable this young aboriginal girl to express her thoughts in a meaningful way. Her extensions of the model suggested that she engaged readily with the metaphor of the river. The use of the Kawa model provided important information about her family context and her perceptions of activities. It was significant that she identified relationships (good and bad) as central to her health and wellbeing. The findings suggested that to improve Jacinta's health or increase her engagement in occupations, any intervention would need to first focus on strengthening her relationships and her stress levels.

The Kawa model has potential to be culturally safe. The opportunity to allow this young girl to add to her river (by allowing her to insert her flowers, fish, and eels) certainly appeared to be key in gaining a true understanding of her context and the ways in which she viewed her life.

Collective occupations flowing powerfully

Erin Hanrahan, occupational therapist, Class of 2009, Program in Occupational Therapy, University of Minnesota, Minneapolis, USA

University of Minnesota Occupational Therapy Commencement Ceremony – *Excerpts from the Student Address, 13 December 2008*

Today is a day for us all to celebrate together. And ... it is fitting that we are gathered today in this beautiful space overlooking the Great Mississippi River (see Fig. 27.5).

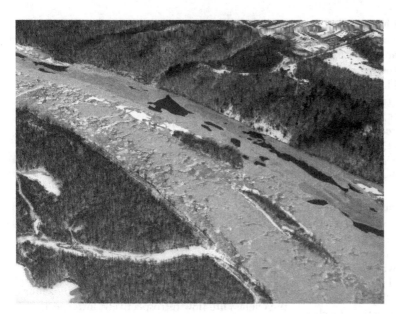

Fig. 27.6 • Aerial view of the Mississippi river in winter, near Minnesota, one day before the graduation ceremony. (Photograph by M Iwama.)

In one of our courses (we) explored various theoretical models in our profession that included writing, and thinking critically about the Kawa model. According to the Kawa model, life is like a river, flowing through time and space. Wellbeing occurs when people live in harmony with the circumstances in their life and their river flows, unimpeded, even in the face of strife.

For the past 16 months, my classmates and I have shared a journey together through this Masters in Occupational Therapy program. In many ways our journey can be compared to the river in the Kawa Model. The flow of the water in the river is affected by the river wall and floor, the rocks, and driftwood. These are all metaphoric elements of the Kawa Model and they can be used to illustrate our experiences in the occupational therapy program.

First there is the River Wall and Floor. In the Kawa model this represents the social and physical environment. The social environment consists of people – and it's the relationships with classmates that have made this program memorable. Our memories include lots of labs and studying together, especially for practical exams.

As one of my classmates shared in a wiki for one of our courses, 'Although we all seem to be very different people, we really banded together to get to the end'. This is reflective of our sense of interdependence and the importance of the River Wall and Floor to our success.

And there were also Rocks. In the Kawa model, Rocks represent problems or difficulties. . . . Rivers – and people's lives – have rocks of varying size, shape, and number. There have been pebble-sized problems – and much larger ones. Difficulties have also surrounded time management, and people have needed to make tough choices regarding priorities over the past four semesters. And there has been fear, such as before the practical examinations and other formal tests. And some classmates have lost loved ones before and during the program. The Rocks have affected us, yet we are here because the rocks gave us strength.

And then there is Driftwood. In the Kawa model, driftwood represents Assets and Liabilities. Simply put, driftwood is our personal character and the special skills that each of us possess. There are many examples that demonstrate the character of individuals in the Class of 2009. All of us have spent three semesters, and at least 72 hours each, being involved with community organizations. This includes planning and staffing CarFit events. Participating with the Rebuilding Together organization. Working with the Kids on 2 Wheels Bike Camp. And volunteering in many other groups that serve people with disabilities.

Driftwood is also represented by our strong commitment to learning. As someone shared in a wiki for one of our courses, 'I have so much respect for the high level of work that my classmates put into each class and it has been an honor to be a part of this group'. This comment speaks to our character. The Class of 2009 is filled with compassionate, dedicated, honest, sincere, and hard working people.

So it is the River Walls and Floor, Rocks, and Driftwood that give shape to our river of life. The river runs through time and space, and there will be times when the river has some rocks and the current is rough. And there will be other times when the river is rushing mightily into the future – such as now, as we are ready to embark on Level II fieldwork.

I hope you have enjoyed reminiscing about our journey together in the river. Let us not forget that the Kawa model was inspired by occupational therapy practitioners who realized that current theoretical frameworks were out of sync with their clients' life experience. The Kawa model was developed out of courage and out of leadership to see new connections between theory and practice, to challenge the status quo, and to create new explanations. I challenge all of us to display such leadership in our future careers. We will lead in different ways. Some will lead with their kindness and optimism. Some will lead with their knowledge and expertise. Others will lead with their laughter. We need all types of leaders to address the great challenges faced in today's world. Leadership is difficult to describe, yet easy to see. Leadership is not always on your résumé, but it remains in the hearts of those you have inspired. Let us use the knowledge gained during this program, the strength from our rocks, and the character of our driftwood to shape the river of our future. Thank you and good luck!

Conclusion

Occupational therapists practicing and learning across diverse cultural spaces are finding the Kawa model to be useful in a number of ways; as a mental framework to help organize the client's occupational issues in client-centered context, as an assessment tool, and as a modality of treatment by itself or in combination. The client can be a single person or a group, or even a process. In all of the vignettes, however, the occupational performance issues that the model helped to illuminate transcended matters of medical pathology into the dynamic realm of client daily life contexts. The case studies demonstrate the flexibility and ability to respond to and appreciate the needs and experiences of people from all walks of life, across diverse contexts. The Kawa metaphor enables both therapist and client to examine the client's life flow retrospectively, introspectively, and prospectively. It is a novel approach in occupational therapy that views the whole person(s) integrated inseparably in context and yields a wide array of occupational therapy possibilities and interventions that will potentially enable the clients' life to flow more fully and powerfully. This chapter was devoted to briefly demonstrating some practical and potential applications of the Kawa model in a variety of cultural contexts. More information and literature relating to the Kawa model's theoretical and philosophical underpinnings can be accessed in greater detail in a growing number of publications and internet resources. For further information, see the Kawa model website (http://www.kawamodel.com).

References

Hasselkus B: *The Meaning of Everyday Occupation*, Thorofare, New Jersey, 2002, Slack Inc.

Iwama M: The issue is ... toward culturally relevant epistemologies in occupational therapy, *Am J Occup Ther* 57:217–223, 2003.

Iwama M: Revisiting culture in occupational therapy research; a meaningful endeavour, *Occupational Therapy Journal of Research* 24:1–2, 2004.

Iwama M: Situated meaning; an issue of culture, inclusion & occupational therapy. In Kronenberg F, Algado SA, Pollard N, editors: *Occupational Therapy Without Borders – Learning*

Through the Spirit of Survivors, Edinburgh, 2005a, Elsevier/Churchill Livingstone, pp 127–139.

Iwama M: The Kawa (river) model; nature, life flow & the power of culturally relevant occupational therapy. In Kronenberg F, Algado SA, Pollard N, editors: *Occupational Therapy Without Borders – Learning Through the Spirit of Survivors*, Edinburgh, 2005b, Elsevier/Churchill Livingstone, pp 213–227.

Iwama M: *The Kawa Model: Culturally Relevant Occupational Therapy*, Edinburgh, 2006a, Churchill Livingstone/Elsevier, pp 242.

Iwama M: The Kawa (river) model: Client centred rehabilitation in cultural context. In Davis S, editor: *Rehabilitation; The Use of Theories and Models in Practice*, Oxford, 2006b, Elsevier, pp 84–93.

Iwama M: Culture and occupational therapy: meeting the challenge of relevance in a global world, *Occup Ther Int* 4:183–187, 2007.

Lau A, McKenna K, Chan C, Cummins R: Defining quality of life for Chinese elderly stroke survivors, *Disabil Rehabil* 25:699–711, 2003.

Lim KH, Iwama M: Emerging models – an Asian perspective; the Kawa (river) model. In Duncan E, editor: *Foundations for Practice in Occupational Therapy*, ed 4, Edinburgh, 2006, Churchill Livingstone/Elsevier, pp 161–189.

Munoz J: Culturally responsive caring in occupational therapy. In Iwama M, editor: *Special Issue on Culture and Occupational Therapy. Occupational Therapy International*, vol 4, 2007, pp 256–280.

Ramsden I: *Kawa Whakaruruhau- Cultural Safety in Nursing Education in Aotearoa: Report to the Ministry of Education*, Wellington, 1990, Ministry of Education.

Human occupation as a tool for understanding and promoting social justice[1]

28

Gary Kielhofner   Carmen Gloria de las Heras
Yolanda Suarez-Balcazar

OVERVIEW

This chapter discusses how the Model of Human Occupation (MOHO) can be used to understand and address social injustice. It highlights how oppression can be internalized and reflected in persons' volition, habituation, and performance capacity. The chapter presents strategies for empowering individuals and discusses how these must be coupled with careful assessment of environmental realities and possibilities. Guidelines and case examples illustrate the potential ways in which MOHO can empower individuals experiencing social injustice and contribute toward structural change that begins to reverse the processes of oppression.

Introduction

The Model of Human Occupation (MOHO) was introduced in 1980 by three occupational therapy practitioners to articulate concepts that guided their practice (Kielhofner et al 1980). Since then, the contributions of practitioners and researchers throughout the world have contributed to the development of this model, which is used internationally (Bowyer et al 2008, Haglund et al 2000, Law & McColl 1989). Its development, in a wide range of contexts, has contributed toward MOHO being a multilevel and cross-cultural model. A number of authors have described the use of MOHO as a theoretical framework for addressing both individuals and groups who were victims of social injustice. Some examples are:

- Legally defending a family's rights which were taken away because of social prejudice and laws directed at persons with intellectual impairment.
- Supporting adolescents with developmental disabilities to move toward employment in a post-communist society with severe economic problems.
- Challenging and changing mental health systems, structures and procedures to better meet the occupational needs of persons with severe and chronic mental illness who were marginalized by the very systems ostensibly designed to help them.
- Developing interventions with homeless people including those facing prejudice because of histories of substance abuse and human immunodeficiency virus (HIV) diagnosis (Aravena & de las Heras 1999, de las Heras 2004, 2006, Kielhofner et al 2008, Penjeam & de las Heras 2000, Porras 2002, 2005, Todorova 2008, Valdés 2000).

As these examples illustrate, the application of MOHO to address issues of social justice are varied in their contexts, circumstances, and methods.

Characteristics central to all these applications are exemplified by a MOHO-based project to empower blind adults in a poor rural community in South Africa (Du Toit 2008). These adults were disadvantaged not only by their visual impairment, but also by poverty, social prejudice (even within their own families),

[1] A number of fields studying issues of oppression, marginalization, social inclusion, and apartheid have placed these concepts in the context of social justice. In this chapter, we use the term social justice to refer to circumstances when individuals are prevented from occupational engagement by virtue of poverty, political oppression, and other social and cultural forces.

and outright discrimination. As a result they were marginalized, alienated, and deprived of meaningful occupations. The program supported clients to develop self-respect and self-worth, to gain new skills, to enact new habits and engage in new roles. It also supported them to have more control over their lives and their environments. These goals were achieved through enabling clients to engage in a range of occupations including those that generated income and contributed to the community. At the same time the program sought to build social support for the participants and to increase community awareness of the participants and what they could contribute to society.

As illustrated by this example, the use of MOHO-based services to address social injustice require careful attention to people's thoughts and feelings about themselves, to their everyday roles and habits and to building critical skills. All these elements are addressed to empower individuals toward greater control over their own lives and their environments. Importantly, MOHO-based services also recognize that it is critical to address barriers and supports in the environment.

This chapter examines MOHO concepts and their utilization to address problems of individuals and groups who experience situations of social injustice. After examining the relationship between MOHO and concepts of social justice, we will discuss how MOHO is used to understand and empower people who have been oppressed.

The model of human occupation and social injustice

Social justice refers to political, social, and economic rights of individuals in a given society (Fondacaro & Weinberg 2002). At the core of social justice is the concept of human rights (Bowring 2002). According to Austin (2001), 'the central assumption of the rights paradigm is that every person can make certain claims based solely on their humanness' (p. 184). However, individuals living in situations of oppression are not allowed to make such claims (Braveman & Suarez-Balcazar 2009).

Social justice has been discussed within occupational therapy as it relates to systematic limitations to engage in occupation and participate in society (Abelenda et al 2005, Kronenberg & Pollard 2005, Townsend 2003, Wilcock 1998, Wilcock & Townsend 2000). Such discussions underscore that societies should provide opportunities for people to engage in meaningful occupations that allow them to develop their potential and participate in their communities (Jakobsen 2004, Wilcock 1998, Wilcock & Townsend 2000). Occupational therapy discourse on social justice underscores that meaningful employment, resources, and opportunities to sustain oneself and one's living environment, and access to play and leisure are among the forms of occupational participation that societies should provide to their members. MOHO was the first occupational therapy model to incorporate the environment as a critical factor in occupational performance; this model's emphasis on the influence of the environment makes it suitable for understanding social justice as it relates to occupation. The most recent edition of the MOHO text explicitly recognizes social, political, and economic conditions as part of the environmental context that affects occupational participation (Kielhofner 2008).

According to MOHO, people's lives are sustained and shaped by what they do (Kielhofner 2008). What people do, in turn, can be enabled or constrained by social, political, and economic factors in the environment (Kielhofner 2008). A form of social injustice is recognized in circumstances in which doing is constrained by environmental conditions to the point that people are prevented from sustaining themselves and realizing their potentials.

Traditionally, women, people with disabilities, indigenous people, low-income individuals, racial and ethnic minorities, and other marginalized groups are less likely to have the freedom to choose their occupations and/or have fewer choices available to them. A large number of individuals across the globe are not free to choose their occupations. For instance, 30% of the working age population is either unemployed or underemployed in nonindustrialized countries (CARE 2009). Thus, social injustice as it pertains to occupation affects large numbers of people in a wide range of contexts.

Using MOHO to understand the impact of social justice on occupational participation

According to MOHO, the individual is understood as including three components of volition, habituation, and performance capacity. By understanding how the individual may be impacted by conditions of social injustice, we can better recognize how individuals and groups can be empowered.

CHAPTER 28

Volition and oppression

Volition refers to the process of choosing and experiencing occupations and the thoughts and feelings that accompany and influence this process. According to the concept of volition, the human motive for occupation begins with an innate drive to do things. Each individual, based on experience and environmental influences has ongoing thoughts and feelings that influence how he or she chooses and experiences occupation. These thoughts and feelings include values (i.e., what one considers important and meaningful to do), interests (the sense of satisfaction and enjoyment in doing), and personal causation (beliefs about how capable and effective one is) (Kielhofner 2008). Individuals living in situations of social oppression may develop self-constraining volition. That is, hemmed in by limited choices and impoverished experiences of doing, they develop patterns of thinking and feeling that internalize the oppression they experience (Freire 2000). Persons who have internalized oppression may not anticipate possibilities for positive participation in life. They may not perceive themselves as having power to shape their own destinies.

Oppression which is internalized as a volitional pattern of thought and feeling may take on many forms. Consider, for example, a young adult who is drawn to and gifted at math and who does not even imagine pursuing higher education as he ekes out barely a survival wage as a street vendor. When the oppression is fully internalized as part of his volition, he hopes for no more and sees his situation simply as his place in life. He does not recognize his intellectual capacity as a source of improving his life circumstances. His values and goals, instead of carrying him toward realization of his capacities, are focused on survival. In the end his choices and experiences are all within the circumstances created by his oppression.

While there are notable examples of people who are able to sustain a sense of dignity, power, and control despite social injustice, many others do develop volitional thoughts and feelings that serve to keep them within their unjust circumstances. For such people, reversing the effects of oppression must include building a sense of self-worth, personal control, and investment in achieving satisfaction.

Habituation and oppression

Habituation refers to the pattern of people's occupational lives that is sustained by roles and habits (Kielhofner 2008). A role is a socially ascribed status that connects people to their larger social environment, linking their performance to that of others. Roles provide a general blueprint for action and grant a sense of identity. Habits are patterns of action that sustain repetitive daily occupations.

Individuals living under conditions of social injustice are often prevented access to certain roles (e.g., worker or student) while being cast into or only allowed access to marginalized roles (e.g. beggars, street people, squatters, or refugees). They may also find it necessary for survival and safety to engage in roles that are outside the law, subjecting themselves to the possibility of punishment. Even when oppressed people manage to sustain ordinary occupational roles as family members or workers, they are often forced to sustain these roles with extremely limited resources (e.g., lacking adequate plumbing and sanitary conditions for raising children or working in substandard conditions that constitute a health risk) and rewards (e.g., earning subsistence wages).

The contextual support for familiar and comfortable and satisfying everyday routines is often lacking for oppressed people. Those who must scramble for basic resources or who develop compensatory habits to manage life under duress, may experience highly stressed routines of daily life. For instance, people who do not have a steady source of food or whose access to clean water is sporadic must devote tremendous energy to securing the basic necessities of survival. Their routines become preoccupied with managing access to scarce or uncertain resources. In other circumstances people may experience impoverished routines with insufficient meaningful activity because of the lack of access to resources and opportunities for doing.

Consider, again, the example of the young adult who is a street vendor. For long days of labor he receives at best a marginal income. Others perceive him as unskilled and outside the normal workforce. To survive, he may engage in practices that, if discovered, could lead to imprisonment or being barred from vending. Thus, he performs on the margins of society without claiming a legitimate place and adequate reward for his labors. His daily routines, because they are a way of survival, are hard to shake off even if his circumstances were to improve because they may be needed again when things take a turn for the worse. Because sufficient environmental support and resources cannot be trusted, he is prone to hang on to the roles and habits that allow him to survive during the worst of times.

Performance capacity and oppression

The skills for effectively performing occupations are developed as one uses capacity in everyday contexts. Oppressed people are routinely denied opportunities to realize skills that their underlying capabilities would allow (Galheigo 2005, Wilcock & Townsend 2000). They are thus robbed of personal resources that would allow them to control and achieve more in their lives.

Consider, once more, the young street vendor who has innate capacities for learning complex math but has barely learned the necessary addition and subtraction for conducting his street vending business because he had to leave school as a child in order to earn income for his impoverished family. Because he never develops an underlying gift, he is bound to his oppressive circumstances.

The individual and oppression

As the previous discussion illustrates, the consequences of oppression often resonate throughout the person. Victims of oppression may develop a volitional process that internalizes their oppression and constrains them from wanting more of their lives. They may have impoverished or overstressed routines. They may occupy marginal roles or struggle to fulfill traditional roles without adequate preparation or resources. They may fail to realize potentials that their underlying capacities would allow. In this way, the individual and his or her occupations become the locus of oppression.

At the same time, the person who lives under conditions of social injustice must do his or her best to survive both physically and psychologically. The accommodations to living under oppression creep into a person's habituation and volition: being resourceful in order to manage with meager resources, compensating for lack of skill by laboring to the point of exhaustion, learning not to accept a life with limited dignity, expectations, and reward. Which such accommodations may inoculate the oppressed person against being destroyed, they result in lives which, at best, are compromised. Ironically, the resilience of many oppressed people can make the extent of the social injustice they experience less apparent both to themselves and others.

MOHO as a framework for empowerment

On a global level, oppression must be fought by efforts to change the social order. Such change is inherently political and economic. It occurs in a historical time frame as social attitudes, policies, laws, and other institutional factors change. What, then, is the role of occupational therapy which deals in the here and now with individuals or groups experiencing oppression? There is no single or simple answer to this question. Much depends on local circumstances and also on the position of the occupational therapist within the context. We propose that there are three critical and interrelated requirements for the occupational therapist who wishes to address social injustice.

The first requirement in addressing social injustice requires the occupational therapist to reflect on his or her position in the social system. It is possible for occupational therapy to become an extension of oppression, reflecting deeply embedded institutional perspectives that can fault and penalize the recipient of occupational therapy services (Kielhofner 1993). Thus, occupational therapists working within existing systems must be deeply mindful of the ways that oppression may have been institutionalized. When oppressive attitudes and practices are embedded into systems such as healthcare delivery, they are often difficult to recognize and easy to perpetuate.

The second requirement is that the occupational therapists must work hard to know their clients and their situation. As we noted above, oppression is found in the thoughts, feelings, behaviors, and routines of individuals and groups. Thus, one of the most common mistakes made is that of blaming the victim (Kielhofner 1993). Occupational therapists must be astute in recognizing oppression in persons as reflected in their volition (e.g., sense of fatalism, the belief that one is not effective or skilled) and habituation (e.g., unreasonable stressed or impoverished routines, marginalized roles), skills as affected by limited education or training. It is also critical that environmental supports and barriers are identified.

The third requirement is the occupational therapist should address oppression by seeking to empower individuals and small groups to take charge of and change their own lives. Efforts to empower individuals and groups, even within oppressive environments, can mitigate to the extent to which those environments constrain individual lives. In some cases, it also enables individuals to change some of the circumstances of oppression in their environments.

MOHO is most useful as a tool for recognizing oppression, understanding clients, and practicing empowerment (Berdichewsky & de las Heras 1995, du Toit 2008, Ziv 2004). Becoming aware of how oppression is reflected in the volition, habituation, and performance skills of persons is a first step towards a change in occupational injustice situations. Using our previous example, we can recognize how the street vendor makes no attempts to change his situation, because he sees no possibility of changing it and accepts it as his role, and because his habits and skills are organized to maintaining this role.

Only when he is awakened to the possibility that he can change his situation and given internal and external resources to do so, will he be able to make choices for action that may lead to change. At the same time, it is critical that the occupational therapist is able to assess the possible environmental reaction to efforts to throw off oppression. Social injustice does not exist by accident; rather, it exists because certain parties benefit from the social order. These parties are typically powerful and motivated to maintain the social order. When occupational therapists support individuals to change the circumstances of their oppression they may place clients in danger. For instance, the street vendor whose action to change his circumstances interferes with the existing social order may find his permit to vend revoked or worse.

Counteracting the forces of social injustice for individuals requires that opportunities be provided to enable victims to develop a sense of their own capacities, interests, and values. Only when they feel capable to achieve their values and interests can they begin to make change in their own lives. At the same time, realistic appraisal of possibilities and of possible negative consequences must be entered into the equation. Here, the therapist must accept responsibility for assessing what the environment will allow and what consequences may occur along with working responsibly to make changes in the environment whenever possible.

The intervention process

The key elements of using MOHO in the context of social injustice are:

- Using the theoretical concepts to generate questions that will provide a clear understanding of individuals and groups.
- Working collaboratively with individuals and groups to generate a deep understanding of their situation and context.
- Developing opportunities in collaboration with oppressed individuals and groups, which allow them to engage in occupations designed to change their lives and circumstances.
- Working with powerful persons and organizations (who may be part of the oppressive system) to advocate for ways to address oppressive conditions.

MOHO-based intervention begins with formulating theory-based questions to guide our understanding of the person/community. Table 28.1 shows examples of questions that can be derived from MOHO concepts to help understand an individual or group. These questions should be generated and answered in partnership with individuals and groups. The occupational therapist takes on the role of observant-participant who seeks to

Table 28.1 Examples of MOHO-based questions to guide understanding of an oppressed person or group

Volition	What are the values and beliefs of this person or group, and how do they affect their choices for action? What is the sense this person or group has of their individual/collective capacities, and how confident do they feel about their possibilities of using them to produce a change in their own circumstances or environment?
Habituation	What are the roles of this person/group and do they contribute to full occupational participation? Are these roles performed without adequate resources? Who decides which roles are available? How does this person/organization organize daily activities? Does this routine meet personal needs?
Performance capacity and skills	What skills (realized and unrealized) does this person/community have to accomplish his/their goals?
Environment	How does the physical, social, economic, cultural, and political environment in which individuals perform impact their occupations? How are choices made, and by whom? How are the social groups organized in terms of decision making (how are choices made, and by whom)?

facilitate his or her own understanding along with helping individuals and groups to generate a deeper understanding of themselves and their own circumstances.

The occupational therapist, together with those he or she is servicing, then generates an understanding of the situation of the person or group, which is based on theory. It is the role of the occupational therapist to teach MOHO theory in terms that are understandable. By sharing one's conceptual tools and making them accessible, one democratizes the process and provides tools for understanding and dealing with issues in the future. In a final step, everyone collaboratively defines the goals for cooperative interaction, setting priorities and a course of action.

Through their choices for action and what they do, people develop their own volition, habituation, and skills, and to an extent, they shape the occupational world they inhabit. The role of the occupational therapist using MOHO is to promote opportunities for people to make choices and engage in action that will accomplish desired goals such as:

- Understanding and removing environmental constraints that affect occupational performance.
- Discovering environmental factors that enable occupational performance.
- Enhancing the ability for making occupational choices consistent with values, interests, perceived potential, or available resources and goals.
- Discovering and practicing new ways to achieve change.
- Increasing confidence in the ability to produce change.

In all instances, working with oppressed people requires recognizing and understanding the oppressing environment. Often, therapists using MOHO begin by working with persons of power within the oppressing environments. MOHO has proved to be a helpful tool in persuading people in positions of power too; it has been used to successfully negotiate for resources to support interventions and programs and to reverse some situation of social injustice as will be illustrated in the examples that follow.

Examples of using MOHO to address social injustice

As noted earlier in this chapter, MOHO has been used in a number of contexts to address social injustice. The following three examples are all taken from South America; they were selected to illustrate

distinctly different circumstances of social injustice as well as quite different MOHO based-strategies for addressing social injustice.

Defending family rights

The first example was previously described in more detail (Abelenda et al 2005). In the province of Santa Fe, Argentina, a Juvenile Court removed three children from the custody of an extremely impoverished couple because they had intellectual impairments. Ironically, the judge removed three children who were identified as 'normal' while leaving in the parents' custody a child identified as developmentally disabled.

In response to the parents' request for help, an occupational therapist working out of the Ecumenical Movement for Human Rights (EMHR) evaluated the parents using the Occupational Performance History Interview (Kielhofner et al 1998), the Role Checklist (Oakley et al 1986), and systematic observation. She found that the parents worked as traveling street vendors working in alternating shifts to ensure that one of them was always with the children. They took good care of the health of their children and routinely visited the local medical center for check ups. The basic family needs of food and shelter were met. The couple valued their role as parents and workers, and their interests revolved around the care of the home and the children. They had plans for the future, such as improving their quality of life by getting running water and buying new beds for the children. The occupational therapist concluded that their mental impairments did not interfere in their performance of their role as parents, and that their habits and lifestyle was consistent with the cultural environment, history, and origins of the couple. Based on elaborate testimony from the therapist which referred to theoretical concepts and formal assessment tools, the Court of Appeals returned the children to the custody of their parents. Importantly, because the therapist used a well-developed model with established and researched tools, she was able to gain credence in the legal system.

Combating social and institutional discrimination and stigmatization of persons with schizophrenia

When 1995 was declared the year for schizophrenia in Chile, special emphasis was given to neuroscience research to address this problem. As it was originally envisioned the campaign would focus primarily on researchers and professionals who addressed schizophrenia.

Within Chilean society, people with schizophrenia were highly stigmatized and misunderstood. As a result, people with this diagnosis lived at the margins of society with few possibilities for participation and no voice in society. Occupational therapists working in Reencuentros, a community occupational therapy center that served this population, discussed this special year with clients to elicit their reactions (de las Heras 2006, Kielhofner 2002). Clients voiced chronic frustration in trying to participate in productive roles and recounted the attitudinal barriers and discrimination they faced from clinicians, institutions, and society. They also felt that an emphasis on medical solutions and inclusion of only researchers and professionals would mask the fact that people with this diagnosis were systematically discriminated against and disenfranchised. In their view, much of the system that was designed to provide them care mainly served to keep them in their place and did nothing to alleviate their marginalized status.

The group discussions led to a decision to seek to play a central role in the national committee organizing this campaign in order to change some of its emphasis. Two members went with the occupational therapist to the organizing meetings, serving as representatives of clients at the community center and also bringing forth ideas that had been generated by members and therapists at Reencuentros. The occupational therapist presented and defended their proposals using MOHO as a framework. Persuaded by this argument, the national organizers agreed to broaden the campaign beyond training for professionals and research in order to include formal and informal participatory educational events. Moreover, it was agreed that the 'formal educational' events that took place all over the country would be done with active participation of professionals, people with schizophrenia and their families. Finally, it was agreed that the training would be not only about the illness, but also about the occupational lives of persons with schizophrenia, and that it would emphasize how to understand and facilitate participation using MOHO as a theoretical framework.

Professionals, health workers, families and people with schizophrenia attended and participated in formal educational workshops together; these events included dialog between these constituents for the first time. At the end of the campaign a formal course, with special manuals based on MOHO, was given to families and others to facilitate development of

self help groups. The informal education component was organized by the community center and sponsored by private companies. It included three national events, 'Encounter with everybody', 'Art with everybody', and 'Sports with everybody'. The phrase 'with everybody' underscored that these events were for all citizens; they were held in public settings in Santiago.

The first event included talks from representatives from professional groups, government, clients; it also featured diverse classical and folk music and cultural performances. The second event featured different forms of visual and performance art, and the last event featured a variety of sports that allowed full participation from everyone. The three events provided a safe setting in which families and people with schizophrenia could feel comfortable, share their skills, and begin looking to the future with a more positive, active, and participatory attitude. They provided opportunities for people to think of those with schizophrenia as individuals instead of patients by seeing them in humanizing context.

The occupational therapists worked behind the scenes validating, informing, negotiating, and advising clients, their families, and other health professionals (Berdichewsky 1996, Berdichewsky & de las Heras 1995, de las Heras 2007). The active participation of clients and their families in the process of planning and implementing these events led to the founding of 25 family associations in the country and the creation of a National Mental Association of Families. Also, the events during this year led to a number of other ongoing initiatives. One is the development of new MOHO-based projects that empower clients and families to have active participation in the course of their recovery process. Another has been occupational therapy participation in ongoing reform of the Chilean Public Mental Health System. Finally, an outgrowth of the efforts is formation of an ongoing consumer's committee, which evaluates mental health services, advocates for consumer rights, and sponsors empowering initiatives.

Empowering adolescents living in poverty

Ten years ago, in Santa Fe, Argentina, an independent occupational therapist applied for government funding to implement a community project to support adolescents living in poverty and at risk for delinquency, drug abuse, and gang activity. Among other negative environmental factors, these adolescents were under pressure from family members to steal in order to bring home food and other basic resources. The project, which was based on MOHO, was designed to help 15 adolescents explore and develop their occupational identity and competence. The therapist began working with the adolescents as an observant-participant to gain deeper insight into their occupational needs and environmental realities. She began by participating in their most meaningful and enjoyable activity: playing soccer. The adolescents showed energy, pride, and pleasure while playing soccer in the streets in the evenings with a handmade ball of old fabrics and pieces of cloth.

The occupational therapist used MOHO-based observational assessments and informal conversations with the adolescents. She found that they disliked their homes, in part because they had very stressful lives there and were very poor. Nonetheless, they saw their roles as thieves to be an important contribution to their family resources. The majority had not attended school and all felt powerless in comparison with adolescents who had been educated. Because these children had internalized their oppression in their volition and habituation and performance capacity, the therapist realized a long process of exploration would be necessary for them before they were able to develop new occupational identities.

Once the occupational therapist had established a relationship with the adolescents, she invited them to play twice a week at a large natural public space instead of on the street. Eventually, they identified this place as their soccer field. Next, she invited them to form a soccer team and enabled them to play with other local soccer teams. The team identified a captain, who collaborated with the therapist to arrange for games with soccer teams from local schools, fostering interaction with other young adolescents. This generated curiosity about school. Hav-

ing a routine of games with different people who accepted them as soccer players and not as street children helped them to see themselves differently.

Two years later, the therapist applied again to government funds, presenting evidence of the adolescents' progress. The program expanded and the group had its own space for meetings, which included a kitchen and a recreational space. Furthermore, some of the adolescents began to prepare for and eventually attended school. In the coming years, the authorities recognized the importance of having occupational therapy working with these children and gave the occupational therapist a permanent position in the educational system. She and her colleagues continue promoting occupational participation with other adolescents in the same situation (D'Angello 1998, de las Heras 2007, de las Heras et al 2003).

Conclusion

MOHO can be a powerful analytic tool for understanding and addressing social injustice. This model highlights how oppression can be internalized and reflected in persons' volition, habituation and performance capacity. It provides guidance for successful strategies to empower individuals. The case examples in this chapter highlighted different ways in which MOHO can empower individuals experiencing social injustice and contribute toward structural change that begins to reverse the process of oppression. Ultimately, each situation will call for unique strategies that must be informed by a careful understanding of individuals or groups and their environmental context.

References

Abelenda J, Kielhofner G, Suarez-Balcazar Y, Kielhofner K: The Model of Human Occupation as a conceptual tool for understanding and addressing occupational apartheid. In Kronenberg F, Simó Algado S, Pollard N, editors: *Occupational Therapy Without Borders: Learning Through the Spirit of Survivors*, Edinburgh, 2005, Elsevier/Churchill Livingstone, pp 183–196.

Aravena I, de las Heras CG: *Posición del Colegio de Terapeutas Ocupacionales*

de Chile ante el Proyecto de Reforma de los Servicios de Salud Mental en Chile, 1999, Ministry of Health Archives. Chilean Congress Archives. Chilean Association of Occupational Therapists' Archives.

Austin W: Using the human rights paradigm in health ethics: the problems and the possibilities, *Nurs Ethics* 8:183–195, 2001.

Berdichewsky E: *Chilean campaign of schizophrenia: Facing the opportunity of integration.* Paper presented at the

International Congress of Psychiatry, Lido, Venecia, Italy, 1996.

Berdichewsky E, de las Heras CG: *Campaña Internacional de la Esquizofrenia: Una Nueva oportunidad, un mundo de Esperanza.* Paper presented at the National Mental Health Conference, Chile, 1995.

Bowring W: Forbidden relations? The UK's discourse of human rights and the struggle for social justice, *Law,*

Social Justice and Global Development Journal 1:1–17, 2002.

Bowyer P, Belanger R, Briand C, de las Heras CG: International efforts to disseminate and develop the model of human occupation, Occupational Therapy in Health Care 22:1–24, 2008.

Braveman B, Suarez-Balcazar Y: Social justice and resource utilization in a community-based organization, Am J Occup Ther 63:13–23, 2009.

Care (2009), US Annual Report, retrieved from: http://www.care.org.

D'Angello M: La pelota de fútbol. Paper presented at the VII Chilean Congress of Occupational Therapy, Chile, July 6-8, Santiago de Chile 1998.

de las Heras CG: Programa de Integración Comunitaria Reencuentros. Trabajando con la Persona y su Familia en la Promoción de su Satisfacción: Aplicación del Modelo de Ocupación Humana. Paper presented at the VIII Chilean Congress of Mental Health, Chile, August 2-4, Santiago de Chile 2004.

de las Heras CG: Reencuentros: Programas y Protocolos de Intervención, Chile, 2006, Copyright Reencuentros, C R P Limitada.

de las Heras CG: Desarrollo de Programas basados en el Modelo de Ocupación Humana. MOHO Training Manual for Occupational Therapists, Santiago de Chile, 2007, Universidad Andrés Bello.

de las Heras CG, Llerena V, Kielhofner G: Remotivation Process: Progressive Interventions for People with Severe Volitional Challenges. Model of Human Occupation Clearinghouse, Chicago, 2003, University of Illinois at Chicago.

du Toit S: Using the model of human occupation to conceptualize an occupational therapy program for blind persons in South Africa, Occupational Therapy in Health Care 22:51–61, 2008.

Fondacaro MR, Weinberg D: Concepts of social justice in community psychology: Toward a social ecological epistemology, Am J Community Psychol 30:473–492, 2002.

Freire P: Pedagogy of the Oppressed (revised ed), New York, 2000, Continuum International Publishing.

Galheigo SM: Occupational therapy and the social field. In Kronenberg F, Simó Algado S, Pollard N, editors: Occupational Therapy Without Borders: Learning Through the Spirit of Survivors, Edinburgh, 2005, Elsevier/Churchill Livingstone, pp 87–98.

Haglund L, Ekbladh E, Thorell LH, Hallberg IR: Practice models in Swedish psychiatric occupational therapy, Scand J Occup Ther 7:107–113, 2000.

Jakobsen K: If work doesn't work: how to enable occupational justice, Journal of Occupational Science 11:125–134, 2004.

Kielhofner G: Functional assessment: Toward a dialectical view of person-environment relations, Am J Occup Ther 47:248–251, 1993.

Kielhofner G: Model of Human Occupation: Theory and Application, ed 2, Baltimore, 2002, Lippincott Williams & Wilkins.

Kielhofner G: Model of Human Occupation: Theory and Application, ed 4, Baltimore, 2008, Lippincott Williams & Wilkins.

Kielhofner G, Burke J, Heard IC: A model of human occupation, part four. Assessment and intervention, Am J Occup Ther 34:777–788, 1980.

Kielhofner G, Mallinson T, Crawford C, et al: A user's guide to the occupational performance history interview-II (OPHI-II) (version 2.0), Chicago, 1998, MOHO Clearinghouse.

Kielhofner G, Braveman B, Fogg L, Levin M: A controlled study of services to enhance productive participation among people with HIV/AIDS, Am J Occup Ther 62:36–45, 2008.

Kronenberg F, Pollard N: Overcoming occupational apartheid: A preliminary exploration of the political nature of occupational therapy. In Kronenberg F, Simó Algado S, Pollard N, editors: Occupational Therapy Without Borders: Learning Through the Spirit of Survivors,

Edinburgh, 2005, Elsevier/Churchill Livingstone, pp 58–86.

Law M, McColl MA: Knowledge and use of theory among occupational therapists: Canadian survey, Can J Occup Ther 56:198–204, 1989.

Oakley F, Kielhofner G, Barris R, et al: The role checklist: Development and empirical assessment of reliability, Occupational Therapy Journal of Research 6:157–170, 1986.

Penjeam A, de las Heras CG: Hogar de Cristo: Projecto de Integración de Personas de la Calle, Santiago, Chile, 2000, Archivos Hogar de Cristo.

Porras X: Terapia Ocupacional: Trabajando con Mujeres en la Promoción de su Participación Ocupacional, Chile, 2002, Archivos del Departamento de Terapia Ocupacional, Universidad Andrés Bello.

Porras X: Terapia Ocupacional: Trabajo con Familias de Alto Riesgo, Chile, 2005, Archivos del Departamento de Terapia Ocupacional, Universidad Andrés Bello.

Todorova L: Assessing employment needs of Bulgarian youths with intellectual impairments, Occupational Therapy in Health Care 22:77–84, 2008.

Townsend E: Power and justice in enabling occupation, Can J Occup Ther 70:74–87, 2003.

Valdés A: Experiencias Subjetivas de las Madres de Personas con Esquizofrenia acerca del Impacto de Apoyos y Oportunidades Ofrecidas, Chile, 2000, Estudio etnográfico publicado en la Universidad.

Wilcock AA: An Occupational Perspective of Health, Thorofare, NJ, 1998, Slack Inc.

Wilcock A, Townsend E: Occupational terminology interactive dialogue: Occupational justice, Journal of Occupational Science 7:84–85, 2000.

Ziv N: Thinking with and applying theory: The model of human occupation: Review of revised concepts, clinical experience and recommendations, Israeli Journal of Occupational Therapy 13: H147–H168, 2004.

A reflective journey and exploration of the human spirit

29

Grace Patricia Mary Cairns   Candice Joy Mes

OVERVIEW

This chapter will outline the engagement process and outcomes of interactions between a group of community-conscious Phillipi youth and the elderly members of an adult day care centre in March 2007, and how this experience was perceived by two final-year occupational therapy students from the University of Cape Town.

As fourth year occupational therapy students placed at the center for community practice learning, we facilitated the interaction between the youth group *Ulutsha Olukhathalayo* (also known as The Caring Youth) and the elderly. The interaction led to meaningful change as reported by the two groups. What emerged in the series of workshops we ran with the youth group was a strong support for the notion of occupation as a synthesis of 'Doing', 'Being', 'Becoming', and 'Belonging' (Hammell 2004; Wilcock 1998, 2006). Validation as a critical part of enhancing potential and reviving the human spirit was highlighted. This chapter also includes reflections from members of the group themselves.

What was the difference. . .? Many people can be at the right place and time, but something extra is needed. Is it a kindness? A respect for person? Taking time to know their inner spirit?

(K Zangqa, personal communication, 2007)

DEFINITION: 'HUMAN SPIRIT'

The meaning and connection of one to their cultural, ethical and moral system, in which the individual experiences a sense of belonging and purpose
Algado & Burgman (2005)

In the beginning: 'Stuck in Nyanga'

This story begins when we were placed in Nyanga – a peri-urban settlement about 15 km outside of Cape Town. We had been placed at a community center for the elderly, which offered a safe space for them to gather during the day. They were given two warm meals and were able to socialize with others. The center gave some of the isolated elderly a purpose for the day and had been identified by the university as a placement so as to give students an introduction into working with and within communities. The resources available are vastly different from other contexts and therefore it is always a challenging placement.

We had been at the center for a week and were feeling lost and confused about our role as students in this particular context. The elderly appeared comfortably set up and were enjoying their daily routine. We asked ourselves: 'What was the purpose of the service? Who are we as occupational therapy students to step in and just keep the elderly busy with things that don't mean anything to them?' We experienced real feelings of wishing we had been placed at one of the more traditional sites of learning such as Groote Schuur Hospital, where our role as occupational therapists might have been more defined and where a clear difference could be made to the people we would be working with.

Our only means of trying to work out the appropriate role of the occupational therapist in this setting was through building relationships with relevant members of the organization and the community, and assessing needs as they arose. We tried to

DOI: 10.1016/B978-0-7020-3103-8.00038-9

approach this with an open mind to create new opportunities that would impact this community and not just engage them in 'doing' for the sake of keeping people busy. Evidence of previous engagements were present in the center itself and in the community context, where students in the past might have experienced (like us) the pressure to do something perceived as productive, rather than taking the time to seek out other creative outlets that were waiting to be explored. Posters on chronic diseases of lifestyle, exercise and stretching methods, and how to set up daily routines cluttered the walls. All these posters were written in English, most doing more by covering the chipped paint than enhancing the lives of those around them.

A change of perspective

It was important for us to walk in the streets of Nyanga and experience it for all it was – a community where people greet anyone and everyone, where sheep's heads were being cooked in large drums to be sold, where traditional herbs were drying in the windows of the houses, where children played games barefoot in the streets and the music of passing taxis created a deep resonating hum. We wanted to see the day-to-day life in this community so that we could understand the context from which the elderly people came. We didn't want to impose something from outside. We wanted to help something to grow from what was already there. While it is an impoverished community that lacks infrastructure, there was definitely something in the air that made us not want to settle on just doing exercise routines with the elderly.

The thoughts of hopelessness that were felt during our first week were radically challenged the moment we met a high school student who had made an appointment to speak to us. His name was Motlatsi Koyo. Some of our first impressions of him, as noted in our reflective journals (20 March 2007), were as follows:

He's about 17. We're surprised to see him dressed so smartly in his blazer even though it's about 30 degrees outside in this Cape Town summer. He looks smarter than some of the professionals we've worked with. And he's on time!

He's a little taller then us but carries himself so confidently we can't help feeling much, much shorter. He has the skin of a struggling adolescent and yet his eyes burn with something far beyond his years. They are glossy and brown.

That's definitely a nervous smile on his face but his handshake is strong and sturdy. He knows what he wants.

The elderly here have warned us about the teenagers of the township so we better be on guard. We've been told they're just looking for money to satisfy their longing to belong with the lifestyle of drugs, sex, and alcohol. But there seems to be something different about him.

During this first encounter with Motlatsi Koyo, we listened as he told the story of his group *Ulutsha Olukhathalayo* (The Caring Youth).

The background to this setting

To provide some context to the environment in which this group was formed, here are some statistics about the youth of the Western Cape: more than 30% of 19-year-old women in the Western Cape are reported to have given birth at least once (Kaufman de Wet & Stadler 2001). HIV prevalence has been noted to be difficult to measure in this age group, as the stigma surrounding testing is high. However, out of those who are tested an estimated 9.4% of girls and 3.2% of boys are HIV positive (Averting HIV & AIDS 2007). Children between the ages of 13 and 18 are noted to make up the biggest drug-user group, especially with regards to *tik* (crystal methamphetamine). *Tik* has had a devastating effect on the Western Cape community, with a noted impact on increasing drug-related crimes – a shocking 159% over the past five years (Parry et al 2007).

Various programs are being run by the government and nongovernmental organizations (NGOs) in these settings. They are focused on risk reduction, but often show little success (Galvaan 2005) since the problems themselves are said to be multifaceted and often not within a health professional's control.

Breaking free

Although the youth came from the context outlined in the previous section and acknowledged the trials they face every day, they were determined to make a difference. Motlatsi Koyo presented a proposal and told us that his youth group was interested in giving back to the people of his community by running holiday programs at orphanages and old-age homes. They wanted to run a free holiday program for the elderly during the upcoming Easter holiday. As they were just starting off with their community projects, they intended to run them on a volunteer basis and do it in their spare time. They wanted to perform for groups who did not necessarily have money to pay for the entertainment, but who would most probably appreciate it. They were also working on a business plan to hopefully one day attain external funding to arrange for bigger events, as their community leaders had turned their backs on them already.

Ulutsha Olukhathalayo wanted to perform various cultural art forms as entertainment for the elderly, and spend time with the *gogos* or wise elders of their community to connect with them on a personal level and honor their individual and cultural heritage.

Building relationships and workshops

After reading Motlatsi's proposal we arranged a meeting with the main committee members of the youth group to discuss the program. We also took advantage of this opportunity to run a workshop with the youth, focusing on the perceptions they had of the elderly and how their program could be adapted to suit the needs of all the participants. The elderly at our center had a range of needs based on their individual abilities. Some of them were living with hemiplegia and the after effects of cerebral vascular accidents and would therefore be unable to be as physically active as others in the proposed group dances. There were also two members who were visually impaired and so would not be able to engage fully with the youth's proposed mime performance.

Connection through scaffolding

When we met the leaders of The Caring Youth, there was no denying their strong presence. They were enthusiastic and bright. Their energy was contagious. The outcome of this first workshop was that the youth felt a little 'stuck'. Their attempts at running programs at other organizations had been met with resistance. This was mainly informed by the prejudice that exists around teenage behavior as described to us by the youth. Their surrounding community saw them as disrespectful. One of the members, Khanyiswa Zangqa, recalls this as something that first hindered their success within their community:

> Before, when meeting other people, people would think we were just stupid kids who had lame ideas about life . . .

The youth group was seeking guidance and support in the process of planning their program so as not to perpetuate this prejudice. This is how we became involved in a facilitative capacity. The youth knew exactly what they wanted to do. For example, as part of their holiday program, they wanted the members of the youth group as well as the center to introduce themselves not only by name and surname, but also by clan name. The group explained this as a means of connection by representing their roots and not just who they are seen as in today's society. They also wore traditional clothing in their drama and dances to honor their cultural and clan heritage. These actions directly showed respect not only for their elders, but also for the journey their spirits had traveled throughout generations.

This reflected a need by the youth to connect with the elderly through meaningful engagement. Connections that bring about a sense of identity have been described by Max-Neef (1991) as one of the fundamental human needs. Similarly Wilding et al (2005) describe 'connection' as strongly associated with the individual's experience of spirituality. During our second workshop discussion, a member from the youth group remarked that she could connect with the *gogos* due to having the 'same spirit' or 'collective feeling', despite the generational divide. Bearing this in mind, it made sense to us to support the youth group to help them succeed in the program they had planned. Our role, then, was 'scaffolding'. We had to give the necessary support and guidance where it was required in tailoring the program to fit the needs of the elderly, without tampering with the contextually relevant cultural art forms.

As we had already assessed the needs of the elderly during our first few weeks at this placement, we could provoke more discussion around making the youth's program accessible to all members. An example of this was accommodating the visually impaired members through adding song to a part of the performance that was mostly miming.

Guided by adult learning theory as highlighted by Hope et al (1984), we probed thoughts and clarified fears and discomforts, but allowed the youth to own the decisions made during the different workshops we ran, specifically those on perceptions of the elderly, handling techniques for the elderly group, structuring of a program, and leadership within a group. This interaction was a successful one not just as a procedural therapy process, but because it also boosted our motivation to engage with the process as noted in field notes on 29 March 2007:

I can go home today and really feel that we have made a difference. Not by having all the answers, but by setting up a workshop with youth who want to do something and giving them the space and time to actually think clearly about how they can go about it. They thrived on our suggestions, such as doing their drama performance first and then using it as a cue to discuss their feelings of cultural importance and the respect they have for the elderly on a more personal level with them. I hope to have more moments like this where I meet people from and for the community.

The interaction

Both the elderly and youth were filled with anticipation on the day of interaction, which led to a haphazard start. The youth group were feeling nervous and unsure of themselves which caused the leaders of the group to rally their members around and start the morning off with a prayer and inspirational song as well as the offer of reassurance that what was planned for the day was appropriate.

During the drama production the elderly listened attentively, cheered for the performers, engaged in song and were moved to tears over the realities portrayed in the dramas. The youth were full of emotion in character, confident in their speech and aware of their audience.

The show was short, but brought across a powerful message. It began with a burst of drum beats and a reflection of the present community, with youth showing disrespect for their social system. This was represented by youths in drunk and promiscuous states, stealing, violating the rights of others, homeless, and begging. The next scene focused in on one of the teens, who was pregnant and desperate. The teen's thoughts and emotions were expressed through a soliloquy. She then turned to those she thought could help only to be turned away. Lastly she went home and shared her feelings with her grandmother who passes on the knowledge she needs. The last scene showed the broader community again where the enlightened teens shared the knowledge of their elders. The show ended on a high note with all those involved in destructive occupations leaving them, uniting with the other youth and the elderly, and singing the national anthem accompanied by the beating of traditional drums.

After the drama performance, every youth group member identified an elderly member who came from the same clan as they did. With our guidance the youth then sat and shared life stories over refreshments which had we arranged at the center.

This engagement opportunity was negotiated and prearranged by us with the center management team. A shared heritage created the opportunity for a cultivated bond irrespective of the difference in age. Smiles and occasional tears could be seen on both the youth and the elderly faces.

Traditional songs sung collectively, followed by prayers and blessings for the youth, concluded the day. A request for their return was made by the elderly which made the youth, especially the leaders, feel greatly honored.

Reflections of the process

The result therefore was that the holiday program was a successful engagement. The youth group and the elderly and disabled members valued the experience. Narrative reasoning, as described by Polkinghorne (1996), was used as a vehicle to illustrate the things one does, has done, wants to, and could do.

The successful engagement between the youth, elderly, and us was expressed through reflective workshops that we held separately with the Nyanga Adult Day Care Centre members and The Caring Youth. The purpose of these workshops was for the members of both groups to unpack what the holiday program meant. One of the themes that emerged from the reflection workshop with the youth was the importance of validation. They pointed out how we had shown a belief in their capacity by making ourselves available to help them plan the holiday program. The engagement brought not only satisfaction, but a feeling of meaning and purpose (Wilding et al 2005). This in turn helped them to feel validated as members of their community and, more crucially, as occupational beings.

> When we met Candice and Grace we were not quite sure how the whole process was going to go. So we started by having a meeting about the things we were going to do at the adult day care centre with the seniors. It worked well; they listened attentively to our opinions and gave us advice when necessary. So that made us feel more important. . . . Grace and Candice have helped us see the potential we have.
>
> (K Zangqa, personal communication, 2007).

During the reflective workshop with the elderly, members expressed their gratitude to the youth for the time and effort they had taken to put the correct cultural nuances in place, for the inclusion of all members in the show and especially for the time they had spent sharing stories together. Some elders were surprised by the youth's genuine willingness to spend time learning more from their elders. They stated that this was a good example of what youth could be like, although they saw it as a sadly isolated case.

Discourse, as described by Lupton (1995), can be understood as the views that society has about a certain phenomenon, such as youth. These perceptions of youth are often social constructions perpetuated by dominant discourses. These shape collective perspectives and individual actions, as they influence what people expect from individuals (in this case, youth) as well as what the individual expects of their own ability.

Within their community and within South African society, the youth we worked with are seen as 'youth at risk' and are often associated with being both the vulnerable and the trouble makers. Members of the youth group expressed their awareness of how they are defined by society. Often what is expected of them is that they would be 'drunk and lying on the streets' (T Ngwabeni, personal communication, 2007) and not involved in projects such as the one they planned for the center's members. Being turned away from organizations was yet another reflection of how little good is expected from the youth. This had such an impact that the youth expressed how, at times, they felt they were wasting their time doing these kinds of projects. Some members pointed out how not even their parents supported their cause. Their parents hoped that they would rather get more structured jobs that would put food on the table, and battled to see the potential of their performances bringing in an income in the future. One could easily be judgmental toward these parents. However, many of them are in a situation where their priorities center on basic needs. They are concerned with survival and thus fulfilling the need for subsistence that Max-Neef (1991) highlights as a fundamental basic human need.

Therefore although some external validation was received from the community's encouragement, it was limited due to lack of support from family. Internal validation was realized due to the youth's self motivation: 'We can't run away, we need to be part of the change'. Although the youth in this group also need to survive, they seem to strive for other things that speak to community-building and 'collective story-making' (E Ramugondo, personal communication, 2007).

The youth chose both to actively break free of a perceived social construction and embrace a traditional philosophy – the philosophy of *Ubuntu*: *umuntu ngumntu ngabantu*, meaning 'a person depends on others in order to be' (see Chapters 1 and 21). This highlights that belonging and caring for one another is a basic value (Shutte 1993). Watson & Fourie (2005) support this concept by expanding on Wilcock's (1998) theory of 'doing, being and becoming', noting how, in an African context, an Afro-centric view is essential, and therefore proposing that 'belonging' be added to the process explained in this theory.

Reflecting on the experience, Khanyiswa Zangqa described to us how this journey caused a change within her, a change that she cannot ignore, a change that is causing her to mature. This has contributed to a new outlook on her perspectives of the elderly and what her role is in her community. She has gone on to win a few community participation awards acknowledged by the province, and has continued to work with other youth on similar projects.

Conclusions

This chapter concludes with three key points that were learnt through this experience:

* Partnership and connection with human beings on more than one level (i.e., emotional, physical, and spiritual) is needed for holistic health promotion. If therapists are to work within communities, they need to be aware that the people they are working with may not have physical or mental illnesses, but may be healthy individuals who need creative direction and support with regard to sustainable projects.
* Even though the youth group faced many complexities in a particular context, *Ulutsha Olukhathalayo* demonstrated how strength can be drawn from togetherness of spirit and determination to engage.
* External validation came from community encouragement earned through positive engagement. Internal validation was realized by the youth's self-motivation.

As students we helped structure the 'doing' (planning workshops based on their holiday programs) and motivated for 'being' (during their reflection on their doing), and therefore allowed for their 'becoming' (change in future and realization of their important skills).

Similar interactions can take place by utilizing the above core principles: encouraging the identification of participating parties; facilitating workshops by making use of adult learning principles to get to the core of what is needed or what is wanted at the outcome of the interaction; and taking note that connection on different levels is vital for a successful engagement.

This chapter has outlined our experience within a community group. All it took was for us to be open and receptive to the support that was required from us for the youth group to succeed in what they saw as necessary in their own community. Every member fortunate enough to be part of this opportunity took a perspective-changing, life-learning experience away with them.

Acknowledgments

Our sincerest gratitude goes out to the members of *Ulutsha Olukhathalayo* for their wisdom and integrity, especially Khanyiswa Zangqa, Mamukuktu Lehana, Motlatsi Koyo, and Thobisa Ngwabeni; to Elelwani Ramugondo and Frank Kronenberg for their constant support and inspiration; Hanske Flieringa for her encouragement and supervision; our family members who were behind the scenes all the way; and finally to all those who are open to connect with the human spirit.

This chapter is dedicated to the memory of Dr DH Griffiths someone who knew the essence of the human spirit.

References

Algado S, Burgman I: OT intervention with children war survivors. In Kronenberg F, Algado S, Pollard N, editors: *Occupational Therapy Without Borders: Learning Through the Spirit of Survivors*, Edinburgh, 2005, Elsevier/Churchill Livingstone.

Avert statistics website: 2007, Online. Available at: http://www.avert.org/safricastats.htm. Accessed September 10, 2007.

Galvaan R: Engaging with youth at risk. In Watson R, Swartz L, editors: *Transformation Through Occupation*, England, 2005, Whurr, pp 186–197.

Hammell K: Dimensions of meaning in the occupations of daily life, *Can J Occup Ther* 71:296–305, 2004.

Hope A, Timmel S, Hodzi: *Training for Transformation, Book 1– A Handbook for Community Workers*, Zimbabwe, 1984, Mambo press.

Kaufman CE, de Wet T, Stadler J: Adolescent pregnancy and parenthood in South Africa, *Stud Fam Plann* 32:147–160, 2001.

Lupton D: *The Imperative of Health*, Thousand Oaks, 1995, Sage.

Max-Neef MA: *Human Scale of Development*, New York, 1991, The Apex Press.

Parry C, Pluddemann A, Bhana A: *Alcohol and drug abuse trends: July-December 2006 (Phase 21)*, 2006, MRC website, SACENDU update May 2007. Online. Available at: http://www.sahealthinfo.org/admodule/sacendumay2007.pdf. Accessed September 10, 2007.

Polkinghorne DE: Transforming narratives: From victim to agentic life plots, *Am J Occup Ther* 50:229–305, 1996.

Shutte A: *Philosophy for Africa*, Cape Town, 1993, UCT Press.

Watson R, Fourie M: Occupation and occupational therapy. In Watson R, Swartz L, editors: *Transformation Through Occupation*, England, 2005, Whurr, pp 19–32.

Wilcock AA: Doing, being and becoming, *Can J Occup Ther* 65:248–257, 1998.

Wilcock A: *An Occupational Perspective of Health*, USA, 2006, Slack Incorporated.

Wilding C, May E, Muir-Cochrane E: Experience of spirituality, metal illness and occupation: A life sustaining phenomenon, *Australian Occupational Therapy Journal* 52:2–9, 2005.

PAR FORE: a community-based occupational therapy program

Alexander Lopez   Pamela Block

OVERVIEW

Engagement in healthy occupations is contingent on performance skills and contextual demands. Resiliency and vulnerability are distinctive personal characteristics that are influenced by sociocultural and environmental contexts. Adolescents from underprivileged communities experiencing occupational apartheid are often deprived of opportunities to participate in occupations that are pleasurable and build generalizable skills for social and economic advancement. PAR FORE (Perseverance, Accountability, Resilience, Fellowship, Opportunity, Respect, Empowerment) addresses these occupational disparities through a grassroots occupation-based golf mentor program serving at-risk and gang-affiliated youths on Long Island, New York. It capitalizes on personal abilities while building community and advancing health-promoting occupations. PAR FORE provides new ways for at-risk and gang-affiliated youths, their parents, student mentors from occupational therapy and related disciplines, and community mentors to learn from each other and combat occupational deprivation and alienation across the varied contexts of education, community service, and leisure.

Introduction

PAR FORE (Perseverance, Accountability, Resilience, Fellowship, Opportunity, Respect, Empowerment) is a grassroots, occupation-based mentoring program to address the occupational disparities experienced by gang-affiliated or at-risk adolescents from several low-income communities on Long Island, New York (Kronenberg & Pollard 2005). 'Gang-affiliated' youths engage in gang-related activities or have a sibling or friend actively involved in gang activities. 'At-risk youth' live in communities with higher incidences of gang activity. They are alienated from and deprived of valued occupations because of dangerous gang activities in their neighborhoods. PAR FORE uses golf to combat occupational apartheid, and capitalize on personal abilities, environmental resources, and participation in health-promoting occupations (Kronenberg & Pollard 2005). It was born out of first author Alexander Lopez's personal life experiences, passions, and current research interests. PAR FORE is a medium for experiential service learning in which students of healthcare professions (occupational therapy, physical therapy, and nursing students), community members (local school teachers, community youth advocates, and local residents) and at-risk youths explore environmental/contextual demands and methods of adaptation. Adolescent participants engage in golf, a sport that fosters positive social interaction. Occupational therapy students gain insights about occupational injustice – the many inequities in distribution of resources and opportunities faced by members of underrepresented communities (Mitchell & Wright 1992, Scaletti 1998). Students gain insight into entrepreneurship and develop the resolute courage and fortitude to move beyond clinical institutions and into the community (Lopez 2006, Scaletti 1998) (Box 30.1).

Golf provides a forum for dialog. PAR FORE golfers spend hours on the golf course, exchanging ideas and breaking down traditional divides between clinical service provider and service recipient, without

DOI: 10.1016/B978-0-7020-3103-8.00039-0

Box 30.1

Reflection of occupations and contexts

Alex Lopez

Few children growing up in the depressed areas of Newark, New Jersey, realize their dreams, which seem like storybook fantasies only illustrated on music and sports networks. Inner city youth have little understanding of what it really takes to make their dreams come true. I was one of those youth who credulously believed that I would someday find my way, never contemplating the energy, hindrances, and demands of social and economic advancement. Like many other youth living in Newark, I was unprepared for the journey to success. I was not blessed with an aptitude for scholarship, a talent for music, or the capabilities of a star athlete, nor did I have the resources to acquire the knowledge and skills to excel in any way. Moreover, Newark was not an environment that would easily cultivate success. Polluted and impoverished, it was a volatile and dangerous physical environment further complicated by human adversity. My social context included prostitutes, gangs, and drug dealers. Like the youth of Brentwood, I played in empty school yards and abandoned buildings where homeless squatters and heroin addicts lived. I broke windows, tagged walls, and rode on the top of subway trains for fun. I sought immediate gratification. I occupied my time with activities that satisfied my short-term needs for friendship, protection, and play. My occupational pursuits were shaped by my social and physical contexts. I ingenuously followed the same path of destruction and poverty as my friends and family. Fortunately, I had the opportunity to be mentored by an adult in the community. I was introduced to new contexts, occupations, and affiliations free of crime and despair. Ultimately I developed passions for golf and occupational therapy which resulted in the PAR FORE program. My dreams were no longer unreachable fantasies but tangible visions for my future.

friendship. There are no referees, umpires, or officiates. Participants are expected to play with honesty and integrity, governed by concrete rules and behaviors. Each member of the group is expected to perform in accordance with rules of etiquette, modeling commonly accepted notions of civility and good citizenship, and resulting in positive behaviors and social skills that can be generalized elsewhere (e.g., to create favorable impressions during job or scholarship interviews) (United States Golf Association (USGA) 2009).

In addition to golf, youth, and mentors participate in service learning projects, providing opportunities to give back to their community. Fellowship is a core principle in PAR FORE: understanding the value of community building and social reciprocity in building character, developing social interaction skills, self-respect and respect for others. For example, adolescents participate in an intergenerational program called the 'Junior and Senior Tour', where they visit local nursing homes and assisted-living communities and teach the residents golf in an intergenerational dialog, learning social interaction skills, and developing an appreciation for older adults. They also attend life skills sessions (i.e., resiliency training, gang prevention, social skills building, and bully prevention) at Stony Brook University and apply academic skills to solving real-world issues, linking established learning objectives with genuine community needs. The university experience provides a vehicle for discovery. Adolescents gain insight and greater awareness of occupational and educational pursuits they had never considered. Through campus tours, student presentations, and interactive lectures, PAR FORE allows the youth to learn about a world foreign to them (PAR FORE 2009).

The setting

The town of Brentwood in Suffolk County, Long Island, is one of the largest and most diverse school districts in New York State. It is a context of occupational apartheid, with one of the highest poverty indices in New York State. Over 80% of its community live in poverty. The Brentwood School District has one of the largest Hispanic enrollments in the state outside of New York City, with a large percentage of immigrant students attending district schools. The school district reports approximately 200 homeless students, a 50% mobility rate among the student population, and the highest number of

the time limitations of conventional intervention sessions. Traditionally, when healthcare providers, educators, and law enforcement professionals reach out to these adolescents, the interaction is inhibited by time and space. Temporal and physical boundaries reinforce power disparities and limit the free flow of dialog. Institutional walls are unnatural and create an atmosphere of constraint and inequality. A round of golf comprises a foursome: two gang-affiliated or at-risk youths, one college student volunteer mentor, and one older community mentor. This social configuration breaks down hierarchies of (generational, class, racial, ethnic, and educational) difference and promotes informal dialog, rapport, and juvenile offenses, arrests, and juvenile delinquents placed on probation in Suffolk County. Gang-related activity has increased in recent years. Law enforcement officers estimate that there are as many as 10 000 gang members in Suffolk and Nassau Counties. Currently, local law enforcement estimates that there are approximately 42 gangs on Long Island (Wiley et al 2004). These gangs are affiliated with national and international gangs, but are somewhat different, in that the loyalties to specific gangs are not as significant. In fact, there is some evidence of crossover. Gangs in Long Island are said to be more business oriented, with drug trafficking as their main source of activity.

Induction into youth gangs, a direct result of occupational deprivation and alienation, has been equated with the extreme end of high-risk 'deviant' adolescent behaviors. All youth in this community have life experiences that either necessitate or prevent gang involvement. Such affiliations do not occur instantaneously. They require time, space, and engagement in certain occupations. Adolescents are exposed to the dynamic interaction between their level of performance skills (cognitive, emotional, and physical skills) and the contextual demands of their environment (American Occupational Therapy Association 2002). Curry & Decker (1998) posited that, when the social contexts fail to meet the needs of adolescents, then high-risk 'deviant' behaviors result. Adolescents who choose to engage in gang activities may believe that they have no reasonable alternative. It might be said that gang participation and drug use is a functional response to a dysfunctional environment. In a context of blatant occupational apartheid, the presence of gang occupation is ubiquitous; it touches all who live in Brentwood. In some neighborhoods, gang activity has become the dominant and prevailing culture. Children often feel compelled to join gangs or engage in delinquency because of the lack of alternatives in their environment.

Unfortunately, once engaged in gang activity or delinquency, adolescents often progress to more dangerous and illegal behaviors. Klein (1995) reported that youth already participating in such activities are less likely to benefit from psychosocial interventions. For this reason, it is important for programs such as PAR FORE to identify and target individuals who are at-risk or who are in the early stages of gang activity. It is within this environment that young adolescents construct their occupational identities. They can choose the occupation of gang member or they can choose alternative occupations that will promote future success and wellness.

Adolescents in Brentwood are barred from opportunities to engage in health promoting activities or occupations. Health-promotion activities support and encourage social, sensorimotor, emotional, and cognitive growth. They allow adolescents the opportunity to develop skills for a safe and successful transition into adulthood. Such activities include sports, tutoring, and play. For example, while other surrounding communities in the Brentwood area send their children to private schools, receive tutoring for math and science, have tennis and music lessons, many children in Brentwood are spending their free time in empty lots and on the street. Hanging out and getting into fights is how they occupy their time. They play in empty school yards with broken basketball hoops. They break windows, and tag walls and fences with graffiti. Abandoned buildings, homes blackened and charred by arsonists, and vacant lots are the contexts for their occupations. Hope is a cognitive process shaped by contextual form and environmental demands. Hope for future goals and aspirations surface when an individual has knowledge of opportunities, can formulate a plan to acquiring a goal, and has the perceived capacity achieve success (Snyder et al 1999). In the context of such grave occupational disparities, these youths do not dream of someday going to college. Instead, they are living in a world where their past, present, and future orientation have merged to satisfy their immediate needs.

Temporality is context and resource driven. Orientation to time is dependent on available resources. Live for today and not tomorrow. The long-term consequences of health compromising activities are of little concern to many adolescents in Brentwood. Instead, they engage in activities that satisfy short-term needs, bullying or avoiding bullies. Given the scarcity of opportunities, social, and institutional resources, adolescents living in impoverished communities fail to recognize their potential for engaging in healthy occupations. Instead, they engage in health compromising occupations that provide immediate safety and security for their present-day experiences, and a sense of belonging. However, such activities do nothing to correct occupational injustices and may have a lasting negative effect on their lives.

Gang membership provides an occupation that is meaningful and purposeful within the immediate context, offering a means of attaining social status, power, and self-worth. It provides safety and security when there are no other alternatives. Perceived self-worth is validated through gang-related occupations.

However, these short-term gains only satisfy the adolescent's immediate need for purpose and meaning. Gang participation and other health-compromising activities do not provide tools to fight or escape systemic injustices, and can harm their long-term potential to acquire adult occupations that are meaningful, purposeful, and productive.

Person, context, occupation

Individuals should be examined in the contexts of the environments where they actually and potentially perform. Contextual factors, such as sociocultural, environmental, economic, political, institutional, and virtual influences, provide the settings in which individuals act. The context provides both location and motivation for the expression of occupational performance skills (Dunn et al 1994). When resources are scarce and contextual demands exceed occupational capacities, the potential for dangerous and illegal activities increases. A context of occupational apartheid, void of opportunities to practice satisfying and health-promoting occupations, may lead youth to choose ways to maximize occupational potential that are ultimately destructive to self and community.

Social support and coping styles are important to the development of resiliency (Garmezy & Rutter 1985, Seiffge-Krenke & Shulman 1990, Werner & Smith 1982). Adolescents' immediate influences include family members, peers, religious leaders and educational professionals. Additional influences may include, television, the internet, movies and any interactions they or family members may have had with the criminal justice system. Adolescents inclined to destructive or unhealthy behaviors may lack positive peer mentoring influences that can help to establish healthy norms, role expectations, and social routines (American Occupational Therapy Association 2002). The presence of social support increases the chances that they will learn and use problem-solving techniques to resolve conflict and demonstrate resiliency. Adolescents with social support demonstrate greater resilience to unhealthy or destructive activities or occupations. Social competency, which also includes critical thinking skills, motivation, and decision making, also influences resilience (Schmeelk-Cone & Zimmerman 1993). It is through participation in occupations that individuals develop social competence. Occupational and social competence are dependent on an adolescent's resilient capacities, supportive familial and community networks, and the context in which they function. PAR FORE members participated in a series of group activities on diversity and disability. After the members completed the sessions, they participated in community activities that supported members of their community who have experienced marginalization (Veteran's Home and Walk for Mental Illness) (PAR FORE 2009). Through such activities, adolescents gain critical perspectives on cultural perceptions and socioeconomic structures.

Resiliency and vulnerability are distinctive personal characteristics influenced by sociocultural background and environment. They are not absolutes, but are psychosocial constructs on a phenomenological continuum. A resilient individual is not invincible to all life events. Resiliencies and vulnerabilities are temporally, contextually, and subjectively oriented (Santon-Salazar & Spina 2000, Spina 1998). Psychosocial factors associated with resiliency include positive temperament, coping styles, positive self-esteem, and problem-solving skills (Werner & Smith 1982). Adolescents who demonstrate the greatest resiliencies may flourish even in high stress, disadvantaged, or harmful contexts (Anthony 1991). Resilient individuals are able to overcome adversity through healthy adaptation (Fine 1991). Contrarily, vulnerability is described as an individual's propensity to engage in self-destructive or harmful behaviors (Garbarino et al 1992, Santon-Salazar & Spina 2000). Counterproductive means of coping with occupational injustice do not eliminate individual or community-level problems. They offer only temporary escape and are likely, in the long run, to increase difficulties. Social contextual factors associated with resilience include: positive reinforcement from significant individuals; positive parenting; encouraging occupational competence and self-esteem; having supportive adults who foster trust, and; having opportunities to engage in healthy occupations (Markstrom Marshall & Tryon 2000) (Box 30.2).

Discussion

Unfortunately, Marie's adolescence (Box 30.2) is not extraordinary. Millions of people in the United States have similar stories. This society is rooted in the idealistic belief that 'all men are created equal,

Box 30.2

Marie's narrative

Marie (name changed), an adolescent girl, was introduced to the harsh realities of adulthood prematurely. At the age of 14, she added the occupation of mother to the already complicated repertoire of roles and expectations of adolescence. She lives in Brentwood, Suffolk County, New York on Long Island, a context of occupational apartheid where few healthy occupational opportunities and resources are available to residents. Growing up, Marie regularly fought with her parents. By the age of 12, she had run away from home, lived in foster homes, juvenile detention centers, and on the streets of New York City, until she met a 27-year-old man and moved in with him in Queens, New York. Now 15, Marie described her relationship with the 27-year-old as 'abusive and bipolar'. At age 14, she became pregnant and he vanished. She decided to keep the baby, believing that keeping it would help her in the long run. Marie moved into a home for young mothers in upstate New York.

After two years of living in homes and detention centers, Marie returned to her parents' home in Brentwood with her 2-year-old son. Upon returning, she discovered that her occupational roles and routines had changed dramatically. Family life was very different than in the past, for now Marie was responsible for her son. She parented her child while being parented by her own mother and

father. Struggling with adolescent needs and adult responsibilities, she had little time for play and self-care, and the consequence was a rising level of tension in her home. She began to exhibit the same problematic behaviors she enacted when she was 12. She had returned to an environment that had brought vulnerability and compromise to her life two years previously. Having returned, she found that her life was now even more complicated. Although she was mature beyond her years, she had periods of regression and a propensity to engage in health compromising behaviors.

In the summer of 2007, Marie joined the PAR FORE program, where she was mentored by Stony Brook University students. At first, she was reluctant and uneasy with the program, but eventually Marie became one of the most active PAR FORE participants. Her parents have seen positive changes in her attitudes, behavior, and occupational performance since she joined the program. Marie realizes that having a son changed her life, and that she is missing out on the 'usual' teen activities, but she also knows that having a son has turned her life around for the better. With the help of the mentors in the PAR FORE program, she has showed increased maturity and become more goal-oriented and responsible.

that they are endowed by their creator with certain inalienable rights that are among these are life, liberty, and the pursuit of happiness' (United States Constitution, article 1 section 2). Many United States citizens genuinely believe equality has been achieved in their society. Yet is this a reality? Equality is both perceptual and contextual. The pursuit of happiness is supported by the philosophical assumption within occupational therapy that everyone seeks meaningful existence through valued occupations. The concept of occupational justice implies that the ability to do so is a basic human right. In American society, such rights are often experienced by individuals with socioeconomic means. However, what is meant by 'life, liberty, and the pursuit of happiness' is relative to person and context. In contexts of occupational deprivation and alienation, where all you know is despair, strife, and distress, your occupational potential may be limited in scope and value. The basic necessities – food, shelter, and security – are of more significance then education or recreation. A high school diploma may offer little to an individual from the inner city. Employment opportunities immediately available are menial and do

not require a high school education, so why bother pursuing a diploma or higher education? Therefore, the cost of higher education outweighs the benefits of employment. Why put off years of earnings while attending school, and engaging in recreation or leisure pursuits? The context gives rise to sense of inadequacy, pessimism, and vulnerability. How are individuals to break the cycle of poverty when they have learned that poverty and violence are normal, and there are no available alternatives to the lifestyles they see in their community (Dahlberg 1998, Markstrom et al 2000)?

When Marie described her story of hardship and misfortune, she did so with very little regret. At first glance, she looked like every other young adolescent girl from her community. She wore an innocent smile with her baggy clothes. She was good-humored and sociable. However, when asked to describe herself, she portrayed someone unlike the person her mentors came to love and appreciate. She characterized herself as intolerant and angry, a common theme among adolescents who participate in our program. However, consider how her adolescence was transformed when she moved in with her boyfriend, became pregnant, and experienced homelessness. We see the epitome of resilience in her ability to acknowledge her boyfriend's abusive behavior, accept the occupation of motherhood, and eventually return home to live with her parents. Marie watched her friends and fellow program participants live as 'typical' adolescents. In her past she endured trauma, distress, and sorrow, but today she has purpose. Together with the help of PAR FORE, mentors, and parents, Marie has maintained her chosen course. Pre and post measures on resiliency and behavioral scales indicate that she has demonstrated improved resiliency, academic performance, social interaction skills, and optimism (Battle 2002, Beck et al 2005, Embury 2007). Prior to joining PAR FORE, she was suspicious and distant. Now she has greater appreciation for her family and engages in community service activities by supporting older adults in nursing homes and assisted-living communities.

A reviewer, misunderstanding the intent of the program and oversimplifying the complex processes at work, suggested that the PAR FORE program encourages adolescents to conform to Euro-American values and mores, as articulated by the sport of golf (Chung 2007). PAR FORE promotes values considered important in many cultural contexts (Perseverance, Accountability, Resilience, Fellowship, Opportunity, Respect, and Empowerment), and offers adolescents skills, options, and opportunities for increased social inclusion. It is not a process of assimilation, but rather of learning how to cross cultural and class boundaries with the potential outcome of individual and systemic transformation. The adolescents gain exposure to institutions of higher education, healthcare, and community. They do not surrender their cultural identity simply by choosing to play golf in clubs located within their own communities. Playing golf provides opportunities to feel and be treated as equals and to build on their self-esteem and social competency.

PAR FORE also serves a transformative function for the sport of golf. Golf organizations are broadening their definitions and understanding of the communities where they are located. By participating in PAR FORE, their relationships with community members have changed. The youths are players rather than threats or nuisances. On a larger scale, the USGA has repeatedly expressed recognition, praise, and funding for the PAR FORE program and its participants. In the long term, what might it mean for the sport, that these adolescents have made it their own? What will happen as they begin to join high school and college golf teams, seeking competitive sporting and educational opportunities such as trophies and scholarships? To the participants, golf is not only a sport, but an occupation that is rich in resources and opportunities.

PAR FORE uses a collaborative model that identifies intrinsic needs of youth participants while capitalizing on the intrinsic strengths that can advance health promoting behaviors. We identify Brentwood youth at-risk for gang participation or other health compromising behaviors, work with community members to better understand these youth's needs, and have developed a dynamic program for health promotion that meets them. Research has shown that resiliency can provide the emotional and mental strength to overcome adversity within a hostile environment (Masten & Coatsworth 1998). Building on an adolescent's ability to master healthy occupations encourages resiliency. PAR FORE offers individualized life-skills training (i.e., anti-bullying, gang prevention, and goal orientation), and community-based service learning (intergenerational activities in nursing homes and assisted-living communities, participation in charity events, and neighborhood beautification). PAR FORE participants have been given service awards by local politicians, been praised by community activists, and recognized by local and national media for their community service (PAR FORE 2009). They view their participation in PAR FORE with high esteem and pride.

Conclusion

Occupational therapy is both logical and abstract. Models, paradigms, and theories guide our practice; however, we are all driven by the overwhelming convictions that occupations are the basis of meaningful existence. Occupational potential is limited only by our perceptions of our practice and its broader potential for systems change. Whether our perceptions are rooted in reductionism or holism, they must be challenged and expanded to include community relationships that extend beyond the traditional client–clinician dyad. If we do this, then occupational therapy becomes uniquely prepared to address the community-based needs of many populations. We must find what drives us and then drive the profession. We must challenge existing social realities and perceptions of practice, and infuse our beliefs, assumptions, and skills within socially responsible community-based practice. In the case of PAR

FORE, the explicative process of resiliency, adaptation, and occupation is manifested through healthier transitions from adolescence to adulthood. Through participation in pleasurable and productive occupations adolescents engage in exploration, skill building, and healthy occupations (Santon-Salazar & Spina 2000).

PAR FORE was designed to address occupational apartheid in the Brentwood community. Most practitioners would identify the at-risk adolescents in our program as 'the client'. However, in reality, it is the entire community, including the golf organizations, that is at risk. Through community participation, PAR FORE participants transform their occupational identities, improve occupational performance, and strive to transform their existing communities. Their participation in community service provides them an opportunity to give back to their troubled community. By confronting and counteracting the inequalities and occupational injustices experienced in their own lives, the youths develop a sense of empowerment. Learning how to adapt to new social, cultural, and physical contexts builds new skills and promotes social participation while developing a more clearly defined sense of self, a better understanding of one's place in the world, and what can be done to challenge occupational apartheid and social and economic disparities. By entering the previously closed world of the golf and by volunteering in assisted-living facilities, youths may end up transforming social contexts and relationships. Community service, positive modeling from mentors, and exposure to healthy alternatives allow adolescents choices they did not have before and an opportunity to explore and participate in potentially transformative occupations and environments.

References

American Occupational Therapy Association: Occupational therapy practice framework: Domain and process, *Am J Occup Ther* 56:609–639, 2002.

Anthony EJ: Risk, vulnerability and resilience. In Anthony EJ, Cohler BJ, editors: *The Invulnerable Child*, New York, 1991, Guilford, pp 3–48.

Battle J: *Culture Free Self-Esteem Inventories*, ed 3, Austin, Texas, 2002, PRO-ED.

Beck A, Beck J, Jolly J, Steer R: *Beck Youth Inventories Second Edition for Children and Adolescents*, San Antonio, Texas, 2005, Harcourt Assessment.

Chung J: 2007, Golf program for at-risk youth approved, *Newsday* June 26. Online. Available at: http://newsday.com/ny-ligolf0627. Accessed June 26, 2007.

Curry GD, Decker SA: *Confronting Gangs: Crime and Community*, Los Angeles, California, 1998, Roxbury Publishing.

Dahlberg LL: Youth violence in the United States: Major trends, risk factors, and prevention approaches, *Am J Prev Med* 14:259–272, 1998.

Dunn W, Brown C, McGuigan A: The ecology of human-performance – a framework for considering the effect of context, *Am J Occup Ther* 48:595–607, 1994.

Embury S: *Resiliency Scales for Children and Adolescents: A Profile of Personal Strengths*, San Antonio, Texas, 2007, Harcourt Assessment.

Fine SB: Resilience and human adaptability: Who rises above adversity? 1990 Eleanor Clarke Slagle Lecture, *Am J Occup Ther* 45:493–503, 1991.

Garbarino J, Dubrow N, Kostelny K, Pardo C: *Children in Danger: Coping with the Consequences of Community Violence*, San Francisco, 1992, Jossey-Bass.

Garmezy N, Rutter M: Acute reactions to stress. In Rutter M, Hersov L, editors: *Child and Adolescent Psychiatry: Modern Approaches*, ed 2, Oxford, 1985, Blackwell Publishing, pp 152–176.

Klein MW: *The American Street Gang: Its Nature, Prevalence, and Control*, New York, 1995, Oxford University Press.

Kronenberg F, Pollard N: Overcoming occupational apartheid: A preliminary exploration of the political nature of occupational therapy. In Kronenberg F, Algado SS, Pollard N, editors: *Occupational Therapy Without Borders: Learning Through the Spirit of Survivors*, Edinburgh, 2005, Elsevier/Churchill Livingstone, pp 55–86.

Lopez A: Occupational advocacy and therapeutic justice for the older driver.

AOTA Continuing Education Article. *OT Practice* 11:CE1–CE8, 2006.

Markstrom CA, Marshall SK, Tryon RJ: Resiliency, social support, and coping in rural low-income Appalachian adolescents from two racial groups, *J Adolesc* 23:693–703, 2000.

Masten AS, Coatsworth JD: The development of competence in favorable and unfavorable environments: Lessons from successful children, *Am Psychol* 53:205–220, 1998.

Mitchell S, Wright M: Community development. In Baum F, Fry D, Lennie I, editors: *Community Health Policy and Practice in Australia*, Bondi Junction, 1992, Pluto Press Australia Ltd, pp 149–163.

PAR FORE: 2009, Online. Available at: http://www.parfore.org. Accessed 17 November 2009.

Santon-Salazar RD, Spina SU: The network orientations of highly resistant suburban minority youth: A network analytic account of minority socialization and its educational implications, *Urban Rev* 32:227–256, 2000.

Scaletti R: A community development role for occupational therapists working with children, adolescents and their families: A mental health Perspective, *Australian Occupational Therapy Journal* 46:43–51, 1998.

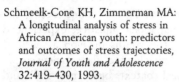

Schmeelk-Cone KH, Zimmerman MA: A longitudinal analysis of stress in African American youth: predictors and outcomes of stress trajectories, *Journal of Youth and Adolescence* 32:419–430, 1993.

Seiffge-Krenke I, Shulman S: Coping style in adolescence, *Journal of Cross-Cultural Psychology* 21:351–377, 1990.

Snyder CR, Cheavens J, Michael ST: Hoping. In Snyder CR, editor: *Coping: The Psychology of What Works*, New York, 1999, Oxford University Press, pp 205–231.

Spina SU: A review of Haggerty RJ, Sherrod LR, Garmezy N, Rutter M (eds) Stress, risk, and resilience in children and adolescents: processes, mechanisms, and interventions, *Mind, Culture and Activity* 5:235–239, 1998.

United States Golf Association: *Golf Etiquette 101*, 2009, Online.

Available at: http://www.usga.org/Etiquette.aspx?id=7790. Accessed 17 November 2009.

Werner EE, Smith RS: *Vulnerable but Invincible: A Longitudinal Study of Resilient Children and Youth*, New York, 1982, McGraw-Hill.

Wiley M, Christeson W, Newman S: *Caught in the crossfire: Arresting Long Island gang violence by investing in kids. Fight Crimes: Invest in Kids in New York*, 2004, pp 1–26.

Section 3

Education and research without borders

Eastern European transition countries: capacity development for social reform

31

Hanneke van Bruggen

OVERVIEW

This chapter is aimed at providing a deeper insight into the complex issues related to capacity development and partnership between occupational therapy educational institutes in Western Europe and university faculties in health and social sciences in Eastern and Central Europe, local governments, and other stakeholders. One of the outcomes of the ENOTHE projects have been the establishment of four occupational therapy schools – each with their own identity and functioning under the jurisdiction of different universities and faculties. The chapter concludes with a discussion of the results of a survey on the impact of these projects on the participation of disadvantaged groups in their communities and the contribution to social reform.

Our lives are too short not to share what and who we know so the world can profit and the journey to sustainability can be shorter.

Robert Davies (2007)

Introduction

One year after its foundation, the European Network of Occupational Therapy in Higher Education (ENOTHE) made the enlargement of Europe and collaboration with the so-called 'new' accession countries a specific objective in its policy plans for the following reasons: (i) the social action and cohesion strategy of Europe, that is, the capacity to ensure the welfare of all its members and minimize

disparities, and building cohesion – the fundamental commitment of the European Union to human rights and democracy (Commission on Social Determinants of Health (CDCS) 2004); (ii) the Bologna process (Communiqué Berlin 2003), which calls for the realization of one European higher education area with compatible degrees and the effective sharing of knowledge, research and expertise; and (iii) the strategy of the European Commission to tackle health inequalities between and within countries in the European Union (Closing the Gap 2004–2007). Within the framework of these policies ENOTHE applied successfully for grants from the European Commission to undertake several projects, whose aims are to facilitate the participation of disadvantaged groups in Eastern and Central European countries and to contribute to social and educational reform. This need to be achieved by developing occupational therapy education and practice. The aims and objectives of ENOTHE and some of the characteristics of the European transition countries will first be discussed in order to understand the projects in the Eastern and Central European region in more detail.

The process of strategically developing occupational therapy's contribution to policies and the clarification of political choices has challenged old ways of thinking and created scope for new ideas. This brings us to the central tenet of this chapter, which should be borne in mind each time you are about to embark on a new dialog: that a good dialog should unite people, create opportunities, and foster understanding.

The chapter will lay particular emphasis on the process of partnering, capacity development,

DOI: 10.1016/B978-0-7020-3103-8.00040-7

and the dilemmas encountered. Strategies from United Nations Developmental Programs (UNDP) and the European Centre of Development Policy Management (ECDPM) have contributed to a methodology in capacity development of a full range of stakeholders, universities, disability organizations, practitioners, students, etc., including lecturers from the ENOTHE site. There is a growing sense that the process of improving abilities and capacities, as opposed to achieved results, needs systematic thought and action. Many practitioners and observers, both in donor and partner institutions/countries, are developing greater insights into the dynamics of people coming together to get things done and of developing the skills and the willingness to act in collaborative ways for the common good. Before developing or building the new profession and education, it is important to build good partnerships, through which important strategic concerns can be addressed. Occupational needs can be defined as essential determinants of health and wellbeing (Commission on Social Determinants of Health (CSDH) 2008), and the need for education can be determined to develop an occupational therapy curriculum and services in the transition countries. These countries usually include the Eastern and Central European countries which have moved from a socialistic style of economy to one that is market driven. It is also important to clarify the quality or standards to be used in practice and education, who is evaluating and what is monitored. Finally, the outcomes of recent reflections of local teachers, students, clients, and other stakeholders will demonstrate the results and impact of the developmental process. This will address some of the most important lessons learned in the journey to achieve social reform through occupational justice.

ENOTHE

The general aims of ENOTHE are to enable European educational institutes, professional associations, and other stakeholders to liaise in order to develop, harmonize, and improve standards of professional practice, education, and research as well as advance the body of knowledge of occupational therapy and occupational science throughout Europe. ENOTHE also aims to facilitate the participation of people with disabilities in an enlarged Europe through the development of high-quality occupational therapy education, research, and practice (ENOTHE

Constitution 2007). The last aim is further elaborated as follows in ENOTHE's policy plan: 'to facilitate interaction and integration with occupational therapy education institutes in the Eastern, and Central European regions by supporting and developing new projects for European grants and funding' (ENOTHE Policy Plan 2008–2011).

Over the past 12 years, ENOTHE has developed three major projects: in the Czech Republic; in Georgia and Armenia; and in Bulgaria, Hungary, and Romania. A fourth project is under development in Poland. All are aimed at contributing to social change as well as reforming higher education through the introduction and implementation of occupational therapy education and services. These projects are based on two general principles:

- The occupational therapy curriculum needs to be developed partly by a participatory action approach including the future local occupational therapists in partnership with a wide range of stakeholders.
- The education of occupational therapy students needs to focus on facilitation of occupational participation of marginalized populations, persons with disabilities, their carers and families in their physical and social environment within a framework of occupational justice and human rights.
- ENOTHE members collaborate with local staff and students, with the direct involvement of client groups and their carers and families, to develop education modules, after each of which a small project is implemented. Since ENOTHE is acting on behalf of the European Community (EC), as an economic 'aid' donor it is important to make sure that aid works and it is effective, as well as to know to what extent the development cooperation makes a difference for the disadvantaged, disabled, and poor people.

Transition countries and social reform

The transitional states are those that, prior to 1989, formed part of communist countries and the former Soviet Union, and shared considerable similarities in health and social care systems based on a common ideology. The historical changes in the socioeconomic system in ex-communist European countries greatly affected the quality of life of their populations.

These changes have been analyzed within a framework of sustainable development and quality of life components: economic, social, political, environmental, cultural, and human. While some components within certain social strata saw improvements, others deteriorated. A major aspect of the changes was the enlargement of human choices in all of the components, and to different extents in different transitional countries (Matutinović 1998).

The transitional countries had well-developed social sectors before the onset of transition. However, their institutional arrangements – which provided 'cradle-to-grave' protection to the entire population – had been designed for a very different economic system. They were incompatible with the incentive mechanisms of a market economy and ill-prepared to cope with the enormous pressures that emerged in the transition to a market economy. Existing social sector institutions and policies were significantly eroded and severely affected by the process. As such, there is a need for these countries to reform their social sectors so as to promote the welfare of their citizens and spur economic growth. In part, this means building up and redesigning social safety nets and addressing problems in such areas as social insurance, budgetary transfers, healthcare, education, labor markets, and tax administration. Reform should also focus on reducing the number of beneficiaries and cutting some privileges (Heller & Keller 2001).

Since the enlargement of the European Union (EU), poverty and cohesion problems have increased, 16% of the EU population currently lives at risk of poverty (Wolff 2009). It is expected that this number will rise, not least as a consequence of the financial crisis and the effects this will have on the labor markets and the society. The reduction of poverty is a process that goes far beyond material and financial assistance. It needs to include strategies to diminish vulnerability, occupational injustice, and discrimination, and to promote social inclusion and participation in all occupational performance areas. In order to adequately address the specific occupational needs of disabled people and vulnerable groups who are deprived from occupations, the strategy needs to be grounded in a comprehensive analysis of poverty issues, social determinants of health (CSDH 2008), and community development approaches.

A European survey has provided evidence that an absolute majority of the people in transition countries view social injustice as the main driver of social exclusion processes (Böhnke P 2004). Health, poverty and unemployment issues of vulnerable groups cannot only be solved by individual solutions, but also need social solidarity and community solutions. This reinforces the need for the occupational therapist to:

- Increase awareness about the relationship between poverty, disability, health inequalities, occupational deprivation, etc.
- Apply an individual as well as a community-development approach
- Develop competencies for poverty reduction.

The developmental process

> Development is a process of expanding the real freedoms that people enjoy.
>
> (Sen 1999, p. 366)

Developing occupational therapy education in order to contribute to social and higher education reform is not a single disciplinary or professional action, but needs complex and widespread cross-sector collaboration to ensure that sustainable development initiatives are coherent and integrated enough to effectively tackle the most intractable problems. When occupational therapists work as individuals in a separate setting in transitional contexts their work can contribute to improvement of care through direct treatment or through providing caregivers or health workers informal education. However, because it is not a cross-sector collaboration between education and health, and the social and labor sector these benefits do not result in structural changes in society. A cross-sector partnership provides an opportunity for doing development better – by recognizing the qualities and competencies of each sector and finding new ways of harnessing these for the common good. The 'core business' of each sector – whether the public sector, business sector or civil society – leads to quite different priorities, values and attributes.

Establishing partnerships: with whom, when, and why?

> Partnership development is easy to talk about but quite hard to undertake. It requires courage, patience, commitment and determination over time. Partnerships enable different groups of people and agencies to collaborate, cooperate and coordinate in order to solve problems and to exchange resources.
>
> Curtin et al (2010, p. 303)

A partnership is a cross-sector collaboration in which organizations work together in a transparent, equitable and mutually beneficial way towards a sustainable development goal and where those defined as partners agree to commit resources and share the risks as well as the benefits associated with the partnership

Tennyson (2003)

Cross-sector (business, not-for-profit organizations, government, academia, media) partnering is an important mechanism for addressing critical and sustainable development issues such as health, employment, social inclusion, post-conflict resolution, and enterprise development (International Business Leaders Forum (IBLF) 2008). 'The United Nations once dealt only with Governments. By now we know that peace and prosperity cannot be achieved without partnerships involving governments, international organizations, the business community and civil society. In today's world, we depend on each other' Kofi Annan, UN Secretary-General (IBFL 2008). For the partnership development in the ENOTHE projects, Tennyson's Partnering Toolbook (2003) has been used. This identifies a 12-step process. The first three steps, scoping, identifying, and building partnerships will be discussed in detail for the project in Romania, Bulgaria, and Hungary.

Developing occupational therapy education for social reform is not just a matter of implementing a 'good' curriculum or training teachers nor simply a question of allocating skills and roles between the right persons, but there must be a significant opportunity for organizational engagement and systems' willingness to change. From the start it is important to consider how the partnership will use its experiences and programs to positively influence each sector and support system change, where necessary. The appropriate partners need to be identified who will have the responsibility for carrying it out. Sufficient time should be taken to check out the motivation and commitment of potential partners as well as finding the right combination of partner organizations. For example, since 1999 one Romanian rehabilitation doctor, who was very committed to the development of occupational therapy education, had made requests to ENOTHE several times for support to establish occupational therapy in Romania. This, however, was an insufficient basis on which to develop a new discipline in a university and to generate social reform in a region or country. Over the next three years potential partners in

different sectors such as higher education, health, social welfare, city councils, government, and client and funding organizations were explored.

In May 2002, about 50 lecturers from different universities, medical doctors, therapists, social workers, representatives at regional and county level, disabled peoples' associations and ENOTHE representatives met over a two-day workshop to discuss the need for occupational therapy in Romania and to find ways to start occupational therapy education at a level compatible with the rest of Europe. The meeting strongly recommended the development of occupational therapy practice and education in Romania in order to enable persons with disabilities and other occupational deprived groups to be self-reliant and agreed a letter stating the importance of occupational therapy in the process of social reform. This was sent to the ministries for education, health, and social affairs.

It was proposed to start a postgraduate course in 'specialization in occupational therapy' for clinicians and lecturers in medicine, psychology, physiotherapy, and social work at the universities at Bacau, Oradea, and Timisoara, where staff already had some knowledge of the profession. The first group of fully trained occupational therapists would become lecturers in occupational therapy in these three universities and (clinical) supervisors in practice.

One of the dilemmas which concerns the development of the profession in a new country is the choice of the appropriate faculty in the appropriate universities. Several options need to be considered, such as whether it is favorable for occupational therapy to be connected with a medical faculty, if this means that it will then be easily recognized and have a high status, or whether instead it will be dominated by the medical model and have less chance to become an autonomous profession? Will it be better off based in a faculty for social sciences or psychology, where a number of subjects offer the potential to share education modules (or curriculum components) with occupational therapy? This will enable it to be developed on a basis of equal standing with these subjects, positioning it to be able to contribute to social reform. Or does occupational therapy need to be developed in the same faculty as physiotherapy under sports and education, or will it be advisable to establish a new faculty in health sciences? What will be then the conditions and requirements for such a faculty? The choice of faculty has consequences for graduate employment chances, for the regulations of the profession and for compatibility with the rest of Europe. This is a serious process of considering political, academic, professional arguments in the local, national, and international contexts and needs time. It may take 10 years before local people can tell if it was the right decision.

During this period much had been described in the media about the living conditions of the disabled in Eastern Europe, particularly in Bulgaria and Romania. Due to this wide publicity measures had been taken mainly concerning disabled and otherwise deprived children under 18. The 'National, Strategy for special protection and social reintegration of disabled in Romania' was set out by the Romanian government. The Bulgarian and Hungarian strategies more or less stress the same issues, and a first step has been taken towards a structural improvement of the position of (young) adult persons with disabilities. Two leading principles of this strategy are the deinstitutionalization and reintegration of persons with disabilities into the community. Subsequently, the overall objective was elaborated in the following sub-objectives:

- Training and employment of persons with disabilities and promoting active participation in society on all levels and in all spheres of daily life, in accordance with EU legislation
- Special attention to the closure of large old-style institutions by developing alternative social services and small scale residential care
- Strengthening of the associations of persons with disabilities
- Establishing a system of community-based services which enables persons with disabilities to live their lives as independently as possible, assisted by a supportive network of qualified people and provisions

The sense of urgency of changes is clearly presented in this National Strategy (RO) and confirmed by experts Het Nederlands Institut voor Zorg en Welzijn (NIZW), final report and National Action Plan, Utrecht/Bucharest, 28 February 2003. The Bulgarian and Romanian national strategies for equal opportunities also discussed the need for adequate education and training of professionals. The question was whether to establish occupational therapy along traditional paths or take risks and identify a responsible and political role centered on the clients.

In the partnership we had found the public sector (different ministries, city councils and different faculties of universities, and the private sector – centers

for rehabilitation, nongovernmental organizations for social inclusion, etc.) had the commitment to solve problems but lacked the answers. But we missed the business sector or funding for establishing occupational therapy. In principle this should not be volunteering work, or a demonstration of charity but occupational therapists, in this case ENOTHE, should fight for the rights of disadvantaged groups and find a strategic moment to apply for a grant and to receive the approval of the national government for a sustainable development of the profession. In 2003, the European Commission and the EU Disability Forum organized the European Year of People with Disabilities to highlight barriers and discrimination faced by disabled people and to improve the lives of those who have a disability. It was about raising awareness of the rights of disabled people to full equality and participation in all areas.

As another important policy issue at this time was the enlargement of Europe through the inclusion of former communist states, this was an excellent opportunity for ENOTHE to ask for a grant to contribute to social reform by establishing occupational therapy education and practice in Romania. Since the policy applied to more than one country we decided to find universities and other stakeholders in Bulgaria and Hungary who might also be interested. Finally an agreement was officially confirmed with 43 partners, consisting of universities, disabled people's organizations, city councils, government and foundations and 'Centers for Rehabilitation and Integration'. In June 2003 the proposed postgraduate program in occupational therapy was approved by the University of Timisoara, and 24 students from Romania, Bulgaria, and Hungary were selected for the academic year 2003/2004.

A group of ENOTHE members developed and implemented the detailed content of the modules in close cooperation with the local universities, clinical and social institutions, and users' associations.

The second phase in the process of partnering is capacity development

Capacity is defined as 'that emergent combination of individual competencies and collective capabilities that enables a human system to create value' (Baser & Morgan 2008, p. 34). The issue of capacity of the project partners including ENOTHE itself is critical and the scale of need is enormous, but appreciation of the problem is low. There is a growing sense that the process of improving abilities and capacities needs systematic thought and action more than the eventual results. Morgan identifies five core capabilities that enable a system to perform and survive. All are necessary, yet none is sufficient by itself (Baser & Morgan 2008):

1. **To commit and engage**: volition, empowerment, motivation, attitude, confidence
2. **To carry out technical, service delivery, and logistical tasks**: core functions directed at the implementation of mandated goals
3. **To relate and attract resources and support**: manage relationships, resource mobilization, networking, legitimacy building, protecting space
4. **To adapt and self-renew**: learning, strategizing, adaptation, repositioning, managing change
5. **To balance coherence and diversity**: encourage innovation and stability, control fragmentation, manage complexity, balance capability mix.

Crucial to capacity development is the energy and the commitment of all partners to engage in a process of change. In the Georgian and Armenian project ENOTHE asked the partners to appoint local project leaders, select appropriate universities that could demonstrate interest in educational and social reform, and select motivated students who could become in the future ambassadors for occupational therapy (point 1).

Implementing education in occupational therapy was not just about service delivery and transferring knowledge and skills. It needed a lot of logistical tasks to bring together students from two neighboring countries who spoke different languages and had different cultural backgrounds and teachers from Western European countries. It took a month merely to arrange transport and prepare the translation of documents for customs (point 2). The need for legitimacy made us seek involvement, support, and approval from other groups, such as clients, local practitioners, and employers in building and executing the program of occupational therapy education (point 3). Furthermore modules were devoted to setting up new projects to meet clients' occupational needs, such as inclusive employment and to apply for grants. At the core of capacity development is the practice, in some form, of learning and adaptation (point 4). Capacity development has to take account of politics and power relations, the process is much about negotiation and accommodation as well as

about 'occupational literacy, that refers to the capacity to make sense of, i.e. read or interpret, human occupations. As a literacy it provides a set of navigation skills which enable the user to explore and make use of contextual factors in order to access occupations of need and choice' (Pollard et al 2008, p. 39). Finally a balance needs to be struck between seeking opportunities for quick wins and keeping an eye on the long term (point 5).

The project in Georgia and Armenia has faced several dilemmas within capacity development. From the beginning when we talked about the foundations of the profession the term occupation has been problematic and still is. Is it wise to use the word occupation in countries which have a history of being occupied by foreign forces? Just a small anecdote from my own experience – Once when I arrived in Armenia and customs asked me 'What is your profession', I answered 'I am an occupational therapist'. The next morning representatives from the Ministry of Defence came to the university to enquire what this 'occupier' was coming to do. After a long conversation with the dean they left. However, the next day they returned, having discovered that this occupier was training occupiers in Europe. And some months later ENOTHE received an email with an offer for military uniforms (Fig. 31.1).

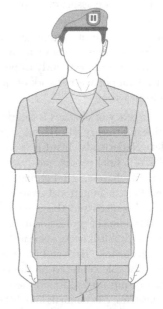

Fig. 31.1 • Uniforms for your occupiers.

So the Armenian occupational therapists have chosen to call themselves ergotherapists, what is the title for the profession in most European countries (ENOTHE 2000). However, the Georgians chose occupational therapy for academic reasons, first, because occupational science underpins the discipline, and, second, to belong to the World Federation and the Council of Occupational Therapists for the European Countries. Recently the president of Georgia stated that Georgia will not be happy until it is no longer occupied and the last invading soldier leaves its territory (Georgian Press 2 April 2009). The term occupational therapy is particularly problematic after the war in August 2008 in Georgia.

The biggest challenge in capacity development is to find ways to resolve the tensions between the focus on results, pressures from standards, grant deadlines, and solutions, and the focus on the more participatory process, collective skills, culture and mindset, and responsiveness to context. The priority is not action and delivery but support and facilitation, and an emphasis on joint learning and partnership through networking.

> As an example of responsiveness to context last August 2008, I received the following email:
>
> > UN agency aid effort tries to link in Georgian volunteers who want to help with the big UN agencies and their activities. So what we need right now is volunteers who are capable in English and/or Russian, obviously Georgian speakers, who can accompany UN teams into the buffer zone around Gori to do assessments. The Georgian volunteers will hopefully be sent out, in teams in their vehicles, into villages in the buffer zone around Gori, to do rapid needs assessments. They will only be going into areas which have been declared safe and will be accompanied by HCR care/ Save the Children/ WFP/ World Vision people.
> > And sorry I have another specific request: I am also looking for volunteers to participate in a psycho-social camp for Internally Displaced Children for two weeks; they need volunteers to work with the kids doing various activities. This will be good experience as well as really worthwhile to help. Maybe some of the students you have been in contact with would be interested?
>
> As temporary head of occupational therapy education I quickly supported the idea but requested the Global Initiative's preparatory course on disaster management and asked the dean's office to provide official academic credits for practicing in these camps, which they agreed to provide.

Last phase of partnering; impact measurement or evaluation

Although the capacity development and sustaining phase is still going on in the different projects, last December 2008 a survey was conducted among students, academics, different client organizations, and employers to receive feedback on the impact of occupational therapy practice and/or education in Georgia and Armenia. Making a systemic impact may not be the immediate task but it should be seen as an indirect but essential outcome. Some reflections from the survey follow:

The founder and first employer of occupational therapists in the Caucasus project said:

> From the very beginning we wanted occupational therapy to facilitate the process of participation and inclusion and as a result many of our children go now to schools, kindergartens and parents have adopted necessary skills and are happy seeing their children more active and integrated.
>
> What really has increased is public awareness and the number of nongovernmental organizations acting in the field of disability. There are also quite clear positive changes in the legislation in respect of definitions, 'equal rights', and 'discrimination'.

Colleagues from Georgia, Armenia, and Bulgaria, who went through the first accelerated bachelor course in occupational therapy stated:

> It was a challenge for me to act as an ambassador of the profession and I found working in a rights-based job most satisfying and being involved in national advocacy of disability issues.
>
> The chief impact of this education is in the reasoning skills that students learn: not to swallow the information until you've not chewed it and to justify thoughts and decisions.
>
> One of the strong aspects was the diversity of the teaching staff and the student group; it was an excellent chance to experience cultural diversity.

Students who are now in the BA course in Armenia see their career in occupational therapy contributing to:

> Promoting public awareness for the recognition of persons with disabilities as equal citizens
>
> To enable people to make decisions
>
> To learn to listen
>
> (Armenian people like to talk)

These kind of projects are intent on providing a strong impetus to set long-term goals and the development of new initiatives throughout a 'wider' Europe.

Conclusion

For an external organization such as ENOTHE it may be useful to summarize what we have come to realize about providing assistance, particularly with respect to capacity development in Eastern and Central European transition countries. We accept that the process of change, both personal and organizational, is mainly a self-generated one; without a strong and committed local team nothing will happen. While 'expert' opinion can obviously be valuable in certain limited technical areas, what matters more is for outsiders to help put in place an open learning environment in which people can sort through and make sense of their own experience. From this perspective, local energy, commitment, and expertise are the critical factors that drive capacity development. But outsiders still can play an important role in facilitating a learning environment that allows participants and stakeholders to build the collaborative and technical skills which the wider community needs. Such partnerships should be seen as a space and an opportunity to create new meaning and engage in collective inquiry rather than simply as a technique to use existing skills or fix old problems.

Organizations such as ENOTHE do not have much to give in the business of development; they have little money, a limited capacity, and can only work in a few places during short periods. These engagements are not going to solve the problems of poverty and exclusion in a country, or conquer problems such as hunger and discrimination. At the best, what we have are experiments in policy that allow us to learn from certain ways of doing practice and to talk to people about new ideas around how to do things better or more efficiently. So, it is the process that is crucial, not the solutions or outcomes, and the recognition of human and occupational rights in combination with poverty-reduction strategies allow us to think about process more intelligently and much more critically. To take on board human and occupational rights raises the bar of developmental practice.

> We have to continue even if it is not always the case that everything goes well. We must face the difficulties and go further, as long as I can see continuous progress. One day we will be really very proud of what we did.
>
> Zaza Kakushadze (initiator of occupational therapy in Caucasus)

References

Baser H, Morgan H: *Capacity, change and performance, study report.* ECDPM Discussion paper 59B Maastricht, 2008.

Böhnke P: *Perceptions of Social Integration and Exclusion in enlarged Europe European Foundation for the Improvement of Living and Working Conditions,* Dublin, Ireland, 2004 European Foundation for the Improvement of Living and Working Conditions.

Bologna Process: *'Realising the European Higher Education Area' Communiqué of the Conference of Ministers responsible for Higher Education,* Berlin, September 2003 Communiqué of the Conference of Ministers responsible for Higher Education.

CDCS: *A New Strategy for Social Cohesion, approved by the Committee of Ministers of the Council of Europe,* Brussels, 2004, Council of Europe workshop.

Commission on Social Determinants of Health (CSDH): *Closing the gap in a generation: health equity through action on the social determinants of health. Final Report of the Commission on Social Determinants of Health,* Geneva, 2008, World Health Organization.

Curtin M, Mollineux M, Supyk-Melsson J: *Occupational Therapy and Physical Dysfunction, Enabling Occupation,* London, 2010, Churchill Livingstone/Elsevier.

Davies R: Founder and Chief Executive of the IBFL, http:thepartneringinitiative. org/what_is_partnering/ When_to_partner_jsp. Accessed July 11, 2010.

ENOTHE: *Occupational Therapy Education in Europe: an Exploration,* Netherlands, 2000, Hogeschool van Amsterdam.

ENOTHE Charter: 2007, Online. Available at: http://www.enothe.hva. nl/org/charter-eng.htm. Accessed July 11, 2010.

ENOTHE Policy Plan: 2008–2011, Online. Available at: http://www. enothe.hva.nl/org/workplan-eng.htm. Accessed July 11, 2010.

European Public Health Programme: *Closing the Gap; Strategies for Action to Tackle Health Inequalities in the EU,* 2004–2007, Online. Available at: http://ec.europa.eu/health/ ph_projects/2003/action3/ action3_2003_15_en.htm. Accessed July 11, 2010.

Heller PS, Keller C: *IMF Working Paper, Social Sector Reform in Transition Countries,* USA, 2001, IMF WP01/35.

International Business Leaders Forum: 2008, Online. Available at: http:// thepartneringinitiative.org/ what_is_partnering/ Partnering_in_Context.jsp. Accessed July 11, 2010.

Matutinović I: Quality of life in transition countries: Central East Europe, *Social Indicators Research* 43:97–119, 1998.

Pollard N, Sakellariou D, Kronenberg F: *Political Practice of Occupational Therapy*, Edinburgh, 2008, Elsevier Science.

Press Office, of the President of Georgia: 2009, Online. Available at: http://www.president.gov.ge/index.php?

lang-id:GEO&SEC id ang_id·ENG Accessed July 11, 2010.

Sen A: *Development as Freedom*, Oxford, 1999, Oxford University Press.

Tennyson R: *Partnering Toolbook*, London, 2003, International Business Leaders Forum.

Wolff P: *Population and Social Conditions Eurostat Statistics in Focus 46/2009*, Luxembourg, 2009, Office for Official Publications of the European Communities.

Empowering learning environments for developing occupational therapy practice in the UK

32

Joan Healey

OVERVIEW

This chapter looks at the potential for learning in voluntary sector placements where students are not supervised on-site by occupational therapists. It draws on the experiences of students on the MSc preregistration occupational therapy course at Sheffield Hallam University. The chapter looks at how the placement environment can be a transformational tool in students' awareness of the potential of our profession rather than a means to define it. Having no professional role models or processes to refer to, students develop their creative, entrepreneurial and leadership skills to open up new possibilities for professional activity. Without the usual hierarchical relationships between service users and statutory service providers, students can forge new relationships with service users and communities that can enrich their understanding of the potential of occupational therapy outside of the borders of government-funded health and social care provision.

Introduction

Historically over the past 40 years occupational therapy students in the United Kingdom have undertaken courses at colleges and universities to prepare them for their future roles within the National Health Service (NHS) and Social Care Services. Governments have commissioned student places to fulfill the needs of the health and social services workforce planning. Occupational therapists in the United Kingdom until very recently have been able to go into secure working environments where their roles and remit have been well defined and their career path mapped ahead for them, supported by secure pay structures and pensions to retire on. This is no longer the case. It is evident to anyone, whether they are an employee of the UK health and social services or a service user that the health and social care community is undergoing the most radical change since its inception in 1945 (Department of Health 2000, 2001, 2005, 2008). The fundamental changes to the way the services are commissioned, delivered, and staffed have implications for everyone. There is no such thing as a secure stable working environment or fixed roles and remits anymore; everything is being questioned. As the hospital-based occupational therapy services become pared down to acute provision and as the government's concepts of health, health promotion, and wellbeing become redefined and retargeted, occupational therapy's traditional sphere of activity is shifting. Occupation may be a concern for some of the acute services but often their focus is on physical function and adaptation. The issues of wellbeing, occupational engagement, and health promotion are being taken up by the voluntary and private sector services whose roles are being expanded each year.

A person qualifying as an occupational therapist in the United Kingdom in the 1970s could apply for a range of posts within the health and social care services which would be theirs for life if they so wished. They could if they wished, expect to be able to stay in the same place doing more or less the same job just updating their knowledge as necessary and adopting new processes as they were developed. They could expect to be able to work with the same sorts of other professions and to expect that their relationships and professional responsibilities would remain the same.

DOI: 10.1016/B978-0-7020-3103-8.00041-9

They could expect a professional supervision and managerial structure to enable them to develop into the experienced and expert roles within a given service.

A person qualifying *today* as an occupational therapist in the United Kingdom can no longer be sure they will find employment in the NHS or social services at all. This trend has been highlighted in UK *OT News* (2007/2008) and several issues have been devoted to exploring new avenues for employment for occupational therapists. If new graduates do secure employment in the NHS or Social Care services they may be part of a flexible work force asked to cover any part of the service according to management needs at any one time. They may be on temporary or short-term contracts or be directly employed by an agency rather than the public body and have little opportunity for supported continuing professional development. They may have little or no professional supervision and be working alone within a multiagency team. They may be asked to market their profession and bid for their post, justifying their input as opposed to that of another professional.

If they cannot find posts within the traditional spheres many newly qualified occupational therapists may go to work for private or voluntary sector organizations in positions that may or may not be referred to as occupational therapy posts but which demand the skills of an occupational therapist nevertheless. There have been many new initiatives for instance in the independent sector for older people for community support workers whose remit is about social engagement and activity with individual older people. In other posts newly qualified staff may be asked to set up occupational therapy services or programs within existing service provision for instance in independent sector provision for adults with learning difficulties where individual budget holding systems are redefining the services. Newly qualified occupational therapists may have to bid for grants and funding to support their posts and new services. They almost certainly will not have any on-site professional supervision if any at all. These posts are often temporary and dependent on funding and may have no career structure attached to them at all.

These are not necessarily negative aspects for our profession and I will look at some of the positive aspects about these changes later in the chapter. What then for occupational therapy education? How does the education and learning that students experience as part of their courses prepare them for the real world environment where roles and power relationships are not fixed but shifting and where the needs of communities are defined by them rather than professional opinion?

As a profession, occupational therapy has never sat comfortably within what has always been a medical-model based service (Wilcock 2004). The history of the development of the profession in the United Kingdom is witness to the ways and means occupational therapists have adapted their ways of working to fit within such a system; the focus on functionality and environmental adaptation of the 1970s and 1980s being the most obvious one (Hocking 2007, Wilcock 2002). Now as the health and social care are changing their focus, occupational therapists are revisiting their occupational roots and capitalizing on the shift in direction to redefine the profession and its roles in these new and changing services.

The challenge for occupational therapy education is to ensure that we give students the opportunity to develop the skills they will need to thrive in this new community and take the profession forward.

Practice placement learning as part of occupational therapy education programs

The UK university-based occupational therapy programs incorporate a range of learning environments – some university based, some practice based and some a variety of project based initiatives which may include community settings. All these environments demand different things from students and promote different aspects of learning. The types of learning in university and the traditional practice education environments are defined and confined by the demands of the curriculum and the practice competencies required for registration by the Health Professions Council in order to ensure the qualified practitioner is fit for practice in the NHS and Social Care. The independent and voluntary sector placement, however, can provide a less constrained learning environment where students can be responsive to local needs in a much less confined context. Such learning environments can have an empowering effect on both students and their practice.

The role of placement learning in an occupational therapy education is pivotal (Healey & Spencer 2008). It is on placement that students have the chance to learn from doing, seeing, experiencing, reflecting, testing out their knowledge and skills, revising the theory they have learnt, developing questions about the theory, and refining their knowledge as it relates to practice. It is here that they engage with professionalism (Bonello 2001). It is also the place that students engage with occupational therapy as it is experienced by service users and where the students have to bring their whole selves to the experience. It is undoubtedly the most challenging and most rewarding part of any occupational therapy education program.

In the usual placements, students are placed with an occupational therapist who is designated their practice placement educator; they have a structured assessment which usually means demonstrating specific competencies at specific levels of the program. The roles of and relationship between educator and student are clearly understood and involve the placement educator providing learning opportunities for the student to be able to experience and 'do' occupational therapy specific tasks and more generic processes involved in health and social care. Usually but not always, it is the placement educator who assesses the student's level of competence at the end of the placement. The university provides support for students on placement usually with one visit to the placement site. Although strenuously denied by many academics involved in placement learning, informal student feedback and my own observations in the field over many years have demonstrated to me that this pattern of placement learning fosters a type of 'apprenticeship' model of learning.

However self-aware and open-minded a placement educator is, students perceive there is an inevitable bias towards expectations which match the educator's own ways of working. Students regularly feedback in placement de-briefs about how important it is to 'fit in' in a department, sometimes to the extreme of being criticized if they choose not to socialize with colleagues during lunch breaks! There is certainly an unofficial culture within organizations which is a powerful dictate of student behavior during placements and as such impacts on the student's ability to express themselves and develop their own learning. From the best possible motives the placement educator often sees it as his or her role to convey as much of their specialized knowledge to the student placed with them as they possibly can in the time given. In many cases placement educators can see it as a two-way exchange of knowledge and can be open to learning from the student and their experience but this is not by any means always the

case and the assessment structures and placement processes do not always foster this at all and indeed they actually be instrumental in impeding this.

This is in no way to undervalue the learning that takes place on traditional placements; they are a vital part of the education and acquisition of professional knowledge, skills and attitudes. However, the environment and culture within which they take place are imbued with notions of hierarchies of knowledge and power, and this cannot but influence and impact the type of learning that can take place there. The student behavior and remit is closely defined by the service provision. The service is closely audited and monitored to ensure that professional practice is of a particular definition and conforms to given protocols. This socialization element of learning is just one aspect of the overall learning experience (emotional learning being another) that university courses tend to overlook.

Practice learning in voluntary sector placements

University occupational therapy programs have been introducing students to voluntary sector placements for many years now. Where they were largely seen as a solution to placement shortages in the early 1990s, their modernizing influence on the profession was also acknowledged (Alsop & Donald 1996, Fisher & Savin-Baden 2002a, b, Friedland et al 2001, Huddleston 1999a, b). They have recently become much more mainstream in programs throughout the UK – either for whole cohorts of students or as options for specific students and their unique learning opportunities and their role in modernizing the profession are much more widely acknowledged (Thew et al 2008, Wood 2005). They have been part of occupational therapy courses in many other countries for instance the University of Alberta, Canada have included 'Independent community placements' as part of their courses for many years (Mulholland & Derdall 2005). Similarly other professions in the UK such as social work and nursing are developing placements in the voluntary sector (Butler 2007, Hunt 2007). They are not new and they are not profession specific to occupational therapy.

The MSc preregistration occupational therapy program at Sheffield Hallam which began in 2006 has one voluntary sector practice experience designed into it. The students go out in pairs on a

13 week part-time placement at the start of their second year. It follows two earlier practice experiences in the more traditional areas of statutory health and social care services. This practice experience has been a central part of the design of the course which aims to prepare students for employment in a changing community environment. It complements and adds to the experience in the more usual health and social care placements. What are the differences in learning that students may expect to experience in these placements?

The first and most obvious difference in the learning environment is the absence of an occupational therapy role model, educator on the placement and this can be one of the issues which occupational therapy students are most wary about to begin with. The other side to this is that students are exposed to a range of different role models and 'educators' who will be involved in their learning – most important arguably being the service user, whose participation in the service is on a completely different basis from that of service users within most NHS or Social Services provision. The usual hierarchies of the statutory service placements are not the same in this sector; there may well be hierarchies between service users, paid workers, and volunteers but they will not be the same as within the health service for example, where title and uniforms delineate the status of individual professions and students have to conform to strict boundaries of behavior and role. The organizations and management of the voluntary sector services involve very different systems of accountability to funding bodies and service users and these in turn impact working relationships.

The student/educator roles and responsibilities are negotiated rather than prescribed in this learning environment and this gives the students the chance to try to define their own roles within the needs of developing services. The placement provider service's lack of in-depth knowledge of occupational therapy as a profession can actually be helpful in that it again opens the possibilities of creativity and innovation for the student on placement. The students are free to use their occupational therapy knowledge and outlook in new and individual ways that are appropriate to the needs of the service users. On a day-to-day level students are required to make decisions and discuss them with their on-site supervisors, taking the lead rather than following their practice educator's example as is usually the case. The set procedures do not exist; the students have to develop these for themselves in conjunction with the service

users and service providers, developing their own learning objectives in a more autonomous way than is possible in usual placement (Bossers et al 2002). These new ways of working encourage the student's self-confidence and self-belief (Griffiths 2003). Instead of receiving wisdom from an expert practitioner, they are exploring the whole concepts of our professional knowledge for themselves.

In the private sector entrepreneurship is encouraged as students have to question where the occupational therapy input can be most usefully applied. In all these areas funding and financial considerations are bound to be paramount. Students have to consider how an intervention can be funded, if it is going to be supported by financial backers, and if it is going to be financially viable where funding is a priority issue. In this way they start to learn basic project management skills (Fortune et al 2006). This aspect of planning is one which is often missing in the more statutory services where the financial aspects of service provision are taken on a much grander scale and by occupational therapy managers who then decide the types of interventions available.

Integrating learning: the role of supervision and support

All the above sounds laudable in promoting the development of professional skills in our students but it can also sound very daunting to a second-year student. One of the most important aspects of creating these learning environments is about supporting the students in developing the skills to process their learning. Reflective practice (Higgs & Titchen 2001) (see Chapter 8) is always one of the core metacognitive skills to developing and integrating practice-based learning and it takes on even more of an important role in this type of placement. Reflective practice is something that students most often develop in placement learning during the process of supervision with their practice educator. Not having an occupational therapist on-site to reflect on the day's/week's events can be a disadvantage and there are a variety of ways in which universities address this – by providing 'long-arm' supervision by occupational therapists working in related services or by university placement tutors providing individual and/or group supervision. This latter approach was used by us in supporting the MSc preregistration students on their voluntary sector placement in 2007. The experience of facilitating these group supervision sessions was an exciting and sometimes daunting one. These sessions encouraged the students to share their experiences and open themselves up to challenge from their peers, to bring ideas, successes and failures, analysis, and support. During these sessions we explored some fundamental issues around occupational engagement with groups of people who have been marginalized from mainstream society. The usual fallback of one's role in a statutory service was not there to 'encourage' the service user to participate.

Participation was a key theme that students in each service brought up. What they realized was that from the very first stage of contact they had to work from the service user and their needs, rather than from accepted occupational therapy practice or an occupational therapy process, and it led to much more of a focus on empowerment and social engagement. This involved a lot of creative thinking particularly where the client group was not fixed and where no one knew from day to day who would turn up to the service and what they would want to do. The skills the students have learnt from thinking this through and using an action learning style approach were shared across the group and will be useful wherever they choose to work in the future. This process was mirrored in the group reflective supervision sessions where as facilitators we had to think on our feet as new issues arose each week and where tried and tested solutions did not exist. The relationship between tutor and student, theory and practice, became more fluid as the group explored avenues and challenged each other in the process.

Whichever way supervision and reflective practice are done, developing the student's ability to make sense of and process their learning is even more critical in this environment. The task is to bring together learning from a variety of environments and domains and make professional sense of it and in this case it may mean bringing a much wider base of learning and integrating the approach or values of other professional and nonprofessional sources, particularly those from social and community work. In doing this it may well be that previously accepted parts of professional knowledge are challenged and critical thinking about the role of occupational therapy becomes central. As an occupational therapist and an educator this is perhaps one of the most exciting aspects of this type of placement learning – that it has the power to help transform the profession itself by opening up the perspectives we have of ourselves and our communities (Higgs et al 2004).

Communication skills, team working, and interprofessional working are all required in any placement an occupational therapy student undertakes. In the nonstatutory environment, without the hierarchical confines of prescribed behavior the student has the chance to develop these skills in more relaxed and open ways: the placement can be empowering for the student and their learning. This very freedom, however, can be a challenge to some students who prefer more structured environments. If occupational therapy courses can embrace diversity and encourage students to challenge orthodoxy in a positively critical way, then placements in the nonstatutory sector may not be seen as so threatening but rather as part of that wider possible practice zone for our profession.

Finally one of the most important aspects of student learning on these type of placements is that students are exposed to their own communities, are encouraged to play a part in their own communities and establish a relationship between themselves and the community that are not based on rank and title or legal requirements of services. In this way these placements can contribute to personal and social development of our students and the way they see themselves in relation to the people they are working alongside.

Kit Sinclair then President of the World Federation of Occupational Therapists in that organization's 2006/2008 biannual report declared that: 'Fundamental issues facing healthcare professionals and occupational therapists are based in human rights and participatory involvement in occupation and development for clients (and people everywhere)'. This type of learning environment encourages these issues to be addressed by our occupational therapists of the future.

To finish I would like to share some of our experience here at Sheffield Hallam University. The first cohort of our MSc preregistration occupational therapy students went out on placements in a variety of settings including a city farm, and a city center project for homeless people. Their feedback shortly after the experience and at the end of the course was very thought provoking. There is no doubt that they found the experience a great challenge. As students they had only completed one year of the occupational therapy program and they were plunged into environments where they were the only occupational therapy presence and were expected to engage with the service users and design and implement an occupation-based intervention with them.

Here are some notes from one student when after she finished the course, talking about her experience on the city farm where she worked with a group of people with learning difficulties. The student sums up what can be the most important, empowering and transformational nature of learning on these placements:

> So much scope and potential, no hierarchy . . . back down to earth working with people not uniforms, black pen, bleeps or titles.

> I was sadder to leave on my last day there than any other placement. It was a whole different way of working. People are there with passion and fire and belief in the organization. No matter whether they understood what an OT was, they were up for positive action! If they had offered me a job I would never have left.

Identifying some of the ways in which she learnt to work, the student went on to list the following advice for students going into these community-based placements:

> Good for confidence, bit wary but go for it, be creative, imaginative, beg steal or borrow, self-direct, self-manage . . .

> So much scope and potential, utilize the community; great group work, use every opportunity you can grasp; free-spirited and fun; fresh air and the natural environment. Working with people with learning disabilities, helping people to enjoy their lives more. Fun, banter, rapport in a more real setting; enabling fun!

I have never read such enthusiastic and inspiring feedback from a placement before.

Empowering learning environments to empower the profession

In the early sections of this chapter I described a health and social care service in flux and discussed the role of our profession within that. I think it is obvious that moves out to the voluntary and private sector may allow us to become the occupational therapists we have always wanted to be. It is up to us to ensure that the occupational therapists of the future have the skills and awareness to thrive in this climate so that our professional skills are available to everyone in the community and not just those referred through the health and social services. New practice experiences in the voluntary and independent sector enable our emerging new professional occupational therapists to develop different skills: a sense of self-efficacy; creative thinking and action; social responsibility; entrepreneurship; negotiation and project management to name but a few. These are the skills they will need not just to meet the challenge of the rapidly changing face of health and social care in the United Kingdom and across the world, but to be able to shape and influence them alongside the service user.

References

Alsop A, Donald M: Taking stock and taking changes: creating new opportunities for fieldwork education, *British Journal of Occupational Therapy* 59:498–502, 1996.

Bonello M: Fieldwork within the context of higher education: a literature review, *British Journal of Occupational Therapy* 64:93–99, 2001.

Bossers A, Miller L, Polatajko H, Hartley M: *Competency Based Fieldwork Evaluation for Occupational Therapists*, Albany, 2002, Delmar.

Butler A: Students and refugees together: towards a model of practice learning as service provision, *Social Work Education* 26:233–246, 2007.

Department of Health: *The NHS Plan*, 2000, Online. Available at:http://www.dh.gov.uk/en/Publicationsandstatistics/Publications/PublicationsPolicyAndGuidance/DH_4010198. Accessed August 2009.

Department of Health: *Shifting the Balance of Power in NHS*, 2001, Speech by the Rt Hon Alan Milburn MP, Secretary State for Health, 25 April 2001. Online. Available at: http://www.dh.gov.uk/en/News/Speeches/Speecheslist/DH_4000938. Accessed August 2009.

Department of Health: *Independence, Wellbeing and Choice: Our Vision of the Future of Social Care for Adults in England*, 2005, Online. Available at: http://www.dh.gov.uk/en/

Publicationsandstatistics/Publications/PublicationsPolicyAndGuidance/DH_4106477. Accessed August 2009.

Department of Health: *High Quality Care For All*, 2008. Online. Available at: http://www.ournhs.nhs.uk/?page_id=915. Accessed August 2009.

Fisher A, Savin-Baden M: Modernising fieldwork, part 1: realising the potential, *British Journal of Occupational Therapy* 65:229–236, 2002a.

Fisher A, Savin-Baden M: Modernising fieldwork, part 2: realising the new agenda, *British Journal of Occupational Therapy* 65:275–282, 2002b.

Fortune T, Farnworth T, McKinstry C: Project-focussed fieldwork: core business or fieldwork fillers?

Australian Occupational Therapy Journal 53.233–238, 2006.

Friedland J, Polatajko H, Gage M: Expanding the boundaries of occupational therapy practice through student field-work experiences: description of a provisionally-funded community funded community development project, *Can J Occup Ther* 68:301–307, 2001.

Griffiths S: *Teaching and Learning in Small Groups. A Handbook for Teaching and Learning in Higher Education*, London, 2003, Kogan Paul.

Healey J, Spencer M: *Surviving Your Placement in Health and Social Care: A Student Handbook*, Maidenhead, 2008, Open University.

Higgs J, Titchen A: *Practice Knowledge and Expertise in the Health Professions*, Boston, 2001, Butterworth -Heinemann.

Higgs J, Richardson B, Dahlgren MA: *Developing Practice Knowledge for*

Health Professionals, London 2004, Butterworth-Heinemann.

Hocking C: Early perspectives of patients, practice and the profession, *British Journal of Occupational Therapy* 70:284–291, 2007.

Huddleston R: Clinical placements for the professions allied to medicine, part 1: a summary, *British Journal of Occupational Therapy* 62:213–219, 1999a.

Huddleston R: Clinical placements for the professions allied to medicine, part 2: placement shortages? Two models that can solve the problem, *British Journal of Occupational Therapy* 62:295–298, 1999b.

Hunt R: Service learning: an eye-opening experience that provokes emotion and challenges stereotypes, *J Nurs Educ* 46:277–281, 2007.

Mulholland S, Derdall M: A strategy for supervising occupational therapy

students at community sites, *Occup Ther Int* 12:28–43, 2005.

Thew M, Hargreaves A, Cronin-Davis J: An Evaluation of a Role-Emerging Practice Placement Model for a Full Cohort of Occupational Therapy Students, *British Journal of Occupational Therapy* 75:348–356.

Wilcock A: *A Journey from Prescription to Self-Health*, London, 2002, British Association and College of Occupational Therapists.

Wilcock A: 2004 CAOT Conference Keynote Address, *Can J Occup Ther* 72:5–12, 2005.

Wood A: Student practice context: changing face, changing place, *British Journal of Occupational Therapy* 68:375–378, 2005.

World Federation of Occupational Therapists Bi Annual Report: 2008, Online. Available at: http://www.wfot.org/office_files/Bi-Annual%20Report_06_08%20final.pdf. Accessed August 2009.

Nature of political reasoning as a foundation for engagement

33

Jo-Celéne De Jongh   Farhana Firfirey   Lucia Hess-April
Elelwani Ramugondo   Neeltjé Smit   Lana Van Niekerk

Overview

Political reasoning as a concept has been a topic of discussion, yet, its application has not been fully explored in occupational therapy to date. This is particularly so with regards to occupational therapy education. As educators we often expect students to grasp the significance of this concept in practice, without having experienced the process ourselves. This chapter reports on a collaborative process in which we, occupational therapy educators from three universities in the Western Cape, South Africa, reflected on our collective experience of political reasoning. It will elucidate how explicit acknowledgment of power issues is central to engagement with the purpose of meaningful collaboration in practice.

Introduction

The process of engagement pervades every human experience; it is about exploring and holding vulnerability, about power issues and what happens when these are not acknowledged. The process involves making explicit the relationship that one has to build in order to engage.

Description (history) of the three universities

Historically, due to apartheid, education policy in South Africa was created to implement and maintain racially divided higher education institutions, with different institutions for each racial group namely blacks, coloreds, Indians, and whites. To this end current universities in South Africa are often categorized as historically white universities (HWU) or historically black universities (HBU). For example, the Universities of the Western Cape, Cape Town and Stellenbosch were created for colored, English-speaking, and Afrikaans-speaking students respectively.

Stellenbosch University

Stellenbosch is the oldest town in South Africa and played an important role in the history of education in South Africa, which is linked with the founding of the Dutch Reformed Church in 1685. The church initiated school instruction and by the 1840s Stellenbosch was recognized as a regional center with a further development of the forming of the Theological Seminary of the Dutch Reformed Church in 1859. After several name changes and passing of the Education Act of 1866, and Higher Education Act of 1874, the Arts Department was formed and received its charter as a College in 1881. The name was changed to the Victoria College of Stellenbosch in 1887. The University Act saw to the transformation of this institution from college to Stellenbosch University in 1916. During the Apartheid era, Stellenbosch University only admitted white Afrikaans-speaking students. The first student of color was only admitted around 1976 (Stellenbosch University 2009a).

The Faculty of Health Sciences (formerly Medicine) was established in 1956 and in 1961 the first group of occupational therapy students

© 2011, Elsevier Ltd.
DOI: 10.1016/B978-0-7020-3103-8.00042-0

was admitted to Stellenbosch University – the first allied healthcare training in the Faculty of Health Sciences. The introduction of this program was sponsored by the National Council for the Care of Cripples and Cape Province Hospital Services (Shipham 2010). Stellenbosch University has always been regarded as a university with strong traditions and excellent training and still attracts many applications, to the extent that only approximately 14% of applicants can annually be admitted to the occupational therapy program. A stratified admission policy is implemented for applicants from diverse backgrounds. The rector of Stellenbosch University, Professor Russel Botman during his speech in 2008, emphasized the importance to accelerate diversity of academic staff and students and reported that 31.3% of the total student population comprised black, colored, and Indian students (Botman 2008, P. 3). Although this number is higher in the Faculty of Health Sciences (47.3%) (Stellenbosch University 2009b) it is significantly lower in occupational therapy (Table 33.1) and recruiting students from a diverse background remains a challenge and priority. No lectures are presented to the students on political reasoning, but students are gradually exposed to different practice settings in communities from their first year. In their fourth year students are expected to take responsibility for a community based service delivery project, providing opportunity for experiential learning and service delivery.

University of the Western Cape

The University of the Western Cape (UWC) has a history of creative struggle against oppression, discrimination, and disadvantage. Among academic institutions it has been in the vanguard of South Africa's historic change, playing a distinctive

academic role in helping to build an equitable and dynamic nation. The university's key concerns with access, equity, and quality in higher education arise from extensive practical engagement in helping the historically marginalized participate fully in the life of the nation.

In 1959, Parliament adopted legislation establishing the university as a constituent college of the University of South Africa for people classified as 'colored'. The first group of 166 students enrolled in 1960. In 1970 the institution gained university status and was able to award its own degrees and diplomas. Protest action by students and black academic staff led to the appointment, in 1975, of the first black rector. In the mission statement of 1982, the university formally rejected the apartheid ideology on which it was established, adopting a declaration of nonracialism, and 'a firm commitment to the development of the Third World communities in South Africa'. In 1983 the university finally gained its autonomy on the same terms as the established 'white' institutions. One of UWC's primary concerns for the future is to use its mandate to create and maintain a sense of hope for the nation while helping to build an equitable and dynamic society (UWC n.d.).

The Department of Occupational Therapy focuses on community-based education and community-based rehabilitation. A strength of the department is that students are representative of diverse cultures. In 2007, UWC final-year students started to engage with political dimensions of human occupation and occupational therapy to critically explore how occupational therapy can be a more relevant resource.

University of Cape Town

Along with three other universities, the University of Cape Town (UCT) can be classified as an HWU for English speaking students. Its formation stems

Table 33.1 Permanent academic appointments and undergraduate student numbers for 2008

	Permanent academics					Undergraduate students				
	Total	Black	Colored	Indian	White	Total	Black	Colored	Indian	White
University of the Western Cape	8	0	4	1	3	126	27	74	13	12
University of Cape Town	7	1	2	1	3	193	16	28	12	137
Stellenbosch University	9	0	1	1	7	127	2	9	1	115

from the upgrading of one of the eight colleges established under British colonial rule in the 1800s. In 1918, the South African college became the University of Cape Town, while one other college became the University of Stellenbosch (De la Rey 1999). While there is some indication that 'nonwhite' students may have been admitted into UCT when it was still a college, there are no records specifying either their first enrollment or the numbers of such students (Ritchie 1918). It must be mentioned here that although 'nonwhite' appears to have been the preferred term used for people other than white during those days, until recently 'black' at the UCT referred to African, Indian, and colored people. It appears that along with the University of the Witwatersrand, UCT chose a more liberal approach to the admission of black students, compared with other HWUs. These two universities were thus regarded 'open' universities. De la Rey (1999) however argues that the term 'open' is misleading given that racial integration at those universities did not extend beyond the classroom. Student residences, sport, and recreation remained segregated. When the apartheid government began to enforce racial segregation across levels of education in 1959, UCT was one of the institutions opposed to it. In open defiance of the policy, UCT increasingly enrolled black students from a proportion of less than 10% of the student body in the 1970s, to over a third in 1993 (Luescher 2009). Over the years, this number increased to the point that in 2005 the overall student body was 50–50 black and white (University of Cape Town, 2005). While the general student body at UCT can be regarded as diverse, the same cannot be said about those students who register to study occupational therapy. Efforts to recruit students across all racial lines, with specific attention to black students, have not yet yielded the desired outcome, except at postgraduate level. While the commitment to recruit a diverse student body at the undergraduate level continues, the occupational therapy program at UCT has made significant gains in transforming the curriculum. Students are placed in diverse fieldwork settings where they have an opportunity to engage with marginalized groups, and are guided in confronting and unraveling various forms of oppression and occupational injustice.

Table 33.1 illustrates the permanent academic appointments and undergraduate student numbers for the three universities for 2008.

Background to this collaboration

Lecturers from the three universities have had good relationships, yet, never found ways to make real collaboration possible. Logistic and practical difficulties make collaborative projects difficult, even though most lecturers in the three universities have shown an openness to collaboration over the years, believing that this would yield a positive outcome. A recent example of collaboration between social work and occupational therapy from UWC and psychology from Stellenbosch University is an indication that logistical and practical difficulties are not insurmountable (Rohleder et al 2008).

The existing dynamics between the universities have never been fully explored or understood. The current project was the first time we jointly engaged in such a way as to explore issues of conflict and cooperation as described by Van der Eijk (Kronenberg & Pollard 2005). When the process started, with the purpose of the chapter being to explore an educational framework for political reasoning, some authors participated in a mandated capacity. This changed when the writing process required sharing of a more personal nature. As authors we acknowledge that we have a long way to go towards fostering a 'political practice orientation' in each of our programs.

The process

The process we followed unfolded in ways that we did not plan upfront. It evolved in a manner that we now believe mirrors the essence of political reasoning as it applies to occupational engagement. What follows is a description of this process from which themes emerged, that will be discussed later.

During our initial meetings, we immediately launched into the intellectual aspects of writing a chapter such as this, in other words, we took a safe route. This purely academic endeavor meant our personal experiences and perspectives initially were not acknowledged. Given all this, it was therefore not surprising that feedback from the editors, as well as from colleagues, challenged us to engage more authentically. A pivotal point had been reached, we needed to take stock and revisit our own points of conflict and cooperation. Our discussions were emotionally charged, honest and energizing, characterized by candid expressions that yielded new insights. How we all confronted each other and ourselves became a valuable part of what we are offering here. We were then confronted with the task of distilling a coherent chapter from this engagement. We individually took time to reflect on the process in writing. These reflections were shared and analyzed, yielding the content that is shared here.

The process of reflection comprised the following:

1. Acknowledging the history of involvement UWC/UCT/Stellenbosch University have in regard to offering a socially responsive occupational therapy curriculum
2. Exploring what place political reasoning has in our respective curricula, if at all
3. Acknowledging occupational therapy education's origins in apartheid South Africa where universities were segregated and curricula were controlled by professional boards who, through inaction, perpetuated apartheid policies. This thinking is in line with Duncan (1999) and Watson (2008)
4. Identifying the obstacles or opportunities this history presented, for example, consideration of the impact of injustice on the health of people and the skills people need to take charge of their lives
5. Acknowledging that, historically, occupation was not seen as a political issue in South Africa and as a result occupational therapy education did not foster this understanding in graduates
6. Recognizing the diverse nature of our students and enhancing our understanding of who they are
7. Identifying where and how our curricula could be better aligned with our country's needs
8. Exploring skills that graduates would need to successfully address these needs
9. Beginning to define the skills and attributes of educators in our context
10. Acknowledging our vulnerability in dealing with these issues and our 'not knowing' how to better prepare our students for political practice.

Themes that emerged

Reflections on the process were done both individually and collectively. They were then analyzed through content analysis and resulted in the following themes.

Not having the answers – what did we miss?

This theme captures a strong sense, shared by all, that when we embarked on the process of writing this chapter, we did not know what it would entail. We doubted that we had the necessary resources to produce a meaningful chapter that tackled issues related to political reasoning adequately. This is depicted in the following quotes:

> Knowing the involved nature of tackling the topic chosen for this chapter, I had a sense that the process would not be easy. I had no idea though on how it would unfold.

> The process that was followed turned out to be the opposite to which I usually approach a similar task. I would normally gain all the possible background information to provide a context and understanding of the content matter, and after 'setting the scene' I would zoom in to the specifics of the differences/examples, backed by literature. I asked for references on 'political reasoning', but the group decided to write first and then go back to the theories.

Anxiety – is this process going to be okay for us – are we going to be okay in the end?

We did not have previous examples of working together on a similar project successfully. Furthermore the topic of political reasoning itself brought forth discomforts linked to having lived through apartheid and continuing to experience its legacy. The individual differences we brought into the group are peppered with political nuance that we knew would emerge if we were to truly engage.

> This was a major source of anxiety (still is). Previous experiences of writing always involved reporting on literature published or on the experiences of other people (captured through data collection, then analyzed). This time the content felt personal – an active process of constructing the answer to questions that involved me and the group of people I was to write with.

> I became intensely aware of my own ignorance, other persons' convictions and insights and I felt inadequate to contribute anything, because I was truly in an unknown world.

> I remember feeling apprehensive and choosing to immediately distance myself as much as possible from the process – meaning the actual process of getting to a point where all these three departments agreed to the writing.

Experience of vulnerability: safety as a trap

This theme captures two major aspects of our experience. The first was a heightened sense of vulnerability that led to us finding safety in taking an academic approach. We came to understand that our vulnerability was linked to a realization, at some level, that in order to participate, we would have to draw on our personal experiences. The second was a recognition that we were not ready to confront what was real for us.

> The focus (of the first draft) was very academic (maybe this was a safe and easy way for everyone to do it) using different examples from the three universities.

> The truth is that I initially felt much more anxious than with other publications I did. This one seemed more personal and I felt I did not have the answer to the question . . .

> I could see ourselves immediately get bogged down with the intellectual aspects of writing a chapter such as this. I must say that I started feeling quite safe.

> Reflections scare me because I really have to look into myself and then say what is inside me, which I feel could come back to haunt me. I therefore tend to be careful with what I write and say, and over think things at times which makes me lose the plot in the process.

Commitment to honesty – building trust

This theme captures our deepening understanding of the level of honesty required to build real engagement that instills trust. Bringing the personal into the conversation was key to this.

> This experience deepened my understanding that as occupational therapy educators we ourselves have to overcome certain obstacles to our occupational potential as educators, of which personal ones seem to be the most important.

> Because I was not 'politically oriented' I felt exposed and constantly had to reflect on my own feelings.

> Hmmm . . . meaningfully connect. I connected with the material in a small way, but in no way was I connected with the authors. As I said, I felt like a student and Lucia and J-C were my lecturers and Elelwani was my 4th yr external examiner.

Journey of finding our voices

Finding our voices was a difficult and important journey for us, as shown in the following quotes:

> This whole process has been a lovely learning experience for me. I was looking forward to working with new people, but this also brought to the fore a feeling of 'don't say something silly, this is an important chapter.'

> The 'finding our voice' journey is taking time in this project. Maybe because the need to do it was not explicitly acknowledged at the onset – maybe because this is just the way it works – maybe because I tried to influence the process away from this type of journey.

> We would not have succeeded in finding our voice if we were not challenged by colleagues, the editors of this book, and ourselves. We now also recognize that writing our reflections was a crucial step in finding our personal voices. The honesty of individuals in the group, gave others the encouragement to do the same.

> My feeling was that although the debate became a bit warm under the collar for some, one should still be sensitive towards different opinions and find ways to deal with it. Is this not what we want our students to do too? Just the fact that one of us admitted that they do not implement political reasoning and questioned whether she should still be part of the process, I felt this took a lot of guts admitting it. This is why being part of this process is so important for all of us.

> I sat here and reflected on honesty and wondered what the difference is between honesty and trust. I thought political reasoning has something to do with both these concepts . . . because I can be very honest with a group of people without sharing any vulnerability – so where is that then, at what level? For me it is the foundation. I think we kind of realized that there is a foundation level for engagement and that foundation for engagement is the relationship that you have to build in order to be able to engage and for me these things are about that . . . its not just the academic project or the teaching project or any of those, so for me it was about when do you have a true collaboration? Such a collaboration can only be when you no longer have separate entities at the table.

Zooming in on the differences

This theme reflects the value and benefit of first acknowledging and then exploring the differences and dynamics between the universities that we knew existed. This includes individual histories, educational foci and approaches, and political orientations.

> The existing dynamics between the universities (that I have never fully explored/considered/understood – but that I know exist) made me feel that I would need to be careful. I felt the relationship that we would rely on to

work on the article as 'not yet consolidated' – I don't want to use words tenuous or precarious – relationships that exist seem stronger than this, but I did not have previous examples of working together on a similar project (successfully) to build anticipation of success on. I felt I should be careful not to overplay our institution's position because of my assumption that our institution has (at times) been seen to be operating from a 'know it all' position.

Participating in this project forced me to consider the reasons why three universities have not worked closer together. This is something that I found curious when I initially started to work in the Western Cape Province. However, I became desensitized over time and took it as the way things are. New reflection on the matter confirmed for me that our situation is not natural – it would have made sense to work much closer together and therefore the reasons for not doing so are deeper than generally recognized.

My own process of dealing with whiteness in relation to politics – this has been a point of vulnerability for a long time. At a personal level, I worried that as an OT and as a white person I lacked significant insights into the subject and that I certainly did not have anything new or specific to contribute.

Maybe from a racial perspective we come in with a particular position. When you said that black people are more politically astute … it made me think 'is that really true?' because one can also come in, being black and arrogant about one's racial credibility.

The question 'why are you doing what you are doing'? is key, I mean … is it culture or is it politics? … I don't think it is based on 'political', its based on my cultural insecurities.

Discussion

Kronenberg & Pollard (2006) highlight the fact that meaningful engagement requires truthful interchange between actors that have allowed for the dialectical triangle of the personal professional and political to inform the conversation. This then becomes a resource for working with communities.

> The basis for 'good practice' in occupational therapy is the possibility for all the actors involved to meaningfully connect with one another, a process akin to conversations that allow people with different views of a topic to learn from each other. The actors are invited to engage in '3P archaeology' – an honest conversation with one's self – which explores interrelated personal, professional and political perspectives of whom one is (to be) and what one is (to) do.
>
> Based on a workshop presented by Kronenberg (2007)

The process we went through mirrors what Kronenberg and Pollard refer to in the above. Our honest uncovering of the conflicts and cooperations while holding onto our collective vulnerabilities meant that we moved from being superficial to a deeper level of engagement. This gave us the foundation on which we could build our still unfolding relationship. This process led to our separate entities dissolving, ultimately resulting in a true collaboration.

Kronenberg & Pollard (2006) also critique the occupational therapists' tendency to ask what they can gain from their occupational therapy practice rather than to ask what it is they are willing to give up. As authors coming from institutions of higher learning where intellect is revered, the hardest aspect for ourselves to let go of in this process was taking an academic approach. This meant that we had to give up our positions of power. We struggled with having to attend to the personal and make this a key part of this endeavor. Discussion of these issues highlighted the fact that we all have power sources and all have vulnerabilities and that these, in fact, are not very different.

The realizations taken from our process of engagement gave us an actual experience of how conceptual frameworks applied in practice. It illuminated the interrelatedness between concepts of power, politics and relationships; power is within politics and politics is unavoidably in each and every engagement.

The next step for us would be to ensure that this engagement continues. We have laid the foundation for a unity of understanding about shared educational and/or professional goals and a willingness to take risks together. We arrived at the understanding that political engagement is about being forced by circumstances and taking up the challenge to collaborate where energy goes into explicating the issues of power and privilege that impact on the layers of people involved in making the project happen.

Conclusion

Often we fall into the trap of needing step-by-step guidelines to address issues surfacing when we are working with people and communities. Incorporating political reasoning into occupational therapy education does not mean incorporating concrete recipes in a 'how to do it' manual for our students. As facilitators of political reasoning we should ensure that political education is not situated within separate courses as it may undermine its importance. Beyond transmitting knowledge, politics in occupational therapy practice should first and foremost focus on exploring and changing attitudes, and increasing awareness of personal biases that we hold. We hope that sharing what we went through will illuminate the dynamic process involved in collaboration and political engagement. We believe that students will understand political reasoning and what it entails through real experiences and reflecting on that experience. Educators can set examples by being open, honest, and authentic in sharing reflections of their own experiences of conflict and cooperation with their students. The role of educators is therefore to facilitate similar opportunities for students.

References

Botman R: *Stellenbosch University Reports: Report of the Rector and Vice-Chancellor*, Stellenbosch, 2008, Stellenbosch University. Online. Available at: http://www.sun.ac.za/university/jaarverslag/verslag2008/pdfs/eng/report_rector.pdf. Accessed August 20, 2009.

De la Rey C: *Career narratives of women professors in South Africa*, Cape Town, 1999, University of Cape Town.

Duncan EM: Our bit in the calabash, *South African Journal of Occupational Therapy* 29:3–9, 1999.

Kronenberg F: *OTWB II Orientation Workshop Session 'Education Without Borders'*, 29 November, 2007, UWC, UCT and Stellenbosch University.

Kronenberg F, Pollard N: Overcoming occupational apartheid. A preliminary exploration of the political nature of occupational therapy. In Kronenberg F, Simó Algado S, Pollard N, editors: *Occupational Therapy Without Borders: Learning Through the Spirit of Survivors*, Edinburgh, 2005, Elsevier/Churchill Livingstone, pp 58–86.

Kronenberg F, Pollard N: Political dimensions of occupation and the roles of occupational therapy, *Am J Occup Ther* 60:617–625, 2006.

Luescher TM: Racial desegregation and the institutionalisation of 'race' in university governance: The case of UCT, *Perspectives in Education* 27:415–425, 2009.

Luescher TM: Student governance in transition: university democratisation and managerialism. A governance approach to the study of student politics and the case of the University of Cape Town, Phd dissertation, Cape Town, 2008.

Ritchie W: *The History of the SA College: 1829–1918* (2 volumes), Maskow Miller, 1918, Cape Town.

Rohleder P, Swartz L, Bozalek V, Carolissen R, Leibowitz B: Community, self and identity: participatory action research and the creation of a virtual community across two South African universities, *Teaching in Higher Education* 13:131–143, 2008.

Shipham E: Reunion of Occupational Therapy at Stellenbosch University, e-mail to N Smit [online], 11 June 2010. Available estellesh@webmail.co.2a.

Stellenbosch University: *Some Historical Notes: A University in the Making*, n.d. Online. Available at:a http://www.sun.ac.za/university/history/history.htm. Accessed August 20, 2009a.

Stellenbosch University Statistical Profile, n.d., Online Available at: http://www.sun.ac.za/university/Statistieke/statseng.html. Accessed August 20, 2009b.

University of Cape Town, *Annual Report*, 2005, Cape Town.

University of the Western Cape: *History*, n.d., Online. Available at: http://www.uwc.ac.za/index.php?module=cms&action=showfulltext&id=gen11Srv7Nme54_8987_1210050562&menustate=about Accessed May 1, 2010.

Watson RM: South African occupational therapy values: 1997 submission to the truth and reconciliation commission, *South African Journal of Occupational Therapy* 39:18–22, 2008.

Research, community-based projects, and teaching as a sharing construction: the Metuia Project in Brazil

34

Denise Dias Barros   Roseli Esquerdo Lopes
Sandra Maria Galheigo   Débora Galvani

OVERVIEW

This chapter aims to present the work being done by the Metuia Project, developed by occupational therapy lecturers in two universities in the state of São Paulo, Brazil for the past 10 years. Through the research, teaching, and development of occupational therapy practices, Project Metuia works on the theoretical basis of the elaboration of occupational therapy programs into the social field. The chapter presents Metuia's principles and objectives and illustrates how teaching, research, and practices have been developed in an intertwined way and describes how Metuia has moved forward from its early strategies of constructing a field to the point of seeking a different quality of reflexivity. Metuia's current work is leading to the diversification and deepening of research themes.

Introduction

The Metuia Project developed from a particular social and political context, within which occupational therapists in Brazil began to develop open-setting initiatives such as community and *territorial* projects. (To better understand the difference in concept and approach between community intervention and territorial intervention, see Chapter 22.) To achieve more inclusive interventions, two lines of action were pursued. First, the adoption of a critical standpoint from which to analyze services and implement actions, which was in favor of an agenda through which social policies could make people's needs and demands their primary concern, disregarding the previous top-down approach to policy

making. Second, encouragement of an academic debate on the impact of the division of knowledge which gave precedence to specialized knowledge and resulted in reductionist strategies. This approach simply focused on people's physical symptoms, disabilities, and disadvantages, and therefore overlooked the complexity of the issues involved in their life conditions (Barros 1991).

The Metuia Project was created in 1998 in Brazil by occupational therapy lecturers and students from three universities in the state of São Paulo. Metuia means *friend* or *companion* in the language of the Bororo people. At the beginning, the Metuia Project was organized at two branch sites: Universidade de São Paulo/Universidade Federal de São Carlos (USP/UFSCar) and Pontifícia Universidade Católica de Campinas (PUC-Campinas). In the subsequent years, the following changes occurred: the USP/UFSCar branch expanded its projects and was further divided into two branches while the PUC-Campinas branch closed in 2005. At the same time, some of the students and occupational therapists who had previously taken part in the project continued with their graduate studies and carried on contributing to the notion of social occupational therapy both within and outwith the Metuia Project.

The objectives of the Metuia Project are

1. To develop and disseminate knowledge in the field of social occupational therapy
2. To develop a critical awareness of the social role of occupational therapists through the characterization of the population assisted by them, with emphasis on territorial or community attention

3. To study the features and living contexts of the population undergoing a breakdown in social support networks, namely: deprived children and youths, homeless and unemployed adults, among others

4. To study the issues of identity and cultural diversity and the new challenges concerning the constitution of subjectivity and the complexity of social demands in the contemporary world

5. To develop theoretical and practical knowledge about the role that human activities – social and culturally embedded, locally contextualized – play as a means of production of personal/social meanings and development of self-confidence and emancipation

6. To develop theoretical and practical knowledge about occupational therapy actions that address social contradictions and cultural confrontations, through the use of conflict resolution strategies

7. To make occupational therapy students and professionals aware of the importance of work in the social field

8. To contribute to the qualification of the practice of professionals and students, providing elements for their action in the territorial and community programs and in social institution

9. To enable professionals and students to develop a practice where the people's and communities' stories are heard, and the solutions for their own needs are fostered in an action that is jointly built and historically contextualized.

Promoting and sustaining teaching of occupational therapy in the social field

Occupational therapy is a field of knowledge and practice applied in health, education, and social care settings. It combines procedures oriented toward the development of autonomy and the emancipation of people who, for different reasons, are experiencing temporary or permanent difficulties in being included in and participating in social life. The members of the Metuia Project share the belief that working in the social field requires an understanding of the circumstances and living conditions of people who are usually placed in a position of social disqualification. We also agree that education of occupational therapists should take place through direct contact

with these people and their life perspectives. Through the exchange of experiences and knowledge, occupational therapists can enable the people they work with to take on a protagonist role.

Metuia's São Paulo branch has been developing a collaborative teaching setting, where the collaborator is seen as someone who has knowledge and life views to share and not someone who is reduced to a receiving position. In the past few years some of the collaborators have been invited to contribute to practical and theoretical classes, such as urban itineraries, specific policy making and the street people social movement, for example, John the Guitar, who has worked with us since 2001 (Box 34.1).

These learning experiences take place in Brazilian public university system, which considers community service to be an integral part of teaching and research. Project support and funding may come from any one of these three activities. Further, interventions taken by the Metuia Project follow the principles of the occupational therapy schools involved in the project and the daily needs of the people and realities of the places where the programs operate. In the past 10 years many partnerships with governmental and nongovernmental organizations have been established with the intention of promoting cooperation, consultancies, and the development of future projects, for example the UFSCar Branch (see Box 34.2).

Integrated research, community-based projects, and teaching

Working with vulnerable young people: the Casarão Project

The Casarão Project – Centre for Culture and 'living together' Celso Garcia – was a six-year community-based project for children and adolescents. It was a result of a partnership between the local Metuia's branch with the Casarão's Association of Building by Mutirão, and was mediated by the residents of a former apartment block, part of the Social Movement for Urban Housing in the city of São Paulo. Their struggle for decent housing led to the establishment of an agreement with the local government for support to build houses by self-managed collective action (a social organization called *Mutirão* in

Box 34.1

John the Guitar: retrieving personal experiences and teaching social life in street context

João da Viola (John the Guitar – a *viola* is a folk guitar in Brazil) is an artist going through difficult times, looking for support, an audience, and market recognition. He has been receiving support from a nongovernmental organization (NGO) known as My Street, My Home Association (AMRMC), which provides him help with basic activities of daily life, such as getting meals, self-care, and doing his laundry, and also provided him a place to keep his belongings. Through the workshops and cultural events developed by occupational therapists in the collective areas of the center, João has achieved his ambition. His dress style and way of relating to other people indicates a folk-singer identity. Indeed, João enjoys composing, singing, and playing folk songs.

João started to play the guitar when he was 13 years old. Later, he met an experienced musician and they started to do shows and recorded some albums together. They toured around Brazil for a long time, but on one of these trips, João's partner died in a car accident. After that, João did not play music for nine years. He said he suffered during the period of the country's economic recession, split up from his wife, and arrived in São Paulo as a street person. He went back to playing the guitar and writing songs eight years ago. The lyrics of his songs tell the story of his life, his thoughts, and his affinity with music. He says that the best way to interview him is through his lyrics; he likes to explain their meanings and the source of his inspiration.

The Metuia's strategy has been to give him support that includes accompanying him to shows, helping him to produce a video, looking for ways to widen his social networks, recognizing the important places of his life, producing a website to promote his work, and seeking places where he can perform beyond the support network of street people.

While he engages in the activities which have meaning for him, João has carried on collecting garbage from the streets in order to survive. Over the years, a collaborative partnership has been established between João and Metuia. While Metuia supports his work and artistic projects, João, along with other Metuia partners, assumed a teaching role in the social context, by introducing students to the debate on the complexity of São Paulo city's life. In 2006 along with other people from AMRMC, João joined Metuia in its efforts to create a new project – the Meeting and Culture Point – supported by an NGO called OCAS (see Chapter 22 and website http://blogdaocas.blogspot.com/2009/07/joao-da-viola-lanca-novo-cd-de-musica.html).

On one occasion, João demonstrated to professionals and students his typical working day as the driver of a cart that collected recyclable rubbish from across the city of São Paulo. His day usually starts at 4 am but on this particular day as we were with him, it started at 6 am. We left his residence at Don Pedro Park and went across to downtown. João collected several garbage bags, checking if there was any recyclable materials inside them. He gathered material such as paper (including toilet paper), cardboard, aluminum, iron, and plastic. At the beginning of the circuit another rubbish collector complained that João had trespassed in his area. The tension was quickly alleviated when João offered to return everything he had mistakenly taken. However, this was not necessary since the other collector replied that it was just a warning. Disputes about territories among collectors, the weight of the load in the cart, the risks posed by the traffic, and the possibility of contamination from the garbage are some of his daily challenges. The cart, appropriately equipped with a broom, garbage bags and traffic signs (to reflect light in the dark), soon filled up. We then stopped in a park under a huge tree so that João could select the material that was worth selling. While he was selecting the objects he told us some stories of his past and talked about music and its importance to him.

The choice of the spot where João did the selecting was something important to him. For João, this has to be a quiet place, since he enjoyed thinking and observing people. He said: 'We need a lot of peace and meditation. It's worthless to do something when the mind is in turmoil. This comes to nothing. Everything we do comes to nothing. So, you need to do something conscious, with love, perfection, in order to make people understand that you are a person, a concrete person, honest, who knows how to live'.

We observed João's work, and how he left everything organized the way it was before. After selecting all the sellable material, he put everything that was not recyclable inside a garbage bin, leaving the square clean again. The separation of the white paper (toilet paper and others) from the other colored paper was the most time-consuming process although it was also the most well paid on this workday. Having completed approximately six hours of work, João earned 20 Brazilian reals, from which 14 Brazilian reals came from the sale of paper. When João talked to the garbage men, other collectors, and private security guards we noted the camaraderie among them. Having done this work regularly for some time, he is now respected in this community. After finishing this work João goes to collect recyclable material that some people had saved for him, and he gets a moment to speak of his music and to sell some of his CDs. Every day, after selling the objects he has collected, João comes back home, takes a bath, cleans his nails, has lunch and then he has a rest. When he feels well or in need of some more cash, he makes a night trip as well.

Box 34.2

Education, research, and practice/service learning projects in the territory: the experience of the Metuia's UFSCar Branch

The Metuia/UFSCar has two lines of action that are interconnected and share the purpose of setting up practices in social occupational therapy while offering education and developing research and thinking on related subjects. These are: the 'Practice and Service Learning Program' and the research group 'Occupational Therapy and Education in the Social Field'. They have in common the perspective that this field employs a specific theoretical and methodological framework through which it is possible to develop projects and means for the interpretation of personal-social reality and practice in complex contexts. Further, they both address the technical and political roles of professionals and their contributions in confronting contemporary Brazilian social problems.

The Practice and Service Learning Program is understood as a way of integrating education and research activities with social demands. To this end, cooperative agreements have been established with social projects organized by government and nongovernment associations. This has enabled the dialog between university and society and democratization of academic knowledge. Also, it is an answer to the continual demand for social, cultural, and professional development created by the joint efforts of undergraduate and graduate

programs and society itself. The projects carried out within this program allow data collection for research which has been developed at various levels: introduction to research (with undergraduate students), master, doctoral and post-doctoral studies. Although most of the students come from the occupational therapy program, the program's interdisciplinary approach has connected people from different knowledge disciplines, namely, education, multimedia, and psychology.

This approach comes from our understanding that practicing in the social field implies the use of interdisciplinary and multisectoral practices and principles which value the connections between health, social welfare, culture, and education. Practice in this field requires professionals to confront important social problems that are the outcome of Brazil's extreme social inequalities. It also calls for technical, ethical, and political competence which can nurture the ongoing social interventions designed to address people's experiences of social vulnerability and disaffiliation, and backed up the search for strategies for the creation and/or strengthening of social support networks to enable autonomy and social inclusion. To sum up, this approach has helped build a practice whose principles are the exercise of democracy and citizenship (Kowarick 2002).

Portuguese). A housing estate was built for 182 families, most of them people under 21 years of age.

The Casarão Project developed territorial intervention, consisting of collective activities on the estate and individual follow-up. These activities were undertaken at the same time as other Metuia activities were taking place, such as research and occupational therapy education. For an example of an individual follow-up, the story of Bianca, see Box 34.3.

Research has been part of either the development of practices and/or education projects. In the case of Casarão, it was triggered by a community request for a social intervention for youth. The research intended to capture the community's way of life, the social support network, and the health, education and social care provisions. Also, to provide a detailed view, every community household – adult, children and young people – was interviewed. The results were presented back to them and enabled the development of a joint project. This research was also the subject of a master's dissertation (Malfitano 2004) and several articles published by Metuia

(Barros et al 2007b, Barros et al 2008, Lopes 2002, Lopes et al 2001a,b, 2002, 2006).

Research in the Metuia projects has been constantly linked to the Brazilian context and the population's needs. One of the most important youth issues, violence, was the main research and practical concern of the PUC-Campinas branch from 1998 to 2005, such as presented in Box 34.4. Violence continues to be a relevant matter for research and intervention at both Metuia branches.

Concluding remarks

Metuia is a 10-year old project which started with the implementation of social projects in the context of occupational therapy education. Over the years the challenges have been changing due to the development of the various programs of intervention, teaching, and research. Consequently, Metuia has moved from the initial phase of constructing a field to a point of seeking a different quality of reflexivity (see Chapter 6).

Box 34.3

The story of Bianca

Bianca is the daughter of 20-year-old Taís, who could not take care of her since Bianca's birth due to health problems. They lived in a flimsy dwelling, without sanitation, electricity, etc. When Bianca was born her father was in jail and her mother had tuberculosis and was involved in drug trafficking. For safety reasons, the Guardianship Council decided that Taís could only take care of her daughter if she got a job, a place to live, and improved her health. It was within this context that Vera – one of the leaders of the local housing movement – got to know Taís and Bianca and offered to temporarily take care of the child by applying for custody. As is often observed among social movement activists, identification with similar living conditions facilitates the establishment of solidarity bonds between people.

The child, despite occasional visits from her mother, started to develop affection for Vera and her family. Meanwhile, Vera's 17-year-old daughter became pregnant, creating a financial challenge to the family's ability to look after two babies at same time. Vera had a support network of neighbors and friends who donated clothing and food for Bianca but this was not enough. Vera started to consider relinquishing her guardianship of Bianca to support and take care of her coming grandson. This was when she asked for our assistance. We facilitated Bianca's acceptance at a local day nursery, helping to make her application a top priority because there was a huge demand for places. This removed the responsibility

of child daycare from Vera and reassured her that should Bianca's guardianship be returned to Taís, she could still monitor the child from the distance.

Bianca returned to her mother some time later but her situation worsened. The nursery coordinator informed us that Bianca had gradually stopped attending and that they suspected her mother of negligence. At the same time, Vera reported her concern about Bianca, noticing during her visits that the child was constantly hungry, losing weight, and crying during sleep. Taís was then arrested for armed robbery and Vera was given back custody of the child. We continued to follow up Vera's family, and Bianca in particular, although it took us some time to find her another nursery place. Neighbors and friends continued to support Vera and she was selected to be health community agent in the new governmental Programme of Family Health, an achievement that helped her to support her family financially. The intervention with Vera sought to identify assistance that would have been significant for Bianca's development, that is, to build a social and affective support network. The aim was to help enhance life possibilities within the presented context, since Bianca was a child with twofold vulnerability. Thus the community activities – collective and territorial – and a focus on individualized care by the program can help acquire qualitative knowledge about children, such as Bianca, in the family. The interventions are intended to provide life alternatives and create or increase the support for the social and personal development of the local children.

The current stage of Metuia shows the diversification and deepening of research themes in three major fields of concern. The first has an epistemological and methodological frame and it seeks to develop strategies and key-concepts which may guide both theory and practice in social occupational therapy (Barros et al 2007a,b). These bases have been created by dialoging with authors in Social Sciences, Humanities and Education.

The second stream is guided by concerns connected to political and institutional challenges, related to social care, education and their interface with health. The third is constituted by crosscutting themes such as cultural diversity, the coexistence of different social practices, displacement, religiosity, social movements, youth and violence.

The current most important challenge is to increase our ability to publish and preparing new younger researchers who have been producing some interesting master's dissertations and doctoral theses (Borba 2008, Costa 2006, Galvani 2008, Malfitano 2004, 2008,

Rafante 2006, Reis 2008, Silva 2007, Stort 2007, Takeiti 2003). Further, we have taken the challenge of developing methodologies of knowledge shared with people and social groups whom we work with.

Acknowledgments

The researchers of Metuia/UFSCar are occupational therapists Roseli Esquerdo Lopes, Ana Paula Serrata Malfitano, Ariane Machado Palma, Beatriz Akemi Takeiti, Beatriz da Rocha Moura, Carla Regina Silva, Diana Basei Garcia, Eni Marçal de Brito, Iara Falleiros Braga, Patrícia Leme de Oliveira Borba, Patrícia Miola Gorzoni, Paula Giovana Furlan, Sara Caram Sfair, Soraya Diniz Rosa, Tatiana Doval Amador e Vanessa Carolina Domingues Rosseto; historian Heulalia Charalo Rafante; social worker Maria Christina Dória Costa; psychologist Daniela Ribeiro Stort; educators Adriana de Castro and Débora Monteiro do Amaral; and biologist Natália Trajber.

Box 34.4

Understanding violence: the development of practice and research projects at the PUC-Campinas branch, 1998–2005

The PUC-Campinas branch began by developing projects for vulnerable young people. Most of the projects were in community-based programs, but there were also some in shelters for abused children and in programs for young people in conflict with the law. The tragic effects of violence on the lives of those we were working with soon became indisputable. As a consequence, a line of research on violence was established and many students were involved in different research projects throughout the period. The first two focused on the identification and characterization of a service network for children and adolescents in Campinas.

Other projects studied children's and youth's views about their daily life in different situations. Violence appeared as a constant theme in their lives. From this, it was possible to understand their views, the perspectives they developed and their involvement in violent events. As violence was always present they accepted it as part of their lives. Also, it was possible to address occupational aspects that might (or might not) give meaning and satisfaction to their lives and the possibility of making connections between a satisfactory and meaningful occupational life and reduction in violence.

In 2003 a major umbrella project to study violence prevention was started: 'Preventive Action against Violence: a study of the guidelines, recommendations and strategies proposed by international organizations and the Brazilian Federal government from 2000 to 2003'. One of its objectives was to study the guidelines for violence prevention set up by international organizations such as the World Health Organization (WHO) (Krug et al 2002, Galheigo 2008, WHO 2002) and UNESCO (United Nations 1998,1999). Another was to study Brazilian policies for violence prevention, especially the federal government's 'Project Youth Agent' that was set up to develop a youth agency for the prevention of violence in local communities. The third objective was to evaluate its implementation in the city of Campinas, getting to know the views of both the local NGO managers of the Project Youth Agent and the youth included in the program. We focused on youth's views on the results of the community programs they attended and their suggestions for violence prevention. According to local NGO managers and young people, community initiatives and engagement in meaningful activities were both recognized as having significant benefit for social cohesion and violence reduction. The managers organized parties in the community, created a drama club and presented plays at local schools, helped other children to learn how to use computers, and develop activities for children at local nurseries. The endpoint was a better understanding of violence, youth, and occupation in the local communities. The results of the research corroborated with international organizations' recommendations, as follows. There is a need to foster a culture of peace and to promote educational initiatives to prepare people, since early age, to enter in dialog for consensus-building actions and nonviolent conflict resolution. However, educational aims cannot be detached from the higher aspirations of respect for human rights and the promotion of gender and social equality. To enable this, we need to work toward eradication of poverty, wealth redistribution, promotion of sustainable economic and social development and, democratic participation.

As a complex, cross-cultural, multidimensional, and transdisciplinary theme, violence prevention projects seem to achieve better results in local, community-based programs. For occupational therapists, a community-based program presents several opportunities to foster bonding and social ties. Community-based collective action makes possible exchange and reciprocity, which are essential elements in social relations; it also helps encourage solidarity, tolerance to difference, and the resolution of conflicts. Occupational therapists' roles should engage in a committed practice taking into account some important considerations as follows: (i) occupation is at the core of culture – it provides life meaning and the sense of belonging to those engaged in all sorts of occupational projects; (ii) occupation plays a major role in the learning process of doing and creating, along with communication, which is essential in human interaction; and (iii) social roles are dependent on learned cultural practices and on how people establish their sense of belonging. Consequently, culture, education, communication, and social interactions are not supplementary, or rather, secondary to occupational therapy programs. On the contrary, they should be central points in occupational therapy practices.

References

Barros DD: Operadores de saúde na área social, *Revista de Terapia Ocupacional da USP* 1:11–16, 1991.

Barros DD, Lopes RE, Galheigo SM: A Terapia ocupacional social: concepções e perspectivas. In Cavalcanti A, Galvão C, editors: *Terapia Ocupacional: Fundamentação & Prática*, Rio de Janeiro, 2007a, Guanabara Koogan, pp 347–353.

Barros DD, Lopes RE, Galheigo SM: Novos espaços, novos sujeitos: a terapia ocupacional no trabalho territorial e comunitário. In Cavalcanti A, Galvão C, editors: *Terapia Ocupacional:*

Fundamentação & Prática, Rio de Janeiro, 2007b, Guanabara Koogan, pp 354–363.

Barros DD, Lopes RE, Galvani D, et al: Territoires de l'enfance au Brésil, *Revue ErgoThérapies* 31:47–56, 2008.

Borba PLO: *Educadores sociais e suas práticas junto a jovens: cotidiano de ONGs na cidade de Campinas/SP*, Master's dissertation, São Carlos, 2008, UFSCar.

Costa MCD: *Bolsa escola e inclusão educacional em Jaboticabal – SP*, Master's dissertation, São Carlos, 2006, UFSCar.

Galheigo SM: Notes on the prevention of violence by the health sector, *Saúde e Sociedade* 17:181–189, 2008.

Galvani D: *Itinerários e estratégias na construção de redes sociais e identidades de pessoas em situação de rua na cidade de São Paulo*, Master's dissertation, São Paulo, 2008, USP.

Kowarick L: Viver em risco: sobre a vulnerabilidade no Brasil urbano, *Novos Estudos CEBRAP* 63:9–33, 2002.

Krug EG et al (ed): 2002 *World Report on Violence and Health*, Geneva, 2002, World Health Organization.

Lopes RE, Barros DD, Malfitano APS, et al: Terapia ocupacional no território: as crianças e os adolescentes da Unidade do Brás – movimento de luta por moradia urbana, *Cadernos de Terapia Ocupacional da UFSCar* 9:30–49, 2001a.

Lopes RE, Barros DD, Malfitano APS, et al: Espaço do brincante – a construção de um espaço de brincadeiras na atenção a criança na busca do fortalecimento das redes sociais de suporte – a experiência do Projeto Casarão, *Revista de Terapia Ocupacional da USP* 12:48–51, 2001b.

Lopes RE, Barros DD, Malfitano APS, et al: História de vida: a ampliação de redes sociais de suporte de crianças em uma experiência de trabalho comunitário, *O Mundo da Saúde* 26:426–434, 2002.

Lopes RE, Barros DD, Malfitano APS, et al: O vídeo como elemento comunicativo no trabalho comunitário, *Cadernos de Terapia Ocupacional da UFSCar* 10:61–67, 2002.

Lopes RE, Malfitano APS, Silva CR, et al: Terapia ocupacional social e a infância e a juventude pobres: experiências do Núcleo UFSCar do Projeto Metuia, *Cadernos de Terapia Ocupacional da UFSCar* 14:5–14, 2006.

Malfitano APS: *Políticas Públicas e movimentos sociais: atenção à infância e o Programa de Saúde da Família*, Master's dissertation, Campinas, 2004, UNICAMP.

Malfitano APS: *A tessitura da rede: entre pontos e espaços. Políticas e programas sociais de atenção à juventude – a situação de rua em Campinas, SP*, PhD Thesis, São Paulo, 2008, USP.

Rafante HC: *Helena Antipoff e o ensino na capital mineira: a Fazenda do Rosário e a educação pelo trabalho dos meninos 'excepcionais' de 1940 a 1948*, Master's dissertation, São Carlos, 2006, UFSCar.

Reis TAM: *A terapia ocupacional social: análise da produção científica de São Paulo*, Master's dissertation, São Paulo, 2008, USP.

Silva CR: *Políticas públicas, educação, juventude e violência na escola: quais as dinâmicas entre os atores envolvidos?* Master's dissertation, São Carlos, 2007, UFSCar.

Stort DR: *Terceiro setor, educação e juventude: um estudo sobre as práticas da Instituição de Incentivo à Criança e ao Adolescente (ICA) de Mogi Mirim – SP*, Master's dissertation, São Carlos, 2007, UFSCar.

Takeiti BA: *O adolescente e a violência: uma análise da configuração de sentido do adolescente sobre o fenômeno da violência*, Master's dissertation, São Paulo, 2003, PUC.

United Nations: *General Assembly Resolution A/RES/53/25: International Decade for a Culture of Peace and Non-Violence for the Children of the World*, New York, 1998, United Nations.

United Nations: *General Assembly Resolution A/RES/53/243: Declaration and Programme of Action on a Culture of Peace*, New York, 1999, United Nations.

From altruism to participation: bridging academia and borderlands

Anne Shordike   Shirley Peganoff O'Brien   Amy Marshall

OVERVIEW

Occupational therapy as a discipline has a long history of service to persons and communities marginalized by social, economic, political, and occupational injustice. For the past several decades the Department of Occupational Therapy at Eastern Kentucky University has actively and consciously sought to support our community through educational resources while instilling values of community engagement and service in our students. This chapter discusses some of the political, economic, and social environments that impacted and shaped our process, as well as the evolution of our understanding of our work and our contexts through the programs we created. We began our service in the way of the time, from a position of academic privilege, bringing what we understood as needed resources to underprivileged individuals and communities. As we have grown to better understand the borderlands of our communities we have moved from the altruism that comes from that place of privilege to more collaborative and participatory involvement with the communities we serve.

The call

The Occupational Therapy Department at Eastern Kentucky University (EKU) has a 30-year history of involvement with socioeconomic and cultural borderlands through faculty dedication in provision of education and service. As the occupational therapy faculty has developed intensive outreach initiatives to serve the local and Appalachian regions, these values of community engagement and service have been instilled into occupational therapy students.

EKU is classified as a comprehensive university, therefore teaching is the primary emphasis with secondary emphases of service and scholarship. The institution historically has been a college of opportunity for many Kentuckians (Ellis 2005). Delivery of occupational therapy education is influenced by institutional focus (Grant & Masagatani 1986). In teaching-based universities, as at EKU, service agendas are valued (Finnegan & Gamson 1996, US Department of Education 2001). Comprehensive universities historically provide professional education programs, such as occupational therapy, which prepare for workforce entry (Harcleroad & Ostar 1987).

EKU's mission to provide education to underserved areas in its service region fits well with the values and agendas of the occupational therapy department. Persons with disabilities and persons of Appalachian culture were initially designated by the occupational therapy department as underserved populations who would benefit from occupational therapy programs. The occupational therapy faculty appreciated that education of students in these cultural contexts would foster public service values and commitments.

Occupational therapy in the borderlands

Although our long history of community engagement with underserved areas and populations has come from a shared need to provide service, we now understand our work through the evolving concept of borderlands. According to Anzaldua (1999), borderlands

© 2011, Elsevier Ltd.
DOI: 10.1016/B978-0-7020-3103-8.00044-4

exist wherever cultural differences exist; it demar-cates 'us vs. them' (p. 106). They are 'unnatural boundaries' (Blackburn 2005, p. 91) where people are 'denigrated, ignored, and misunderstood' (Gee 1992, p. 147). Borderlands may also exist where two or more cultures occupy the same territory (Chang 2000).

Borders traditionally distinguish physical terri-tories, but as Chang (2000, p. 1) highlights, this essentialist view of a border 'makes assumptions that a culture is separate, distinguishable, and homoge-neous'. Appalachia has a distinct cultural history, however, defining it solely by cultural characteristics is an essentialist view that ignores individual agency and analysis of power dimensions, 'subtle mechan-isms of hegemony which define non-dominant cul-tural practices as deviant and marginal' (Keefe 2005, p. 5).

Borderlands marginalize certain people and ideas over others (Blackburn 2005). European migration to Appalachia occurred early in United States history and included persons driven by political and religious discrimination, poverty, and famine, primarily from Ireland, England, Wales, Scotland, Germany, Switzerland, and France, displacing the native Cherokee and Shawnees. Current Appalachian culture contains a mix of the descendents of the European immigrants, African slaves, and Native Americans (Keefe 2005). Appalachian people have experienced a century of cultural and economic domination imposed by the outsider interests of the affluent middle class and corporations (Lewis 1999). Social reform volunteers, beginning with the 1960s War on Poverty and continuing with Volunteers in Service to America came to Appala-chia, to help persons marginalized by poverty and stereotypical cultural concepts. This created tensions due to the coexistence of the culture-privileged, altruistic aid workers and those who lived in the Appalachian cultural borderlands (Barney 2000, Barrett 2000).

Although borderlands are often sites of depri-vation, they are also sites of 'radical possibility' (Blackburn 2005, p. 108). While deprivation limits the voices of persons living in borderlands, opportu-nities for discourse can position people as agents and support individuals to construct their social identities (Chang 2000). Inclusion of multiple voices in dis-course can subvert oppression by those with the power to define the borders. Borderland discourse (Gee 1992) deterritorializes master narratives (Giroux 1988) of those in power, producing a

'counter-hegemonic discourse that asserts agency and is found in not just words but in habits of being and the way one lives' (Blackburn 2005, p. 109).

Although there is little reference to borderlands in the occupational therapy literature, Jeannie Jackson's 2004 Ruth Zemke Lecture in Occupational Science provides an entrée for occupational thera-pists to frame their work within a borderlands context. She refers to borderland occupations incorporating intermingling differing worldviews, leading to possible transformations of individuals and communities. Jackson discusses the importance of agency, creating authentic occupational lives and constructing identity inside or outside of the domi-nant culture. Borderlands can occur anywhere in practice. Mattingly (2008, p. 140) considers the clinic a border zone describing 'border activities of healthcare professionals where structural conditions of health care are routinely produced and embodied through cultural scripts that influence how profes-sionals and clients understand each other'. Many occupational therapists within the United States practice in borderlands. These include homeless shelters, prisons, battered women's shelters, alterna-tive schools for troubled children and adolescents, after-school programs, and more. Occupational therapists' involvement with community-based pro-grams that increasingly integrate practice, education, and research is supported by the American Occupa-tional Therapy Association's Centennial Vision, which states that 'by the year 2017, we envision that occupational therapy is a powerful widely recog-nized, science-driven, and evidence based profession with a globally connected and diverse workforce meeting society's occupational needs' (AOTA 2007).

As occupational therapy educators at EKU have embraced working in Kentucky's borderlands, our understanding of structural and personal factors affecting the individuals we serve has transformed educational philosophy and delivery. We have had to increase our own and our students' awareness of the impact of power and privilege on health and well-being. As Urbanowski (2005, p. 302–303) says, 'Being able to practice without borders means being able to understand and act on the marginalization forces that affect occupational therapy service reci-pients'. Our particular challenge with working with Appalachian people in our region is to ensure that their voices are included in the collaborative dis-course regarding health, wellbeing, and service provi-sion (Keefe 2005). We are inspired by radical possibilities of borderlands work identified by community partners and faculty, illustrated in the programs described below.

Initial outreach to Kentucky's Appalachian region

The United States Congress created the Appalachian Regional Commission (ARC) in 1965 to advocate for a 13-state, impoverished area of the eastern United States. Of the 51 Appalachian counties of Kentucky, 42 are classified as distressed, an indicator of low per capita incomes and high unemployment rates (ARC 2001). Most of our students come from EKU's service region in these distressed mountain communities of Appalachian Kentucky.

Stereotypic images of Appalachia have been prevalent in the popular culture in the United States, since its description as a 'strange land and peculiar people' in 1873. Appalachia has been viewed as a homogeneous region, resulting in a pathologizing 'culture of poverty' that precludes economic development by isolation and perceived backwardness. Such stereotypes, however, misrepresent historical realities (Eller 1999). The 'myth of Appalachian otherness facilitates absentee corporate hegemony' (Lewis 1999, p. 22). The coal industry has dominated the Appalachian region since the early twentieth century, but as large-scale strip-mining becomes more widespread, fewer mining jobs exist. Those who remain in the region are largely unemployed, poorly educated, and disabled (Keefe 2005). Years of corporate abuses have squandered public and private resources, as individuals leave their homes and communities in search of work elsewhere. Environmental destruction has resulted from the irresponsible practices of absentee landowners; 633 miles of the Kentucky River have been classified as unsafe for human use (Cole & Siegel 2001).

Despite this, there is a rich cultural heritage in Appalachia, expressed through music, art, and exceptional craftsmanship. Certain core characteristics are often attributed to persons living in Appalachia, including a strong sense of place, ties to family, neighborliness, and independence. All of these impact Appalachian individuals and communities' responses to well-meaning outsiders' attempts to influence their health and wellbeing. A powerful example of this is documented in the film *Stranger with a Camera* (Barrett 2000), describing the murder of a well-meaning liberal social activist and photographer, killed because of portrayal of Appalachia as an economic and culturally impoverished area.

It is essential for health professional students to be educated in order to provide culturally sensitive healthcare. EKU provides culturally sensitive education drawing on Appalachian scholarship as well as creative literature and the arts in the classroom to familiarize students with the 'social, political, and economic realities of the society in which they will eventually live and work' (Blakeney 2005, p. 108). There must also be a critical analysis of power that has been brought about by globalizing forces of domination (Keefe 2005).

The EKU occupational therapy department was formed with federal funding to develop health professions in underserved areas. Twenty-one of 22 counties in EKU's service region are designated Appalachian. At the inception of the EKU occupational therapy program, no occupational therapists practiced in the Kentucky Appalachian region. The department's mission was to train students from the area so they could return as practitioners to their rural home-places, providing services for their neighbors and families. A series of rural service grants supported the student experiences, which involved staying in eastern Kentucky for up to a month at a time. Students and faculty involved provided traditional occupational therapy as well as education to stakeholders in specific and rich cultural contexts (Rydeen et al 1995).

These Appalachian-based outreach experiences occurred over a 20-year period. Community agencies partnered with EKU to provide immersion in Appalachian culture and enhance service delivery. Student preparation included a healthcare in Appalachia course, a book club with literature reviews specific to Appalachia, and cultural and health-related education by community partners. Cultural immersion continued throughout the experience with ongoing literature review and collaboration with the local public radio station, a hub of Appalachian culture and political activism. Student fieldwork sites included residential facilities, educational programs and alternative schools, hospitals, nursing homes, and community mental health agencies.

This long-term commitment and collaboration had positive results for the region and occupational therapy. The number of occupational therapists in eastern Kentucky rose from four to 38. These occupational therapists provide services and educational opportunities in many settings (Blakeney 2005).

Expansion of the EKU occupational therapy service mission

This time was highlighted by a return to the primacy of occupation in occupational therapy (AOTA, 2002). As the EKU occupational therapy department continued to grow during the final decade of the twentieth century, faculty and students were attracted to the university with broader public service interests and agendas. Borderlands initiatives moved from a regional focus to population based services. This time was highlighted by a return to the primacy of occupation within occupational therapy. Programs were developed and negotiated in response to the needs of persons marginalized by ability, culture, and society in several venues in and beyond the Appalachian region.

Sensory integration camps

Attending summer camp is a traditional occupation of childhood in the United States (Florey 1999). Camps take many forms: day camps, residential sleep-over camps, theme-related, etc. It is through engagement in camps that children learn and reinforce skill development in the truest sense of bio-psychosocial occupations. Children with disabilities often have not had the opportunity to participate in camp experiences, because of their conditions and related behaviors, safety, availability, and costs. Barriers continue to exist for individuals with special needs that interfere with their ability to participate in typical occupations of childhood, such as sporting activities, camps, and other community events (Baum 2000, Cohn 2001).

Day camps were developed with several community partners addressing needs for sensory processing and sensory integration through occupational experiences. Programming consisted of play opportunities, both as means and end, fostering development of interests, skills, and social interaction. Therapists, staff and students coordinated and implemented culturally relevant camp activities. Treatment in naturalistic environments was extremely successful, meeting the needs identified by children and families. Programs were an initial step in answering the call to create community experiences providing safe environments to negotiate and mediate the degree of occupational challenge necessary for

achievement. Key to successful implementation was collaboration among various professionals, families, organizations, and academic institutions. Faculty and students educated numerous public and professional stakeholders. Outcomes for this experience were powerful; 75% of students went on to offer similar experiences in practice.

Although these camp experiences increased participation and accessibility for children, challenges remain. Although lauded by parents and professionals, cost has limited sustainability in this rural area. Successful programs relied on expert volunteerism by faculty, students, and community therapists. Given the economic environment, efforts have been scaled back in this area.

Urban homeless shelters

Homelessness is a complex social condition with multiple causes and contributors. At least 3.5 million persons experience homelessness in the United States every year (Burt 2001). Personal factors contributing to homelessness include mental and physical health problems, addiction disorders, being veterans, domestic violence, and abuse. Structural contributors include poverty, eroding work opportunities, declining public assistance and affordable housing, lack of affordable healthcare, incarceration, and living in foster care as children (Burt 1999, National Coalition for the Homeless 2002a,b, Petrenchick 2006). These physical, mental, and social conditions contribute to marginalization of many individuals and families, creating a substantial borderland named homelessness in the United States.

Occupation-based programs were developed and implemented over a 10-year period in two urban homeless shelters bordering EKU's service region. Students and faculty worked with persons experiencing all of the structural and personal contributors to homelessness listed above, facilitating development of a garden, a woodworking shop and many self-care, instrumental activities of daily living (ADLs), prevocational/vocational and leisure programs (Scaffa et al 2001). Numerous in-service and program manuals were created. Faculty and students were involved in many state, regional, national, and international presentations, explicitly integrating teaching, service, and scholarship. Students consistently reported positive experiences on their fieldwork evaluations, noting that they had 'made a difference' and that they valued working with these individuals, from whom they had 'learned a lot', particularly the application of occupation across socioeconomic levels and the impact of limited resources (Shordike & Howell 2001). They often stated that they would like to continue working in this type of setting. Staff members valued the programs greatly, but were not available to continue them, generally due to the agencies' emergency response priorities and rapid turnover of personnel.

Although measured outcomes of these programs have been positive for all stakeholders (Shordike & Howell 2001), the programs are not sustained when occupational therapy faculty and students are not present (Scaffa et al 2001, Shordike & Howell 2001). Faculty consulted with both homeless shelters to include occupational therapist positions and program as applications for funding were written. The positions were deleted and money redirected once the grants were funded. The agencies tried to hire occupational therapists in staff positions at staff wages, but therapists would not accept the salaries offered. Even as faculty found funding to provide needed programs and skills training, participants who transitioned out of the shelters continued to find themselves losing the battle for independence with a society that creates functional dependence (Mosby 1996) for many of its members.

Youth at risk

There is a disproportionate representation of youth with disabilities in alternative educational settings. Youth receiving special education services in juvenile justice facilities is about four times higher, at 33%, than in public schools. Of these, 48% are diagnosed with emotional disturbance (Quinn et al 2005). These students are underserved by school-based occupational therapists due to lack of awareness, lack of funding, and stigma (Beck et al 2006). Youth with emotional disturbance are also underserved by community agencies in Kentucky (Kentucky Department of Mental Health and Mental Retardation Services 2003).

Providing Rural Interdisciplinary Services to Youth with Mental Health Needs (PRISYM) was a federal training grant preparing occupational therapy, social work, and psychology students to provide culturally sensitive services to youth with mental health needs. PRISYM partnered with 16 underserved counties in Appalachian Kentucky from 2004 to 2006. Student training occurred through internships at innovative regional community mental health

agencies. Coursework focused on Appalachian culture, historical impact of poverty, and economic issues. Occupational therapy students in PRISYM developed occupation-based modules for practice with youth at risk. PRISYM was discontinued prematurely due to unexpected Congressional budget cuts at the start of the Iraq War. However, thousands of hours of services were provided to youths and their families in the partnering regions by PRISYM students, and a significant number of these students were hired by their internship sites on graduation. Following the grant, the occupational therapy department developed a partnership with the Kentucky Educational Collaborative for State Agency Children to provide occupational therapy services in Kentucky's alternative educational settings and is engaging in research on the transition needs of adolescents in state agencies exiting or aging out of these programs.

Expansion of EKU's conception of occupation-based education and service: moving from altruism to participation

As the twenty-first century began, and the educational requirement for occupational therapy in the United States changed to post-baccalaureate entry, EKU developed a bachelor of science program in occupational science to support the master's program. As faculty became educated in occupational science, EKU's concept of occupationally relevant involvement in community grew, resulting in a more transformational approach to education, service delivery, and scholarship for students and faculty. Philosophically, faculty began moving from their roots in altruism, that is, providing services to those in need, to participation, co-creating programs with multiple stakeholders for positive health and wellbeing.

The Headwaters Project

The Headwaters Project was a partnership between the EKU Center for Appalachian Studies and Letcher County, an Appalachian county in the heart of the coal-mining region of Kentucky. The county is classified as distressed due to high rates of poverty and unemployment. In Letcher County, a strip-mining method called mountaintop removal

Fig. 35.1 • Mountaintop removal site encroaching on community below. (photograph courtesy Appalachian Voices)

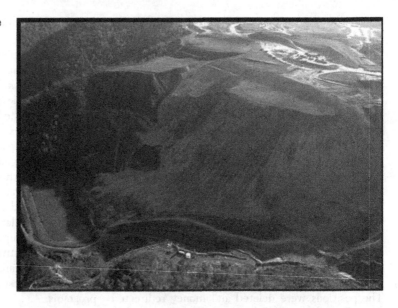

(MTR) is a common method of coal extraction which blasts off up to 243 m (800 ft) of the mountaintop to scrape out the coal, dumping the overburden – or former mountaintops – into narrow adjacent valleys, thereby creating valley fills (Ohio Valley Environmental Coalition n.d.). People's homes are located in these valleys as well as hundreds of rivers and streams used for drinking water. As a result of MTR, the watershed in Letcher County no longer provides safe water for its residents (Fig. 35.1).

The Headwaters Project was a multi-year effort based on a participatory action research framework. Students and faculty from occupational therapy, anthropology, sociology, and geography were involved (Banks et al 2003). Letcher County citizens approached the EKU Center for Appalachian Studies to ask for assistance as they struggled to cope with the impact of MTR on their water supply. The first research phase involved a data visualization project, in which large maps and graphs were made to fit existing water quality data and then were presented at community forums so that residents could see the exact type and location of water contaminants. In the second phase, students surveyed healthcare professionals in Letcher County about their beliefs and practices in relation to poor water quality. In response to concern created by the first two phases as well as suggestions made by the advisory committee, the next research phase explored how poor water quality impacted residents' ability to engage in valued occupations. The continual blasting that destroyed the mountains and polluted

water continues to cause deaths by flooding, collapsing structures, and mudslides. Fifteen students conducted 40 semi-structured interviews over the semester, finding that there was indeed a significant impact on people's daily occupational lives. Occupational therapy graduate students wrote master's theses on the findings, including the pollution's effect on ADLs such as bathing, cooking, and home maintenance, as well as the impact on children's development after it was no longer safe for them to play outdoors, and on increased stress levels of residents (Blakeney & Marshall 2009). One of the most important contributions to the Headwaters Project was recognition of the impact of the physical as well as sociopolitical context on human occupations. The county used the Headwaters research report to secure millions of dollars for the development of improved water systems.

Health and wellbeing for migrant farm workers

The Latino population of Fayette county, an area bordering EKU's service region, grew 235% (compared with an overall population increase of 16% in the United States) between 1990 and 2000, in response to the need for labor in the tobacco and horse industries. The labor market insertion of the immigrants is now past the initial, transient, seasonal stage with many workers and working families employed in low-wage service jobs, especially in the hospitality industry, construction industry, or in factories.

The majority of the primarily Mexican immigrants are living with family and relatives, including children (Rich & Miranda 2005). Health access and resources are a primary concern for Latino migrant farm workers in Kentucky and the United States. The Latino migrants in Fayette County experience the same problems as Latino immigrants throughout the United States, such as availability of culturally, linguistically, and financially appropriate and accessible healthcare services.

A partnership was developed with the Bluegrass Farmworkers' Health Center, an agency formed to respond to the health needs of the Latinos particularly the migrants and immigrants in the area. The first students to be involved here were occupational science seniors, creating their capstone integrative projects. The students reviewed and archived literature related to culture, politics and health of migrant workers. Then they created bilingual, occupationally oriented *fotonovelas*, picture books, to address the areas prioritized by the staff and the literature: pesticide safety, safe body mechanics for working in the tobacco fields, and dental hygiene. The *fotonovelas* are distributed at the center and in the migrant community, and used as in-house educational materials by the center staff. Students in the occupational therapy program have been involved in creating and conducting health needs assessments with homeless and marginally housed horse industry workers, as well as designing occupation-based health classes for the center. This collaboration is ongoing and has potential for long-term sustainability due to the center's connection with EKU and its strong federal funding (Fig. 35.2).

The oral history project

Living with Difference: Oral Histories of Life and Disability in Kentucky is a project funded by the Kentucky Oral History Commission. It will create a bank of oral histories of persons constrained from participation in society secondary to disabilities that will be housed both with the Kentucky Historical Society and EKU. Disability is defined as 'an umbrella term for impairments, activity limitations or participation restrictions' (World Health Organization 2001, p. 3). Persons who consider themselves disabled, or may be considered disabled by others, will share their life stories in the form of oral histories that will be made publicly accessible. As occupational

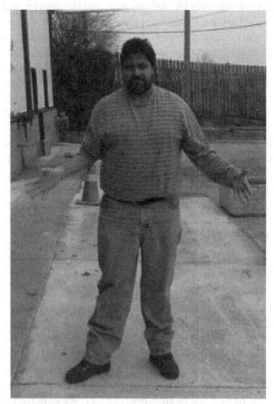

Fig. 35.2 • Page from *fotonovela*. Miguel is a farmworker who often works around pesticides. As working with pesticides can be dangerous, he wears special gloves to protect himself.

therapy recognizes that narrative is one essential means for making sense of experience (Mattingly & Fleming 1994, Precin 2002), this project serves occupational therapy as well as the discipline of oral history by facilitating discourse. Faculty, students, and community partners are gathering these histories. Interviewers use open-ended questions to explore interviewees' life participation – what they do and have done – in relation to their experiences of disability.

The borderland contexts for this project include Kentucky's status as second-highest in the nation for population rates of disability (Ungar 2007), with 22.6% of Kentucky adults experiencing physical, mental, or emotional disability that limits activity (Centers for Disease Control and Prevention 2005), and society's ongoing trend towards inclusiveness in the United States, marked by the deinstitutionalization movement, the passage of the

Americans with Disabilities Act, and the genesis and growth of the Independent Living Movement. As the project collects stories about participation in life in Kentucky, and how this may be impacted by disability, it will inform the historical record with the voices of those who may be constrained by disability thus mitigating the constraint. It will provide a resource for students, families, community, researchers, and any interested parties. This project, the first of its kind in the nation, may provide opportunity for understanding and discourse regarding the experience of living with disability. The dream for this project is that it will grow, with renewed funding and continued partnership with the Kentucky Oral History Commission, inspire more community involvement, and become self-sustaining.

Conclusions

Since its founding, the occupational therapy department at EKU has prioritized efforts to directly impact participation, health, and wellbeing for underserved citizens in its region. Inherent values of EKU supported faculty initiatives, recognizing service as an important component of faculty roles. Moving into the twenty-first century, we experience a variety of constraints and ambiguous expectations from the university, profession, and external stakeholders.

The current climate within higher education in the United States emphasizes austerity, doing more with less, while continuing delivery of quality education by increasingly credentialed faculty. Nationally, state financial support for public higher education continues to decline (Hebel & Selingo 2001), resulting in fewer positions and increasing pressure for external funding. State governing bodies have instituted significant changes in hiring, tenure, and other policies that may limit academic freedom and expression (Honan & Teferra 2001, O'Meara et al 2003, Rice 2006). These factors are evident at EKU, as teaching and service requirements increase in the context of research and funding expectations

Research associated with our service priorities is invariably qualitative in nature, to best capture outcomes related to participation for individuals and communities in our region. The valued hierarchy of research in the United States is driven by Western-based scientific methodologies. This prioritizes large quantitative studies of discrete components that may be related to health (AOTA 2008), creating tension between the service and research values of faculty and funding bodies. As the evidence-based medicine focus of reimbursement has practitioners scrambling for credible data to support practice (Holm 2000), our qualitative and participatory research methods to date are less recognized and rewarded by the medical community as well as our profession.

Despite external constraints, our service agendas have been successful and, for the most part, sustainable. The projects we have developed benefited persons in multiple borderlands while fostering skills and values in our students. We have successfully integrated teaching, service, and scholarship even with our high teaching requirements and labor intensive projects. We have often found funding for our initiatives, particularly through training and small foundation grants. EKU faculty continue to be inspired by the radical possibilities (Blackburn 2005) and negotiate support to provide opportunities for participation and discourse regarding health and wellbeing for students, persons, and communities of Kentucky's borderlands.

This chapter has shared our long-term vision, commitment, and program development. We hope that this brief discussion of our methods and outcomes may be of help to other universities and individuals seeking to work in a rich, relevant, and occupational manner. We offer our experiences and reflections to enter discourse regarding the complexity of educators' responsibility and involvement in broader venues of occupation, health and wellbeing.

Acknowledgments

The authors gratefully acknowledge Doris Pierce, Joy Anderson, and Anne Blakeney for their initial contributions to this chapter, as well as the many EKU faculty and students who created these experiences and brought them to life.

Further reading on Appalachian history and culture

Beagan B: Experiences of social class: Learning from occupational therapy students, *Can J Occup Ther* 74:125–133, 2007.

Billings DB, Blee KM: *The Road to Poverty: The Making of Wealth and Hardship in Appalachia*, Boston, 2008, University of Cambridge Press.

Billings D, Norman G, Ledford K, editors: *Backtalk from Appalachia:*

Confronting Stereotypes, Lexington, KY, 2000, University Press of Kentucky.

Cunningham R: *Apples on the Flood: The Southern Mountain Experience*, Knoxville, 1987, University of Tennessee Press.

Eller R: *Uneven Ground: Appalachia since 1945*, Lexington, KY, 2008, University Press of Kentucky.

Fisher SL, editor: *Fighting Back in Appalachia: Traditions of Resistance and Change*, Philadelphia, 1993, Temple University Press.

Keefe SE, editor: *Appalachian Cultural Competency: A Guide for Medical, Mental Health, and Social Service Professions*, Knoxville, TN, 2005, University of Tennessee Press.

References

American Occupational Therapy Association: *Centennial Vision*, 2007, Online. Available at: http://www.aota.org. Accessed May 5, 2008.

American Occupational Therapy Association: *Evidence-Based Practice and Research*, 2008, Online. Available at: http://www.aota.org. Accessed May 29, 2008.

American Occupational Therapy Association: Occupational therapy practice framework: domain and process, *Am J Occup Ther* 56:610–639, 2002.

Anzaldúa G: *Borderlands/La Frontera: The New Mestiza*, ed 2, San Francisco Ca, 1999, Aunt Lute.

Appalachian Regional Commission: *Distressed Counties in the Appalachian Region*, Washington DC, 2001, Author.

Banks A, Jones A, Blakeney A: *Final Report: The Headwaters Project*, Richmond, KY, 2003, Eastern Kentucky University.

Barney SL: *Authorized to heal: Gender, class, and the transformation of medicine in Appalachia, 1880–1930*, Chapel Hill, 2000, University of North Carolina Press.

Barrett E (Director): *Stranger With a Camera*, Whitesburg, KY, 2000, Appalshop Films.

Baum CM: Reinventing ourselves for the new millennium, *OT Practice* 12–15, 2000.

Beck AJ, Barnes KJ, Vogel KA, et al: The dilemma of psychosocial occupational therapy in public schools: The therapists' perceptions, *Occupational Therapy in Mental Health* 22:1–17, 2006.

Blackburn MV: Agency in borderland discourses: Examining language use in

a community center with queer black youth, *Teachers College Record* 107:89–113, 2005.

Blakeney AB: Educating culturally sensitive health care professionals in Appalachia. In Keefe SE, editor: *Appalachian Cultural Competency: a Guide for Medical, Mental Health and Social Service Professionals*, Knoxville, TN, 2005, University of Tennessee Press, pp 161–178.

Blakeney AB, Marshall A: Water quality and human occupation, *Am J Occup Ther* 63:46–57, 2009.

Burt MR: *What Will it Take to End Homelessness?*, Washington, DC, 2001, The Urban Institute.

Burt M, Aron L, Douglas T, et al: *Homelessness Programs and the People They Serve*, Washington DC, 1999, Interagency Council for the Homeless.

Centers for Disease Control and Prevention: *Behavioral Risk Factor Surveillance System Survey Data*, 2005, Online. Available at: http://apps.nccd.cdc.gov/brfss/display.asp?cat=DL&yr=2005&qkey=4000&state=KY. Accessed February 2, 2007.

Chang H: *Re-examining the Rhetoric of the 'Cultural Border'. 2000*, Online. Available at: http://www.edchange.org/multicultural/papers/heewon.html. Accessed April 17, 2008.

Cohn ES: Parent perspectives of occupational therapy using a sensory integration approach, *Am J Occup Ther* 55:284–294, 2001.

Cole L, Siegel E: *State of Kentucky's Environment: A Report on Environmental Trends and Conditions*, Frankfort, KY, 2001,

Kentucky Environmental Quality Commission.

Eller RD: Forward. In Billings DD, Norman G, Ledford K, editors: *Confronting Appalachian Stereotypes: Back Talk from an American Region*, Lexington KY, 1999, University of Kentucky, pp ix–xi.

Ellis WE: *A History of Eastern Kentucky University: The School of Opportunity*, Lexington, KY, 2005, University of Kentucky Press.

Finnegan DE, Gamson ZF: Disciplinary adaptations to research culture in comprehensive institutions, *Review of Higher Education* 19:141–177, 1996.

Florey LL: Transformations in a summer camp: The role of occupations, *Mental Health Special Interest Section Quarterly* 22:2–4, 1999.

Gee JP: *The Social Mind: Language, Ideology, and Social Practice*, New York, NY, 1992, Bergin & Garvey.

Giroux HA: Border pedagogy in the age of postmodernism, *Journal of Education* 170:162–181, 1988.

Grant HK, Masagatani GN: Managing an academic career, *Am J Occup Ther* 40:83–88, 1986.

Harcleroad F, Ostar AF: *Colleges and Universities for Change: America's Comprehensive Public State Colleges and Universities*, Washington, DC, 1987, AASC Press.

Hebel S, Selingo J: For public colleges, a decade of generous state budgets is over, *Chronicle of Higher Education* 47:32, 2001.

Holm M: The 2000 Eleanor Clarke Slagle lecture – Our mandate for the millennium: Evidence-based practice, *Am J Occup Ther* 54:575–585, 2000.

Honan JP, Teferra D: The US academic profession: key policy challenges, *High Educ* 41:183–203, 2001.

Jackson J: *Occupation at the center: creating authentic lives in social worlds*, 2004 Ruth Zemke Lecture. USA, 2004, Society for the Study of Occupation.

Keefe SE: Introduction. In Keefe SE, editor: *Appalachian Cultural Competency: A Guide for Medical, Mental Health and Social Service Professions*, Knoxville, TN, 2005, University of Tennessee Press, pp 1–26.

Kentucky Department of Mental Health and Mental Retardation Services (KDMHMRS): Community Mental Health Services Performance Block Grant Application: Fiscal Year 2004, Frankfort, KY, 2003, KDMHMRS.

Lewis RL: Beyond isolation and homogeneity: Diversity and the history of Appalachia. In Billings DD, Norman G, Ledford K, editors: *Confronting Appalachian Stereotypes: Back Talk from an American Region*, Lexington, KY, 1999, University of Kentucky, pp 21–43.

Mattingly C, Fleming MH: *Clinical Reasoning: Forms of Inquiry in a Therapeutic Practice*, Philadelphia, 1994, FA Davis.

Mattingly C: Reading minds and telling tales in a cultural borderland, *Ethos* 36:136–154, 2008.

Mosby I: A guide to the responsibilities of occupational therapists and their managers in regard to homeless people who use their services, *British Journal of Occupational Therapy* 59:557–560, 1996.

National Coalition for the Homeless: *Who is Homeless?*, 2002a, NCH Fact sheet #3. Online. Available at: http://www.nationalhomeless.org. Accessed July 6, 2007.

National Coalition for the Homeless: *Why are People Homeless?*, 2002b, NCH Fact sheet #1. Online. Available at: http://www.nationalhomeless.org. Accessed July 6, 2007.

Ohio Valley Environmental Coalition: *What is Mountaintop Removal?* n.d., Online. Available at: http://www.ohvec.org/issues/mountaintop/removal/articles/mtr_fact_sheet.pdf. Accessed March 1, 2004.

O'Meara K, Kaufman RR, Kuntz AM: Faculty work in challenging time: Trends, consequences and implications, *Liberal Education* 89:17–23, 2003.

Petrenchik T: Homelessness: Perspectives, misconceptions, and considerations for occupational therapy, *Occupational Therapy in Health Care* 20:9–20, 2006.

Precin P: *Client-Centered Reasoning: Narratives of People with Mental Illness*, Woburn, MA, 2006, Elsevier Science.

Quinn MM, Rutherford RB, Leone PE, et al: Youth with disabilities in juvenile corrections: A national survey, *Except Child* 71:339–345, 2005.

Rice RE: From Athens and Berlin to LA: Faculty work in the new academy, *Liberal Education* 92:6–13, 2006.

Rich BL, Miranda M: The sociopolitical dynamics of Mexican immigration in Lexington, Kentucky, 1997 to 2002: An ambivalent community responds. In Zuniga H-L, editor: *New Destinations of Mexican Immigration in the United States*, New York, NY, 2005, Russell Sage Foundation Publications.

Rydeen K, Kautzmann L, Cowan M, et al: Three faculty-facilitated, community-based level I fieldwork programs, *Am J Occup Ther* 49:112–118, 1995.

Scaffa ME, Brownson CA, Shordike A: Implications for professional education and research. In Scaffa ME, editor: *Occupational Therapy in Community-Based Practice Settings*, Philadelphia, PA, 2001, FA Davis, pp 367–390.

Shordike A, Howell D: The reindeer of hope: An occupational therapy program in a homeless shelter, *Occupational Therapy in Health Care* 15:57–68, 2001.

Ungar L: Kentucky 2nd-Worst State in Disabilities, *Courier-Journal* 2007. Online. Available at: http://www.courierjournal.com/apps/pbcs.dll/article?AID=/20070205/NEWS0102050439/1008. Accessed February 18, 2007.

Urbanowski R: Transcending practice borders through perspective transformation. In Kronenberg F, Simó Algado S, Pollard N, editors: *Occupational Therapy Without Borders: Learning Through the Spirit of Survivors*, Edinburgh, 2005, Elsevier/Churchill Livingstone, pp 302–312.

US Department of Education: *National Center for Education Statistics. Digest of Education Statistics, 2000*, Washington, DC, 2001, Author.

World Health Organization: *International Classification of Functioning, Disability and Health*, 2001, Online. Available at: http://www3.who.int/icf/intros/ICF-Eng-Intro.pdf. Accessed February 18, 2007.

An occupational justice research perspective

36

Pamela K. Richardson   Anne MacRae

OVERVIEW

Theoretical and philosophical discourse in the field of occupational therapy has deepened the commitment to the founding principle of occupation while simultaneously increasing awareness of the significance of environment and social inclusion, as well as the devastating effect of disparities on the health of individuals and communities. Nevertheless, approaches to research that are commonly taught in our educational programs and supported in our clinical practices may limit our ability to address disparity. It is our position that research in occupational therapy should not only create knowledge, but also in so doing it should empower and enable those who participate to create change. An occupational justice research perspective can be a driving force in the continuing evolution of knowledge in occupational therapy while facilitating participation in meaningful and dignified occupations for individuals, groups, and communities. We propose four broad areas of occupational justice research; worldview, context, action, and evaluation. These areas are not mutually exclusive and each encompasses a range of research methodologies. The unifying characteristics within this perspective are the inclusive, participatory orientation of the researcher, and the need for highly developed interpersonal and performance skills, as well as extensive content and process knowledge of the contexts under consideration.

Introduction

Medical and social science research has created knowledge that has improved the health and quality of life of people around the world. However, the benefits of research have not been equally distributed, and in many marginalized communities, research epitomizes the practice of the privileged mining the lives of the powerless to advance their own wellbeing and reinforce existing power relationships (Smith 1998). Currently, ethical principles and regulations govern the conduct of research in most countries (World Medical Association 2003). However, even research that is conducted in accordance with ethical principles can reinforce societal oppression and exclusion of marginalized groups if the voices of the group members are not represented in the research process (Kielhofner 2005). This chapter explores a research perspective that is dedicated to the application of the principles of occupational justice within the parameters of occupational therapy and occupational science.

Research is a key to the advancement of knowledge and the evolution of practice in occupational therapy (Kielhofner 2006). Expectations for evidence-based practice are accelerating, and occupational therapists are under increasing pressure to demonstrate that interventions are both effective and cost-efficient. Kronenberg & Pollard (2006) have criticized the evidence-based practice movement for its lack of concern with social responsibility, and challenge occupational therapists to employ a process of critical self-reflection in order to ensure that their practice is socially responsible as well as evidence based. Townsend & Wilcock (2004) urge researchers to expand their scholarly perspective to include critical analysis of social and political structures that influence the ability of individuals and communities to engage in meaningful, dignified, and health giving occupations. The evidence-based practice movement

© 2011, Elsevier Ltd.
DOI: 10.1016/B978-0-7020-3103-8.00045-6

and the occupational justice movement create challenges for researchers that may appear to be incompatible. We contend that an occupational justice perspective on research can be both rigorous and socially responsible. An occupational justice perspective in research can achieve the desired synergy between scholarly inquiry and everyday practice: it can be a driving force in the evolution of knowledge in occupational therapy while facilitating participation in meaningful and dignified occupations for individuals, groups, and communities. We propose a broad research agenda in occupational justice and discuss specific knowledge and skills that contribute to an occupational justice research perspective.

An evolving global context for research and practice

The conceptualization of health and disability is undergoing an evolution. This paradigm has been influenced by many social, political, and scientific ideas. Two influential documents include the *International Classification of Functioning, Disability and Health* (ICF), approved by the World Health Organization (WHO) in 2001 and the *United Nations Standard Rules for People with Disabilities*, adopted by the UN General Assembly in 1993. The ICF, an outgrowth of the 1980 *International Classification of Impairments, Disabilities, and Handicaps*, conceptualizes disability as having social aspects, expanding the definition of disability beyond medical or biological dysfunction. The inclusion of Contextual Factors in the ICF encourages consideration of the impact of the environment on an individual's function. The UN Standard Rules were developed as an instrument for policy development and program implementation and address equal participation for people with disabilities in all aspects of life.

Further broadening this conceptualization of health, a growing body of evidence suggests that the social environment is a major contributor to health of people around the world, and that disparities in health and mortality both within and between countries can largely be attributed to social factors such as: poverty; drugs; working conditions; unemployment; housing quality; social support; social structures such as law enforcement, places of worship, and schools; food quality; public transportation; and the presence or absence of violence in the community (United States Department of Health and Human Services 2000, Wilkinson & Marmot

2003). The WHO Commission on Social Determinants of Health (CSDH 2007) defines the social determinants of health as 'the fundamental structures of social hierarchy and the socially determined conditions these structures create in which people grow, live, work and age' (p. iii). The CSDH proposes a global movement to improve health and reduce health inequities by addressing them at a societal level, creating empowerment through change and enabling people to participate and flourish in society. A central purpose of this movement is accumulation of evidence on health disparities and needs that will create a basis for action by policy makers, researchers, and practitioners. Healthcare disciplines are re-examining their philosophies, interventions, and research methodologies in light of this changing paradigm of health, focusing on the social, environmental and justice issues of not only individuals but also of communities (Kilbourne et al 2006, London 2005, Schim et al 2006).Within occupational therapy the World Federation of Occupational Therapy (WFOT) has issued position papers on community-based rehabilitation (2004) and human rights (2006) that articulate a vision of empowerment and enablement of all people.

Clearly, an occupational justice perspective of research is consistent with this movement. Social and environmental awareness have been a part of occupational therapy from its inception (Schwartz 2005), however, for many years the practice of occupational therapy has been dominated by the biomedical perspective. This uncomfortable alignment began to be called into question by occupational therapists in the United States, where the medical model was the most deeply entrenched, as early as the 1970s (Kielhofner & Burke 1977, Shannon 1977). However, quite appropriately, a major impetus for change has come from outside the profession, by the people whose experiences are most affected by disability and injustice. The Independent Living Movement (Gill 1987) and the Disability Rights Movement and concurrent advancement in the field of disability studies (Kielhofner 2005) are continuing to shape not only how occupational therapists practice, but also how we forge our future research agenda. Occupational therapy researchers are encouraged to explore the philosophical underpinnings of research designs (Kielhofner 2006) and with a renewed focus on the influence of societal factors on health, they are now more likely to identify with a critical or postmodernistic research philosophy rather than the traditional positivist approach to research.

The occupational justice perspective on research

A key principle of occupational justice is the recognition of differences between individuals and communities in their occupational needs and strengths, and an acknowledgement that they require different forms of enablement in order to achieve full occupational and social participation (Townsend & Wilcock 2004). Researchers who use an occupational justice perspective incorporate the inclusive, participatory vision of occupational justice into their inquiry. They ask what must be done to create occupational opportunities for different individuals and groups (Townsend 2003). Creation of knowledge within this perspective empowers and enables participants to create change.

This perspective also implies establishment of a contract between the researcher and the participants/collaborators. The researcher assumes a responsibility to insure, to the best of her/his ability, that the approach to the research respects cultural and community values and practices, that the research is rigorous, that it produces meaningful information that is useful to the participants as well as to a general audience of research consumers, and that the dissemination of the information maximizes the opportunity of the participants to benefit from the outcome. In order to accomplish this, the researcher must have substantial knowledge of the social, political, and cultural contexts of the research environment. Czymoniewicz-Klippel discusses these contexts and their influence on her research on Cambodian children and childhoods in Chapter 40.

In order to engage in research using an occupational justice perspective, specific skills and knowledge are required (Table 36.1). First, the researcher must have a clear understanding of the politics of power in human relationships and how this has been manifested through the biomedical research tradition. A critical or post-modernist perspective provides a lens through which researchers can critique existing research approaches and explore how the knowledge obtained using these approaches is constructed by researcher ideologies and context (Kielhofner 2006). One important outcome of scholarship conducted using the critical or post-modern perspective has been an evolution in how the nature of knowledge is understood (see Chapter 14). The concept of knowledge as a social construct informs many contemporary research methods and traditions, emphasizing the importance of understanding the lives and perceptions of those who experience occupational injustice. This has led researchers to re-conceptualize the roles of the researcher and the research subject. Increasingly, participants contribute as collaborators in the process of knowledge generation (Table 36.1).

Table 36.1 Knowledge and skills needed for an occupational justice research perspective

Content knowledge	Process knowledge
Cultural values and beliefs	Proposal writing/obtaining funding
Political systems and functions	Scholarly writing
Institutional review protocols	Methods for advocacy and sustainability
Broad range of research methodologies	Multiple human and technological resources
Mastery of scholarly literature	Clinical reasoning
Interpersonal skills	**Performance skills**
Reflexivity	Development of trustful relationships
Openness and sensitivity	Consensus building
Bracketing of bias	Negotiation
Ability to yield control; role release	Facilitation of shared power
Respectful engagement	Fair dissemination of research results

A second area of contextual understanding for researchers is the politics of power in research and program development in the context where they work. This consists of an understanding of the processes involved in obtaining funding, receiving approval to conduct research, disseminating results, and achieving program sustainability. Knowledge and skills in grant/proposal writing, completing institutional review board (IRB) applications, and scholarly writing are necessary. The researcher may additionally need to be able to use the research evidence to advocate for services or programs for the participants/collaborators. Occupational therapy researchers may work within an interdisciplinary research team or alone. In order to be successful in either situation the researcher must be aware of funding and program priorities, how individual research interests and community needs may or may not align with these priorities, and how to effectively communicate research objectives, methods, and outcomes to a variety of stakeholders, both verbally and in writing.

Third, researchers must understand the politics of power in empowerment; in other words they must know how to create equal partnerships in research in order to enact the socially informed values of occupational justice. These techniques are embedded within participatory research processes, but must be incorporated into all types of research. Researchers must be able to work with individuals and communities who possess a broad range of characteristics and skills. They must be able to negotiate their roles in the research process, stepping back when needed to allow others to take leadership roles and facilitating the process whereby the individual/community takes responsibility for the outcomes of the research. This entails the ability to yield control of some aspects of the research process and a respect for the capacity of the group to engage fully in the decision making process that is central to participatory research approaches (Taylor et al 2006).

Finally, the researcher needs to develop a specific set of skills in order to effectively participate in occupational justice research and to bring results to fruition. These skills include knowledge of specific research methodologies and the ability to determine which methodologies are the most appropriate for a particular situation. Since few of the research areas in occupational justice dictate a specific methodology or research design, the researcher must have a strong generalist knowledge of research methods and a willingness to seek qualified assistance in areas where her or his knowledge base is weak. The researcher must

also be able to make difficult decisions about how to balance her or his desire to conduct a study in the most rigorous manner possible with the needs and desires of the research participants. Compromise is often necessary, and it is important that this process be discussed and documented. In addition the researcher must have skills in critical self-reflection in order to acknowledge and bracket assumptions and biases through all steps of the research process. See Galvaan's discussion of the bracketing process that she engaged in prior to initiating her study of domestic workers (Chapter 37).

Areas of focus for occupational justice research

We propose four broad areas of occupational justice research that encompass a range of research methodologies. These areas represent methodologies that are explicitly participatory as well as those that represent a more traditional/empirical orientation. The unifying characteristic is the inclusive, participatory orientation of the researcher, which influences all aspects of the research from the underlying assumptions, to the questions asked, to the methodology chosen, to how information is collected, analyzed, and interpreted. The areas of occupational justice research are summarized in Table 36.2 and discussed in more depth in the following sections. Examples of studies that illustrate each area of research are included in the table. This is not intended to be an exhaustive list of research conducted using an occupational justice perspective. In some cases the authors do not explicitly discuss occupational justice, but the orientation towards the research is consistent with this perspective. The research categories are not meant to be rigid or mutually exclusive; some studies could be represented in more than one area but are presented in one place for simplicity and clarity (Table 36.2).

Worldview

Research in this area seeks to understand the experiences and occupational needs of individuals and communities. Worldview can be defined as a set of commonly held values, ideas, and images concerning the nature of reality and the role of humanity within it, that shapes one's emotional, cognitive, and physical (action) responses. Being aware of alternative

Table 36.2 Areas of research within an occupational justice perspective

Research Area	Areas addressed	Methodologies	Examples of studies
Worldview	Experiences, perceptions, beliefs, and practices of individuals, groups, communities	Phenomenology Ethnography Critical analysis Grounded theory	Gerlach 2008 Martins & Reid 2007 Nelson 2007 Sakellariou & Simó-Algado 2006
Context	Policies, systems, contexts, environments	Critical analysis Descriptive analysis Ethnography Population-level analysis Historical analysis Content analysis Grounded theory	Bryant et al 2004 Hemingsson & Borell 2002 Jakobsen 2004 Magasi & Hammel 2009 McColl 2005 VanLeit et al 2006 Vik et al 2007
Action	Community or group needs	Participatory action research (PAR) Community-based participatory research (CBPR) Consensus methods	Blakeney & Marshall 2009 Brodrick 2004 Lorenzo et al 2002 Simó-Algado et al 2002 Stewart & Bhagwanjee 1999 Suarez-Balcazar et al 2005 Townsend et al 2000
Evaluation	Program outcomes Community outcomes Individual outcomes	Experimental group or single case design research Qualitative methods Empowerment and participatory evaluation	Suarez-Balcazar 2005 Taylor 2003 Taylor et al 2004

worldviews does not require one to adopt or agree with them. However, without an appreciation of differing worldviews it is difficult to identify the meaning of the experiences of others and there is great potential for misinterpretation. Throughout this book are poignant stories representing differing worldviews. We suggest that a phenomenological attitude be embraced in order to grasp the full meaning of these stories.

The phenomenological attitude 'is understood as the process of retaining a wonder and openness to the world while reflexively restraining pre-understandings' (Finlay 2008, p. 1). Sokolowski (2000) contends that all human beings do this sort of reflective philosophy from time to time but a true phenomenological attitude is conscious and a person shifts into this type of thinking explicitly. Developing this reflective attitude is quite difficult and may be best mastered by working with an experienced mentor. Giorgi (1983) recommends engaging in a workshop format in order to work through the difficulties and best learn phenomenological research methods. Mentorship, practice, sometimes years of study, and certainly self-reflection are also required to master the knowledge and skills needed

for the occupational justice research perspective that we suggest in Table 36.1. For example, Bailey & Cohn (2001) developed an occupational therapy course using various forms of interactive clinical reasoning with the express purpose of 'understanding others' (p. 31). The knowledge and skills listed in Table 36.2 are not only prerequisites to understanding worldview, they are necessary to gain access to communities as a welcomed and invited member of a group and to be able to conduct and disseminate research in a way that is fair and beneficial to all participants.

The specific methods used for understanding worldview come from varying philosophical schools of thought and have differing degrees of researcher participation and immediate application. The commonality of these research traditions is the acknowledgment that the perception of the participants' experience is paramount in understanding the phenomenon under study. Examples of the various research methodologies that address worldview can be seen in Table 36.2. As previously mentioned, the four categories outlined in this table are not meant to be mutually exclusive. We recommend that all occupational justice research, including studies focused on context, action, and evaluation, begin with an understanding of the participants' worldview.

An argument can be made that the misunderstanding of differing worldviews and the misinterpretation of experiences is best minimized by designing studies in which the primary researcher is of the same background as the other participants (Smith 1998). In many ways, this is ideal and a model to be encouraged. However, it is not always practical due to limitations in training and funding. Furthermore, even when the primary researcher is a member of the same cultural, ethnic or geographic group, there may still be differences in experiences, education and socioeconomic status that can lead to unconscious bias and erroneous assumptions. Table 36.3 lists a variety of factors that can influence an individual's worldview. Although worldview is generally considered to be shared by a particular group, it also must be acknowledged that individual differences arise and unique variations can be found within an overarching cultural or group worldview (Table 36.3).

Context

Research in this area includes the study of the political contexts, policies, systems, and environments that contribute to occupational injustice. This ranges from studies of the environments experienced by individuals to analysis of broader contexts and policies that create occupational injustice for groups of people. A variety of quantitative and qualitative methodologies can be used. The most salient aspect of this area of research is that the focus extends beyond the individual or group of interest to evaluate the interaction between the individual and the context and/or the impact of the context on the ability of the individual or group to engage in meaningful occupations.

Some of the research in this area uses qualitative methodologies with small sample sizes. Qualitative studies can elicit in-depth descriptions of how individuals experience and interact with physical, social, and political environments, and how these environments may create or contribute to occupational injustice. Interpretation and analysis can identify the types of policies and practices that create social and institutional support to enable individuals to engage productively in self-selected occupations. Quantitative studies using large samples complement qualitative research by providing broad-based data identifying regional or national patterns. Research conducted at the population-level affords researchers a 'systemic, structural view of the relationship between persons with disabilities and society' (McColl 2005, p. 516). The data obtained provides information for policy makers about the healthcare needs of a particular group, and provides evidence to support advocacy efforts. Occupational therapy researchers conducting inquiry in this area can do so individually or as part of an interdisciplinary team. In either case, the focus of inquiry in this area is solidly in line with international priorities in health-related research (CSDH 2007).

Action

Research in this area includes action-oriented and participatory approaches initiated in collaboration with individuals and communities to develop initiatives to empower change and transformation. Participatory action research originated through community activism work in Africa, Asia, and South America (Borda 2001). Consciousness raising, social critique and social change are actions undertaken to transform oppression into empowerment (Townsend et al 2000). An underlying assumption of participatory research is that change will occur as knowledge is developed through the research process (Letts 2003). The research takes place in the context where the knowledge is expected to be applied, and empowers the participants by allowing them to define and shape the research agenda (Taylor et al 2006).

Table 36.3 Factors affecting worldview

Age	Lifestyle
Authority structure	Personal experience
Citizenship status	Political system
Cultural traditions	Race/ethnicity
Education	Religious affiliation
Family structure	Sexual orientation
Gender	Socioeconomic status
Geographic region	Spatial awareness
Health status	Time sense
Infrastructure	Values and beliefs

Participatory action research is characterised by three major principles (Taylor et al 2004). First, consumers and service providers have the opportunity to actively engage in the creation, delivery, and refinement of services (Taylor 2003). This insures that services are relevant and meaningful for the consumers. Second, a strengths-based approach is used, where participants identify, use, and build on their resources to accomplish goals. This approach is crucial in empowering marginalized and oppressed communities to take an active role in determining how services will be configured. Third, traditional roles of researcher and subject are eliminated. The researcher often functions in an advisory or consultative role while individuals and groups within the community take on decision making and leadership roles (Brodrick 2004). The researcher may take on other roles such as a meeting facilitator, community advocate, or organizer. This process of role release creates learning opportunities for all participants (Taylor et al 2004). Dialog is a key part of the process, and is implemented through strategies such as listening sessions, focus groups, public forums, and ongoing team meetings (Taylor et al 2006). Through the dialog process information is exchanged and critical reflection occurs, creating new awareness for all participants.

Participatory action research (PAR) and community-based participatory research (CBPR) are two of the most commonly used action approaches. Within these approaches a variety of data gathering techniques are used. The commonality is that the data gathering and evaluation processes are chosen by the participants. The participatory research process is cyclical, with the knowledge generated through the research process informing practice, and practice informing subsequent data collection. This creates a closer link between research and practice, as clinicians and consumers have a more active role in determining what is studied (Taylor et al 2006). In occupational therapy, participatory approaches have been used with a variety of communities and consumer groups. See Bryant et al's discussion in Chapter 39 of how their participatory action research process unfolded and the decisions that were made along the way.

Evaluation

Research in this area includes evaluation of program effectiveness and generation of information that can be used to advocate for administrative and financial support of programs and initiatives. Studies of programs and interventions conducted using an occupational justice perspective that collect specific outcome data are less frequently found in the literature; however, program evaluation should be an integral component of any program development process. This category of research is presented here to emphasize the importance of obtaining and documenting information on the outcomes of interventions. In a participatory research approach, evaluation is embedded in the research process. However, not all outcomes will be based on a participatory process. This is an area of inquiry where researchers must be highly cognizant of the outcome data requirements of external stakeholders such as funding sources, sponsoring organizations, and legislative bodies. To some extent the type of evaluation data collected may be dictated by these outside bodies. If a participatory process is being used, the evaluation components specified by the stakeholders must be discussed and negotiated with the participants. The participants may also identify different types of desired outcome measures, and the researcher should work with them to incorporate these outcome measures in the design of the program. Some examples of outcome data collected include quality of life, symptom severity, functional capacity, service utilization, resource acquisition, and coping (Taylor et al 2004), client monitoring of goal attainment, ongoing participant reflection (Taylor 2003, Taylor et al 2004), perceived control, neighborhood cohesion, and specific actions taken (Suarez-Balcazar 2005).

Challenges and considerations

For occupational therapy researchers trained in traditional empirical research methods, an occupational justice perspective on research may require a reconceptualization of the roles and responsibilities of the researcher. The inclusive, participatory orientation requires a sharing of power between researcher and research participant. This may be uncomfortable for both. The researcher may be reluctant to give up control, and the participants may not feel confident in their ability to take on a more active role because of differences in power due to education and/or cultural issues. The researcher may need to assume a variety of roles within the scope of the research project, and may need to tailor the specific research methodologies used as a result of participant input. This input can change the direction of the project, moving the focus away from the researcher's original vision (Letts 2003).

Procedural and practical challenges also exist. Participatory methodologies are often not well understood by IRB committees. Malone et al (2006) discuss the significant challenges they experienced in attempting to obtain university IRB approval for a community-based participatory research project. Issues of informed consent for participatory methodologies often do not fit neatly into conventional IRB procedures and may require different consent processes at different points in the research. Additionally, cultural values of individuals and communities may dictate that consent is handled in specific ways. These issues may also affect the willingness of funding sources to fund studies using participatory methodologies (Letts 2003).

The complexity of the social and health problems addressed in an occupational justice perspective of research, and the collaborative nature of the research methodologies used requires a broad skill set for researchers. Researchers working in this area must be prepared to work under timelines established by the community collaborators and do so using consensus processes. Research conducted using these processes is rarely tidy or quick. This may create conflict with timelines and outcomes expected by funding sources, universities, and other stakeholders, and researchers will need to anticipate and have a plan for addressing potential tensions between the various constituencies. A solid research knowledge base, a commitment to the concepts of empowerment and occupational justice, strong communication skills, cultural competence, patience, and flexibility are some of the key skills needed.

Conclusion

There are dramatic changes occurring in how we conceptualize and study health issues on an individual, community, and worldwide level and there are exciting opportunities for occupational therapists to be engaged in this process (Frank & Zemke 2008, Kronenberg & Pollard 2006). In this evolving paradigm, healthcare and research must be grounded in the principles of inclusion, respect, and participation within multiple worldviews. Although all healthcare and social service professions are aiming to incorporate these principles into their practice and research, it is our position that the core occupational therapy concepts of enablement through client-centered practice provide a solid foundation for occupational therapy and occupational science researchers to approach their inquiry using inclusive, participatory principles.

The goal of this chapter is to explore the developing occupational justice research perspective and to encourage occupational therapy researchers to incorporate the values imbedded in occupational justice in all forms of research. It is not possible within the confines of this brief chapter to fully explore the background, principles, or methodologies needed to fully understand and incorporate this perspective. Rather we view this chapter as part of an ongoing dialog and invite readers to explore additional resources and engage with researchers and practitioners around the world to continue to refine the conceptualization and practice of occupational justice through research.

Acknowledgment

We wish to express our heartfelt thanks to the clinicians, professors, researchers, clients, community members, students, and friends from around the world, who have challenged our thinking with critical dialog and insights. Many years of these conversations have formed the basis of the research perspective presented in this chapter.

References

Bailey D, Cohn E: Understanding others: a course to learn interactive clinical reasoning, *Occupational Therapy in Health Care* 15:31–46, 2001.

Blakeney AB, Marshall A: Water quality, health, and human occupations, *Am J Occup Ther* 63:46–57, 2009.

Borda OF: Participatory (action) research in social theory: origins and challenges. In Reason P, Bradbury H, editors: *Handbook of Action Research*, Thousand Oaks, CA, 2001, Sage, pp 27–37.

Brodrick K: Grandmothers affected by HIV/AIDS: new roles and occupations. In Watson R, Swartz L, editors: *Transformation Through Occupation*, London, 2004, Whurr, pp 233–253.

Bryant W, Craik C, McKay EA: Living in a glasshouse: exploring occupational alienation, *Can J Occup Ther* 71:282–289, 2004.

Commission on Social Determinants of Health: *Achieving Health Equity: From Root Causes to Fair Outcomes Interim Statement*, Geneva, 2007, World Health Organization.

Finlay L: A dance between the reduction and reflexivity: explicating the 'phenomenological psychological attitude', *Journal of Phenomenological Psychology* 39:1–32, 2008.

Frank G, Zemke R: Occupational therapy foundations for political engagement and social transformation. In Pollard N, Sakellariou D, Kronenberg F, editors: *Political Practice in Occupational Therapy*, Edinburgh, 2008, Elsevier Science, pp 111–136.

Gerlach A: 'Circle of caring': a First Nations worldview of child rearing, *Can J Occup Ther* 75:18–25, 2008.

Gill C: A new social perspective on disability and its implications for rehabilitation, *Occupational Therapy in Health Care* 4:49–55, 1987.

Giorgi A: The importance of the phenomenological attitude for access to the psychological realm. In Giorgi A, Barton A, Maes C, editors: *Duquesne Studies in Phenomenological Psychology IV*, Pittsburgh, 1983, Duquesne University Press, pp 209–221.

Hemingsson H, Borell L: Environmental barriers in mainstream schools, *Child Care Health Dev* 28:57–63, 2002.

Jakobsen K: If work doesn't work: how to enable occupational justice, *Journal of Occupational Science* 11:125–134, 2004.

Kielhofner G: Rethinking disability and what to do about it: disability studies and its implications for occupational therapy, *Am J Occup Ther* 59:487–496, 2005.

Kielhofner G: The aims of research: philosophical foundations of scientific inquiry. In Kielhofner G, editor: *Research in Occupational Therapy: Methods of Inquiry for Enhancing Practice*, Philadelphia, 2006, FA Davis, pp 10–19.

Kielhofner G, Burke JP: Occupational therapy after 60 years, *Am J Occup Ther* 31:675–689, 1977.

Kilbourne AM, Switzer G, Hyman K, et al: Advancing health disparities research within the health care system: a conceptual framework, *Am J Public Health* 96:2113–2121, 2006.

Kronenberg F, Pollard N: Political dimensions of occupation and the role of occupational therapy, *Am J Occup Ther* 60:617–625, 2006.

Letts L: Occupational therapy and participatory research: a partnership worth pursuing, *Am J Occup Ther* 57:77–87, 2003.

London AJ: Justice and the human development approach to international research, *Hastings Cent Rep* 35:24–37, 2005.

Lorenzo T, Saunders LC, January M, et al: *On the Road of Hope: Stories Told by Disabled Women in Khayelitsha*, Cape Town, 2002, Division of Occupational Therapy, University of Cape Town.

Magasi S, Hammel J: Women with disabilities' experiences in long-term care: a case for social justice, *Am J Occup Ther* 63:35–45, 2009.

Malone RE, Yerger VB, McGruder C, et al: 'It's like Tuskegee in reverse': a case study of ethical tensions in Institutional Review Board review of community-based participatory research, *Am J Public Health* 96:1914–1919, 2006.

Martins M, Reid D: New-immigrant women in urban Canada: insights into occupation and sociocultural context, *Occup Ther Int* 14:203–220, 2007.

McColl MA: Disability studies at the population level: issues of health service utilization, *Am J Occup Ther* 59:516–526, 2005.

Nelson A: Seeing white: a critical exploration of occupational therapy with Indigenous Australian people, *Occup Ther Int* 14:237–255, 2007.

Sakellariou D, Simó-Algado S: Sexuality and disability: a case of occupational injustice, *British Journal of Occupational Therapy* 69:69–76, 2006.

Schim SM, Benkert R, Bell SE, et al: Social justice: added metaparadigm concept for urban health nursing, *Public Health Nurs* 24:73–80, 2006.

Schwartz KB: The history and philosophy of psychosocial occupational therapy. In Cara E, MacRae A, editors: *Psychological Occupational Therapy: A Clinical Practice*, ed 2, Clifton Park NY, 2005, Thomson Delmar, pp 57–79.

Shannon P: The derailment of occupational therapy, *Am J Occup Ther* 31:229–234, 1977.

Simó-Algado S, Mehta N, Kronenberg F, et al: Occupational therapy intervention with children survivors of war, *Can J Occup Ther* 69:205–217, 2002.

Smith LT: *Decolonizing Methodologies: Research and Indigenous Peoples*, London, 1998, Zed Books.

Sokolowski R: *Introduction to Phenomenology*, Cambridge, UK, 2000, Cambridge University Press.

Stewart R, Bhagwanjee A: Promoting group empowerment and self-reliance through participatory research: a case study of people with physical disability, *Disabil Rehabil* 21:338–345, 1999.

Suarez-Balcazar Y: Empowerment and participatory evaluation of a community health intervention: implications for occupational therapy, *Occupational Therapy Journal of Research* 25:133–142, 2005.

Suarez-Balcazar Y, Martinez LI, Casas-Byots C: A participatory action research approach for identifying health service needs of Hispanic immigrants: implications for occupational therapy, *Occupational Therapy in Health Care* 19:145–163, 2005.

Taylor RR: Extending client-centered practice: the use of participatory methods to empower clients, *Occupational Therapy in Mental Health* 19:57–75, 2003.

Taylor RR, Braveman B, Hammel J: Developing and evaluating community-based services through participatory action research: two case examples, *Am J Occup Ther* 58:73–82, 2004.

Taylor RR, Suarez-Balcazar Y, Forsyth K, et al: Participatory research in occupational therapy. In Kielhofner G, editor: *Research in Occupational Therapy: Methods of Inquiry for Enhancing Practice*, Philadelphia, 2006, FA Davis, pp 620–631.

Townsend E: *Occupational justice: ethical, moral and civic principles for an inclusive world*, Keynote presentation at the Annual Conference of the European Network of Occupational Therapy Educators. Czech Republic, Prague, ; 2003.

Townsend E, Wilcock AA: Occupational justice and client-centred practice: a dialogue in progress, *Can J Occup Ther* 71:75–87, 2004.

Townsend E, Birch DE, Langley J, et al: Participatory research in a mental health clubhouse, *Occupational Therapy Journal of Research* 20:19–44, 2000.

United Nations General Assembly: *The Standard Rules on the Equalization of Opportunities for Persons with*

Disabilities, 1993. Online. Available at: http://www.un.org/esa/socdev/enable/dissre00.htm. Accessed January 6, 2009.

US Department of Health and Human Services: *Healthy People 2010: Understanding And Improving Health*, ed 2, Washington, DC, 2000, US Government Printing Office.

VanLeit B, Starrett R, Crowe TK: Occupational concerns of women who are homeless and have children: an occupational justice critique, *Occupational Therapy in Health Care* 20:47–62, 2006.

Vik K, Lilja M, Nygård L: The influence of the environment on participation subsequent to rehabilitation as experienced by elderly people in Norway, *Scand J Occup Ther* 14:86–95, 2007.

Wilkinson R, Marmot M, editors: *Social Determinants of Health: The Solid Facts*, ed 2, Copenhagen, 2003, World Health Organization.

World Federation of Occupational Therapy: Online. Available at: *Position Paper on Community Based Rehabilitation*, 2004. http://www.wfot.org/office_files/CBRpositionFinalCM2004(2).pdf. Accessed June 5, 2009.

World Federation of Occupational Therapy: Online. Available at: *Position Statement on Human Rights*, 2006. http://www.wfot.org/office_files/HumanRightsPositionStatementFinalNLH(1).pdf. Accessed June 5, 2009.

World Health Organization: *International Classification of Functioning, Disability and Health: ICF*, Geneva, 2001, Author.

World Medical Association: Online. Available at: *World Medical Association Declaration of Helsinki: Ethical Principles for Medical Research Involving Human Subjects*, 2003. http://www.wma.net/e/policy/b3.htm. Accessed May 26, 2008.

Domestic workers' narratives: transforming occupational therapy practice

37

Roshan Galvaan

OVERVIEW

This chapter introduces my research into South African live-in domestic workers' experiences of occupational engagement. It explores the process of problem identification and the careful navigation of the ethnographic method. The four study participants' occupational profiles elucidated the multiple challenges and barriers that they experienced. An interpretation from occupational therapy perspective suggests how occupational therapists may contribute to working with domestic workers to facilitate change.

Introduction

The application of occupation in occupational therapy has predominantly been in relation to its therapeutic application within health institutions. However, occupational therapy theorists (Molineux & Whiteford 1999, Townsend & Whiteford 2004) have argued that the application of concepts of occupation has more than just therapeutic value. Practice accounts of occupational therapy with street children (Kronenberg 2005) and writers' groups (Pollard & Smart 2005) are two examples of the many instances where occupational therapists have reinterpreted their understanding of how concepts of occupation can be applied to benefit marginalized groups in society. The occupational therapy profession's extension of its borders holds the potential for addressing communities' socio-political demands through addressing occupational needs. This requires an appreciation of what the needs are, how to address these in a relevant

manner, and a sense of how policy can guide contributions to change. The shift in practice from traditional clinical settings necessitates that research is extended in a similar way.

This chapter presents research into the experiences of occupational engagement for live-in domestic workers in Cape Town, South Africa. It highlights the potential role of research in making the needs and rights of marginalized groups explicit. The chapter reflects on prior ethnographic research (Galvaan 2000) and suggests ways for occupational therapists to begin to identify research needs.

Problem identification: domestic workers as marginalized

Clinical practice has traditionally been the source of most research topics in occupational therapy. This has led to research often focusing on occupational performance components and improving an individual's function. My research interest began in a similar way, that is, while working with clients who had performance component deficits, presenting at a psychiatric hospital. I worked as an occupational therapist in a psychiatric unit for women at a tertiary (specialist) level hospital. During this time, I encountered young, 'live-in domestic workers' who had developed psychiatric diagnoses such as substance-induced psychosis, depression, and bipolar mood disorder. A domestic worker is someone who carries out household work in private households in return for

DOI: 10.1016/B978-0-7020-3103-8.00046-8

wages (Sharma 2003). The term 'live-in' refers to the form of accommodation where the domestic worker lives on the employer's property. The domestic workers whom I saw in the psychiatric unit were all black women, of rural origin, and under the age of 35. During therapy sessions, they shared how stressful it was for them to be away from 'home' and how they struggled to adapt to the work environment. It appeared that their difficulty in adapting to their work contributed to the development of their diagnoses. Their descriptions alerted me to the fact that much of what they did was work related. They had little access to alternative occupations that were more restful.

As a black South African living in a home and a community where domestic workers were routinely employed, I was conscious of the popular discrimination based on socioeconomic inequalities and racial injustices that often existed between the worker and employer (and employer's family). As an occupational therapist committed to equity and transformation in South Africa, I considered the rights of these clients in terms of the South African constitution (Constitution of the Republic of South Africa 1996). Discrimination was unconstitutional, a violation of human rights, and unethical. The evidence of human rights violations expressed by domestic workers exposed instances of dysfunction and possible occupational injustice. This context-bound experience led me to a theoretical exploration of the macro environmental factors before returning to conduct direct research with domestic workers. Exploring the macro factors allowed me to appreciate a comprehensive view of the extent of the phenomenon of domestic work.

Domestic work was most common among black female South Africans and originated during apartheid (Lessing 1994). Black women were coerced by poverty in rural areas to do domestic work. Currently domestic workers account for 8% of all formal and informal employment in South Africa (Stats 2007). However, they are regarded as easily replaceable, low skilled, and of little economic value to their employers (Grossman 1997). Employers undervalue their work, so that it is viewed as unskilled, women's work (Budlender 1997). The trend for domestic workers to be black women whose work is undervalued continues in post-apartheid South Africa (Hertz 2004, South African Department of Labour 2001, Woolman & Bishop 2007). A submission by domestic workers to the Employment Conditions Commission (South African Department of Labour 2001)

described the complaint that the workers were required to look after the welfare of guests who visit the household where they were employed without additional remuneration. There was no arrangement regarding the worker's responsibilities towards guests or her entitlement to some form of remuneration for the additional workload. This caused conflict, and employers were not always approachable to discuss concerns in this respect. The contract stipulated in the Basic Conditions Of Employment Act for domestic workers (Department of Labour 1997) could be used as the mechanism to dispute such 'unfair' requests. However, most domestic workers are often only notionally free to alter their conditions of employment (Woolman & Bishop 2007). Effective implementation of the basic conditions of employment remains elusive (Tweedie 2007). The vulnerability of domestic workers is not limited to the interpersonal relationships between the employer and domestic worker. Factors such as educational achievements, labor legislation, familial arrangements, and unemployment ratios all bear weight on the power differentials between domestic workers and their employers (King 2007).

Devaluing domestic work is not unique to domestic workers in South Africa. Similar concerns have been raised for domestic workers in urban India (Dickey 2000) and Canada (Barber 2000). In fact the problematic nature of domestic work is a global problem. Many domestic workers in the European Union are skilled professionals (Anderson 2000). When migrating to Europe, their expertise may not be formally recognized and so they cannot realize the professional status that they previously had. Their invisible, low status, and low earning positions as domestic workers exacerbates this. However, driven by poverty in their original countries, they may have to accept domestic work as migrants (Anderson 2000). Despite that, their work continues to be devalued (Casco 2006). A small scale study in north London found that domestic workers were a hidden, but growing sector of the informal economy (Cox & Watt 2002). The American economy relies significantly on Latina immigrant labor (Hondagneu-Sotelo 2001). It is of significance to note that issues of domestic work are intricately related to political and economic factors associated with transnational migration (Blackett 2000).

Appreciating the socio-political concerns associated with domestic work helped frame the research. It supported the view that the factors contributing to domestic workers' occupational experiences are not limited or even unique to their individual work environments. The lack of diversity of opportunities (Human Rights Watch World report 2003) and occupations experienced by this marginalized group in their daily occupational lives seemed reflective of this category of workers. This perspective shaped my approach to the research. Literature, within the domains of labor and human rights has highlighted that domestic workers' poor work environments endanger their health (International Labour Organization 2008a,b). Consequently I decided to conduct a qualitative, ethnographic study into live-in domestic workers' experiences of occupational engagement.

Ethnographic data collection with domestic workers

The majority of live-in domestic workers in South Africa are isolated and not affiliated to trade unions. Initially gaining access to the scarce minority of 'organized' domestic workers was essential to ensuring the credibility of the research. Subscribing to the principles of ethnography (De Poy & Gitlin 1994) allowed me to further ensure credibility. These included becoming accustomed to domestic workers' circumstances and engaging in the research field for a prolonged period in order to establish trust with the participants. I sought opportunities to become more accustomed to the circumstances experienced by domestic workers. Establishing contact with key informants, attending workers' forum meetings, and reading domestic workers' narratives contributed to achieving this. I was aware of how I was different from live-in domestic workers. I also noticed the diversity and similarities between domestic workers' social histories, socioeconomic class, and use of language.

I gained access to three key informants (Hettie, Karen, and Patsy – pseudonyms used for confidentiality) through a social scientist who worked with local labor unions. Interviews and discussions with the key informants created the opportunity to explore personal accounts of what is was like to be a domestic worker and how this influenced what they did. Hettie was a proud domestic worker who was actively involved in the South African Domestic Workers Union. Karen had experience as a domestic worker. Patsy had recently left her job as a domestic worker and was hoping to find an administrative job

instead. I met with each key informant to discuss my research ideas and hear their opinions. They were skeptical of my concern with domestic workers given the differences in social class, but affirmed the need for a study with domestic workers and highlighted some of the problems that they experienced as domestic workers. During discussions with them, they agreed to contribute to accessing potential participants and to remain available for consultation. From discussions with the key informants, I started to consider how the issues of gender and power related to domestic workers work and subsequently their occupational engagement. Their skepticism shifted as they became clearer on how the research could inform current policies that affected domestic workers and as I continued to attend their forum meetings.

I attended workers forum meetings at the local parliament constituency advice office. These meetings offered domestic workers and those working in the hospitality industry an opportunity to voice their labor-related grievances and obtain advice or support from each other. This was a nonunionized forum where workers motivated each other. Discussions at these forum meetings confirmed that these workers' work and living conditions had a profound impact on their choices of occupations. It also allowed me to observe the unrestricted but respectful manner in which workers interacted and shared their stories, affirming that rich data could be collected through interviews.

My research explored domestic workers' experiences of occupational engagement from their perspective. I intentionally made no contact with the employers. Research into the employer–domestic worker relationship in post-apartheid South Africa revealed that conflicting relationships which disempowered domestic workers often existed between employers and domestic workers (King 2007). Of particular significance was employers' prejudiced attitudes toward domestic workers. Direct contact with domestic workers prevented potential distrust that I may be in alliance with potentially prejudiced employers. Furthermore, it affirmed and recognized their power as opposed to having the employer 'consent' to or 'order' the domestic worker's participation.

The following criteria were set for selecting four participants using snowballing sampling: they were able to communicate in English or Afrikaans; were between the ages of 22 and 35 and of rural origin (including small towns close to urban areas, but poorly resourced); should have been in their place of employment for at least three months; and have been working as domestic workers in Cape Town for a maximum of two years. Snowball sampling refers to a technique of sampling where the researcher selects participants who meet the necessary characteristics and through their recommendations finding other subjects with similar characteristics (Gobo 2004). Informed consent was negotiated and received verbally and in written format from each participant.

Each of the four participants contributed to an interview which was audio-taped. Interviews were transcribed verbatim and participants were assigned pseudonyms. The data were managed using the QSR NUD*ST Vivo computer software package. Content analysis was applied in order to identify, code, and categorize the primary patterns within the data (Patton 1990). Through content analysis, codes emerging from the data inductively were then labeled. Similar codes were grouped together to form subcategories. These subcategories were then incorporated into the dynamic systems theory (Gray et al 1996). The dynamic systems theory suggests that systems change with time and are complex, non-linear, and random. The concept of complexity was useful to this study because it emphasizes that levels of variables exist within the passage of time (Gray et al 1996). It provided a manner for analyzing how environmental factors interacted with other variables to form patterns of occupational engagement.

The participants' occupational profile

The four participants were Emma, Victoria, Nomfundo, and Eliza (pseudonyms used for confidentiality). Their occupational profiles highlight some of the main challenges that domestic workers experience.

Emma

Emma appeared as an energetic, 25-year-old, Afrikaans-speaking woman. I met her at her employer's luxurious double-storey home. The house was empty as her employers had emigrated to America earlier that month. Emma proudly related that she had completed high school and a secretarial diploma course.

She described occupational experiences of triumph and joy that she had had during this time. One such experience detailed the creative manner in which she initiated and organized a netball tournament between different hostels while at college. Through these stories it became clear that Emma was a person who thrived on meeting challenges and had been a leader at school and college.

After completing her diploma, Emma was unable to find work in her home (rural) town. She thus resorted to work as a domestic worker. After doing this for one year she returned to home, hoping to find secretarial work. Unable to secure employment there, she went to work in Cape Town instead. Emma had been working in her place of employment for 10 months at the time of the study. She had the responsibility of minding her employers' house until the weekend of the interview, when the house was being sold.

Emma was to start a new job on the day after the interview. Her employer had arranged that Emma could work for a friend. She made it very clear that she had to be interviewed before she started her new job, since she would no longer be allowed any outside contact or visitors. She vividly described the restrictions that she anticipated she would experience in this new job. This alerted me to the reality of 'restricted choice' when working as a domestic worker.

Victoria

Victoria was a pleasant, 26-year-old, Xhosa-speaking woman with a 4-month-old baby, Temba. She initially came to Cape Town to work as a 'pamphlet distributor' and 'tea-girl' for estate agents. When the company closed down, she started work at a restaurant in Sea Point. Continuous conflict with the patrons and management of the restaurant about the multiple tasks she had to complete simultaneously made this job too stressful, leading her to the decision to become a domestic worker.

Victoria sadly described how emotionally painful her first months as a domestic worker had been for her. She recalled missing her rural home and being especially concerned about her mother's health, who passed away soon after Victoria started domestic work. Victoria had worked for her employer for two years when Temba was born. Her employer would allow Temba to live with Victoria until he was a year old. Victoria felt unable to negotiate this condition and was very distressed because she wanted to be with her child. Also, since her mother died, she did not have anyone at home who could care for her baby. Victoria illustrated the price that she pays for having Temba with her. She worked with her baby on her back or by her side. She had to constantly fulfill roles as a mother and worker at the same time.

Victoria's work circumstances and her role as a mother impacted on the information gathering process. She did not arrive for the first meeting because her employer had given her extra tasks to do. She was late for the second meeting because she had to use her short time off to meet me as well as buy nappies for her baby. The third meeting was only half an hour because she had to fetch her employer's shoes. Victoria consistently apologized for being late and seemed genuinely embarrassed. Temba, who accompanied his mother, was cared for by Karen (a key informant) during the interviews. This led me to reflect on the impact that dual roles and rigid working conditions could have on an individual.

Nomfundo

Nomfundo was a 27-year-old, smartly groomed, Xhosa-speaking woman from a local, historically black township called Khayelitsha. She was eager to participate in the interview, saying that domestic workers needed to speak out. However, she also needed much reassurance about the way in which the information would be presented. Her concern was about being exposed and that this could lead to her losing her job. She explained that she had not completed her secondary education and had started to do a nursing certificate. She stopped when the college could not fund her any longer because of government retrenchments. Nomfundo had three young children, who lived with her mother in Khayelitsha.

Nomfundo expressed distress about the nature and consequences of her job. She felt that her employers ill-treated her, but that she had no choice because she needed the job. She related these experiences to her suffering physical symptoms of illness, such as headaches and ulcers. She attributed these symptoms to her experience of stress at work and her concern about her family's welfare. She also related how difficult it was to adapt to living and working in a new area.

Eliza

Eliza was a 26-year-old, Afrikaans-speaking woman from Bloemfontein with a 3-year-old daughter. She was recruited for domestic work by an agent who fetched 'girls' (as she refers to domestic workers) in her hometown. We met at a shop close to where she works and proceeded to her acquaintance's home for the interview. She was late for the interview because her employer insisted that she performed some trivial tasks (in Eliza's opinion) before she left – for example, having to do a few arbitrary articles of laundry and wake the employer's husband in order to make his bed before she left. She expressed immense irritation and resentment about these trivial tasks.

She had been at her current place of employment for two years. She expressed her frustrations regarding working long hours, not being given sufficient time off, and having to comply with her employer's whimsical demands. She also spoke of her sadness regarding not having had 'annual leave' in the two years. This meant that she hadn't seen her 3-year-old daughter for all this time. She hoped to go home for a week's holiday at the end of July, and she was worried that her daughter would not recognize her.

Live-in domestic workers' experiences: an occupational perspective

Domestic workers' occupational engagement was described as a tension existing between occupational engagement that was restricted and attempts to make the best of their situation and aspire toward a different future. The theme describing the experience of occupational restriction will be elaborated upon here, following which occupational therapists' potential contribution will be discussed.

Occupational restriction

The domestic workers felt that they had no choice but to sacrifice their education and endure separation from their families in order to earn a living. The restraining work environment controlled their living, working, and socializing environments (Galvaan 2000). These domestic workers had little or no opportunity to apply or develop their repertoire of skills. The environment was organized to match the employer's needs. Occupational restriction referred to the experience of occupational engagement that was significantly restrained by internalized oppression together with forces in the external environment. That is, the domestic workers' limited agency within their occupational engagement together with their orchestrated external environment, restrained their occupational engagement. This was consistent with the conceptualization of domestic work as a form of servitude (Woolman & Bishop 2007).

'Servitude is about caste or status. Persons in conditions of servitude occupy a social station that does not allow them to alter the conditions of their existence: their station makes it appear that they work "voluntarily" for those above them' (Woolman & Bishop 2007, p. 595). Immigrant domestic workers in America (Hondagneu-Sotelo 2001), Kuwait, United Arab Emirates, and Saudi Arabia have also been compared to bonded laborers, where employers may confiscate their passports (Rassam 1999). The devaluing of domestic work is perpetuated by the employers. Employers use expected personal distance to maintain the illusion that the domestic worker does not know the intimate details of the household. On the other hand, given the nature of the work, the domestic worker is very familiar with the details of the household. The employer denies this knowledge by exercising personal distance between themselves and the domestic worker and in this way is able to better exercise control (Hondagneu-Sotelo 2001). National policies in countries such as Thailand have supported the migration of women as it serves as a source of revenue (Nadeau 2007). Despite migrant work being encouraged since the workers help develop the host country's economy and help out in the service sector, they still face negative attitudes and have few support services (Ariffin 2001, Parrenas 2001). Furthermore, the majority of live-in domestic workers are exploited and are not affiliated to trade unions. The servitude experienced by domestic work becomes a violation of workers' human rights.

Towards equitable work for domestic workers

Domestic workers do not experience equitable access to opportunities or resources and experience occupational injustice in the form of occupational deprivation, occupational imbalance (Galvaan 2000) and occupational restriction. Underlying occupational determinants such as the division of labor, the employer–worker relationship and the historical context of domestic work perpetuated their way of being and doing.

Given that an occupational perspective of domestic workers' experiences borrows from other disciplines, it is imperative that the response to the issues raised in this chapter occurs as complementary to and in conjunction with other disciplines. Occupational therapists can collaborate with non-governmental organizations, such as Kalayaan, which works for justice for domestic workers in the United Kingdom (Kalayaan 2009), or trade unions (for example, SA Domestic Service and Allied Workers Union (SADSAWU)) in educating domestic workers and lobbying for change. This, together with encouraging domestic workers to unionize and organize themselves as workers is particularly important. This is especially so since they are a group which has had little positive experience with succinctly articulating their needs. One of the suggested strategies is for domestic workers to form cooperatives that provide domestic services (International Labour Organization 2008a). Occupational therapists could contribute to labor initiatives, such as the Unity Housecleaners Co-operative (Workplace Project 2009). Occupation-based support could involve the application of participatory and organizational development approaches to developing domestic workers' entrepreneurial capacity. This would complement the skills development that they may already have access to through various training facilities. Opportunity exists to contribute to the International Labour Organization, which has recognized the need for and has programs dedicated to fair globalization of and decent work for all (International Labour Organization 2008a). These focus on creating opportunities for social, economic, and political empowerment and rights, and dignity. Working toward this means working against poverty and for justice. Furthermore, the global presence and extent of domestic work presents the possibility for international collaboration between international occupational therapists working with domestic workers.

This chapter has illustrated that domestic workers' marginalization is reflected in their occupational engagement. It has raised awareness of the global presence of this phenomenon and made suggestions for future research and practice to promote equity for domestic workers.

References

Anderson B: *A Foot in the Door: The Social Organization of Paid Domestic Work in Europe. Doing the Dirty Work? The Global Politics of Domestic Labour*, London, 2000, Zed Books.

Ariffin R: *Domestic Work and Servitude in Malaysia*, Hawk Institute Working Paper Series, Adelaide, 2001, University of South Australia.

Barber P: Agency in Philippine women's labour migration and provisional diaspora, *Women's Studies International Forum* 23:399–411, 2000.

Blackett A: *Making Domestic Work Visible: The Case for Specific Regulation. Social Dialogue, Labour Law and the Labour Administration Department*, Geneva, 2000, International Labour Organization.

Budlender D: *The Second Women's Budget*, 1997, Cape Town, Idasa.

Casco RR: Lighting a torch for empowerment – 'We matter,' say Filipino domestic workers, *World of Work Magazine* 58:12–15, 2006.

Constitution of the Republic of South Africa: Government Gazette, *Government Gazette* 1–147, 1996.

Cox R, Watt P: Globalization, polarization and the informal sector: the case of the paid domestic workers in London, *Area* 34:39–47, 2002.

De Poy E, Gitlin LN: *Introduction to Research: Multiple Strategies for Health and Human Services*, St Louis, 1994, Mosby.

Department of Labour: Basic Conditions of Employment Act, *Government Gazette* 18491:1–79, 1997.

Dickey S: Permeable homes: domestic service, household space and the vulnerability of class boundaries in urban India, *American Ethnologist* 27:462–489, 2000.

Galvaan R: *The Live-In Domestic Worker's Experience of Occupational Engagement. Occupational Therapy*, MSc (OT), Cape Town, 2000, University of Cape Town.

Gobo G: Sampling, representativeness and generalizability. In Seale C, Gobo G, Gubrium JF, Silverman D, editors: *Qualitative Research Practice*, London, 2004, Sage.

Gray J, Kennedy M, Zemke R: Dynamic systems theory: an overview. In Zemke R, Clarke F, editors: *Occupational Science: The Evolving Discipline*, Philadelphia, 1996, FA Davis Company.

Grossman J: *Summary of Submission on Basic Conditions of Employment*, Cape Town, 1997, University of Cape Town.

Hertz T: *Have Minimum Wages Benefited South Africa's Domestic Service Workers? African Development and poverty Reduction: The Macro-Micro Linkage*, Lord Charles Hotel, 2004, Department of Economics American University.

Hondagneu-Sotelo P: *Domestica: Immigrant Workers Cleaning and Caring in the Shadows of Affluence*, Los Angeles, 2001, University of California Press.

Human Rights Watch World Report: 2003, Online. Available at: http://www.hrw.org/wr2k3/americas6.html. Accessed October 1, 2003.

International Labour Organization: *Decent Work for All*, 2008a, Online. Available at: http://www.ilo.org/global/About_the_ILO/Mainpillars/WhatisDecentWork/lang–en/index.htm. Accessed May 3, 2010.

International Labour Organization: *Working Out of Poverty*, 2008b, Online. Available at: http://www.ilo.org/global/About_the_ILO/Mainpillars/Workingoutofpoverty/lang–en/index.htm. Accessed May 3, 2010.

Kalayaan: *Kalayaan: Justice for Migrant Domestic Workers*, 2009, Online. Available at: http://www.kalayaan.org.uk. Accessed May 3, 2010.

King AJ: *Domestic Service in Post-Apartheid South Africa: Deference And Disdain*, Aldershot, England, 2007, Ashgate Pub Co.

Kronenberg F: Occupational Therapy with Street Children. In Kronenberg F, Simó Algado S, Pollard N, editors: *Occupational Therapy Without Borders: Learning Through the Spirit of Survivors*, Edinburgh, 2005, Elsevier/Churchill Livingstone.

Lessing M: *South African Women Today*, Cape Town, 1994, Maskew Miller Longman.

Molineux M, Whiteford G: Prisons from occupational deprivation to occupational enrichment, *Journal of Occupational Science* 6:124–130, 1999.

Nadeau K: A maid in servitude: Filipino domestic workers in the middle east, *Migration Letters* 4:15–27, 2007.

Parrenas RS: *Servants of Gobalization: Women Migration and Domestic Work*, Stanford, 2001, Stanford University Press.

Patton M: *Qualitative Evaluation and Research Methods*, London, 1990, Sage.

Pollard N, Smart P: Voices talk and hands write. In Kronenberg F, Simó Algado S, Pollard N, editors: *Occupational Therapy Without Borders: Learning Through the Spirit of Survivors*, Edinburgh, 2005, Elsevier/Churchill Livingstone.

Rassam Y: Contemporary forms of slavery and the evolution of the prohibition of slavery and the slave trade under Customary International Law, *Virginia Journal of International Law* 39, 1999.

Sharma K: In the name of Servitude. India Together 2003 (cited 3 July 2008). Available from: www.indiatogether.org/2003/sep/Ksch-domestic.htm.

South African Department of Labour: *Employment Conditions Commission report on the Domestic Workers Sector*, 2001, South African Department of Labour.

Stats SA: *Labour Force Survey*, 2007, Online. Available at: http://www.statssa.gov.za/publications/P0210/P0210September2007.pdf. Accessed May 10, 2008.

Townsend E, Whiteford G: A participatory occupational justice framework: Population based processes of practice. In Kronenberg F, Simó Algado S, Pollard N, editors: *Occupational Therapy Without Borders: Learning Through the Spirit of Survivors*, Edinburgh, 2004, Elsevier/Churchill Livingstone.

Tweedie D: *SADSAWU and COSATU Gauteng meet at Booysens Hotel*, 2007, Online. Available at: http://groups-beta.google.com/group/COSATU-Daily-News/web/sadsawu-and-cosatu-gauteng-meet-at-booysens-hotel-23-july-2007. Accessed April 28, 2009.

Woolman S, Bishop M: Down on the farm and barefoot in the kitchen: farm labour and domestic labour as forms of servitude, *Development Southern Africa* 24:595–606, 2007.

Workplace Project: *Unity Housecleaners Cooperative: Creating Alternatives to Exploitation*, 2009, Online. Available at: http://www.workplaceprojectny.org/index_files/Page840.htm Accessed May 3, 2010.

Universities and the global change: inclusive communities, gardening, and citizenship

38

Salvador Simó

OVERVIEW

The Project Miquel Martí i Pol integrates education, research, health, and the construction of inclusive communities. The project is based on a garden that was created jointly by occupational therapy students at the University of Vic and those who for many years have lived far away from town in situations of social exclusion, with mental health, poverty, and immigration survivors. The project is based on the integration of reality-grounded education with research. Universities must be a school for democracy and citizenship (Dewey 1969). The clients learn a profession and simultaneously they develop a meaningful occupation with a powerful therapeutic value. A key element of the project is to educate society about the value and potential of excluded people: they are citizens who are contributing to society. The outcome of the research is a contribution to the knowledge of human beings as occupational beings and the contribution of meaningful occupation to the wellbeing and the construction of inclusive communities and citizenship. The art of politics and partnerships is central to the process of creating a society based on the values of justice, equality, freedom, active respect, and solidarity.

Introduction

The poet and master Miquel Martí i Pol (Martí i Pol 1999), who lived for more than 30 years with multiple sclerosis, wrote (p. 70):

Beauty is your heritage
but you prefer
the sad and routine laziness

of a cardboard box ...
Let me say that it's time to love,
it's time to believe in miracles,
some day
there will be flowers in the garden and wind in the trees ...
Those, who for many years lived far away from town,
will be called to return.

These words inspired the decision to develop the Miquel Martí i Pol project: to transform an abandoned and sad space into a space of beauty, the garden. The garden was created jointly by occupational therapy students at the University of Vic and those who for many years have lived far away from town in situations of social exclusion, with mental health, poverty, and immigration survivors. The various dimensions of the project are described below.

Construction of inclusive communities

Poverty is avoidable (Sachs 2007), a sign of the lack of morality of our unfair societies (Pogge 2005). Occupational therapists concerned with social transformation are interested in the promotion of occupational justice (Townsend & Whiteford, 2006) and the creation of inclusive communities (Grady 1995). The author understands inclusive communities as those where all people can participate as equal citizens (Cortina 2005) despite any kind of occupational dysfunction. In this uncertain or 'liquid' time (Bauman 2005, 2007), it is extremely important to recover the sense of community, a place where we use the pronoun 'we' (Sennett 1998). The neoliberal

DOI: 10.1016/B978-0-7020-3103-8.00047-X

economy promotes individual atomism by breaking up natural and familiar communities. Governments that yesterday protected individuals through the welfare state now abandon them, psychiatrizing their problems despite their social and economic origin (Alvarez Uría 2006, Rendueles 2006). To have a job is a 'must' in our society, a condition of being socially accepted. When women and men lose their jobs they are also losing their life projects and their confidence in their ability to control their own lives. They are dispossessed of their dignity as citizens, their self-esteem, and the feeling of being useful to society (Linhart 2002).

The project has the objective of raising public awareness about the potential of these formerly socially excluded persons, breaking prejudices and stigmatic attitudes through their acquisition of a worker's role: the gardeners' work has given a garden to the community. We believe that the garden produces a powerful message, that has been spread widely through the mass media (TV, radio, newspapers, web), which in turn has helped the local community to understand that these formerly excluded people are citizens.

Education

While Dewey (1969) argued that the universities must educate citizens as a foundation of democracy, Harkavy (2006) denounces today's universities as being marked by commercialization (becoming dependent on and influenced by the interests of enterprises), Platonism (elitism and living in 'ivory towers'), and disciplinary ethnocentrism (interdepartmental conflict). Rachel Thibeault (2006) has suggested that our occupational therapy students are passing through university without gaining awareness about the global problems that determine their futures. In the face of the weakening of democracy, of the 'proletarianization' of the teachers (Tostado 2006), Tocqueville (2007) alerted us to the dangers of soft despotism, a political control based on persuasion and manipulation.

The project is also confronting the ecological crisis. We were told by Ann Coffey (cited in Houghton 2003): 'There cannot be a better place than our educational centers to begin the greater task of Humanity, to re-connect with our natural world' (p. 23). While the students have participated in reality-grounded learning about occupational therapy, they also have understood the connection between human

occupation and the ecological crisis (Boff 2000, Suzuki 2002). Gardening can be considered as an ecopation (Persson & Erlandsson 2002, p. 93), a term denoting occupations that are performed with concern for the ecological context at a pace that gives room for reflection and experience of meaning.

Health

Gardening enables human beings to reconnect with nature, and emerge from their immersion in a cyber-world dominated by the instrumental reasoning which orders people to fit the rational economy of its design (Taylor 1994) and the consequent ethics of the machine society (Persson & Erlandsson 2002). It enables the capacity of introspection, to connect with oneself as well as promoting a feeling of relaxation and wellbeing, developing motor skills as well as cognitive and affective. In a time of atomism (Taylor 1994) gardening is a social occupation that allows people who may have acquired a sick role and may feel socially excluded to adopt the new roles of carer and gardener. It is an esthetic experience, a ritual of creation of beauty and life, which confers an artistic gaze or perspective on the participant, to work listening to the water falling, seeing the colors of the plants, smelling the scent of the flowers, touching the bark of the trees. The garden is a metaphor for the process of recovery. During the winter we must work hard although we do not see the results, in the hope that they will arrive in the spring.

Gardening has a deeper sense in this liquid modernity (Bauman 2005, 2007), it gives roots to the human being, a place of meaning and belonging (see Chapter 23).

Research

This project has generated new knowledge about the human being as occupational being, the therapeutic impact of gardening, the potential of meaningful occupation to the creation of more inclusive communities and the promotion of citizenship, and the political art of partnership (Fig 38.1).

The project

The two key questions at the beginning of the process were: Where will the users come from? How will we be able to finance it? Thus, coordinated by the

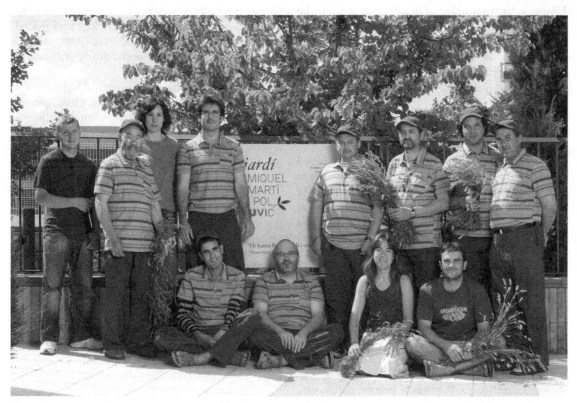

Fig. 38.1 • The gardening team.

occupational therapy university school, the project has involved a group of political, social, and business institutions, and showed the need for occupational therapists to develop political skills. Occupational therapists need to be proactive and ready for leadership and entrepreneurship in order to develop transformative social projects.

The clients, referred to later on as the gardeners, came from Caritas Arxiprestal and Osona Mental Health Foundation. The inclusion criteria were that participants should be persons experiencing social exclusion, mostly related to mental health issues, poverty, and the motivation to be engaged in gardening. Funding for the project was obtained through Caixa de Sabadell Foundation (bank), Rotary Club Osona, Provincial Government of Osona, Vic City Council and the University of Vic.

Gardening sessions took place two days per week from 9.00 to 11.00 am. The process of creating the garden took 18 months, from March 2005 to September 2006. Not only did the participants become gardeners, but they have also acquired the role of conference speakers, talking about the project

at the Universities of Vic (Simó Algado et al 2007), Granada and Valencia. Educational tours were developed, with a masterclass for all the team at the gardens of Alhambra in Granada, and in some of the best gardens of Spain. The project continues, since the garden needs continual maintenance. On average eight gardeners attend the program at any time. Four of our gardeners have placements in local companies. A webpage has been created, and we are filming a social documentary.

Currently we are negotiating a formal contract with the University of Vic to be responsible for all the green spaces of the campus, to eventually realize the author's vision of converting the whole university into a garden that also will be an art exhibition space. When today's cities are becoming spaces of segregation (Bauman 2005, 2007), it is so important to ensure that universities promote public spaces in which citizenship can be built and enjoyed.

The garden has been included in the project 'A European Learning Partnership: Empowering Learning for Social Inclusion through Occupation', which has just been approved by the European

Union, with the participation of partners from the Netherlands, Greece, Belgium, and Spain. It is part of the project for 'Competences for poverty reduction', with 14 European partners, funded by European Union and led by Hanneke Van Bruggen, also approved during the writing of this chapter.

Research

The research did not seek neutrality; it was developed within a critical ideology. One cannot forget what was seen in the valleys of suffering. The personal journey of the author, as a human being and as professional in Bosnia, Guatemala (Simó Algado 2004a, Simó Algado et al 1997), Kosovo (Simó Algado 2004b, Simó Algado et al 2002) and in Spain, working with prisoners (Simó Algado et al 2003) and immigrant survivors, profoundly influenced this research. Functionalist and structuralist interpretations of social exclusion must be confronted with chaos and social conflict theories to gain a fuller understanding of them (Galheigo 2004), otherwise we are just blaming the victims for their situation. This research was intended to give voice to persons silenced by our society's obsession with physical beauty, narcissism, appearing youthful, and efficiency. This was a transformative project within a critical paradigm inspired by Participatory Action Research (PAR) (Cockburn & Trentham 2006). Marx (1970) pointed out that philosophers had been only concerned with understanding the world, whereas the real need is to transform the world and make it better. Mounier (cited by Esquirol 2001) compared this cycle of reflection and action with the movements of systole-diastole in the human heart, close to the cycles of PAR.

The theoretical basis for the project is transdisciplinary, influenced by Morin's (1999) and Ira Harkavy's (2006) denunciation of disciplinary ethnocentrism. A complex problem must be confronted through a complex vision, so the theoretical base of the research was based on political, psychological, sociological, ecological, educational, philosophical, and occupational perspectives.

Antecedents and motives for investigation of this issue

Sempik et al's (2003) scientific literature review about the therapeutic application of gardening concluded that evidence for its effectiveness as a

therapeutic tool was scarce. The most rigorous studies came from an environmental psychology background. Sempik et al (2005) developed an in-depth research evaluation of therapeutic horticulture, studying 24 projects, with diverse users.

In their study with elderly people Milligan et al (2003) reported that the major benefit from gardening activity was the feeling of mental wellbeing. Frumkin (2004) called for investigations into the impact of the nature on human beings. Yamane et al (2004) and Son et al (2004) tried to control all the variables to be able to replicate the studies and utilized electroencephalograms and electromyograms to test whether the work with plants had an influence on relaxation.

Anitha Unruh (2004) utilized in-depth interviews to examine the meaning of gardens and the practice of gardening for survivors of cancer. She concluded that gardening has a deep meaning for people who face critical illnesses. Our research adopted this qualitative orientation to explore the meaning of the gardening project for its protagonists.

Participatory action research

PAR (Cockburn & Trentham 2006) is a process by which questions are systematically examined from the re-lived perspectives and experiences of those community members who are especially affected by the issues under review. What meaning did the creation of the Martí i Pol garden have for the participants?

Due to the group's characteristics, with basic education, language, and communication problems and no experience in previous studies, the project team leaders felt that it would be difficult for the group to develop the investigative questions, although this was not ruled out. The purpose of the investigation was proposed and explained to the participants, who were then asked whether they considered it important to continue. With their assent we went on to agree research questions, but as the group did not make any proposals it was decided to base these on the theoretical framework already elaborated by Sempik and colleagues (2005). Having agreed the themes for the investigation, the participants gave written consent.

The investigation was based on ethical criteria. It was decided that, to have a more global understanding about the experience, the investigation would gather not only the voices of the gardeners but those voices of all the institutions represented by the persons involved in the project or representatives and students involved in the project. The main means of collecting the information were in-depth interviews based on the theoretical framework and the investigation of Sempik; the interviews were undertaken with the representatives of the University of Vic (Rector of the Universitat de Vic, Director of Health Sciences School), social (President of Caritas NGO, Occupational Therapist Osona Mental Health Foundation), public, and business (President of Rotary Club) institutions (City council, Osona Provincial Government), students and gardeners.

The results of the research

It was extremely important to give voice to those silenced by society because they have mental health or other issues, developing a sociology of emergences (Sousa Santos 2005). Different themes were identified through the comparison of the narratives in each group with those of the others to develop a dialog. This approach was inspired by the discursive ethics of Habermas (1999), as it defends a morality of equal respect and solidaristic responsibility for everybody. Based on the in-depth interviews all 14 voices were internally analysed and cross-referenced (five gardeners, two students, and seven institutions) to define categories which related to the questions of the investigation. The process considers a thematic analysis to ascertain how the individuals create meaning according to their experience. The transcribed interviews were read both in a complete and in a segmented way many times, and the investigator was immersed in the data. This allowed themes to be identified and their interrelations to be established. The compilation and the analysis of the data did not take place in a linear fashion, but simultaneously.

In this section I present the themes and some narratives that are representative of each one of these themes. Paco, Plácido, Mustapaha, Benaissa, Eli, and Rafa are the gardeners and students; 'Vic' represents the person in charge of the social affairs department at the Vic City Council; 'Rector' is for the Rector of the Universitat de Vic; 'Director' is the Director of the Health Sciences University School; 'Osona' represents the person in charge of the social affairs department at the Osona Provincial Government; 'Rotary' stands for the president of the Rotary Club; 'Caritas' is for the president of Caritas; and 'FCMPPO' represents the occupational therapist at this mental health foundation.

BUILDING MEANINGFUL OCCUPATION

We start from a situation of occupational deprivation and from the difficulty of being integrated in the labor market:

> 'We do not have spaces where these persons can occupy their time in a meaningful way, we lack work rehabilitation projects' (Vic)

Occupations have to be meaningful occupations:

> 'it is important for these people to occupy their time in a meaningful way ...' (Vic)

The project influenced the transition from the sick person's role to that of caregiver, gardener and citizen:

> 'the role of caregiver ... to know that the plant is alive thanks to you, you feel better about yourself...' (Plácido)

The project has increased the possibility of finding work:

> 'All the people that have left the project have found a job, they are in a normalized life, they fly alone now' (Caritas)

GARDENING AS A SOURCE OF HEALTH AND WELLBEING

Meaningful occupation promotes health and physical wellbeing:

> 'Yes, yes, it makes you to do exercise, if not you would be at home doing nothing' (Plácido)

And psychological wellbeing:

> '...because you have an occupation your mind is clear, and you have no paranoid thoughts' (Plácido)

This wellbeing is translated into a feeling of happiness:

> 'Yes, when you come here you find happiness' (Mustapha)

Participants show an improvement in their self-esteem:

> 'You can achieve a higher degree of self-esteem'.

And a feeling of being useful:

> 'because before I was a non-useful person. But now, working here, I feel useful' (Paco)

And social wellbeing:

> 'I was not going out home before. Here I find company that is very important when you live alone, because solitude is very bad' (Paco)

Its impact has a spiritual dimension:

> 'Yes, yes, I recognize the garden as a part of myself. It will last with me, apart from the medical visits it is the most important part of my life' (Paco)

And the sense of contributing to humanity:

> 'I have contributed to the kindness between mankind' (Benaissa)

The garden becomes a spiritual sanctuary, offering a religious experience:

'my soul likes all that I do here ... it helps me to open my heart' (Benaissa)
'This job will help us to open the gate to paradise' (Benaissa).

Contact with nature has had a therapeutic impact:

'When I see the plants I feel alive, because 'through them I see life' (Mustapha)
'When I am in a closed space for a long time I feel bad, anxious, but in the garden I feel as if I'm at home' (Paco).

THE DIGNITY OF CITIZENSHIP

Participants see that their work changes social perceptions:

'they are used to news such as that a schizophrenic has killed someone, and now they see that mentally ill persons can contribute to society with a garden ...' (Plácido)

Despite the persistence of stigma:

'We are in a society where people who do not fit the standards are stigmatized ...' (Rector)

The gardeners demanded to be heard and to have more opportunities:

'They do not listen to us ... they should understand what it means to have a mental illness, a bipolar disorder ...' (Paco)
'persons with mental health problems [need more opportunities so they] can contribute more to their communities (Plácido)

They gained experiences of empowerment. The gardeners saw that they were able to influence their own lives:

'What Martí'i Pol wrote was very nice [your hands will be made of wind and light] ... that if you want, you can. Although you are ill, you can do important things in your life' (Paco)

THE CONSTRUCTION OF INCLUSIVE SOCIETIES

Social inclusion has been promoted by facilitating the creation of inclusive communities:

'I am known by more people in Vic in two years than in 15 years in Centellas ... the garden helped me to enter the community' (Paco)

There was social recognition for the gardeners:

'If you have shaken the hand of Rector of university and he's given you a diploma, this has as much meaning for me ... as I've got married again ...' (Paco)

It is shown to be vital that their voice was heard:

'Look, we went to Granada to give a conference. I felt myself as important as Mr Zapatero' (Paco)

A UNIVERSITY AT THE SERVICE OF THE HUMANITY: A NEW EDUCATIONAL PRAXIS

The purpose of the University is to educate compromised citizens, aware of the socio-ecological reality:

'To educate so students possess the spirit to contribute to the improvement of world and the society' (Rector)

This mission is in danger:

'The University should help the society to avoid dying [from indifference]. If the term University only implies knowledge, it wouldn't serve anything ...' (Caritas)

We cannot ignore the risk of commercialization of the University, the increasing pressure to generate economic benefits:

'Each time the University is expected to educate according to the demands [of graduates'] employers ...' (Vic)

The project has been a school for citizenship through the transformation of educational praxis:

'It has been more meaningful than all the talk around citizenship that a politician can give me' (Eli)

It has materialized the relationship of the University to the community:

'... what I would emphasize more is that this project opened the University to the socially disadvantaged' (Osona)

The project integrates education, investigation, and social intervention:

'It already has an extraordinary value, if only for this integration between education, research, and the compromise with the territory' (Rector)

It enabled learning grounded on reality, a transition from theory into practice:

'I have had the opportunity to see people achieve their own bio-psycho-social and spiritual equilibrium through meaningful activity', (Rafa)

The students have looked beyond the diagnoses to discover the person and his or her potential:

'each of them has shown excellent potential for humanity, generosity, sympathy, commitment, friendship ...' (Eli)

The garden has been a place to encounter the Other, enabling students to develop their empathy:

'It made me see the world from the other perspective; from the point of view of those socially considered as the 'others' (Eli)

THE ART OF THE STRATEGIC ALLIANCES AND SYNERGIES

The public, social and business institutions, and the University have recognized the need to develop strategic alliances. It was important to also recognize the contribution of the third sector in maintaining wellbeing:

'To maintain wellbeing, it's important to take account of the public and the Third Sector's powers, as these strategic alliances are indispensable' (Vic)

The project can serve as a model or an example of good practice to be continued at both university level and at the broader level of social policy, influencing the meso and exo as it has already been replicated by Caritas and FCMPPO and it is being disseminated in Europe via the European Network of Occupational Therapy in Higher Education as 'Example of good OT practice in Europe' and Grundtvig and Competences for Poverty Reduction projects:

'It could be an example for others, with perspectives for other professions or groups ...' (Rector).
'FCMPPO has evaluated the possibility of reproducing a similar project ...' (FCMPPO)

Discussion

A 'job' is a 'must' for social integration in our modern capitalist societies, where a huge part of humanity is considered just superfluous, a 'residue' of the economic system. Neo-liberalism imposes individual atomism, job precariousness, and is destroying the social welfare society. It assumes the appearance of a judicial state, based on personal security and the policy of fear. We must go further than our naive analysis if we want to promote occupational justice. We must develop our political dimension, not just talking about politics, but doing politics. The art of strategic alliances with political, social and business sectors forms a basis for the construction of a society, based on the values *justice, equality, active respect, freedom,* and *solidarity*. We must begin from micro and meso levels, growing toward the macro levels. From the author's practical experience, political activism means a vision, partnership, leadership, entrepreneurship, courage, compromise, determination, resilience, empowerment, and to inhabit a space of 'magic realism', balancing the utopian vision that guides us with the hard reality we are confronting.

The project Miquel Martí i Pol is generating knowledge about the human being as an *occupational being*. It is demonstrating more than the link between gardening and the health and wellbeing of the people

at the physical, psychological, social, and spiritual level. The connection between occupation and health is especially relevant as a medium to empower the person and the experience of meaning in life while avoiding paranoiac thoughts. *Meaningful occupation* is a powerful instrument for the creation of more inclusive communities where all the members can participate as citizens with equal rights, recovering the dignity of citizenship and the sense of belonging and common interdependence. The education of society is a basic role for occupational therapists, converting stigma and prejudice into social recognition, and making it possible for 'the Other's' voices to be heard, in a sociology of emergences (Sousa Santos 2005). Qualitative research (based on in-depth interviews or life histories) and use of mass media (the project has appeared on TV, newspapers, and radio) and audiovisual communication (we have a website and we are making a social documentary film), and active participation of the clients in the promotion of the projects (the gardeners have given conferences at several universities) have a critical role in this purpose. A PhD research study 'Health, citizenship and sustainability through new educational praxis' is currently being developed by the author, to increase the knowledge of occupational being and the power of meaningful occupation.

Universities have to transcend the 'ivory tower' and deconstruct the walls that separate them from society. The moral independence of a university is dogged by the pressures of *mercantilization, platonization*, and by *disciplinary ethnocentrism* (Harkavy 2006). Remembering Dewey's guidelines (1969), university students have not only gained knowledge about contemporary reality, but also are working for social and ecological change, 'doing' the change, and becoming social and ecological activists. This project demonstrates a new educational praxis adapted to the New European Space of Higher Education, which provides the transition of theory into practice and puts students in contact with the Other, transcending diagnoses. It not only transmits the knowledge of occupational therapy in a reality-grounded context but also promotes the ecological education of our students through being in contact with green spaces and developing their own reflections as a result. Such education is basic for the survival of the planet (Houghton 2003). In the face of the soft despotism (Tocqueville 2007) and the 'proletarianization' (Tostado 2006) of university teachers, we must revitalize universities as the foundation for citizenship and democracy. Once again it has proved the potential, value, and generosity of those 'who have lived for long time outside the village'. It is time to call them back, as they are the 'majority world' (Thibeault 2006) and it is our indisputable responsibility. As the poet said 'all is still to be done, but all is possible' (p. 174), working together with our clients 'our hands will be of wind and light' (p. 60).

It seems difficult to summarize more than two years of experiences, after so many moments of struggle, of exhaustion, of hope … so many visions and moments shared. Miquel Martí i Pol (1999, p. 207) wrote some verses that express the perfection we have experienced in the garden:

It is thanks to love that

Roses are growing from our fingers

And we apprehend all the mysteries

And in love all is fair and necessary.

Acknowledgments

This research was conducted for the Bachelor's Degree in Advanced Studies at the PH doctoral program in *Inclusive education and socio-educative attention through the life span*. The resulting work received unanimous outstanding merit marks from the academic tribunal. The PhD study *Health, citizenship and sustainability through new educational praxis* has already received an honorary mention by the Ferran Salsas Research Awards.

A photo exposition and a DVD on the development of the project is available from Salvador Simó (salvador.simo@uvic.cat). Universitat de Vic. Escola Universitaria de Ciències de la Salut, Sagrada familia 7, 08500 Vic (Spain).

References

Alvarez Uría F: *Pensar y Resistir. La Sociología Crítica Después de Foucault*, Madrid, 2006, Ediciones Ciencias Sociales.

Bauman Z: *Vidas Desperdiciadas: la Modernidad y Sus Parias*, Barcelona, 2005, Paidós.

Bauman Z: *Tiempos Líquidos: Vivir en Una Época de Incertidumbre*, Barcelona, 2007, Ensayo Tusquets Editores.

Boff L: *La dignidad de la tierra. Ecología, mundialización, espiritualidad. La emergencia de un nuevo paradigma*, Madrid, 2000, Editorial Trotta.

Cockburn L, Trentham B: Investigación Acción Participativa: Creando Conocimientos y Oportunidades Para la Involucración Ocupacional. In Kronenberg F, Simó Algado S, Pollard N, editors: *Terapia Ocupacional sin Fronteras: Aprendiendo Del Espíritu de Supervivientes*, Madrid, 2006, Editorial Médica Panamericana.

Cortina A: *Ciudadanos Del Mundo: Hacia Una Teoría de la Ciudadanía*, Madrid, 2005, Alianza Editorial.

Dewey J: The ethics of democracy. In *The Early Works of John Dewey, 1882–1898*1:Carbondale, 1969, Southern Illinois University Press.

Esquirol J: *Què es el Personalisme? Introducció a la Lectura d'Emmanuel Mounier*, Barcelona, 2001, Editorial Pòrtic Panorama.

Frumkin H: White coats, green plants: clinical epidemiology meets horticulture, *Acta Horticulturae* 639:15–25, 2004.

Galheigo S: Occupational therapy and the social field. In Kronenberg F, Simó Algado S, Pollard N, editors: *Occupational Therapy Without Borders: Learning Through the Spirit of Survivors*, Edinburgh, 2004, Elsevier/Churchill Livingstone.

Grady AP: Building inclusive community: A challenge for occupational therapist, *Am J Occup Ther* 49:300–310, 1995.

Habermas J: *La Inclusion Del Otro*, Barcelona, 1999, Paidós.

Harkavy I: *The Role of the Universities in Advancing Citizenship and Social Justice in the 21st century. Education, Citizenship and Social Justice 1:1. Descargado el 5 de enero de 2007 desde*, 2006, Online. Available at: http://esj.sagepub.com. Accessed January 5, 2007.

Houghton E: *A Breath of Fresh Air: Celebrating Nature and School Gardens*, Toronto, 2003, Learnxs Foundation.

Linhart D: *Perte d'emploi, perte de soi*, Paria, 2002, Erès.

Martí i Pol M: *Antología Poética a càrrec de Pere Farres*, Barcelona, 1999, Edicions.

Marx K: Theses on Feuerbach. In Arthur CJ, editor: *The German Ideology*, New York, 1970, International Publishers.

Milligan C, Bingley A, Gatrell A: *Cultivating Health: Study of Health and Mental Well-Being Among Older People in Northern England*, Lancaster, 2003, Institute for health research. Lancaster University.

Morin E: 1999, *Los siete saberes necesarios para la educación del futuro, Online. Available at:*http://unesdoc.unesco.org/images/0011/001177/117740so.pdf. Accessed October 15, 2005.

Persson D, Erlandsson LK: Time to revaluate the machine society: post industrial ethics from an occupational perspective, *Journal of Occupational Science* 9:93–99, 2002.

Pogge T: *La pobreza en el mundo de los derechos humanos*, Barcelona, 2005, Paidós estado y Sociedad.

Rendueles G: *Pensar y resistir. La sociología crítica después de Foucault*, Madrid, 2006, Ediciones Ciencias Sociales.

Sachs J: *El fin de la pobreza*, Barcelona, 2007, deBolsillo.

Sempik J, Aldridge J, Becker S: *Social and Therapeutic Horticulture:*

Evidence and Messages from Research, Reading/Loughborough, 2003, Thrive/Centre for child and family research.

Sempik J, Aldridge J, Becker S: *Health, Well-Being and Social Inclusion*, Bristol, 2005, The Policy Press, University of Bristol.

Sennett R: *The Corrosion of the Character*, New York, 1998, WW Norton & Company.

Simó Algado S: The return of the corn man. In Kronenberg F, Simó Algado S, Pollard N, editors: *Occupational Therapy Without Borders: Learning Through the Spirit of Survivors*, Edinburgh, 2004a, Elsevier/Churchill Livingstone.

Simó Algado S: Children survivors of war. In Kronenberg F, Simó Algado S, Pollard N, editors: *Occupational Therapy Without Borders: Learning Through the Spirit of Survivors*, Edinburgh, 2004b, Elsevier/Churchill Livingstone.

Simó Algado S, Gregory JMR, Egan M: Spirituality in a refugee camp, *Can J Occup Ther* 61:88–94, 1997.

Simó Algado S, Mehta N, Kronenberg F, et al: Occupational therapy intervention with children survivors of war, *Can J Occup Ther* 60:205–217, 2002.

Simó Algado S, Pollard N, Kronenberg F, et al: Terapia ocupacional en el mundo penitenciario, *Terapia Ocupacional* 33:10–20, 2003.

Simó Algado S, Carrillo B, Bourkha, et al: *Un Jardín Donde Confluyen la educación, la investigación y la ciudadanía*. Presentación audiovisual presentada en el V 'Congres de Educació en Valors' Vic. Spain, 2007.

Son KC, Song JE, Um SJ, et al: Effects of visual recognition of green plants on the changes of EEG in patients with schizophrenia, *Acta Horticulturae* 639:193–199, 2004.

de Sousa Santos B: *El Milenio Huérfano: Ensayos Para Una Nueva Cultura Política*, Madrid, 2005, Editorial Trotta.

Suzuki D: *The Sacred Balance*, Vancouver, 2002, Greystone Books.

Taylor C: *La ética de la autenticidad*, Barcelona, 1994, Paidos.

Thibeault R: Globalisation, universities and the future of occupational therapy: Dispatches for the majority world, *Australian Journal of Occupational Therapy* 53:159–165, 2006.

Tocqueville A: *La democracia en America*, Madrid, 2007, Akal.

Tostado G: El papel del académico en la construcción de la democracia. Reflexiones a partir del pensamiento de John Dewey, *Reencuentro* 46:96–104, 2006.

Townsend E, Whiteford G: Un marco de referencia de la justicia ocupacional participativa: Procesos y práctica centrados en la comunidad. In Kronenberg F, Simó Algado S, Pollard N, editors: *Terapia Ocupacional sin Fronteras: Aprendiendo del espíritu de supervivientes*, Madrid, 2006, Editorial Médica Panamericana.

Unruh AM: The meaning of gardens and gardening in daily life: a comparison between gardeners with serious health problems and healthy participants, *Acta Horticulturae* 693:67–73, 2004.

Yamane K, Kawashima M, Fujishige N, Yoshida M: Effects of interior horticultural activities with potted plants on human psychological and emotional status, *Acta Horticulturae* 639:37–43, 2004.

An occupational perspective on participatory action research

39

Wendy Bryant   Elizabeth McKay   Peter Beresford
Geraldine Vacher

OVERVIEW

To improve services, a significant resource of
expertise could remain unexplored if people are
only asked about the services they have received.
The participatory action research described in this
chapter valued doing things together: to explore
personal perspectives, have new experiences, and
imagine future possibilities. Critical ethnography
deepened appreciation of what shaped the actions
of everyone involved (Madison 2005, Thomas 1993).
The findings confirmed that there were valuable and
important aspects of the local mental health day
services, which were being modernized.
Occupational therapy knowledge of participation
and occupation was a key resource, including the
person-environment-occupation model (Law et al
1996). This model shaped the research design,
which included various methods, such as
photography. These methods were used to
facilitate participation and dialog for mutual benefit.
An occupational perspective enhanced existing
social and political understandings of participation
(Beresford 2005, Cooke & Kothari 2001, Wilcock
2006) and occupational therapists are urged to
develop this work for the benefit of all.

Drawing on direct experiences raises questions about
how representative those experiences are, particularly when people give verbal accounts, synthesizing
experiences with thoughts and beliefs. Without an
occupational perspective, valuing the actions behind
the words, those who are unable, unwilling, or unin-
vited to contribute would not be included. This is as
important for research as it is for practice. In this
chapter, we describe how an occupational perspective shaped the design and implementation of a
participatory research project. The direct experiences in this chapter were those of people using
and working in mental health services. The services
were being modernized, in response to government
policy, generating anxiety and resistance. Critical
ethnography was used alongside participatory action
research, to directly engage with questions being
asked locally about interpretations of the policy.
The research involved collaborative phases of consultation, action, and evaluation. It was agreed that
three strands of the main action phase should focus
on social networking in contrast to other local initiatives in employment and volunteering.

Setting the scene: mental health day services and social inclusion

Prior to this research, in 2002, we conducted an independent review of local services using focus groups:
Wendy Bryant and Elizabeth McKay were researchers, and Geraldine Vacher a participant (Bryant et al
2004, 2005). Findings indicated that day services
could develop to provide a better experience for service users. In 2003, Geraldine was appointed to take
the findings forward for day services and approached
us for further involvement. This evolved into Wendy's PhD, with Elizabeth and Peter Beresford as
supervisors (Bryant 2008).

Although the initiative was local, the modernization of day services was driven by a United Kingdom
national agenda to promote social inclusion for marginalized groups, including people with mental health

© 2011, Elsevier Ltd.
DOI: 10.1016/B978-0-7020-3103-8.00048-1

problems (Office of the Deputy Prime Minister 2004). This had direct relevance to occupational therapy, shifting the focus from clinical settings to mainstream community resources (College of Occupational Therapists 2006). The very first day hospitals in the United Kingdom all offered occupational therapy in various forms, being set up to address the occupational (in its broadest sense), medical and social needs of people being discharged from hospital (Farndale 1961). Since then, day services have developed in partnership with social care and voluntary providers (Catty et al 2005). Locally, people could become involved in initiatives such as the Green Gym (BTCV 2009), meeting in local nature reserves to work with conservation volunteers. The local health promotion team actively recruited new members through their partnerships with day services staff.

Similar examples have been promoted as illustrations of social inclusion (National Social Inclusion Programme 2008), based on the belief that being included in community life through paid work, leisure activities, and transport is beneficial for everyone. At the time of this research, there was an emphasis on paid employment as a route to inclusion, raising questions about stigma, discrimination, and further exclusion of those who could not work. Critical responses to the focus on social inclusion point to its origins in promoting self-improvement, regardless of the resources available, further excluding those who do not make the effort (Levitas 1998). As an alternative diagnosis in mental health, social inclusion does not offer a sophisticated understanding of motivational problems (Morgan et al 2007). Questions have also emerged about the justification for labeling places such as sheltered workshops, day centers, and supported housing, as socially exclusive (Beresford & Bryant 2008, Parr et al 2004).

However, social inclusion is central to the recovery model, which considers every aspect of life, building therapeutic partnerships, and identifying priorities for positive change (Repper & Perkins 2003). The social model of disability highlights the external factors that create disability, which for mental health service users could be the hostile response of society to a person described as schizophrenic or psychotic (Tew 2005). These models have fostered a growing interest in factors that impact on peoples' lives beyond psychiatric and psychological symptoms (Beresford 2005, Tew 2005). This interest, which has been user-driven, professional and political,

was incorporated in the modernization agenda for mental health day services (National Social Inclusion Programme 2008), generating a strong local and national political significance for the research and for a wider audience (Beresford & Bryant 2008).

National policies also promoted user involvement (Hui & Stickley 2007), and so we started by establishing a forum for dialog and consultation between everyone involved. This forum was concerned with the overall modernization and the research, and so ownership was a complex issue. Conflicts arose occasionally from different understandings of what day services were for, shaping perceptions of personal power to influence service development directly or via the research. External factors, such as the financial crisis in the National Health Service in 2006 (Batty 2006), fueled beliefs that modernization was for economic reasons, undermining and disempowering those involved. There was a dynamic relationship between external factors, the forum, and the research. At the forum meetings, the research would be one agenda item alongside other issues, gradually taking a distinct path focused on social networking and directly involving service users in the separate strands of the action phase. A few people remained involved throughout, whereas others, as their circumstances changed, participated and moved on.

Those involved emphasized the importance of social contact and a safe place, reflecting the previous research (Bryant et al 2004), and to some extent the national government report on social inclusion and mental health, which used the term 'social networking' (Office of the Deputy Prime Minister 2004). At the forum, there was much discussion about this in relation to mental health. Online social networking was just emerging, generating curiosity to understand and define it in relation to shared experience. Experience suggested a continual process of renewing informal and meaningful contact with other people, often friends and family (Capra 2002). Establishing and sustaining social networks was more achievable and meaningful for many than finding a full-time paid job, offering a credible focus for the research. Two 'Social Networks' action days developed ideas, with the first directly influencing the design of the three strands. The second day launched the first strand (strand A), and also focused on developing and promoting local resources for social networking. Ethical approval was given for the three strands from the university and from the local health research ethics committee.

An occupational perspective on research design: the research topic

In addition to an occupational perspective on participation, the design of the three strands drew on the person-environment-occupation model to structure approaches to the topic (Law et al 1996). The reciprocal relationship between the forum and the research made this possible, subjecting theoretical perspectives suggested by Wendy to critical appraisal by service users and staff in a very practical way. There was a perceived threat to the resource center social lounges, used for informal social contact and building social networks for peer support. This threat came from the political view that such spaces were socially excluding, limiting opportunities to get involved in the wider community and creating dependence on clinical resources (Spencer 2004). However, no acceptable alternatives were known which could be easily accessed in the wider community, especially at times when mental health problems were overwhelming, and a safe and tolerant environment was needed. From the person-environment-occupation model, strand A focused on the environment of the social lounges, using photography. Like PhotoVoice, an emancipatory research method (Wang et al 2000), a research group captured images of this environment. They were involved in every part of the research process, producing a report calling for a safe space to be protected in day services for those who needed it.

A second concern was about using mainstream community resources for social networking (Office of the Deputy Prime Minister 2004), as these resources meant different things to different people. At the first action day, many different venues for social contact were identified and the information was organized into an index, the 'BITRA', which was essentially a list of places. But the service users wanted to know more about those resources which were valued by other service users. This evolved into the second research strand (strand B), the occupation part of the person-environment-occupation design. A second group developed the BITRA using a systematic approach and producing posters of the findings for local venues.

The final strand (strand C), concerned with the person aspect of the person-environment-occupation model, explored the roles that people played in user-led groups for social networking. A user-led group was defined as being a group organized by service users for themselves, without staff involved. User-led groups in mental health often offer informal social contact and occupation, sometimes alongside advocacy and campaigning. Locally, these groups were valued yet required new roles for service users and staff which were not always clearly understood. Ten members of three user-led groups were interviewed. The interviews were transcribed and analyzed for themes, which were also used for service development.

An occupational perspective on research design: participation and occupational form

People participated in different ways at the action days, forum and research strands, working together in a typical approach to participatory action research (Koch & Kralik 2006). From many perspectives, being physically present or offering a verbal contribution is assumed to be an indication of participation (Cooke & Kothari 2001). Considering participation from an occupational perspective requires a more inclusive and broader view of what participation is, engaging the whole person (Polgar & Landry 2004). Participation was not just an outcome but the primary focus of the process. People were considered to be participating in the research if they were *doing* something related to it: this could be achieved by paying careful attention to what people wanted and needed to do. This required constant review of the occupational forms of the research. These were *the ways of doing* the research, which took different forms to accommodate the various cultures associated with the day services, academic conventions, and personal identities. The research evolved its own specific occupational forms, such as the research groups. These groups resembled the familiar groups in day services and action research groups, but combined the two.

Freire (1970) was an important influence, sustaining an awareness of how acting and reflecting together could be used in research and service development. Ideas and experiences were shared and reflected on together, exploring the significance for individuals and for the services. Immediate and ongoing experience shaped interpretation of ideas as they unfolded. User involvement often means individuals working as a representative for others, and then being undermined as the authenticity and authority of their representative role is questioned (Beresford 2005). Bringing people together sidesteps this possibility of being undermined, and the social context gives an opportunity for people to examine the authenticity and authority of their own perceptions in relation to those of others. Freire described this process in terms of language and power. The potential to abuse power, as an oppressor, is within everyone, not just people designated as leaders. Naming experiences, or giving language to them can not only be an empowering process but also indicates power is being exerted (Freire 1970).

The idea of naming experiences was important, not just the naming process but also generating the experiences to be named. It could have been enough to gather people together and hear their stories. This approach is indicated by the consultative approach to user involvement (Beresford 2005). From a social perspective, people are being included within a restricted role as consultant. However, from an occupational perspective, this approach denies access to many people, for example those who are not comfortable sitting in prolonged meetings or who find it difficult to put their experiences into words. This research took an occupational perspective on research methods, creating varied occupational forms to enable people to share their experiences and ideas in diverse ways.

Strand A: 'The social lounge'

There were several resource centers locally, all with spaces for informal social contact and some of these spaces were called social lounges. One of these lounges was particularly valued by the people who used it, and so the first strand was focused there. A research group was set up, involving five service users, a member of staff, and Wendy, as facilitator. We took photographs of how the social lounge, dining room, and garden at one resource center were used for social networking. The service users believed that at certain stages of their lives it was important to have access to a safe space. This was a space where they were accepted by others present. They were not required to spend money, unless they chose to buy the cheap, hot food available. It was also a space where they could informally access information from each other about surviving the mental health services and recovery, enabling them eventually to plan to move on. As the services changed around them, including staff teams, they could build supportive networks with each other.

These views were synthesized from the photographs taken by the group. Careful and detailed preparation was required to set up the group. People attending the user/staff business meeting were consulted about using photography, which led to the research group taking place weekly on an afternoon when the resource center was not used by other groups. This meant that only those who chose to be involved would be in the photographs. At the first meeting of the group, we explored how people felt about photography, by asking them to show the group which side of the camera they preferred to be on. Some people preferred taking photographs, others preferred being photographed and others did not mind either way. One person was very interested in reading an account of another project using photography (Knowles 2000) and another contributed more significantly to the analysis of the photographs, being unwell and unable to attend regularly initially.

Strand B: 'Getting better by going out'

Strand B developed the index of local social and recreational activities. The research group consisted of four service users, a different staff member and Wendy, again as facilitator. The poster that summarized the findings was named 'Getting better by going out' by the group. To gather the findings, we created a checklist to evaluate the social and recreational activities known and valued by service users, using the questions listed in Table 39.1. The act of creating the checklist, using it, and analyzing the findings all demanded different skills and knowledge, which were shared within the group. One group member had administrative and organizational skills, which were particularly useful, but they experienced a period of mental ill-health requiring in-patient treatment during the middle weeks of the strand. This made participation very difficult, but not impossible, and contact was maintained. Wendy went to the ward to deliver and collect checklists, and another group member visited on a separate occasion. The work of the group extended to include many other day service users. The checklist was distributed to draw on their knowledge and cover a range of activities, resulting in 44 responses.

Table 00.1 Checklist questions for Strand B 'Getting better by going out'

1.	Is this a place you can go to on your own?
2.	The first time you go, how easy is it to get there?
3.	Are there accessible toilet facilities?
4.	How much does it cost to visit this place?
5.	Can you get refreshments at this place?
6.	Do people talk to you at this place?
7.	Would you feel comfortable starting up conversations at this place?
8.	Are there like-minded people at this place? (not just mental health)
9.	How does this place affect your mental health?
10.	Is there anything you do not like about this place?
11.	Is there anything you really like about this place?
12.	Would you visit this place again? And would you recommend this place to other service users?

This process prompted reflection on the barriers to social and recreational activities. Three group members decided to go to the cinema together and spent a meeting planning this, as some had not been to the cinema for many years. They gained valuable shared experience for reflection, particularly on what made social and recreational activities accessible to them and others. They identified a distinction between when it was preferable to conceal their problems, and when being a mental health service user was accepted, and did not have to be hidden. People had to make a choice, where possible, whether or not to reveal their experience (Thornicroft 2006). Places where being a mental health service user was accepted were valuable, because the risk of hostility was so much less.

Strand C: 'A state of flux'

Originally it was intended that the final strand, exploring the roles of service users in user-led social groups, would contrast with the previous two in method. It was planned that the researcher and interviewer would control the process of recruitment and data analysis. However, by this stage of the project, people were very interested in the research, wanting to help with recruitment, and requesting rapid feedback on the analysis. They recruited 10 people from three user-led groups, who described the groups in interviews at the groups' venues. The occupational forms of the groups varied, expressing different priorities and beliefs about mental health. A complex history preceded each of the groups, which suggested the title for this strand, 'A state of flux'. One group met in a large pub, having a hot drink together but otherwise taking a relaxed approach to social contact. Another group held structured meetings in a resource center, having funds for art materials and table games. New members had to agree to ground rules. The third group gathered in a room in a church building, and had frequent contact at other times. They support each other alongside a program of outings and events.

Data analysis indicated that while the location of the groups was important, there were many other factors that were equally important. These groups had to manage a balance between being supportive and not becoming overwhelmed by the many problems associated with life with a long-term mental health problem. For them, this balance meant forming supportive social networks but keeping an occupational focus. Being located in a pub might suggest that the first group were focused on alcohol. However, in the United Kingdom pubs have changed significantly in recent years, offering a social space to eat and meet friends. This group met on Monday mornings, drank coffee, did crosswords together and ate snacks, which were more affordable than in other local venues. Focusing on the roles of people in all the groups revealed issues of leadership, recruitment, retention and dealing with conflict. Being a group leader was demanding and not everyone felt confident about this commitment. In contrast, members of the group were not always aware of people in leadership roles, particularly in the first group. These findings deepened local understanding of how to support user-led groups sensitively.

Sixteen service users and two members of staff made a sustained commitment to these strands, but many more people participated. For example, Wendy was organizing an interview room at a resource center for the third strand and by chance met a person who attended the forum occasionally. She pointed out the new poster displaying the findings of the second strand on a wall nearby. Another person was very involved in debating the focus of the research and promoting the strands with other people, but did not join any of them himself. He believed his experiences were not so relevant because they were less recent, but his support was very valuable. The findings of the research supported his efforts to alert local politicians to how mental health service reform was being undermined by funding restrictions.

Critical ethnography

It was necessary to engage with what was currently happening and consider alternative possibilities. This demanded a critical approach to examining what was sustaining the day services in their particular form at the time. Thomas (1993) proposed critical ethnography as an active way of engaging with a setting, identifying, and exposing assumptions of everyone involved, including the researchers. This process makes space for alternative views. This required constant shifts in perspective: from being a therapist facilitating transformation, to being a researcher analyzing what happened, to being a person engaging with the many views, feelings, and ideas that people brought to the research. The literature on participatory action research offered little insight into how to manage these shifts, and to what extent a facilitator should be a tool and resource for the setting and its participants (Cook 2005, Koch & Kralik 2006).

It was impossible not to engage with the questions people were asking about the modernization of day services, and not to respond to the fact that the action days were heavily supported by service users who wanted to use every opportunity to get their voices heard. There was a danger that energy would refocus on implementing new ideas without question, losing the critical edge provoked by the modernization agenda. The literature on critical ethnography confirmed and enhanced the importance of everybody's critical edge (Madison 2005, Thomas 1993): the right to question without being dismissed, challenged aggressively, or undermined.

Critical ethnography emphasizes how the researcher can respond to the research setting, with particular attention to ethical issues (Madison 2005). Traditionally, ethnography involves a systematic process of uncovering what happens in a particular setting, emphasizing culture (Hammersley & Atkinson 2007). Taking a critical approach involves questioning what is driving those occupational forms or ways of doing things (Thomas 1993), from asking about particular groups or procedures to exploring

the metaphors involved (Madison 2005). At one early forum meeting, the day services were described by Wendy as 'a muddy puddle', to capture the difficulties of working with many different needs with scarce resources. This led to questions about what resources there were and why they were scarce. Later, at the first action day, the metaphor of a fish in a fish-tank emerged, inspired by the film *Finding Nemo* (Stanton 2003). This metaphor was used to convey the restrictions placed on service users, and their sense of alienation from the wider world.

Contrasting the 'muddy puddle', which might dry up at any moment, and a fish-tank, an artificial environment restricting its inhabitants provoked more responses. Critical ethnography is concerned with revealing these different responses and the assumptions which underlie them (Thomas 1993). The modernization project had been initiated in an effort to use resources more effectively and promote social inclusion, whereas the service users sensed the possibility of increased restrictions on their lives as services were reconfigured or reduced. Yet a limitless ocean was not helpful, as unlimited resources could be overpowering, restricting opportunities to develop independence from day services.

Although service users took control of parts of this research, it was not possible for them to take over completely. This was mainly because it was a doctoral study and also because of the complex collaborative partnerships with the statutory and nonstatutory organizations involved. It was necessary to be very honest about what was driving the research at every stage, and to engage in critical reflection about the implications. One of the implications was the ongoing negotiations about ownership, as each stage evolved. This did not appear to be a barrier to people getting involved: it seemed as if they recognized and welcomed an opportunity to participate, knowing they could make autonomous decisions about their own participation but not having to take overall responsibility for the project.

Conclusion

Participation in this research meant doing things in varied ways, emphasizing different occupational choices and capacities, and making the most of resources immediately available in the setting. The most important resources were the people involved. Finding ways of adapting the occupations associated with the research was essential to promote and sustain their involvement. The experience of the research was often fun, challenging, and thought-provoking. Laughing, questioning, and reflecting together were consistent features.

The modernization project challenged the ways staff worked, as much as the service users' way of using the services, and the research offered them a means of exploring what this might mean. Not everyone took this opportunity up. Meaningful participation in any occupation cannot be forced. With a critical ethnographic approach, meaningful and helpful changes could be suggested, by and for the people who receive them. Using an occupational perspective made it possible to involve many different people who used and provided services. A practical and meaningful approach was taken to issues which were directly relevant to their experience. This understanding of participation and occupation is shared by occupational therapists yet not routinely used beyond therapeutic encounters. Occupational therapists could and should use their expertise in designing and using occupation in participatory action research to benefit everyone.

Acknowledgments

Funding was generously given by Brunel University, the Elizabeth Casson Trust, and the Institute of Social Psychiatry.

References

Batty D: The NHS Cash Crisis, *The Guardian*, 2006, Monday 24th April 2006. Online. Available at: http://www.guardian.co.uk/politics/2006/apr/24/publicservices.health. Accessed July 7, 2010.

Beresford P: Social approaches to madness and distress: user perspectives and user knowledges. In Tew J, editor: *Social Perspectives in Mental Health*, London, 2005, Jessica Kingsley, pp 32–52.

Beresford P, Bryant W: Saving the Day Centre, *Society Guardian*, p 5, 2008. Wednesday 11 June. Online. Available at: http://www.guardian.co.uk/society/2008/jun/11/mentalhealth.socialcare. Accessed June 29, 2009.

Bryant W: *An occupational perspective on user involvement in mental health day services*, PhD, West London, UK, 2008, Brunel University. Online. Available at: http://bura.brunel.ac.uk/handle/2438/3365. Accessed June 29, 2009.

Bryant W, Craik C, McKay EA: Living in a glass house: exploring occupational alienation, *Can J Occup Ther* 5:282–289, 2004.

Bryant W, Craik C, McKay EA: Perspectives of day and accommodation services for people with enduring mental illness, *Journal of Mental Health* 14:109–120, 2005.

BTCV: *Green Gym: how a Green Gym works*, 2009, Online. Available at: http://www2.btcv.org.uk/display/greengym_how. Accessed June 29, 2009.

Capra F: *The Hidden Connections*, London, 2002, Flamingo.

Catty J, Goddard K, Burns T: Social services and health services day care in mental health: do they differ? *Int J Soc Psychiatry* 51:151–161, 2005.

College of Occupational Therapists: *Recovering Ordinary Lives. The Strategy For Occupational Therapy in Mental Health Services 2007–2017. A Vision for the Next Ten Years*, London, 2006, College of Occupational Therapists.

Cook K: Using critical ethnography to explore issues in health promotion, *Qual Health Res* 15:129–138, 2005.

Cooke B, Kothari U: The case for participation as tyranny. In Cooke B, Kothari U, editors: *Participation: The New Tyranny?*, London, 2001, Zed Books, pp 1–15.

Farndale J: *The Day Hospital Movement in Great Britain*, Oxford, 1961, Pergamon Press.

Freire P: *Pedagogy of the Oppressed*, London, 1970, Penguin.

Hammersley M, Atkinson P: *Ethnography. Principles in Practice*, ed 3, London, 2007, Routledge.

Hui A, Stickley T: Mental health policy and mental health service user perspectives on involvement: a discourse analysis, *J Adv Nurs* 59:416–426, 2007.

Knowles C: *Bedlam on the Streets*, London, 2000, Routledge.

Koch T, Kralik D: *Participatory Action Research in Health Care*, Oxford, 2006, Blackwell Publishing.

Law M, Cooper B, Strong S, et al: The person-environment-occupation model: a transactive approach to occupational performance, *Can J Occup Ther* 63:9–23, 1996.

Levitas R: *The Inclusive Society? Social Exclusion and New Labour*, Basingstoke, 1998, MacMillan Press Ltd.

Madison D: *Critical Ethnography: Method, Ethics and Performance*, Thousand Oaks, 2005, Sage.

Morgan C, Burns T, Fitzpatrick R, et al: Social exclusion and mental health, *Br J Psychiatry* 191:477–483, 2007.

National Social Inclusion Programme: *From Segregation to Inclusion: Where Are We Now? A Review of Progress Towards the Implementation of the Mental Health Day Services Commissioning Guidance*, London, 2008, Department of Health.

Office of the Deputy Prime Minister: *Mental Health and Social Exclusion*, 2004, Online. Available at: http://www.socialinclusion.org.uk/publications/SEU.pdf. Accessed June 29, 2009.

Parr H, Philo C, Burns N: Social geographies of mental health: experiencing inclusions and exclusions, *Transactions of the Institute of British Geographers* 29:401–419, 2004.

Polgar J, Landry J: Occupations as a means for individual and group

participation in life.
In Christiansen C, Townsend E,
editors: *Introduction to Occupation.
The Art and Science of Living*, New
Jersey, 2004, Prentice Hall,
pp 197–220.

Repper J, Perkins R: *Social Inclusion and
Recovery*, Edinburgh, 2003, Balliere
Tindall.

Spencer A: Everyday Concerns, *NHS
Magazine* 2004. Online. Available at:
http://www.nhs.uk/nhsmagazine/
archive/oct04/feat13.asp. Accessed
May 17, 2005.

Stanton A: *Finding Nemo*, United States,
2003, Walt Disney Pictures.

Tew J: *Social Perspectives in Mental
Health*, London, 2005, Jessica
Kingsley.

Thomas J: *Doing Critical Ethnography*,
London, 1993, Sage.

Thornicroft G: *Shunned: Discrimination
Against People With Mental Illness*,
Oxford, 2006, Oxford University
Press.

Wang C, Cash J, Powers L: Who knows
the streets as well as the homeless?
Promoting personal and community
action through Photovoice, *Health
Promot Pract* 1:81–89, 2000.

Wilcock A: *An Occupational Perspective
of Health*, ed 2, New Jersey, 2006,
SLACK.

Researching to learn: embracing occupational justice to understand Cambodian children and childhoods

Melina T. Czymoniewicz-Klippel

OVERVIEW

Drawing on ethnographic data from a 10-month study on the reconstruction of childhood in Siem Reap, Cambodia, this chapter explores Cambodian children's perspectives on daily practices, or *everyday occupation*, that are meaningful and relevant to their unfolding lives. I begin by reflecting on how my history as an occupational therapist and the emergence of justice-related themes from the data influenced my selection of occupational justice as a conceptual research framework to apply to the research findings. Through this process, I discover a critical role for occupational therapy in childhood: giving visibility and voice to children regarding the enabling and disabling factors that mediate their engagement in everyday occupation. Then, to contextualize the possibilities of the occupational justice concept in the field of childhood studies, I present findings from my own research. By focusing on the occupational opportunities of female children, especially cognizant of their filial duties (whom I term *trying-to-be-good girls*), I confront the 'messiness' of Cambodian children's lives. In so doing I stress the incongruence between *trying-to-be-good girls'* occupational desires and the powerful global ideologies operating on them. I conclude that viewing children's lives through a narrowly focused, neocolonialist lens masks important determinants of children's occupational justice.

Part I: Embracing occupational justice

Over the past 10 years a small but committed global network of occupational therapists has guided the profession to reorient itself beyond the medical model of disability toward a perspective that additionally recognizes the social forces that affect population-level occupational performance (see Kronenberg et al 2005). In so doing, occupational therapy is arguably beginning to better satisfy its disciplinary responsibility toward ensuring all people who experience disabling conditions, not just those who are easiest to access, can collaborate with and benefit from its services (Kronenberg & Pollard 2006). Still, the profession could be achieving more by, inter alia, reframing cases of social exclusion in terms of preclusion from meaningful occupation, i.e. advocating an *occupational justice* perspective (Sakellariou & Simó Algado 2006), and examining the cultural relevance of its constructs (Iwama 2003).

Similarly, the field of childhood studies has recently confronted a directional crossroads in that major conceptual and epistemological challenges have emerged from its failure to enrich itself through greater interdisciplinarity (Prout 2005) and develop methods to better disentangle children's simultaneous vulnerability and agency (Bluebond-Langner & Korbin 2007). Unless further development ensues, 'childhood research risks becoming marginalized once more and will fail to provide an arena within which children are seen as social actors who can provide a unique perspective on the social world about matters that concern them as children' (James 2007, p. 261).

In this chapter, I illustrate the benefits of occupational therapists and childhood studies scholars pursuing closer collaborations. As an occupational therapist conducting research under the rubric of childhood studies, I consider myself not only well placed, but professionally obligated to contribute to greater collaboration between these two fields

DOI: 10.1016/B978-0-7020-3103-8.00049-3

of study. After all, as C Wright Mills (1959) reminds us, in being part of society we are also implicitly part of its problems. When conducting research, each of us unwittingly brings our background and experiences to our work (Ryan & Golden 2006). Therefore, understanding why I engaged the occupational justice framework in this research requires reflection on my professional experiences to date.

Disassociating from occupational therapy

Prior to commencing this research, I was somewhat disassociated from my qualifying profession, occupational therapy. This disengagement was born during the final years of my undergraduate years when, through the completion of one year's clinical interning within the Australian health system, I was taught to engage with occupationally deprived populations in a manner I considered unduly reductionist. That is, I was mentored to develop expertise in enabling clients to compensate for their biomedical deficits, with minimal regard for the social and structural determinants of their disabilities. I felt (then and now) decidedly uncomfortable in doing things *to* or *for* rather than *with* my clients, an approach which inevitably occurs when health professionals are positioned as experts. By the time I had graduated, I had begun to seriously question the models of mainstream occupational therapy.

After qualification, I initially pursued occupational therapy-specific work in Viet Nam (Simmond 2005). Yet, professional isolation and frustration regarding the perceived role of majority world-based occupational therapists soon drew me to seek alternative ways of engaging people who experience occupationally depriving conditions. For several years I worked with marginalized Asian families, first in Vietnam and then Nepal, contributing to projects framed within various development models. Then, on returning to Australia I engaged with refugee and asylum seeker populations through a human rights lens. At this time I attempted to reconnect with the Australian occupational therapy community; I published writings, delivered presentations, and lectures, and put forward innovative ideas for more radical practice. However, paid employment as a *non-traditional occupational therapist* remained elusive. After four years of navigating theoretical and conceptual borders, I found myself knowledgeable on many health and social science paradigms but master of few. It was time to more precisely articulate my professional niche.

Reconnecting with my disciplinary roots

In 2006, I enrolled as a doctoral candidate at Monash University and in noting the need for further research on globalization and children (Kaufman & Rizzini 2002, von Felitzen & Carlsson 2002), decided to research the influence of rapid social change on the social construction of childhood. Given its susceptibility to global influences through continuing dependency on foreign aid (Marston 2002) and rapid modernization (Sodhy 2004), and its especially youthful population – in 2004, over 60 percent of the Cambodian population was aged 24 years or less (National Institute of Statistics 2004) – Cambodia appeared an ideal study site. A village in Siem Reap town, which over recent years has experienced spectacular infrastructural change due to exponential growth in the tourism sector and foreign investment (Brickell 2008), was selected to provide greater understanding of the sociocultural changes accompanying Cambodia's transition to development.

It has been argued that scholars have comparatively obfuscated the more ordinary aspects of majority world children's everyday lives (Punch 2003). Considering my professional grounding in the concept of everyday occupation, tending to Cambodian children's mundane day-to-day experiences rather than a particular children's social problem seemed befitting. I proposed a grounded theory analytic approach to move the research towards theory development (Charmaz & Mitchell 2001); however, given the exploratory nature of the research, theoretical frameworks or models within which the findings could be framed were not able to be designated during the research design phase. Still, in acknowledging the discovery of a grounded theory indeed entails deductive effort (Markovic 2006), I reviewed relevant literature, including that of occupational therapy and science, to sensitize myself to the themes likely to emerge from the data and in doing so reconnected, albeit rudimentarily, with my disciplinary roots.

Discovering occupational justices and injustices

Following entry to the field, interviews and participant observation were commenced with a diversity of children (both boys and girls), as well as with adults of particular importance in their lives. Data collection and analysis proceeded concurrently to enable the identification and interrogation of themes using the constant comparative method (Glaser & Strauss 1967). As the fieldwork proceeded, repetitions regarding children's restrictions from everyday occupation, or *occupational injustices*, were discovered within and across the interview transcripts. Participants were particularly concerned about some children's lack of access to regular schooling, which was not surprising given the high levels of poverty (World Bank 2007) and corruption (Transparency International 2007) that ravage Cambodia, and the fact that attaining both a salary and moral virtue, ideally through individual education and merit rather than social networks (Dy 2004, Tan 2008), is essential for securing social value in the Cambodian context.

Many participants regarded children's failure to study a direct by-product of insufficient household income. Yet, previous research in both Cambodia (Ray & Lancaster 2005) and Cambodian diasporas (Okagaki & Sternberg 1993, Smith-Hefner 1993) indicates that multiple determinants underpin children's school attendance and performance. Acknowledging this, I collected further data to elucidate the factors impeding children's school participation and identified several outlying cases in which impoverished children had successfully assumed the occupational role of student. This confirmed my suspicion that poverty naturalizes and depoliticizes children's preclusion from the occupational right to education by reinforcing the structural inequalities of Cambodian society. Otherwise stated, while participants suggested children's actions were often severely limited by their disadvantaged position within hierarchical structures of social and economic status, opportunities for occupational engagement clearly exist.

I decided to inspect these standout cases within the broader scope of the research to interrogate the means through which participatory spaces are created for and by Cambodian children. Recently, Bluebond-Langner & Korbin (2007) called for the identification of conceptual frameworks through which childhood studies scholars can enhance their understanding of children's everyday, ordinary experiences as social actors. Indeed! Application of an occupational justice framework would accentuate those regular, daily activities that Cambodian children regard as meaningful and the factors that support or impede their engagement in them. Before fixing on an occupational justice framework, however, I needed to validate my selection through reflection on the congruence between the broader missions of occupational therapy and childhood studies, and the core purpose of my research.

Selecting a conceptual framework

While derivative of models of human development (Prout & James 1997), since the early 1990s the epistemologies underpinning the social study of childhood have shifted away from regarding children as mere embodiments of development toward also ascribing them a sense of present value (Christensen & Prout 2005). This has facilitated the now popular pursuit of listening to children to, among other things, inform practitioners and policy makers of the ways in which young people collectively give shape to and build meaning in their everyday lives (Alldred & Burman 2005). While this process is not without its problems and pitfalls (James 2007), if children are to be regarded as articulate spokespeople on matters affecting their lives, then adults must ensure their small, yet powerful voices are heard and respected.

Occupational therapists are, I suggest, ideally positioned to respond to this challenge of channeling children's standpoints. This is because they are masters at the art of developing practical, evidence-based strategies that focus on satisfying the self-identified needs of physically and socially disabled populations vulnerable to occupational injustices (Hasselkus 2002), such as children. And, while the profession has traditionally lacked power and in turn struggled to enable occupation for its consumers (Townsend 2003), its enabling perspective orients occupational therapists to people- or *client-centered* rather than agency-centered approaches. The utility of an occupational justice framework that extends understandings of social justice and human rights, then, lies in the visibility it brings to clients' own analyses of their involvement in everyday occupation rather than other power and justice-related issues, such as equity in resource allocation or access (Townsend & Whiteford 2005).

To this end, selection of an occupational justice framework would clearly promote my analysis of the meanings and dis/enabling factors underpinning Cambodian children's wishes to do, be, and become i.e. guide me to highlight children's desires within competing discourses of childhood. Beyond this, by promulgating justice in living fully as a specific goal for research/practice initiatives, occupational justice frameworks inherently engender action for change (Townsend & Wilcock 2004). Thus, in employing occupational justice to raise awareness of the power relations that influence Cambodian children's everyday activities I would also be well positioned to encourage development practitioners, one of the key audiences to whom this research aimed to speak, to better link global visions of justice with local, culturally determined occupational goals. Given the fact I had couched the research within a critical rather than traditional ethnographic methodology that stresses data production for the purpose of provoking social change (Simon & Dippo 1986), this point was significant.

Part II: Understanding Cambodian children and childhoods

In Part I of this chapter I reflected on the process of selecting a theoretical or conceptual framework that fits the data, supports the research and broader disciplinary aims, and facilitates the application of the research findings. To illustrate the value of employing an occupational justice framework in childhood research, I now present a case study that reflects the fragility of occupational justice in at least some Cambodian children's lives. This case study draws on evidence obtained from participant observation and semi-structured interviews conducted as part of a larger ethnographic project on competing understandings of childhood in post-conflict Cambodia. Girls are case studied because of the widespread belief, and indeed observed reality, that on the whole female children are more likely than male children to comply with the traditional moral code of Cambodian society.

The value of Cambodian children

While many of the participants I interviewed, both local and expatriate, believed that Cambodians chiefly value children for their economic worth, the findings of this and another (Smith-Hefner 1999) study suggest that Cambodian children are principally revered for their social value. Throughout the fieldwork I observed Cambodian babies and infants being admonished daily by young and old, relatives and non-relatives, males and females; they clearly brought immeasurable joy. Participants also

averred that without children a family is incomplete and lacking in 'warmth', the supposed reason for which childless couples often seek to locally adopt. Admittedly, I did observe instances in which structural inequalities pushed, or easy access to money enticed, children to engage in productive activities, thereby heightening financial interdependence within families. Still, adult participants, including those whose children worked, both reported and were observed as championing children's futures over their present earning capacities.

Parents of all social and economic statuses did, however, expect their children to assist them with housework or the running of the family business upon becoming 'a little bit big', i.e., from the age of 8 or 10. For the participants, a child's actions and behaviors underscored not only their own social and economic status in this *and* future lives, but also that of their kin. Given the interdependence of family members, parents reported raising their children to first and foremost appreciate their evolving social position and develop the knowledge and skills to progressively carry out their familial and communal obligations, rather than operate as individuals with rights of their own. From this perspective, childhood in the Cambodian context represents a period during which children mature and are matured in accordance with their inborn attributes and aptitudes so as to assume the position of valuable family member and citizen on coming of age.

Of all their social responsibilities, those that demonstrate children's reverence towards their parents were considered to be of greatest importance. This is because in Buddhist philosophy – Theravada Buddhism is the dominant religion in Cambodia – each birth represents the transmigration of a soul into a new and particular human (or animal) form on the basis of its store of merit, or *kamm* (Hansen 2004). As a local spiritual healer explained to me, upon being afforded life, the soul come child is immediately and forever indebted to those persons who gave it a body and whose flesh and blood it represents, i.e., its parents. Both child and adult participants described children's filial debt as being insurmountable and inalienable. The literature (Pyinnyāthīha 2002, Rahula 1978) states that Buddhist children have five broad duties: they must look after their parents in old age and illness, assist them with their work, revere them, perform their funeral rites after their death, and take care of the family reputation. These duties demand that children simultaneously attend school and work throughout their childhood.

Trying-to-be-good girls

Within the scope of traditional hierarchies of deference that position children inferiorly to adults, Cambodian children have restricted opportunities in which to exercise individual agency. However, through the influence and encouragement of powerful forces stemming from globalization, Cambodian children and youth are resisting adult authority and thereby facilitating a reconstruction of childhood (MT Czymoniewicz-Klippel, unpublished work, 2009). Still, as the local adult population is struggling to adjust to a more modern cultural framework, compliance with the traditional ideals of childhood remains the most effective means whereby Cambodian children can, regardless of their individual characteristics or living environment, negotiate social value.

Here, I refer to those female children living within the study village who were assessed by their families and neighbors as behaving with moral accordance while engaging in occupations that, within the traditional Cambodian view of childhood, are deemed socially worthwhile as *trying-to-be-good girls*. Driven by an internal desire to repay their parents' good deeds and ensure their own future success, these girls readily accepted punishment by their parents and significant others, because of their belief that adults genuinely act toward ensuring their childrens inclusion in society. They were chiefly driven by fear, for example, the fear of being publicly shamed, or creating unnecessary suffering for the family, or of witnessing the death of a parent through excessive work. They also pitied their parents for their commitments towards raising them and their siblings. For *trying-to-be-good girls*, helping their parents was considered 'as important as the whole wide world'.

During the fieldwork, I observed *trying-to-be-good girls* as independently negotiating time and space to achieve and maintain occupational balance. Most reported spending either a half or full day, depending on their school's requirements, tending to lessons. For some, this involved bicycling for 30 minutes into town, whereas others walked only a short distance to the village-based school. Outside school hours, *trying-to-be-good girls* chiefly occupied themselves with domestic duties, such as cooking rice, pumping water, and/or washing clothes. If/when necessary, they assisted their parents with business-related tasks. Some, for example, manned a stall at the local *phsar* (market) while others walked around the village selling seasonal fruits. In the early

evening, many attended the free or minimal cost foreign language classes offered by various Siem Reap-based nongovernmental organizations (NGOs). Bedtime was sometimes preceded by an hour or two of homework. Notably, play featured marginally in these girls' schedules, with most engaging in leisure activities only within the context of study or work. A typical day for Amom (all names used in this chapter are pseudonyms, chosen by the child participants themselves), a Grade 7 student, is illustrated in Box 40.1.

Barriers to occupational justice

During the interviews, both local and expatriate participants consistently cited wealth as the chief factor shaping children's occupational realities. This perception, which is widely represented in the Cambodian-based literature, including NGO reports, newspaper articles, and tourist magazines, creates a particular view of what Cambodian childhoods are: either occupationally deprived (if the household is poor) or occupationally satisfied (if

---

Box 40.1

Typical day of Amom, a 14 year old *trying-to-be-good girl*

- 5.30 or 6 am: Wake up, clean the house, wash dishes from the previous evening
- 7.30 am: Eat breakfast (leftover rice or instant noodles)
- 8.30 am: Buy ingredients from the market for cooking and iced coffee for father, cook rice and lunchtime meal, serve father's lunch, watch television
- 10.30 am: Gather mother and siblings, eat lunch
- 10.50 am: Rest for 10 or 15 minutes
- 11 or 11.15 am: Wash dishes
- 11.30 am: Take a bath, comb hair, change into school uniform
- 12 midday: Cycle to school
- 12.30 pm: Clean the classroom, do homework or review lessons
- 1–5 pm: Attend classes
- 5–6 pm: English lesson at a town-based NGO school
- 6–7 pm: Korean lesson at a village-based NGO school
- 7.15 pm: Cycle home, take a bath
- 8 pm: Eat dinner, watch television
- 9.30 pm: Go to bed

the household is rich). Yet, findings from the research suggest that it is far too simplistic to view children's occupational injustices as a straightforward financial problem. Not all poor Cambodian children fail to study, as the case of Pich, a 13-year old *trying-to-be-good girl* who migrated to the study village with her parents and nine siblings for economic reasons (see Box 40.2), illustrates. Pich, like the other *trying-to-be-good girls* involved in the research, stands out for her success in harnessing those internal (e.g., courage, initiative, determination) and external (e.g., supportive friendships, parental yielding, teacher flexibility) resources to which she has access in order to accrue the cultural power necessary to offset her subordinate social position. In doing so, she defies not only her own *kamma*, which the participants perceived as underpinning her impoverished living conditions but also stereotypes of Cambodian children as powerless victims of poverty.

Furthermore, the findings of both this and previous research (Bearup 2003) indicate that many better off children are also out of school, regularly truanting so as to join with romantic partners and friends, including those comprising gangs. As illustrated in Table 40.1, school enrolment and attendance is determined by myriad individual and environmental-level social and structural factors, including but not limited to class. Importantly, these factors can be combined almost innumerably and which act as enablers to occupational justice in some situations but inhibitors in others. A narrow focus on poverty therefore not only conceals the agency children mobilize in accessing opportunities for occupational engagement but also the complexity of determinants that mold children's occupational realities.

Thus, global forces that seek to ameliorate children's miseries can generate occupational barriers for those Cambodian children who wish to fulfill the traditional cultural ideals of childhood. As mentioned, these data indicate that simultaneous engagement in school- and domestic-related work is critical to Cambodian children's negotiation of a socially

 Box 40.2

Pich's story

At the time of accompanying her family to Siem Reap, Pich occupied herself by assisting her mother to sell cakes, corn, and snails from their home. One day, she queried her parents about the possibility of attending school. She had studied in the first grade in her home province and dreamed of completing Grade 12 and becoming a teacher. After hearing her daughter's request, Pich's mother was silenced for a minute or two and then stated that she was afraid of having to pay a high 'fee' to the teacher for her daughter's registration. While bitterly disappointed, Pich respected her mother's decision and continued to assist her in running the family businesses.

A few months later, Pich's aunt requested she accompany her cousin to study English at a nearby NGO school. Here she met Amom (see Box 40.1) and Chea who, in making small talk, asked Pich in which grade she was studying. Pich shyly replied, 'Nowadays I do not study'. Before entering the classroom, her new friends urged her to enroll to study at the nearby government school. During the English lesson Pich contemplated her situation, and after class dared to ask Amom and Chea whether they knew of how she could go about registering to study. They advised her of the necessary procedures and the small fee involved, suggesting she hurry as the once-yearly sign-up period was soon to close.

Later that evening, Pich spoke with her mother and was delighted when she granted her permission to register to

study. Her mother, however, would not be available to accompany her to the school as she had work and childcare commitments. Instead Pich asked Chea, who lived nearby, to bring her to the school. The next day Pich met the teacher, paid the 1000 Riel ($0.25 US$) registration fee and successfully enrolled to study in the Grade 1 morning class. Later she discovered that the timing of her study proved slightly problematic; her friend with whom she would share transport (a bicycle) studied in the afternoons. So, Pich bravely re-approached the teacher to request a change in class. Upon hearing of Pich's living situation, the teacher happily altered her enrolment and also informed Pich of her exemption from all further school fees.

Today, Pich attends school daily and continues to work in the mornings. She wakes at 3 or 4 am and accompanies her father to the market in the center of town, where they buy fresh produce for Pich to sell in the village. Then, from 6 or 7 am Pich mans a market stall, happily chatting with the other sellers and her customers as she works. On selling all the foods, she returns home and gives her day's earnings (perhaps 4000 Riel or $1 US$) to her mother. If needed, she helps her mother or older siblings with housework before preparing to go to school. After school, she studies English with Chea and her older sister and then bicycles home to turn in for the night.

Table 40.1 Selected reasons cited by the study participants as to why Cambodian children do not attend school

Individual-level factors

Age	Child is perceived by themselves and/or others as being too young or old to study
Cognitive capacity	Child lacks intelligence and/or good concentration and cannot keep up in class, which pushes them to stop studying prematurely
Physical, mental and emotional health	Child suffers illness or injury that prevents them from studying and/or working to finance their study Child is fearful, e.g., of punishment by the teacher, ridicule by other students or of being hit by gangsters while traveling to/from school Child feels discouraged, e.g., by consistent poor grades, lack of parental support, boring classes, knowledge of societal corruption Child is angered by the excessive surveillance, abuse, and neglect they face at home and retaliates by skipping school or running away with friends
Disposition and values	Child is rebellious, fun-loving, and/or easily influenced, which prompts them to engage in socially unacceptable behaviors including truancy Child is lazy, e.g., does not attend class when they do not have access to a motorcycle, but rather only a bicycle to ride to school Child strongly desires modern materials or wants to financially assist their poor parents, which leads them to champion work over school Child is obedient when their elders' request they stop school to begin working full-time Child is complacent towards corruption and aware of the willingness of their parents to pay for their grades, and thereby disvalues their education

Environmental-level factors

Geographical environment	Child lives nearby or far away from the school and is therefore encouraged to truant regularly Child regularly migrates, for example, with or without their family for employment
Financial environment	Child's parents/guardians lack the capacity to purchase school materials and/or pay informal school fees Child's parents/guardians can afford to purchase modern materials (mobile telephone, motorcycle) that encourages the child to truant with their friends Child's family incurs a serious financially disabling event e.g. severe illness or death of a parent
Familial environment	Child's parents/guardians do not emotionally or intellectually support the child in their studies (e.g., they fail to monitor their child's homework, grades or school attendance) Child's parents/guardians engage in blaming behaviors rather than taking individual responsibility for their children's schooling Child's parents/guardians are not aware of how to tend to enrolment paperwork and/or are fearful of having to pay teachers high facilitation fees Child's parents/guardians withdraw the child from school as a form of punishment or because the child brought shame to the family by grossly misbehaving at school
School environment	Child is unable to study because of school rules and regulations e.g., registration criteria, class size limits, rules regarding punishment for arriving late or misbehaving Child's teacher uses teaching methods that children find dispiriting, e.g., they are especially strict, violent, unimaginative or corrupt Teachers are time-starved, meaning they fail to closely monitor children's school attendance
Sociocultural environment	Child's parents/guardians lack the social capital necessary for, inter alia, facilitating school registration Child is discriminated against because of their individual characteristics such as behaviors, age, gender, birth position, class, ethnicity, educational status, physical appearance, perceived cognitive ability, and/or the nature of their familial relationships (e.g., birth versus adopted/stepchild)
	Child is considered as having a particular destiny that is determined by their *kamma* and ultimately cannot be reversed

valued identity. Further, none of the *trying-to-be-good girls* whom I interviewed perceived their work as negatively influencing their studies. Most prioritized their studies, for example, by 'releasing' themselves from certain labor-related tasks if/when necessary. However, all stated they would, albeit reluctantly, adjust their study schedule or temporarily postpone their classes in order to engage in full-time work should their family's financial situation change for the worse. When questioned on how they would feel if unable to assist their parents, several girls remained speechless, some spoke of emotional distress such as 'feeling hard inside' and one cried over her prospective uselessness and shame.

The vast majority (90%) of Cambodia's working children labor for their families in an unpaid capacity (World Bank 2006). In Cambodia, many externally funded development interventions implicitly seek to banish working children from the workforce altogether in spite of their sociocultural obligations, occupational desires, *and* the current labor law, which sets the minimum age of wage employment at 15 years and additionally permits children 12–15 years to engage in nonhazardous work that does not affect regular school attendance (National Assembly of the Kingdom of Cambodia 1997). For many of the expatriates whom I interviewed all forms of child work constituted exploitation. Such a position is comprehensible; from medical and education perspectives, children's working signals potential concerns regarding their health and learning (Waterson & Goldhagen 2007). From an occupational perspective, however, participation in everyday occupation underscores children's capacity to acquire skills and competencies, connect with others, and find purpose and meaning in life (Law 2002). As such, if access to the occupational repertoires which foster meaning in *trying-to-be-good girls'* lives are obscured by global policies and practices imported to eradicate child work/labor, then occupational injustices will certainly arise.

The costs of occupational injustice

Throughout the research, I observed *trying-to-be-good girls* as having their desirable behaviors reinforced by attentive parents, encouraging teachers, admiring neighbors, and supportive friends, which was in turn further motivating. Contrarily, children who voluntarily or because of structural inequalities were denied the opportunity to engage in culturally valued occupations provoked parental anxiety, which consistently resulted in some form of discipline. This and previous studies (Save the Children Australia 2006, Save the Children Norway 2006) document cases of children being beaten, blamed, physically confined or restrained, treated with indifference, disowned, and/or imprisoned as means of re-education, actions which overwhelmingly satisfy the Western definition of child maltreatment. Further, children perceived as failing to learn the moral code of Cambodian society were observed as being progressively marginalized from participation in mainstream society.

Needless to say, such disciplinary regimes incite physical and especially emotional injury, and for those subjected to occupational injustices over a prolonged period, risk occupational deprivation. The wider, long-term impact of Cambodian children's prolonged preclusion from engagement in everyday occupation is beyond the scope of full exploration here. According to Whiteford (2000), possible outcomes include lack of meaningful time use, deteriorating sense of efficacy, truncated identity constructions, maladaptive responses (e.g., suicide), and engagement in nonlegitimated occupational groups such as gangs. Whilst these consequences may sound extreme, my observations of the behaviors of occupationally dissatisfied boys indicates Cambodian children's participation in deviant activities, including community violence and substance abuse, is real and at least in part propelled by occupational deprivation (MT Czymoniewicz-Klippel, unpublished work, 2009). These issues warrant further inquiry as a matter of urgency both within and outside an occupational perspective.

Conclusion

This chapter explored the value of engaging an occupational justice perspective in childhood studies that strive to give greater visibility to children's standpoints. I have demonstrated, via the case of *trying-to-be-good girls*, that exploring children's daily activities through occupational eyes has particular advantages for understanding the perspectives of members of this typically voiceless group. I have also shown that occupationally focused research aids in troubling global discourses that fail to recognize the diversity and complexity of children's childhoods. Studies that exemplify what Hasselkus (2006, p. 627) refers to as the 'delicate layerings' of occupation are therefore critical inasmuch as when interventions, such as those instigated by development partners, fail to draw on nuanced cross-cultural perspectives, they do more than risk ineffectiveness; they raise the real danger of bringing harm to local populations. Confronting the global campaign for the universalization of childhood that opposes child work and so on, to facilitate the development of situated justice frameworks in which both local and global views on childhood are represented *and* respected will be neither easy nor neat. After all, like Cambodian childhoods occupational therapy is also highly gendered, lacking power and status within the professional arena within which it operates (Pollard & Walsh 2000, Sakellariou & Pollard 2008). But, should the profession wish to persist in promoting itself as one of enabling occupation, this is the type of challenge with which it *must* engage.

Acknowledgments

I am indebted to the *trying-to-be-good girls* who stepped outside cultural norms to share the intimacies of their experiences with *Borng Melina/Sophea/Macarena*, my local research team who toiled from morning to night, both in the office and ghost-ridden forests of Angkor, in pursuit of children's own constructions of life; the anonymous reviewers who provided helpful comments on earlier drafts of this chapter; and, my occupational therapy colleagues who, through their insistence on the power of occupation to counter injustice, have collectively facilitated my re-identification as an OTwB practitioner.

References

Alldred P, Burman E: Analysing children's accounts using discourse analysis. In Greene S, Hogan D, editors: *Researching Children's Experiences: Approaches and Methods*, London, 2005, Sage, pp 175–198.

Bearup L: *Paupers and Princelings: Youth Attitudes Towards Gangs, Violence, Rape, Drugs and Theft*, Phnom Penh, 2003, Gender and Development for Cambodia.

Bluebond-Langner M, Korbin JE: Challenges and opportunities in the anthropology of childhoods: an introduction to 'children, childhoods and childhood studies', *American Anthropologist* 109:241–246, 2007.

Brickell K: Tourism-generated employment and intra-household inequality in Cambodia. In Cochrane J, editor: *Asian Tourism: Growth and Change*, Oxford, 2008, Elsevier, pp 299–309.

Charmaz K, Mitchell RG: Grounded theory in ethnography. In Atkinson P, Coffey A, Delamont S, et al, editors: *Handbook of Ethnography*, London, 2001, Sage, pp 160–174.

Christensen P, Prout A: Anthropological and sociological perspectives on the study of children. In Greene S, Hogan D, editors: *Researching Children's Experiences: Approaches and Methods*, London, 2005, Sage, pp 42–60.

Dy S: Strategies and policies for basic education in Cambodia: historical perspectives, *International Education Journal* 5:90–97, 2004.

Glaser B, Strauss A: *The discovery of grounded theory: strategies of qualitative research*, London, 1967, Wiedenfeld & Nicholson.

Hansen A: Khmer identity and Theravada Buddhism. In Marston J, Guthrie E, editors: *History, Buddhism and New Religious Movements in Cambodia*, Chiang Mai, 2004, Silkworm Books, pp 40–62.

Hasselkus BR: *The Meaning of Everyday Occupation*, Thorofare, 2002, Slack.

Hasselkus BR: The world of everyday occupation: real people, real lives, *Am J Occup Ther* 60:627–640, 2006.

Iwama M: Toward culturally relevant epistemologies in occupational therapy, *Am J Occup Ther* 57:582–588, 2003.

James A: Giving voice to children's voices: practices and problems, pitfalls and potentials, *American Anthropologist* 109:261–272, 2007.

Kaufman NH, Rizzini I, editors: *Globalization and children: exploring potentials for enhancing opportunities in the lives of children and youth*, New York, 2002, Kluwer Academic/Plenum Publishers.

Kronenberg F, Pollard N: Political dimensions of occupation and the roles of occupational therapy, *Am J Occup Ther* 60:617–625, 2006.

Kronenberg F, Simo Algado S, Pollard N, editors: *Occupational Therapy Without Borders: Learning Through the Spirit of Survivors*, Edinburgh, 2005, Elsevier/Churchill Livingstone.

Law: Participation in the occupations of everyday life, *Am J Occup Ther* 56:640–649, 2002.

Markovic M: Analyzing qualitative data: health care experiences of women with gynecological cancer, *Field Methods* 18:413–429, 2006.

Marston J: Cambodia: transnational pressures and local agendas, *Southeast Asian Affairs* 95–110, 2002.

Mills CW: *The sociological imagination*, New York, 1959, Oxford University Press.

National Assembly of the Kingdom of Cambodia: *Labor Law*, Phnom Penh, 1997, Royal Government of Cambodia.

National Institute of Statistics: *Cambodia Inter-Censal Population Survey 2004*, Phnom Penh, 2004, Ministry of Planning.

Okagaki L, Sternberg RJ: Parental beliefs and children's school performance, *Child Dev* 64:36–56, 1993.

Pollard N, Walsh S: Occupational therapy, gender and mental health: an inclusive perspective? *British Journal of Occupational Therapy* 63:425–431, 2000.

Prout A, James A: A new paradigm for the sociology of childhood? Provenance, promise and problems. In James A, Prout A, editors: *Constructing and Reconstructing Childhood: Contemporary Issues in the Sociological Study of Children,* London, 1997, Routledge, pp 7–33.

Prout A: *The Future of Childhood,* London, 2005, Routledge.

Punch S: Childhoods in the majority world: miniature adults or tribal children? *Sociology* 37:277–295, 2003.

Pyinnyāthīha U: *The triple gem and the way to social harmony,* Penang, 2002, Triple Gem Publications.

Rahula WS: *What the Buddha Taught,* London, 1978, The Gordon Fraser Gallery.

Ray R, Lancaster G: The impact of children's work on schooling: multi-country evidence, *International Labour Review* 144:189–210, 2005.

Ryan L, Golden A: 'Tick the box please': a reflexive approach to doing quantitative social research, *Sociology* 40:1191–1200, 2006.

Sakellariou D, Simó Algado S: Sexuality and disability: a case of occupational injustice, *British Journal of Occupational Therapy* 69:69–76, 2006.

Sakellariou D, Pollard N: Three sites of conflict and cooperation: class, gender and sexuality. In Pollard N, Sakellariou D, Kronenberg F, editors: *Political Practice in Occupational Therapy,* Edinburgh, 2008, Elsevier Science, pp 69–89.

Save the Children Australia: *Child protection: child abuse, prevention and protection strategies in Cambodia,* Phnom Penh, 2006, Save the Children Australia.

Save the Children Norway: *Children's view on domestic violence: research into physical and emotional punishment of children in Cambodia,* Phnom Penh, 2006, Save the Children Norway.

Simmond M: Practicing to learn: occupational therapy with the children of Viet Nam. In Kronenberg F, Simo Algadó S, Pollard N, editors: *Occupational Therapy Without Borders: Learning Through the Spirit of Survivors,* Edinburgh, 2005, Elsevier/Churchill Livingstone, pp 277–286.

Simon RI, Dippo D: On critical ethnographic work, *Anthropology & Education Quarterly* 17:195–202, 1986.

Smith-Hefner NJ: Education, gender, and generational conflict among Khmer refugees, *Anthropology & Education Quarterly* 24:135–158, 1993.

Smith-Hefner NJ: *Khmer American: identity and moral education in a diasporic community,* Berkeley, 1999, University of California Press.

Sodhy P: Modernization and Cambodia, *Journal of Third World Studies* 21:153–174, 2004.

Tan C: Two views of education: promoting civic and moral values in Cambodia schools, *International Journal of Educational Development* 28:560–570, 2008.

Townsend E: Reflections on power and justice in enabling occupation, *Can J Occup Ther* 70:74–87, 2003.

Townsend E, Wilcock A: Occupational justice and client-centred practice: a dialogue in progress, *Can J Occup Ther* 71:75–87, 2004.

Townsend E, Whiteford G: A participatory occupational justice framework: population-based processes of practice. In Kronenberg F, Simó Algado S, Pollard N, editors: *Occupational Therapy Without Borders: Learning Through the Spirit of Survivors,* Edinburgh, 2005, Elsevier/Churchill Livingstone, pp 110–126.

Transparency International: *Report on the Transparency International Global Corruption Barometer 2007,* Berlin, 2007, Transparency International – International Secretariat.

von Felitzen C, Carlsson U, editors: *Children, Young People and Media Globalization,* Goteborg, 2002, UNESCO International Clearinghouse on Children, Youth and Media.

Waterson T, Goldhagen J: Why children's rights are central to international child health, *Arch Dis Child* 92:176–180, 2007.

Whiteford G: Occupational deprivation: global challenge in the new millennium, *British Journal of Occupational Therapy* 63:200–204, 2000.

World Bank: *Children's work in Cambodia: a challenge for growth and poverty reduction,* Washington DC, 2006, World Bank.

World Bank: *Sharing growth: equity and development in Cambodia,* Washington DC, 2007, World Bank.

Occupational injustioc in Pakistani families with disabled children in the UK: a PAR study

41

Debbie Kramer-Roy

OVERVIEW

This chapter describes both the processes and the findings of a participatory action research (PAR) project carried out with a group of Pakistani families with disabled children living in the UK. The research was conducted in the context of the author's PhD studies and therefore restricted in scope and length. However, it resulted in rich data and its findings are important for occupational therapists and others who work with Pakistani families. First the research process is described, which indicates how PAR can be used successfully with this population, keeping in mind specific cultural and religious characteristics as well as universal aspects. Then the findings of the study that relate to occupational science are presented, with a focus on occupational injustice and on cultural aspects. Key observations relate to the concept of belongingness and how the families experience a lack of this due to negative perceptions of disability in their community. The positive changes in their own faith led to positive perceptions and the ability to accept their disabled child and deal with community attitudes better. The PAR process fostered important life skills, enabling participants to reflect on and deal with the challenges of living with a disabled child better.

In the light of the recent development of occupational science, Wilcock (1999, p. 10) urges occupational therapists to take on the challenge to work not only with people with impairments of various kinds, but 'also with those suffering from the disorders of our time, such as occupational deprivation, occupational alienation, occupational imbalance and occupational injustice ... [in order] to enable occupation for personal wellbeing, for community development, to prevent illnesses and towards social justice ...'. Pakistani families with disabled children are one population that suffers from such 'disorders of our time'.

Pakistani families in the UK with disabled children

The reasons for choosing to conduct research with Pakistani families in the UK are twofold. First, my long previous experience of working in Pakistan (nine years) and with the Pakistani community in the UK (four years) means I have a relatively good understanding of their culture, religion and – importantly – language. The knowledge, skills and attitudes resulting from this experience have been instrumental in building up relationships in the Pakistani community and with the research participants, which have contributed to gaining rich data. Second, the limited amount of previous research paints a depressing picture of the Pakistani community in the UK, especially for families with disabled children. Compared to the total population of the UK, the Pakistani community faces higher levels of poverty and unemployment, poorer housing, prejudice based on both racism and Islamophobia,[1] and a lack of faith/culture appropriate provision of social and leisure activities (Government Equalities Office 2008, Khan 2006, National Statistics Website 2002).

Furthermore there is a higher prevalence of childhood disability in the Pakistani community (e.g. Morton et al 2002) and the families of these

---

[1] The term Islamophobia denotes the prejudice and discrimination against Muslims. In the UK it has been in use for around 20 years and it became more commonly used and understood after the Runnymede Trust, which promotes research and advocacy on issues around ethnicity and cultural diversity, published a report titled *Islamophobia. A challenge for us all* in 1997.

DOI: 10.1016/B978-0-7020-3103-8.00050-X

children face the additional challenges of the high cost of raising one or more disabled children, are less likely to receive benefits at the appropriate rates and face more difficulty in accessing health and social care (Beresford 1995). Although negative attitudes towards disability exist throughout society, some of the specific attitudes met in the Pakistani community, such as blaming the mother for the child's disability, a belief in disability as God's punishment and the subsequent lower levels of support received in the extended family and the community cause high levels of distress in the primary carers of disabled children (Bywaters et al 2003, Chamba et al 1999, Fazil et al 2002, Hatton et al 2004).

The need for critical (social) paradigm research

Although the above has been known from research findings dating as far back as the mid 1990s (e.g. Beresford 1995) more recent studies (e.g. Hatton et al 2004) suggest little progress has been made in either defining the specific support needs of this group more precisely, or in meeting these needs.

A critical social paradigm of research is most likely to be able to start unraveling the complex web of marginalization, made up of issues related to ethnicity, religion, disability and – for most carers – gender, which these families are caught up in. Within the critical paradigm, I have chosen to use participatory action research (PAR) to engage the families actively in identifying and starting to address their support needs within their families, in the community and/or through the service system (see Kramer-Roy 2007).

Participatory action research

PAR can be defined as 'an emancipatory practice aimed at helping an oppressed group to identify and act on social policies and practices that keep unequal power relations in place' (Herr & Anderson 2005, p. 9). A very important principle is that the lived experience and knowledge of the participants are directly valued and central to the process. The aims are to produce knowledge and action that are directly useful to the participants and to empower them through the process of constructing and using their own knowledge (Reason 1994). This approach to research very clearly recognizes that many real-life situations can not be accurately described or addressed by academic knowledge only, and can be seen as the bundling of practical-experiential and academic knowledge in order to improve the situation.

Although PAR is generally considered an approach, rather than a prescriptive method (e.g. Meyer 2006), a helpful way of describing action research is as a spiral of cycles, each of which consists of planning, action, observation of the impact of the action, and reflection on that action and its impact. It is a dynamic process in which these four aspects are not seen as static steps, but rather as moments in the action research spiral, (Kemmis et al 2004). An exploratory phase, in which the research participants identify the key issues to focus on in the research process, precedes this succession of cycles. What makes the process emancipatory is the fact that the participants are not only facilitated to address problematic situations in their lives, but also that they gain important research and problem-solving skills in the process (Fig. 41.1).

Congruence of PAR and occupational therapy

Trentham & Cockburn (2005, p. 440) observe that PAR is

> consistent with the values of occupational therapy and occupational justice' and is therefore a particularly suitable choice of approach to researching occupational aspects of individual's or families' lives.

First, the participants engage in an occupation that helps them 'to develop the skills and knowledge necessary to take greater control over their own lives; in so doing, they promote their own health as well as the health of other community members' (Trentham & Cockburn 2005, p. 446). Second, the approach to working as a team of co-researchers is very congruent with principles of client-centered practice, such as respect for people's skills and insights, taking responsibility for one's own choices, enabling participation, flexibility, and keeping in view the links between the person, their environment, and occupation (Letts 2003).

In both occupational therapy and PAR 'action' and 'collaboration' are central, whether they are implemented with individuals or groups. The successful outcomes of both processes depend much on the therapist or lead researcher's openness to learn from their partners, rather than viewing oneself as the 'expert'.

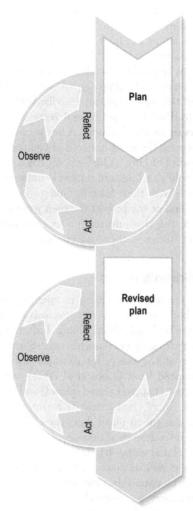

Fig. 41.1 • The action research spiral (Kemmis et al 2004, p. 4) Reproduced with kind permission of Professor Stephen Kemmis.

The study

The central research question for this study was as follows: 'How can families with disabled children be facilitated to identify their support needs and ensure they are met, within the family, in the community and/or through the service system?' Therefore *the process* of facilitating the participants to engage in the research was as important as *the content*, i.e., identifying their support needs. Within this occupational science offered a helpful perspective, but was not the main theme (see Kramer-Roy 2009, for the full thesis).

Six families participated in this study. In the exploratory phase, carried out in each family's home, all family members were involved in constructing their family story. For the main action research phase separate action research groups were formed for the men, women and nondisabled children of the families to engage with the issues in ways most appropriate to them. In these groups they identified key issues and planned, implemented, and reflected on action taken to address these issues. Because it was soon evident that this was the first time that participants were invited to reflect on their situation of living with a disabled child, and because recruitment difficulties led to a shorter period being available for the PAR process (around seven months), the 'action' focused primarily on gaining a better understanding of their specific issues and needs. Some steps were also taken towards meeting those needs, which the participants intended to build on beyond the project. An enormous amount of learning was gained from the process, both by the participants and myself.

The action research groups

Each group had its own unique dynamics and processes. As none of the participants families knew each other beforehand, initial meetings provided opportunities to share some of their stories and experiences. Once group members were comfortable with each other I explained the principles and purposes of PAR, emphasizing that the decisions and actions to be taken needed to be theirs, rather than mine. Even though each group was positive about this in principle, none of them found it easy to act accordingly and frequently asked me to take decisions or actions as I was 'much better at it'. Constant reminders that they were the experience experts, or the ones who had the right to ask questions, encouraged them to take over the reigns gradually. I will now describe how this worked out in each group.

The women's group

For the women the opportunity to come together with other women of their own cultural and linguistic background, who all had a disabled child, was probably the most significant aspect of the project. Introductory activities included making a drawing of an allegory about their child and filling out a worksheet to index their skills. Both these activities led to sharing of very personal stories, which they experienced as a very welcome opportunity for catharsis and mutual encouragement. On considering which issue to focus on in their own action research cycles, they decided that these meetings filled a gap in their local support system, and should therefore not stop when the research project finished. Their key action was to design and distribute leaflets inviting other Pakistani women to join their support group. The women continued to work on this after the project.

The men's group

The men started off by sharing one positive and one negative anecdote from their child's life, which set the tone for much openness in subsequent meetings – much more in fact than I had expected, based on my own experience, and other researchers' as well as Pakistani women's predictions. On reflection I recognize several reasons for this openness. The first reason is my unique position as both insider and outsider. The men realized I knew their country of origin, culture, religion, social issues, and language rather well, and did not feel they needed to hide anything for that reason. At the same time I was not a member of the local Pakistani community and therefore highly unlikely to feedback any 'gossip' into the local grapevines. In addition meetings took place in one of the local mosques, where they felt at ease, as it was a respectable public place and neutral territory.

In terms of their research focus, the men noted that attitudes towards disability in the Pakistani community are overwhelmingly negative, while their own attitudes towards their own and other disabled children are largely positive. As the negative community attitudes are mostly expressed in religious terms, they decided to consult Islamic scholars to find out what the Qur'an and other early Islamic scriptures actually teach about disability, so they could use that knowledge in challenging community attitudes. This information was not at all easy to come by and required much perseverance in getting appointments to see local scholars, emailing those in other countries and searching the internet.

Their search confirmed their expectation that the Qur'an does not provide a basis for negative attitudes towards disability. For example the only place in the Qur'an where disability is directly referred to, the verse serves to remove any stigma experienced in society: 'No blame will be attached to the blind, the lame and the sick. Whether you eat in your own houses, or those of your fathers, ... or any of your friends' houses, you will not be blamed'

(Qur'an, p. 24:61, translation by Abdel Haleem 2004). Eating together in Arabic culture implied a close association at equal footing and this verse is the clearest indication in the Qur'an that no moral judgment is applied to disabled people. Other issues like the concept of God testing believers and the duty to support the 'needy' are not described with explicit relation to disability, but general verses imply positive views on disabled people. A key message is that 'in God's eyes, the most honored of you are the ones most mindful of Him' (Qur'an p. 49:13), i.e., that in Islam people's abilities are relatively unimportant in comparison with their faith in God.

By the end of the project the men were considering how to use this information to encourage more positive attitudes in their community.

The children's group

The children took much time to open up and were initially both superficial and exclusively positive about living with a disabled sibling. I offered a number of activities to encourage more sharing of the other side of the story, for example the 'feelings cube' (adapted from Gibbs et al 2002), which had three positive (happy, excited, proud) and three negative (sad, angry, embarrassed) feelings on its six sides and was rolled like a dice; the child then told a story about a time their disabled sibling had caused them to feel that way or had felt like that themselves.

The children had quite a lot of knowledge about what research entails, but initially did not think children could carry out research themselves. Referring back to their own description of research as 'finding out information', 'observing' and 'asking the right questions' helped them to realize that they did indeed possess the required skills. Once the children were ready to start their research, they had clear ideas about their focus, i.e., to understand their disabled sibling better, so they could make him/her happier. They took a step towards this by writing stories about their sibling. The children indicated that this was the first time anyone had asked about their ideas and feelings about having a disabled sibling, or encouraged them to take decisions and plan and implement activities themselves. Organizing a family party, in which their disabled siblings could be fully included, was a very important opportunity to reflect on their disabled siblings' likes, strengths and limitations, to look for new ways of supporting them and to practice decision-making and planning skills.

Through the processes described above, the participants reflected on and shared with me their individual and family lives in much detail. The next section presents some of the findings from an occupational science perspective.

An occupational science perspective on the findings of this study

When I reflected on what this study has taught me about concepts of occupation relevant to these family's I took as my starting point Wilcock's (2006) 'formula': $d + b^3 = s\, h$. Or, put in words: doing, being, becoming, and belonging equal survival and health. In the women's group I asked the participants to reflect on the relative importance of and interplay between doing, being, becoming, and belonging in their lives, by manipulating four colored paper circles, cut along one radius, to form a pie chart. They found this very helpful. The circle in the picture shows how little one woman felt she was allowed to 'belong', or think about 'becoming'; she felt she was always 'doing' and that that was expected of her. However, her sense of 'being' was very important to her and had been influenced by her strengthened faith and resilience through raising her disabled child (Fig. 41.2). Some key findings related to these aspects of occupation follow, and implications for occupational justice will be pointed out where appropriate.

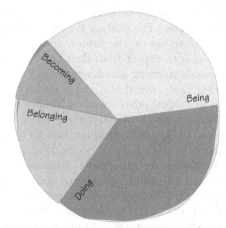

Fig. 41.2 • Paper circle used to explore $d+b^3$.

Belonging

The 'belonging' aspect was vitally important for these families. In the Pakistani cultural context interdependence is very important, in many respects more important than independence. There are advantages as well as disadvantages to this. When a girl gets married, the contract entered into is not just between her and her husband, but between the two families. In most cases the bride moves into her husband's home, but even if they live on their own, she still is responsible for keeping her in-laws happy, as that will also ensure a good relationship with her husband. Intimacy or support are not necessarily expected in the husband–wife relationship, although it is often present. The importance of being a good daughter-in-law also reaches beyond the family, as it affects the family's position in the community. 'Good' entails good housekeeping and cooking, raising respectful children, and avoiding anything that might blight the honor of the family. In a good, supportive family, this can be a very positive and safe situation, but in many cases the woman is constantly aware of having to maintain the family's stability – not an easy task in a culture where gossip and shame have much influence (see Campbell & Mclean 2003).

When a disabled child is born, community attitudes mean that the mother is often made to feel responsible for or guilty of this – the child's disability is seen as a punishment or a 'test' from God. All but one of the families report that this issue caused them much grief in the early months or years of their disabled child's life, but despite this they have all been able to accept their child and gradually come to the opposite point of view of seeing their child as a blessing. However, the contrast between the child's positive sense of belonging within the immediate family and the lack of acceptance in their extended family and community, including the Mosque, is an ongoing source of frustration and grief as it has significantly reduced the social contacts and support the families have.

In this family context, the nondisabled siblings tended to be very loyal to their parents, which meant they willingly shared in the care for their disabled sibling. At the same time, they were initially extremely reluctant to express any negative views about their sibling or parents until they realized that the other children in the group had similar experiences, and acknowledging and dealing with them did not mean a betrayal of their family.

A final observation on belonging is the feeling of 'homecoming' the women experienced in their research group – they strongly expressed how safe and accepted they felt in the group due to the shared background and issues, saying 'we don't need to defend ourselves' and 'it is so uplifting to share each other's problems'.

The significant lack of belongingness within the extended family and community created a situation of occupational injustice for the disabled child as well as the family, as it restricted their choice of occupations significantly. For example, culturally highly valued activities such as attending weddings, visiting relatives and friends, and attending Qur'an classes and religious celebrations at the Mosque were greatly restricted for the families, particularly for those whose children had intellectual impairments or behavioral difficulties.

Being

Parents talked about how their faith had changed through the process of accepting their disabled child. Initial negative reactions from relatives and community members, which implied that the child's disability was a divine punishment for their sins, were distressing, but despite that they started to see their disabled child as a blessing, who brought them closer to God. As the men's group found out through their research, the negative community attitudes toward disability are not based on the religious scriptures, which do not suggest any value or moral judgment on disability (see Bazna & Hatab 2004). However, the Islamic concept that God presents all Muslims with challenges to test or refine their patience and perseverance in faith (e.g. Qur'an p. 2:155), was considered a positive aspect in this process, as expressed by one mother who said that God only tests those He wants to enter into Heaven. The negative connotations that the community appears to have with the idea of disability as a 'test' was turned around into a positive opportunity to become a better human being through the experience. This reasoning and personal growth was expressed by all mothers and several of the fathers and their Muslim faith was central to their sense of identity. It also helped them to accept the child as they are, or in other words to allow them to 'be'.

Doing

In all families the mothers were the main carer of the disabled child, although most fathers also took on a significant role in practical caring and decision making. All mothers indicated that they had no time for themselves and regretted the loss of certain hobbies or relaxing habits. They also all indicated the importance of having something else, such as work or study, to provide balance, distraction, and contact with the 'real world', but not all had actually achieved this. Balancing work and caring tasks was also described as a challenge by several of the fathers.

Most siblings also took on caring responsibilities for the disabled child, which was perceived to have both positive and negative outcomes. On the one hand they had limited opportunities for socializing and engaging in their own play and hobbies. On the other hand they valued the maturity and sense of responsibility their situation caused. Importantly, none of the parents or siblings expressed any resentment towards the disabled child for the resulting occupational imbalance, as they said it was natural to do this for their 'own flesh and blood'. Where dissatisfaction was expressed it was about the division of tasks within the family or about the insufficient level of culturally appropriate respite care facilities.

Caring for a disabled child led to considerable occupational imbalance (one of the aspects of occupational injustice), particularly for the mothers, but to a lesser extent also for the fathers and siblings of the child.

Becoming

To some extent the way family life with a disabled child impacts on each family member's personal development and hopes for the future has already been alluded to in the sections on belonging, being, and doing above. Dominating themes when participants talked about the future, related to not knowing what to expect from their child's abilities in adulthood; worrying about who would care for them after their own death; and a desire to look for ways to support other Pakistani/Muslim parents in the same position. As described above in the section on 'doing' most mothers had no time to think about, or work towards personal future goals. These limitations on participants' sense of becoming were caused mainly by external social factors, and the resulting limited scope for personal development for the disabled child and their family members thus constitutes a form of occupational injustice.

Occupation and culture

Iwama (2005, p. 247) cautions that 'current definitions of occupation demonstrate a valuing that is particularly reflective of Western experience and worldviews' and that the concept of occupation must be redefined in each new cultural context. For this group of Pakistani families with disabled children living in a Western context the aspects of 'belonging' and 'being' were relatively very important and strongly influenced by their cultural and religious background. In meetings of the women's group participants remarked repeatedly that many aspects of family and community relationships were universal, but the way they presented in their own culture was often very different. This illustrates the importance of finding a balance in recognizing the differences in people's cultural background while also expecting many similarities, as it is the latter that are instrumental in creating relationships of trust that enable collaborative work and effective intervention.

This study also illustrates the importance of recognizing that some of the cultural differences are an important positive source of support and inspiration for the families. Examples of this are the role of faith in accepting and allowing the disabled child to 'be', and the way the interdependence or loyalty within the family makes it easier for family members to share the burden of care. Enabling people to build on the strengths in their cultural background in this way can contribute to increased occupational justice.

Conclusion

This project provided the participants with an opportunity to engage in a meaningful occupation – participatory action research – which led to a deeper understanding of their situation, and facilitated the development of valuable skills like problem solving, collaboration, and taking action to improve their situation. Despite the limited scope of a project undertaken for doctoral studies, participants reported a range of positive outcomes for them as individuals (e.g., improved understanding of community perceptions of disability and increased assertiveness to address them) and families (e.g., improved communication between family members). The practical and participatory nature of the project lent itself well to exploring occupational aspects of their experience, giving occupational therapists more insight into the particular strengths and needs of Pakistani families with disabled children, as well as inspiration for working with them in ways that capitalize on their strengths, so that their needs can be met more effectively.

References

Abdel Haleem MAS: *The Qur'an. A New Translation by MAS Abdel Haleem*, Oxford, 2004, Oxford University Press.

Bazna MS, Hatab TA: Disability in the Qur'an: The Islamic alternative to defining, viewing and relating to disability. In *Disability Studies: Putting Theory into Practice*, Conference 26–28 July 2004, Lancaster, Disability Studies Association. Available at http://www.lancs.ac.uk/fass/events/disabilityconference_archieve/2004/papers/bazna_hatab 2004. Accessed July 12, 2010.

Beresford B: *Findings: The Needs of Disabled Children and Their Families*, Social Care Research 76. York, 1995, Joseph Rowntree Foundation.

Bywaters P, Ali Z, Fazil Q, et al: Attitudes towards disability amongst Pakistani and Bangladeshi parents of disabled children in the UK: considerations for service providers and the disability movement, *Health and Social Care in the Community* 11:502–509, 2003.

Campbell C, Mclean C: Social capital, local community participation and the construction of Pakistani identities in England: implications for health inequalities policies, *J Health Psychol* 8:247–262, 2003.

Chamba R, Ahmad W, Hirst M, et al: *On the Edge: Minority Ethnic Families Caring for a Severely Disabled Child*, Bristol, 1999, The Policy Press.

Fazil Q, Bywaters P, Ali Z, et al: Disadvantage and discrimination compounded: the experience of Pakistani and Bangladeshi parents of disabled children in the UK, *Disability and Society* 17:237–253, 2002.

Gibbs S, Mann G, Mathers N: *Child-to-Child: A Practical Guide. Empowering Children as Active Citizens*, London, 2002, Lambeth, Southwark and Lewisham Health Action Zone and Groundwork Southwark. Online. Available at: http://www.child-to-child.org/guide/guide.pdf. Accessed July 12, 2010.

Government Equalities Office: *Ethnic Minority Women in the UK*, 2008, Online. Available at: http://www.equalities.gov.uk/pdf/EthinicMinorityWomen.pdf. Accessed July 12, 2010.

Hatton C, Akram Y, Shah R, et al: *Supporting South Asian Families with a Child with Severe Disabilities*, London, 2004, Jessica Kingsley.

Herr K, Anderson GL: *The Action Research Dissertation. A Guide for Students and Faculty*, Thousand Oaks, 2005, Sage.

Iwama MK: Occupation as a cross-cultural construct. In Whiteford G,

Wright-St Clair V, editors: *Occupation and Practice in Context*, Sydney, 2005, Churchill Livingstone, pp 242–253.

Kemmis S, McTaggart R, Retallick J: *The Action Research Planner*, Karachi, 2004, Aga Khan University Institute for Educational Development.

Khan H: *Working with Muslim Fathers: A Guide for Practitioners*, London, 2006, An-Nisa Society and Fathers Direct.

Kramer-Roy D: Researching the support needs of Pakistani families with disabled children in the UK, *Research, Policy and Planning* 25:143–153, 2007.

Kramer-Roy D: Exploring the support needs of Pakistani families with disabled children: a participatory action research study. Doctoral thesis, London, 2009, Brunel University, Online. Available at: http://bura. brunel.ac.uk/handle/2438/4377. Accessed July 12, 2010.

Letts L: Occupational therapy and participatory research: a partnership worth pursuing, *Am J Occup Ther* 57:77–87, 2003.

Meyer J: Action research. In Pope C, Mays N, editors: *Qualitative Research in Health Care*, London, 2006, BMJ Publishing.

Morton R, Sharma V, Nicholson J, et al: Disability in children from different ethnic populations, *Child Care Health Dev* 28:87–93, 2002.

National Statistics Website: *Ethnicity: Low Income*, 2002, Online. Available at: http://www.statistics.gov.uk/cci/nugget_print.asp?ID=269. Accessed July 12, 2010.

Reason P: Three approaches to participative inquiry. In Denzin NK, Lincoln YS, editors: *Handbook of Qualitative Research*, Thousand Oaks, 1994, Sage, pp 324–339.

Trentham B, Cockburn L: Participatory action research. Creating new knowledge and opportunities for occupational engagement. In Kronenberg F, Simó Algado S, Pollard N, editors: *Occupational Therapy Without Borders: Learning from the Spirit of Survivors*, Edinburgh, 2005, Elsevier/Churchill Livingstone, pp 440–453.

Wilcock A: Occupation and Health: are they one and the same thing? Keynote speech at 5th Occupation UK & Ireland Symposium 'Health Through Occupation. The Evidence', 11–12 Sept. 2006, Northampton, 2006.

Wilcock AA: Reflections on doing, being and becoming, *Australian Occupational Therapy Journal* 46:1–11, 1999.

The occupation of city walking: crossing the invisible line

42

Teresa Cassani Danner   Charlotte Royeen   Karen Barney
Sarah R. Walsh   Matin Royeen

OVERVIEW

Most of the staff and faculty in our building never walk outside of the physical limits of the medical center, i.e., they never cross the invisible line to egress into a world beyond the 'ivory tower'. The purpose of this chapter is to present a pilot study designed to prevent this exclusionary behavior by exposing students to cultural variation by crossing the invisible line. In this pilot study 19 occupational therapy students participated in a walk within the area surrounding the St Louis University Medical Center Campus. Using guiding questions developed by the investigators, students reflected on their experience individually (written responses) and in groups (two focus groups). The data were then analyzed using ATLAS.ti, Version 5.1 and categorized into emergent themes. A major theme that emerged was that the simple act of walking lessened stereotypes and educated students about the community surrounding the campus. It is, therefore, suggested that city walking be considered for implementation into occupational therapy curricula as an introductory activity presenting the concept of culture and cultural variance. Through this combination of learning activities, occupational therapy students can cross the invisible line that separates their way of doing from how people different from them live.

Introduction

Gaining cultural understanding and competence has become increasingly important in the United States as globalization takes hold and the populations of minorities grow (Hamon 2006). In fact, what has been one minority (those of Hispanic origins) will

likely become the majority in the United States by the mid part of our current century (Davis 2001, Denton & Emory 2002, Huntington 2004), thus transforming existing notions of majority, minority, and mainstream cultural values.

We believe that cultural competence cannot be learned from textbooks alone. Cultural competence is a difficult concept to define and has yet to obtain a universal understanding. The United States Department of Health and Human Services defines cultural competence as '… behaviors, attitudes, and policies that can come together on a continuum; that will ensure that a system, agency, program, or individual can function effectively and appropriately in diverse cultural interaction and settings'. Another definition from the American Medical Association states that cultural competence involves 'knowledge and interpersonal skills that allow providers to understand, appreciate, and work with individuals from cultures other than their own. It involves an awareness and acceptance of cultural differences; self-awareness; knowledge of patient's culture; and adaptation of skills'. Cultural competence refers to an ongoing volitional process of personal growth that includes an awareness of one's biases, a willingness to learn about differences among all types of people, and a motivation to apply the reflective insights and new awareness gained to one's personal and professional roles (Black & Wells 2000, Dillard et al 1992).

A number of theoretical models propose that achieving and maintaining cultural competence is a multifactorial process: an interactive product involving one's cognition, behavior, and values (Opp 2007). For occupational therapists and other healthcare service providers, there is a need to continually work to address patients and clients' differences and related needs (Suarez-Balcazar & Rodakowski 2007). When interacting with others, communicating knowledge gained from being culturally competent in a respectful manner is essential (Hamon 2006). Gaining or working towards cultural competence through experience, or 'doing' should begin at the student level and in a meaningful manner so that the student's repertoire of understanding and skills developmentally grow as they transition into a professional. In fact, the Accreditation Council for Occupational Therapy Education (ACOTE 1998) requires the entry-level occupational therapist to have a knowledge base in subjects associated with global concerns, diversity, sociocultural, and socioeconomic issues, as well as lifestyle decisions politically determined within society. These subjects directly relate to one's culture.

It is difficult to leave one's everyday life for an extended amount of time in order to experience different cultural groups and then return home. People would have to rearrange their schedules, which would in turn influence the schedules of those around them. For many, this is not an option. Most working citizens in the United States live by a relatively strict schedule, one where production is idealized and wasted time minimized (Kohls 1984). Alternative methods, therefore, are needed in order to obtain a glimpse of how others live. Even a small glimpse of another culture designed to promote reflection and discussion might be beneficial, possibly leading to a synthesis of information that would not have been obtained from simply reading a textbook or article. City walking is one introductory method, allowing students to experience different surroundings.

Review of relevant literature

Previous research in city walking is limited and is found in various categories of scholarship such as anthropology and sociology, forming a small, but eclectic collection of knowledge.

Human beings tend to emotionally connect to their surroundings, partly based on their culture of origin (Burns 2000). Identity is shaped by one's culture, which in turn contributes to ideas of where one is, and a sense of belonging, and one's experience of health and wellbeing. 'The city is not in other words, merely a physical mechanism and an artificial construction. It is involved in the vital processes of the people who compose it' (Burns 2000, p. 73).

The city is an extension of people of the community. Therefore, part of experiencing a culture involves experiencing the context or area in which the people within the culture originated.

In a study by Brown et al (2007), the environmental features influencing where one prefers to walk were investigated. Participants, both male and female, walked in an urban area that contained diverse features. Some portions of the walk were filled with fountains and plazas, while portions included buildings under construction and in the beginning stages of redevelopment. After the walk, participants completed a questionnaire, rating different walking segments. The study concluded that the students are deterred by places that do not provide a pleasant, aesthetically pleasing, and safe walking environment. Students wanted an area with well maintained sidewalks that lead to a variety of destinations. In addition, if an area is desolate or contains a high flow of automobile traffic, it is deemed unsafe, un-walkable, and out of their comfort zone. Participants also enjoyed walking more if they found a good social atmosphere to connect to within the area.

Another study by Joseph & Zimring, (2007) looked at the factors that influence the walking path choices of older adults in order to determine how the built environment affects people's health. The findings of the study were similar to the study by Brown et al (2007). Paths with numerous destinations and attractive scenery were the most walked. Paths with steps or other movement barriers were, for the most part, avoided. All of these factors in the environment combine to influence where people decide to walk, if they even walk at all. We suspect that people view walking as functional. It is a mechanism to get from one place to another or to keep the body in shape. Thus, people may not avail themselves of all the other benefits that walking can provide. In a manifesto from the realm of performance research by Hodge et al (2006), people are encouraged to get out of their 'pod' and experience places where they have never gone before. This manifesto reveals walking as a way to create a story, experience novel sensations, see what is often hidden, discover unknown paths, and encounter individuals who are often overlooked.

A qualitative study by Jacks (2006) also looks at walking as more than functional, exploring if walking, an 'old' way of experiencing cities, can be used to gain insight into the city of Manhattan, and discover the often unseen benefits of walking. Participants were chosen to walk in Manhattan and reflect on their experiences. One participant viewed the walk as a way to connect the city of the past to the present. Seeing the city evoked memories of when he was younger. Another participant learned that one's surroundings are never truly seen unless people diminish the need for a destination and look around. 'Each such act of walking reconnects us, no matter how temporarily, to where we are and who we are' (Jacks 2006, p. 75). Walking gives meaning and organization to the world outside the home, creating an intimate relationship between people and the environment (Bendiner-Viani 2005), possibly creating a sense of belonging through the act of doing.

Walking is a form of doing and occupational therapy strives to instill meaning in others' lives through implementing and discovering people's occupations, an embedded form of doing. Occupation, as used here, refers to doing with meaning (Royeen 2002). If the profession is based in the act of doing, then the learning process for students entering the field of occupational therapy should also stress engagement or active doing to facilitate more meaningful and lasting, relevant learning.

We believe that walking can be a useful tool to assist students in introductory level or foundational understanding to allow for development of cultural competence before working in the field of occupational therapy. The experience might assist students to become more observant, see how others live, and assist them in future client-centered practice. As a profession, occupational therapy needs to start early to make their professional knowledge base as culturally diverse as the society in which they live. Walking, both urban and rural, depending on a university's location, could be one way to begin to achieve this goal. Therefore, the purpose of this action research project was to introduce occupational therapy students to the surrounding community through the occupation of walking as an introductory method of being exposed to cultural variation. The overarching question is: In an urban setting, what are occupational therapy student's reactions to their community surroundings?'

Methods

Context

The context for our project at Saint Louis University was the midtown section of the City of St Louis, in the Midwestern state of Missouri, United States.

Saint Louis University was established in 1010 by the Society of Jesus, and is known for being the oldest college west of the Mississippi River. The values of the university, reflected in the mission and vision, emphasize 'the whole person' – mind, body, heart and spirit, and service – an excellent fit for the occupational science and occupational therapy department, situated in the Gate District neighborhood. This neighborhood is near the geographic center of St Louis, and was originally developed in 1875 around the railroad yards and a baseball park. The residents have been historically of mixed ethnicity, of which the majority has been African American. The Gate District neighborhood has a recent history of lower income groups, deterioration of properties, poverty, and crime. Within the past 20 years, however, this neighborhood has experienced a number of redevelopment projects that have resulted in new homes and residents of mixed income groups. The extensive development and expansion at Saint Louis University has influenced these neighborhood changes (History of St Louis Neighborhoods 2008).

Description of participants

Eighteen of the participants were female and one was male. All were Caucasian and juniors in the occupational therapy program, aged 19, 20, or 22. They were a cohort of students in a single course.

Process

Students in the spring term of their junior (third) year of the Bachelor of Science in Occupational Science course, 'Occupation in Diverse Communities' were introduced and oriented to the study, as mandated by the Saint Louis University Institutional Review Board. Approval for the city walking study from the Institutional Review Board was received in November of 2006. Prior to the study, students completed assignments that required personal reflection and investigation regarding their own cultural heritage. They presented genograms in class, so that all members became additionally aware of their classmates' cultural heritage.

The students were divided into two groups, each walking at different times during the daylight hours in the middle of November 2006. (Daylight hours were chosen since these are perceived as the 'safest hours' in the neighborhood.) The city walk was a little over 1 mile, taking about 30 minutes to execute.

Box 42.1

Individual reflection questions

1. Approximately how long did your walk take?
2. Describe your walking experience including what you saw, heard, and felt.
3. What, if anything, about the experience surprised you?
4. What, if anything, would you like to know more about after your city walk?
5. Would you take a city talk again? Why or why not?

Box 42.2

Focus group discussion questions

1. Approximately how long did your walk take?
2. Describe your walking experience including what you saw, heard, and felt.
3. What, if anything, about the experience surprised you?
4. What, if anything, would you like to know more about after your city walk?
5. Would you take a city walk again? Why or why not?
6. Do you have any additional comments or questions?

The walk was designed by the second author who had been walking this neighborhood for the past three years. Immediately after the city walk, the students filled out a five-item questionnaire (see Box 42.1). Within two months, they participated in one of two audiotaped focus groups using the guiding questions presented in Box 42.2.

The data were then transcribed and coded into categories using ATLAS.ti, Version 5.1, a qualitative data analysis program.

Results and discussion

Six categories emerged, addressing: the students' stereotypic views, their physical observations of the area, the perceived level of safety during the city walk, the students' feelings after the experience, the students' feelings during the walk, and whether or not they would participate in another city walk. Findings for each will be presented in turn.

1. *The students' stereotypic views.* The surrounding area of the medical center campus is often stereotyped as rundown and dangerous. One occupational science student said 'people do just say that [the university] is in a bubble and really nice and just right outside of it is ghettos and chaos'. Few students ever walk in the surrounding neighborhoods, but had already formulated preconceived notions. Most of the occupational science students were expecting to find houses that were falling apart with broken windows and overgrown yards. In addition, they thought people, mostly African Americans, would be loitering around the area, doing nothing.

2. *Their physical observations of the area.* The city walk, however, surprised the students. Instead of a completely rundown, poor area, they observed new houses interspersed with rundown ones. In front of the middle class houses were middle class cars and paved sidewalks. In front of the houses that were not kept up as much were choppy sidewalks overgrown with tree limbs, causing the students to duck as they walked past. One student described the surroundings, writing, '[T]he cars parked in the streets resembled vehicles of high socioeconomic status ... Portions of the neighborhood contained cobbled sidewalks, overgrown yards, litter, and unraked leaves; this particular area of the neighborhood was merely a blemish on an otherwise beautiful setting.' Most of the houses had one or more satellite dishes, even the houses that were poorly kept. In addition, security appeared high. Many yards were fenced in and over three-fourths of the houses had notices of security systems protecting the house. Few people outside of the student group were seen on the city walk. No kids were playing in the yards and no-one was loitering around. Only the noises of traffic and barking dogs were heard.

3. *The perceived level of safety during the city walk.* The majority of occupational science students felt safe. They said that since it was daylight, in a large group, and close to campus, they rarely felt threatened or in danger. The only time that the students felt unsafe was when there were no traffic signs while crossing a busy street. The participants also considered the safety of those in a wheelchair or using a walker, by commenting on how it would be dangerous for them to travel outside due to the sidewalk being choppy, alternating from smooth to irregular. Finally,

participants wondered how safe the people who lived in the neighborhood felt and if they themselves should be more worried about safety.

4. *The students' feelings after the walk.* After experiencing the city walk, occupational science students recognized error in their past stereotypes, however, new ones were quickly forming. Many began to wonder and some began to assume that the middle class houses had to be government or subsidized housing. In addition, some students assumed that an older population lived there due to the lack of children running around, and the outward appearance of the houses.

5. *The students' feeling during the walk.* Feelings were also evoked during the city walk. Occupational science students felt sad that the new houses had replaced much of the old, and the few old houses that remained were crumbling. To them, part of St Louis history was deteriorating. The students also felt fortunate for what they each had. During their childhood, they could play outside and not need security systems or to lock their doors. One student reminisced, 'I lived out in the middle of nowhere. We don't lock our doors on our cars; we don't lock our house … There was only one park that we saw and it didn't have a lot of play equipment so it was fortunate that when I was younger, we had parks to play in … '. Things are different now, no one is ever truly safe, and kids cannot just go off on their own unsupervised. By walking through the neighborhood, seeing the security systems, the gates around the yards, and the desolate yards with no children, the occupational science students realized how different the inhabitants' lives were from their own.

6. *Whether or not they would participate in another city walk.* Nearly every student said that they would participate in a city walk again. One student even said the walk was enjoyable, stating, '[I]t is kind of fun to peek in and see what's in the different houses and see what kind of houses they are and see the older features'. A few said they would walk again only if they were with someone else. One student thought it would be interesting to compare how it feels to walk in an area farther from campus, where the safety of the university's campus is much more distant. The only student who said 'no' to a second city walk stated that she preferred walking in parks rather than around blocks.

Discussion

The city walking experience proved to be an effective introductory learning activity to expand students' cultural knowledge and traverse the invisible line between campus and neighborhoods. The occupational science students did not come directly in contact with people in the neighborhood, so they were unable to explore communication skills, but the students did gain a greater understanding of the physical context in which others live, as well as become more aware of how they themselves live. The students were exposed to the physical setting of how inhabitants of the neighborhood live, allowing them to compare one way of life to their own. The occupational therapy students personally connected to the place and relived stories of their childhood, such as how they would wander and play outside without supervision or worry. Reflection in the exercises and the focus groups allowed the students to begin to relate how their own occupational choices are directly influenced by cultural elements and the environment, becoming aware of how their own surrounding communities positively and negatively influence the activities in which they engage.

Hodge et al (2006) stated that walking is medium that spurs a search for understanding. This city walking experience provided a learning opportunity outside the confines of the classroom setting, but it also fostered more questions. Many of the participants wanted to know the neighborhood's economic background, who owned the homes, how safe people felt, and the level of crime. These evolving questions indicate a desire to learn and leads to continuing, self-directed education. Occupational therapy embodies the doing. Therefore, if the profession teaches the core concept of doing to its clients, then the doing aspect should be incorporated into how occupational therapists are educated.

Limitations

The first limitation of the city walking study was that the sample size was extremely small in comparison with the number of students in occupational science programs throughout the United States. Also, the study was not longitudinal, thus only assessing one point in time. Also, it is only a pilot investigation that needs replication and additional in-depth analysis.

Conclusion

The occupational therapy profession needs professionals in the field to be as knowledgeable as possible upon entering the field. Students need to become self-aware of their own cultural and physical contexts, so that they can better communicate and understand those with whom they work. City walking is an introductory tool for achieving this goal, which points students toward a greater understanding of themselves and those they will serve.

References

Accreditation Council for Occupational Therapy Education (ACOTE): *Standards for an Accredited Educational Program for the Occupational Therapist (Electronic Version)*, Bethesda, MD, 1998, The American Occupational Therapy Association, pp 1–13.

Bendiner-Viani G: Walking, emotion, and dwelling: guided tours in prospect heights, Brooklyn *Space and Culture* 8:459–471, 2005.

Black R, Wells S: *Cultural Competency for Health Professionals*, Bethesda, MD, 2000, The American Occupational Therapy Association.

Brown B, Werner C, Amburgey J, et al: Walkable route perceptions and physical features: converging evidence for en route walking experiences, *Environment and Behavior* 39:34–61, 2007.

Burns A: Emotion and urban experience: implications for design, *Design Issues* 16:67–79, 2000.

Davis M: *Magical Urbanism: Latinos Reinvent the US City*, New York, 2001, Verso Books.

Denton N, Emory TS: *American Diversity: A Demographic Challenge for the Twenty-First Century*, New York, 2002, Suny Press.

Dillard et al: *American Journal of Occupational Therapy* 46(8): 721–726, 1992.

Hamon RR, editor: *International Family Studies: Developing Curricula and Teaching Tools*, New York, 2006, The Haworth Press Health Resources and Services Administration (HRSA).

History of St. Louis Neighborhoods: 2008, Online. Available at: http://stlouis.missouri.org/neighborhoods/history/midtown/population18.htm. Accessed October 8, 2008.

Hodge S, Persighetti S, Smith P, et al: A manifesto for a new walking culture 'dealing with the city', *Performance Research* 11:115–122, 2006.

Huntington SP: *The Hispanic Challenge*, Washington, USA, 2004, Foreign Policy, pp 30–45.

Jacks B: Walking the city; Manhattan projects, *Places* 18:68–75, 2006.

Joseph A, Zimring C: Where active older adults walk: understanding the factors related to path choice for walking among active retirement community residents, *Environment and Behavior* 39:75–105, 2007.

Kohls R: *The Values Americans Live By*, Washington, DC, 1984, Meridan House International.

Opp A: Becoming a culturally competent occupational therapy practitioner, *OT Practice* 24:12–13, 2007.

Royeen CB: Occupation reconsidered, *Occup Ther Int* 9:112–121, 2002.

Saint Louis University: *Historical Data*, 2008, Online. Available at: http://www.slu.edu/x844.xml. Accessed October 8, 2008.

Suarez-Balcazar Y, Rodakowski J: Practical ways to increase cultural competence, *OT Practice* 24:15–17, 2007.

Index

Note: Page numbers followed by *b* indicate boxes, *f* indicate figures and *t* indicate tables.

Printed in the United States
By Bookmasters